Clinical Disorders of the Endometrium and Menstrual Cycle

Clinical Disorders of the Endometrium and Menstrual Cycle

Edited by

Iain T. Cameron

Department of Obstetrics and Gynaecology,
University of Glasgow, Glasgow, UK

Ian S. Fraser

Department of Obstetrics and Gynaecology,
University of Sydney, Australia

and

Stephen K. Smith

Department of Obstetrics and Gynaecology,
University of Cambridge/School of Clinical Medicine,
Cambridge, UK

OXFORD UNIVERSITY PRESS

This book has been printed digitally and produced in a standard specification in order to ensure its continuing availability

OXFORD
UNIVERSITY PRESS

Great Clarendon Street, Oxford OX2 6DP

Oxford University Press is a department of the University of Oxford.
It furthers the University's objective of excellence in research, scholarship, and education by publishing world-wide in

Oxford New York

Auckland Bangkok Buenos Aires Cape Town Chennai
Dar es Salaam Delhi Hong Kong Istanbul Karachi Kolkata
Kuala Lumpur Madrid Melbourne Mexico City Mumbai Nairobi
São Paulo Shanghai Taipei Tokyo Toronto

Oxford is a registered trade mark of Oxford University Press in the UK and in certain other countries

Published in the United States
by Oxford University Press Inc., New York

Reprinted 2004

ISBN 0-19-262724-4

Antony Rowe Ltd., Eastbourne

Preface

It is 115 years since Moricke first used a curette to obtain endometrial samples from living women. The intervening years, and particularly the last 30, have seen a remarkable advance in the understanding of reproductive medicine. At the time of Moricke's observations, women had fewer menstrual periods than they do today. They had a later menarche, an earlier menopause, and for many the reproductive years were characterized by a series of pregnancies followed by lactational amenorrhoea, with the occasional ovulatory menstrual cycle in between. This pattern has now changed. The widespread availability of effective contraception has led to the acceptance of the monthly menstrual cycle as the norm, and in turn, this has led to the evolution of the common clinical disorders of menstruation, menorrhagia, dysmenorrhoea, and premenstrual syndrome. In addition, while the development of exogenous oestrogens and progestogens for contraception, cycle control, and hormone replacement therapy has been a significant therapeutic advance, irregular, unscheduled bleeding from the endometrium is a considerable threat to compliance.

This book provides an overview of clinical disorders of the endometrium and menstrual cycle. Current knowledge of pathophysiology, investigation, and treatment has been reviewed by leading health professionals and scientists from Europe, Australia, and North America. Basic scientific understanding has been outlined in detail, particularly where advances have led to improvements in treatment, but emphasis has been placed on the practical management of these common clinical conditions.

The text is arranged in five sections. The first section offers a background, comprising a cultural and historical perspective, details of the physiology and practical assessment of the endometrium, and a view of menstruation as a normal every-day event from the woman's perspective. A major section is devoted to menorrhagia, with chapters ranging from definition, epidemiology, and pathophysiology, through to clinical investigation and treatment, both medical and surgical. The third section reviews amenorrhoea, oligomenorrhoea, and irregular bleeding, including postmenopausal bleeding. Often considered separately from menorrhagia, there is considerable overlap in terms of clinical presentation (oligomenorrhoea/anovulatory dysfunctional uterine bleeding) and investigation. The section on dysmenorrhoea describes the underlying pathology and clinical management, with detailed accounts of adenomyosis and endometriosis. Psychosomatic considerations and the relationship between psychiatric morbidity and the menstrual cycle are documented in the next section, along with a description of the aetiology and management of pre-menstrual syndrome. The last section provides a guide to the pathophysiology and practical management of bleeding disorders resulting from the use of intrauterine devices and hormonal delivery systems, contraceptive steroids and hormone replacement therapy. Overlap between chapters is inevitable and indeed necessary. In most situations there is agreement, but this is not always the case, a reflection of either different points of view or a conflicting evidence base, or both!

We are most grateful to all of the authors for joining us in this venture, and for their authoritative and informative chapters. We hope that the quality and diversity of contributions will not only appeal to hospital specialists and family practitioners, but also to many others with an interest in women's health. Finally, we thank Kay Byrne, without whose excellent and willing secretarial help the book might still not be finished.

Iain T. Cameron
Ian S. Fraser,
and Stephen K. Smith
August 1997

Contents

Contributors

Mats Åkerlund Department of Obstetrics and Gynecology, Lund University Hospital, S-221 85 Lund, Sweden

Kerstin Andersson Department of Obstetrics and Gynaecology, East Hospital, University of Gothenburg, S-416 85 Gothenburg, Sweden

David F. Archer Department of Obstetrics and Gynecology, The Jones Institute for Women's Health, Eastern Virginia Medical School, 601 Colley Avenue, Virginia 23507-1627, USA

Christine Bain Department of Obstetrics and Gynaecology, Aberdeen Royal Hospitals NHS Trust, Aberdeen Maternity Hospital, Cornhill Road, Aberdeen AB9 2ZA, UK

Salim Bassil Department of Gynecology, Catholic University of Louvain, Cliniques Universitaires St Luc, Avenue Hippocrate 10, B-1200 Brussels, Belgium

Ivo A. Brosens Department of Obstetrics and Gynaecology, Katholieke Universiteit Leuven, Herestraat 49, B-3000 Leuven, Belgium

Jan J. Brosens Institute of Obstetrics and Gynaecology, Royal Postgraduate Medical School, Hammersmith Hospital, du Cane Road, London W12 0NN, UK

Iain T. Cameron Department of Obstetrics and Gynaecology, The Queen Mother's Hospital, Yorkhill, Glasgow G3 8SJ, UK

Steven Campbell Department of Obstetrics and Gynaecology, Glasgow Royal Infirmary, 10 Alexandra Parade, Glasgow G31 2ER, UK

Angela Coulter King's Fund Development Centre, 11-13 Cavendish Square, London W1M 0AN, UK

Hilary O.D. Critchley Department of Obstetrics and Gynaecology, University of Edinburgh, Centre for Reproductive Biology, 37 Chalmers Street, Edinburgh EH3 9EW, UK

Ann Day University Department of Psychiatry, The Warneford Hospital, Old Road, Headington, Oxford OX3 7JX, UK

Peter Dockery Department of Anatomy, University College, Cork, Republic of Ireland

Jacques Donnez Department of Gynecology, Catholic University of Louvain, Cliniques Universitaires St Luc, Avenue Hippocrate 10, B-1200 Brussels, Belgium

James O. Drife Academic Unit of Obstetrics and Gynaecology, The University of Leeds, D Floor, Clarendon Wing, Belmont Grove, Leeds LS2 9NS, UK

D. Keith Edmonds Department of Obstetrics and Gynaecology, Queen Charlotte's & Chelsea Hospital, Goldhawk Road, London W6 0XG, UK

Stephen Franks Department of Obstetrics and Gynaecology, Imperial College of Science, Technology and Medicine, Imperial College School of Medicine at St. Mary's, Norfolk Place, London W2 1PG, UK

Ian S. Fraser Department of Obstetrics and Gynaecology, Queen Elizabeth Research Institute for Mothers and Infants, University of Sydney, New South Wales 2006, Australia

Dennis Gath University Department of Psychiatry, The Warneford Hospital, Old Road, Headington, Oxford OX3 7JX, UK

Stephane Gillerot Department of Gynecology, Catholic University of Louvain, Cliniques Universitaires St Luc, Avenue Hippocrate 10, B-1200 Brussels, Belgium

Milton Goldrath Department of Gynecology, Sinai Hospital, DMC, Wayne State University, 6767 West Outer Drive, Detroit 48235, Michigan, USA

Abha Govind North Staffordshire Hospital, Thornburrow Drive, Hartshill, Stoke-on-Trent ST4 7QB, UK

David L. Healy Department of Obstetrics and Gynaecology, Monash Medical Centre, 246 Clayton Road, Clayton, Victoria 3168, Australia

Martha Hickey Department of Gynaecology, Central Middlesex Hospital, Acton Lane, Park Royal, London NW10 7NS, UK

Jenny Higham Department of Obstetrics and Gynaecology, Imperial College of Science, Technology and Medicine, Imperial College School of Medicine at St. Mary's, Norfolk Place, London W2 1PG, UK

Changulanda Medappa Joshi North Staffordshire Hospital, Thornburrow Drive, Hartshill, Stoke-on-Trent ST4 7QB, UK

Henry C. Kitchener Department of Obstetrics and Gynaecology, St. Mary's Hospital, Hathersage Road, M7anchester M13 0JH, UK

Britt-Marie Landgren Department of Woman and Child Health, Division of Obstetrics and Gynecology, Karolinska Hospital, P.O. Box 104, 171-76 Stockholm, Sweden

TC. Li Department of Obstetrics and Gynaecology, Jessop Hospital for Women, Leavygreave Road, Sheffield S3 7RE, UK

Mary Ann Lumsden Department of Obstetrics and Gynaecology, The Queen Mother's Hospital, Yorkhill, Glasgow G3 8SJ, UK

Phyllis Kernoff Mansfield Department of Women's Studies, Pennsylvania State University, State College, Pennsylvania, USA

Michelle Nisolle Department of Gynecology, Catholic University of Louvain, Cliniques Universitaires St Luc, Avenue Hippocrate 10, B-1200 Brussels, Belgium

P.M. Shaughn O'Brien University of Keele, School of Postgraduate Medicine, North Staffordshire Hospital, Thornburrow Drive, Hartshill, Stoke-on-Trent ST4 7QB, UK

Viveca Odlind Department of Obstetrics and Gynaecology, University of Uppsala, Akademiska sjukhuset, S-751 85 Uppsala, Sweden

Moses A. Okon Biomedical Research Unit, Jessop Hospital for Women, Leavygreave Road, Sheffield S3 7RE, UK

David L. Olive Reproductive Endocrinology and Infertility, Department of Obstetrics and Gynecology, Yale University School of Medicine, 333 Cedar Street, P.O. Box 208063, New Haven, Connecticut 06520-8063, USA

Oswald M. Petrucco Department of Obstetrics and Gynaecology, University of Adelaide, 1st Floor Queen Victoria Building, Women's and Children's Hospital, 72 King William Road, North Adelaide 5006, South Australia

Roland Polet Department of Gynecology, Catholic University of Louvain, Cliniques Universitaires St Luc, Avenue Hippocrate 10, B-1200 Brussels, Belgium

Margaret C.P. Rees Nuffield Department of Obstetrics and Gynaecology, John Radcliffe Hospital, Headington, Oxford OX3 9DU, UK

Peter Rogers Department of Obstetrics and Gynaecology, Monash Medical Centre, 246 Clayton Road, Clayton, Victoria 3168, Australia

Jan L. Root Utah Health Information Network, Salt Lake City, Utah, USA

Peter Russell Department of Anatomical Pathology, Royal Prince Alfred Hospital, University of Sydney, New South Wales, Australia

Göran Rybo Department of Obstetrics and Gynaecology, East Hospital, University of Gothenburg, S-416 85 Gothenburg, Sweden

Mireille Smets Department of Gynecology, Catholic University of Louvain, Cliniques Universitaires St Luc, Avenue Hippocrate 10, B-1200 Brussels, Belgium

Stephen K. Smith Department of Obstetrics and Gynaecology, University of Cambridge School of Clinical Medicine, The Rosie Maternity Hospital, Robinson Way, Cambridge CB2 2SW, UK

R. William Stones Department of Obstetrics and Gynaecology, Level F (815) Princess Anne Hospital, Coxford Road, Southampton SO16 5YA, UK

Eric J. Thomas Department of Obstetrics and Gynaecology, Level F (815) Princess Anne Hospital, Coxford Road, Southampton SO16 5YA, UK

Ann M. Voda The Tremin Trust, University of Utah College of Nursing, 25 South Medical Drive, Salt Lake City, UT 84112, USA

Beverley Vollenhoven Department of Obstetrics and Gynaecology, Monash Medical Centre, 246 Clayton Road, Clayton, Victoria 3168, Australia

Bo von Schoultz Department of Woman and Child Health, Division of Obstetrics and Gynecology, Karolinska Hospital, P.O. Box 104, 171-76 Stockholm, Sweden

Pamela Warner Department of Public Health Sciences, University of Edinburgh Medical School, Teviot Place, Edinburgh EH8 9AG, UK

Tony G. Zreik Division of Reproductive Endocrinology, Department of Obstetrics and Gynecology, Yale University School of Medicine, 333 Cedar Street, P.O. Box 208063, New Haven, Connecticut 06520-8063, USA

Background

1 Menstruation: a cultural and historical perspective

James O. Drife

Introduction

Attitudes to menstruation have an important influence on the practice of gynaecology. Menstruation is surrounded by myths and taboos in many cultures. Like any physiological process, it can become dysfunctional but doctors and indeed women themselves may find it difficult to define the difference between normal menstruation and pathological bleeding. The dividing line may be strongly influenced by the culture in which the woman and her medical attendants live. The effect of culture has been discussed by Philip Rhodes:

> Culture consists of everything which has ever been accepted as a way of doing or thinking, and so taught by one person to another... The child in her growth learns what is done and what is not done partly by being told explicitly, but more importantly, by observing for herself what actions of herself and others appear to receive approval or disapproval. It is these cultural attitudes which in large measure mould her thinking, and which determine her values and philosophy of life.

Cultural attitudes to menstruation vary between countries and are affected by general attitudes to women in society. The role of women has changed in many countries during the past century, and is likely to continue to change.

There is relatively little historical information about menstruation. The subject has rarely been mentioned by either male or female writers. This chapter will review what information is available and its relevance to present-day attitudes.

Evolutionary perspective

Menstruation

The menstrual cycle occurs only in a few species, including old world monkeys, anthropoid apes, and humans. Reproductive cycles in other mammalian species very widely, with induced ovulation in the rabbit, an annual cycle in the sheep, and oestrous cycles in dogs and cats.

The word 'menstrual' is derived from the Latin words for 'moon' or 'month'. At some point in evolution human ovulation became a monthly event coinciding with the lunar cycle. How this change occurred is unknown. A chronobiologist has suggested that perhaps primitive humans were nocturnal creatures, hunting by the light of the moon: once a month there was insufficient moonlight for hunting so there was selection pressure in favour of women who ovulated on the night of the new moon. This is rather a fanciful theory and the truth may be a simpler link between the visual cortex and the hypothalamus. In annual breeders such as sheep the length of the day controls the reproductive cycle.

In *The women's history of the world*, Rosalind Miles pointed out that the change to a menstrual rather than an oestrous cycle made humans many times more fertile than other primates, and may be the main reason why our species has been so successful. If so, she emphasized, the success of humans has depended on female, and not male, evolutionary adaptation.

Male and female roles

Before leaving the subject of evolution, other aspects of primate 'culture' should perhaps be mentioned. One basic characteristic shared by humans and many other species, primate and non-primate, is that in general the male is larger and physically stronger than the female. In these species, males fight one another and establish a hierarchy, with a 'dominant male' having control over lower males and a group of females. Echoes of this type of social system survive in modern human societies, and some zoologists have suggested that this sexual dimorphism in humans means that we must have evolved as polygamous herd animals. Desmond Morris, however, in *The naked ape*, emphasized the importance of long-term pair-bonding among other primate species as well as our own.

Another point made by Morris was that when humans adopted the upright posture, male genital display – an unusual activity among animal species – became inevitable throughout normal human activity. He suggested that the wearing of some genital cover – a 'fig leaf' – must have been an early event in human evolution. As far as females are concerned, the upright posture meant that the vulva became a hidden organ, along with the organs of excretion. This may have been a factor in beginning the menstrual taboo.

The significance of evolution

These evolutionary concepts may be relevant when considering human cultural attitudes to menstruation. As Desmond Morris wrote nearly thirty years ago, '*Homo sapiens* has remained a naked ape... there is no hope of quickly shrugging off the accumulated genetic legacy of his whole evolutionary past.' Many of the attitudes to be considered in the next section have been determined by 'dominant males' – either religious leaders or, in more recent times, legislators.

Study of other primates also reminds us that the menstrual cycle is arbitrary and is by no means essential to health. This could usefully be pointed out to manufacturers and users of the oral contraceptive pill, which is formulated to give women a monthly withdrawal bleed. This pattern (which is the main reason for the pill's failure rate) has been adopted in part for marketing reasons, because monthly bleeds seem 'normal'.

Cultural attitudes

Menarche

A useful starting point for examining cultural attitudes to menstruation is a paragraph from *The female eunuch*, written by Germaine Greer in 1970:

> The arrival of menarche is more significant than any birthday, but in the Anglo-Saxon households it is ignored and carefully concealed from general awareness. For six months while I was waiting for my first menstruation I toted a paper bag with diapers and pins in my school satchel. When it finally came, I suffered agonies lest anyone should guess or *smell* it or anything. My diapers were

> made of harsh towelling, and I used to creep into the laundry and crouch over a bucket of foul clouts, hoping that my brother would not catch me at my revolting labours. It is not surprising that well-bred, dainty little girls find it difficult to adapt to menstruation, when our society does no more than explain it and leave them to get on with it. Among the aborigines who lived along the Pennefather river in Queensland the little girl used to be buried up to her waist in warm sand to aid the first contractions, and fed and cared for by her mother in a sacred place, to be led in triumph to the camp where she joined a feast to celebrate her entry into the company of marriageable maidens, it seems likely that menstruation was much less traumatic.

Other writers have remarked on the fact that in some cultures menarche is a public event to be celebrated by the whole tribe. Paula Weideger, in her book *Female cycles*, points out that such rites of passage are celebrated even in cultures which observe menstrual taboos. The anthropologist Margaret Mead described a custom in New Guinea: at the first menstruation of a young girl who is already married, her brothers are summoned to build her a menstrual hut (see below) and her female relatives rub her with stinging nettles: after three days her mother's brother makes decorative cuts on her shoulders and buttocks. In South India members of the Brahmin community perform the ritual of Samati Sadang: the girl is given a milk bath by a married male relative and then joins a family feast. Weideger also writes:

> In some families a vestige of more elaborate ritual remains. Among Jewish families, for example, it is customary to slap a young woman's face on the day that menstruation begins. The women I have met who have had this experience say they hadn't the vaguest notion of why their mothers slapped them. Many believed that it was a unique experience and the product of an aberration or a disturbed mother.

Rosalind Miles quotes a ritual among the Kafe of Papua New Guinea:

> When a girl began to menstruate she was shut in a darkened hut for a week, deprived of food, and taught that she was dangerous to herself and to others if she failed to abide by the ritual restrictions: her body and blood would make a man vomit, turn his blood black, corrupt his flesh, addle his wits and waste him to death.

In Western culture the menarche is generally a secret and unwelcome development. Simone de Beauvoir wrote about puberty in her classic book *The second sex*:

> She is proud of becoming a woman and watches the maturing of her bosom with satisfaction, padding her dress with handkerchiefs and taking pride in it before her elders; she does not yet grasp the significance of what is taking place in her. Her first menstruation reveals this meaning, and her feelings of shame appear. ...All the evidence agrees in showing that whether the child has been forewarned or not, the event always seems to her repugnant and humiliating.

De Beauvoir quotes a study reported by Havelock Ellis in 1896 showing that about half of American schoolgirls had either no advance knowledge or only vague knowledge at the time of their first menses, and she suggests that things were much the same in 1946. Instances of attempted suicide are not unknown: Rev Chad Varah founded the charity, The Samaritans, after officiating at the funeral of a girl who had committed suicide after experiencing her first menses.

Some of the information summarized above seems to suggest that negative feelings about menstruation may be innate rather than learned. However, such feelings are strongly reinforced in some cultures by menstrual taboos.

The menstrual taboo

Myths and taboos have been attached to menstruation in many cultures. The word 'taboo' ('forbidden' and 'sacred') comes form the Polynesian 'tabu' which, it is said, originally meant 'menstruation'. Rosalind Miles points out that 'of all human substances, blood is the most highly charged with power and danger'. She cites 'the dietary prohibition against eating blood in force from Jews to Sioux to Hindus'. Primitive fear of blood is still exploited today by the modern film industry.

In many societies menstruation was regarded as unclean. In ancient China menstrual blood was not allowed to touch the ground for fear of offending the Earth spirit. In ancient Egypt ritual cleansing baths were mandatory at the end of menstruation. Hindu teaching according to the Parsi sage Zoroaster was:

> A menstruous woman is the work of Uhremaun, the Devil. A woman in her courses is not to gaze upon the sacred fire, sit in water, behold the sun or hold conversation with a man.

Nowadays in Britain, Hindu women may ask for tablets to delay their periods so that they may take part in religious festivals.

Rosalind Miles points out that some primitive people had profound fear and respect for the power of menstruation. For example, the early native Americans of the Dakota territory believed that the *wakan* (sacredness or power) of a menstrual woman could weaken the *wakan* of all masculine objects of power, both of war and peace.

Paula Weideger quotes numerous examples of how some primitive peoples segregate women during menstruation: 'Special huts are built for menstruating women by the Baikairi of Brazil, the Shuswap of British Columbia, the Guari of Northern India, the Veddas of Ceylon, and the Algonquin of the North American forest.'

In some cultures, the segregation of menstruating women goes further.

> In Uganda, pots which a woman touches while the impurity of menstruation is upon her have to be destroyed; spears and shields defiled by her touch are, however, merely purified. Among the Bribri indians of Costa Rica the only plates she may use for her food are banana leaves, which when she has done with them, she throws away in some sequestered spot; for if a cow were to find them, and eat them, it would waste away. And she drinks out of a special vessel for the same reason: if any one drank out of the same cup after her, he would surely die.

Among the Dogan of East Africa the menstrual taboo is so strong that a woman in this condition brings misfortune to everything she touches. Not only is she segregated in an isolated hut and provided with special eating utensils, but if she is seen passing through the village a general purification must take place.

In the Middle East, women during menstruation must sometimes leave the home and live in a menstruation hut or tent. If the woman is allowed to live in the home, she must not prepare any food or touch her husband. Nor may she enter a house in which there is an ill person. These attitudes form the background to the next section of this chapter, which discusses historical attitudes directly related to present day culture.

Ancient history

Biblical attitudes

Chapter 15 of the book of Leviticus begins by giving rules of hygiene relating to a 'discharge' from a man's body. These rules are an entirely reasonable guide to avoiding infection from, perhaps, an infected wound or an abscess. The chapter then applies the same rules to a discharge of semen, whether or not a man is lying with a woman. Finally, the chapter applies the same rules to regular and irregular 'discharge of blood' from a woman's body. The rules relating to the emission of semen are less rigorous than those relating to discharge or menstruation: with the former, the uncleanness lasts only until the evening, but with the latter, uncleanness lasts for seven days after the end of the discharge or menses.

> When a woman has a discharge of blood which is her regular discharge from her body, she shall be in her impurity for seven days, and whoever touches her shall be unclean until the evening. And everything upon which she lies during her impurity shall be unclean; everything also upon which she sits shall be unclean. And whoever touches her bed shall wash his clothes, and bathe himself in water, and be unclean until the evening. And whoever touches anything upon which she sits shall wash his clothes, and bathe himself in water, and be unclean until the evening; whether it is the bed or anything upon which she sits, when he touches it he shall be unclean until the evening. And if any man lies with her, and her impurity is on him, he shall be unclean seven days; and every bed on which he lies shall be unclean. [verses 19–24]
>
> And if a woman has a discharge of blood for many days, not at the time of her impurity, or if she has a discharge beyond the time of her impurity, all the days of the discharge she shall continue in uncleanness; as in the days of her impurity, she shall be unclean. Every bed on which she lies, all the days of her discharge, shall be to her as the bed of her impurity; and everything on which she sits shall be unclean, as in the uncleanness of her impurity. And whoever touches these things shall be unclean, and shall wash his clothes, and bathe himself in water, and be unclean until the evening. But if she is cleansed of her discharge, she shall count herself seven days, and after that she shall be clean. And on the eighth day she shall take two turtledoves or two young pigeons, and bring them to the priest, to the door of the tent of meeting. And the priest shall offer one for a sin offering and the other for a burnt offering; and the priest shall make atonement for her before the Lord for her unclean discharge.

The second paragraph (verses 25–30) refers to abnormal vaginal bleeding. Atonement by the priest is not required after regular menstruation.

Roman attitudes

The most widely quoted authority for Roman attitudes is the historian Pliny (1st century AD). It is difficult to know if his strictures were typical of the attitudes in his society, but his description of menstruation is so picturesquely phrased that it is reproduced here from O'Dowd and Philip's *History of obstetrics and gynaecology*:

> A fatal poison corrupting and decomposing urine, depriving seeds of their fecundity, blasting garden flowers and grasses, causing fruits to fall from branches, dulling razors… If the menstrual discharge coincides with an eclipse of the moon or sun, the evils resulting from it are irremediable. …Congress with a woman at such time being noxious and attended with fatal effects to man. …Contact with [menstrual blood] turns new wine sour, crops touched by it become barren, grafts die, seeds in gardens are dried up, the fruit of trees fall off, the edge of steel and the gleam of ivory are dulled, hives of bees die, even bronze and iron are at once seized by rust and a horrible smell fills the air; to taste it drives dogs mad and infects their bites with an incurable poison. …Even that very tiny creature the ant is said to be sensitive to it, and throws away grains of corn that taste of it and does not touch them again… Over and above there is no limit to woman's power. First of all, they say that hail storms and whirl winds are driven away if menstrual fluid is exposed to the very flashes of lightning; that stormy weather too is thus kept away. It makes a liniment for gout and by her touch a woman in this state relieves scrofula, parotid tumours, superficial abscesses, boils and eye fluxes.

Mediaeval history

The mediaeval church (which was of course governed by celibate males) declared it sinful for a menstruating woman to enter a church and also forbade sexual intercourse during menstruation.

Nevertheless, negative attitudes were not confined to male priests. In the 12th century St Hildegard, abbess of Rupertsberg convent, wrote that the menstrual flow in virgins was lighter and of a different colour from those who had been deflowered, and said that menstruation was a punishment for the fall of Eve in the garden of Eden.

Modern history

The last three centuries have seen a steady increase in knowledge about anatomy and physiology, as well as changes in attitudes to women and to menstruation.

Eighteenth century

Knowledge

Regnier de Graaf described the ovarian follicle in 1672, but there were relatively few advances in medical knowledge about menstruation during the eighteenth century. In 1775 Percival Potts linked oophorectomy with cessation of menstruation and Cruickshank identified the human oocyte in 1778.

The first edition of the *Encyclopaedia Britannica*, published in 1771, gave the following explanation for the phenomenon of menstruation:

> As soon as a healthy female arrives at her full growth, she generates more blood than can be conveniently contained in the vessels; wherefore the superfluity is evacuated by the uterine arteries, and is called the Menses.
>
> Boerhaave observes, that in a suppression of the menses there is a plethora, with a listlessness to motion; a heaviness, a paleness, a pain in the loins and of the groin; all the functions, whether natural, vital, or animal, are depraved. Sometimes the menses will force a way thro' the eyes, ears, nostrils, gums, the salival ducts, bladder, breasts, skin, wounds or ulcers.

Attitudes

Little is known about the cultural attitudes in Britain towards menstruation in the eighteenth century. The *Encyclopaedia Britannica*'s definition: 'MENSES, Flours, Courses, *catamenia*: in medicine, the monthly evacuations from the uterus of women not with child and not giving suck' reminds us that in eighteenth century Britain, as in primitive cultures, women were commonly either pregnant or lactating. The *Encyclopaedia*'s definition does not include the word 'period' which first appeared in the 1820s.

Nineteenth century

Knowledge

Some scientific investigation of menstruation began in the late nineteenth century.

1863 Pfluger developed the 'German theory' of menstruation: increasing pressure in the Graafian follicle causes reflex irritation of the ovarian nerves, leading to pelvic congestion and menstruation.

1866 J. Marion Sims, the 'father of American gynaecology' wrote in his textbook *Clinical notes on uterine surgery*: 'Menstruation is the sign of ovulation; it is preparatory to reception of the ovum… the ovum reaches the cavity of the uterus two to ten days after menstruation… the uterus itself is the normal seat of conception.'

1882 Moricke obtained endometrial samples from living women, using the curette, which had been developed in the 1850s.

Attitudes

During the Victorian era, women in Britain and America were regarded as delicate, though this attitude probably applied only to the middle and upper classes. The American medical historian Harold Speert quotes Harper's magazine: 'The fact is certain, that the American girl is a very delicate plant… not generally strong in nerve and muscle, and too ready to fade before her true mid-summer has come.' Dr Speert also quotes Edward Clarke, in a popular book published in 1874:

> A girl cannot spend more than four, or, in occasional instances, five hours of force daily upon her duties, and leave sufficient margin for the general physical growth that she must make. …If she puts as much force into her brain education as a boy, the brain or the special apparatus will suffer.

This attitude towards women underlay the advice given about menstruation itself. Speert quotes William Robinson, from a book which was first published in the late 19th century but went through many editions until 1928:

> Rest is just as important during menstruation as cleanliness, if not more so. …It is an outrage that many delicate, weak girls and women must stay on their feet all day or work on a machine when they should be at home in bed or lying down on a couch. …there should be as much rest as possible. For delicate and sensitive girls it is always best to stay away from school during the first and second days… It is best that dancing, bicycle riding, horseback riding, rowing, and other athletic exercises be given up altogether during the means. Automobile riding and railroad and carriage travel prove injurious in some instances.

It would be wrong to imagine that this advice represented the view of all informed opinion in the nineteenth century, but it was widespread enough to merit a challenge from an American woman doctor, Mary Putnam Jacobi, one of the first women to graduate in medicine in the United States. In 1876 she published a report, *The question of rest for women during menstruation*, which began by summarizing the opinions of previous authors:

> Thus one of the most essential apparent peculiarities of the menstrual process, its periodicity, that formerly was supposed to indicate a periodical increase in the vital forces of the female organism, has come to be considered as a mark of constantly recurring debility, a means of constantly recurring exhaustion demanding rest as decidedly as a fracture or a paralysis.

Dr Jacobi then cited data from other countries showing how many women work for a living (including 467 261 women employed in the textile industry in Great Britain). She performed experiments showing that muscular strength did not in fact change during the monthly cycle, and she circulated a questionnaire to 1000 women, of whom 268 responded. The results of this questionnaire showed that 35 per cent did not suffer pain, discomfort, or weakness during menstruation. She concluded:

> Purely spasmodic pain of moderate intensity, may be, and certainly is, tolerated in an immense majority of cases, far better while the ordinary occupations are continued. ...The only cases where rest really cures or prevents menstrual pain, are those where general debility is so marked that the loss of blood at menstruation is sufficient to lower the nutrition of the nerve centres below the level to which they are capable of generating force with ease. ...There is nothing in the nature of menstruation to imply the necessity, or even the desirability, of rest, for women whose nutrition is really normal... The menstrual flow is the least important part of the menstrual process, and the arguments for rest drawn from the complexity of the physiological phenomena involved in this, should logically demand rest for women during at least twenty days of the twenty-eight or thirty. In other words, should consign them to the inactivity of a Turkish harem.

Twentieth century

Knowledge

Understanding of ovarian physiology and menstruation became more complete during the twentieth century. For example:

1908 Hitschmann and Adler published detailed histological pictures of the endometrial cycle

1929 oestrogen and progesterone were isolated

1934 von Euler introduced the term prostaglandin

1939 follicle-stimulating hormone (FSH) and luteinizing hormone (LH) were identified as separate hormones

1940 Markee published his studies of endometrium transplanted into the eyes of Rhesus monkeys.

Attitudes

Our century has seen changes in attitudes to the role of women in many countries. Women achieved electoral equality with men in New Zealand in 1893 and women's suffrage was introduced in the United States in 1918. In Britain, after a violent campaign by suffragettes, wives over the age of 30 years were given the vote in 1918. Nevertheless, even at the end of the twentieth century, women tend to be paid less than men (despite equal pay legislation in some countries) and to be in less senior posts.

The feminist movement, which began in the 1960s, challenged traditional attitudes to women. Most of the rules and customs described in this chapter were developed by male-dominated societies and feminists argue that women were content to live by such rules because they had been conditioned over generations to accept a passive role in society.

Feminists have divided opinions about menstruation. Some celebrate it as an essential part of womanhood. The new feminist comedians enjoy breaking the menstrual taboo and shocking male audiences by describing its details.

Germaine Greer's book, *The female eunuch*, included the following remarks about menstruation:

> Women still buy sanitary towels with enormous discretion, and carry their handbags to the loo when they only need to carry a napkin. They still recoil at the idea of intercourse during menstrua-

> tion, and feel that the blood they shed is of a special kind, although perhaps not so special as was thought when it was the liquid presented to the devil in witches' loving cups. If you think you are emancipated, you might consider the idea of tasting your menstrual blood – if it makes you sick, you've a long way to go, baby.

Dr Greer also commented on the language of menstruation:

> The contradiction in the attitude that regards menstruation as divinely ordained and yet unmentionable leads to the intensification of the female revolt against it, which can be traced in all the common words for it, like the *curse*, and male disgust expressed in terms like *having the rags on*. We have only the choice of three kinds of expression: the vulgar resentful, the genteel ('I've got my period', 'I am indisposed'), and the scientific jargon of the *menses*. Girls are irrepressible though: in one Sydney girls' school napkins are affectionately referred to as *daisies*; Italian girls call their periods *il marchese* and German girls *der rote Konig*.

It is possible, however, that the word 'curse' comes from 'courses' (see above). The reference to 'rags' may be no more than an allusion to the normal method of sanitary protection before the invention of the disposable napkin. Until well into the twentieth century women used rags or pieces of linen which they washed after use. Modern disposable sanitary towels were first marketed in the United States in 1921 under the brand name 'Kotex'. The idea of internal tampons was patented in the United States in 1937, when the Tampax company was founded. Their use did not spread around the world until after the Second World War.

The advertising of sanitary protection on British television was banned entirely until 1979, when a limited range of advertisements was allowed for an experimental period. Advertising was finally allowed in 1986 on Channel 4 and on ITV in 1988. The press release from the Independent Broadcasting Authority (IBA) is quoted by Sophie Laws in her book *Issues of blood: the politics of menstruation*:

> Viewers' attitudes were monitored during the two years both by the ITV companies and by the IBA. The research showed a significant shift in public opinion. In July 1984, 55 per cent of those surveyed had said such advertising should be allowed, 38 per cent said it should not, with 6 per cent don't knows. By March 1988 66 per cent said it should be allowed, 30 per cent that it should not, with 4 per cent don't knows.
>
> A broad picture of increasing acceptance of the advertising over the period emerged. Nevertheless it is recognised that a minority, mainly of older women, remain opposed to it.
>
> A frequent reason given by those who object is embarrassment when watching with their families. The IBA received 889 complaints during the experiment on Channel 4.

Laws also quotes the guidelines to advertisers, which include the advice that 'No commercial may contain anything likely to cause embarrassment or to undermine an individual's confidence in her own personal hygiene standards', 'No advertisement may feature an unwrapped towel or tampon', and 'The use of potentially offensive words like "odour" is not acceptable.'

Feminist commentators have suggested that the decision to allow advertising of sanitary products on television owed more to pressure from large commercial organizations than to any wish for equality of the sexes. The market in the UK is worth at least £179 million a year. Feminists also comment on the fact that the British government charges Value Added Tax (VAT) on sanitary protection, bringing the Treasury at least £30 million a year (Drife 1992). As super-absorbent tampons cost more than regular tampons, a woman with heavy periods pays more tax than a woman with light periods. The fact that sanitary protection is not among the many necessities of life exempt from VAT says much about current attitudes to menstruation. The only pressure to change this anomaly has come from small radical feminist groups: mainstream political parties do not feel it is a suitable topic for a party manifesto.

Conclusion

In spite of feminism, present day Western society is still affected by the taboos that amuse us when we look at primitive cultures. The modern Englishwoman does not mention her periods. She does not campaign to have women's toilets made larger than men's, or to have sanitary protection exempted from VAT. Nevertheless, attitudes are changing and are slowly becoming more rational. Perhaps the last word should go to Germaine Greer: 'Menstruation does not turn us into raving maniacs or complete invalids; it is just that we would rather do without it.'

References

De Beauvoir, S. (1953). *The second sex*. Jonathan Cape, London.

Drife, J.O. (1992). Rags to riches. *British Medical Journal*, **304**, 646.

Encyclopaedia Britannica (1771). Edinburgh. Facsimile published by Encyclopaedia Britannica, London.

Greer, G. (1970). *The female eunuch*. MacGibbon & Kee, London.

Laws, S. (1990) *Issues of blood: the politics of menstruation*. Macmillan, Basingstoke.

Miles, R. (1988). *The women's history of the world*. Michael Joseph, London.

Morris, D. (1967). *The naked ape*. Jonathan Cape, London.

O'Dowd, M. and Philip, E. (1994). *History of obstetrics and gynaecology*. Parthenon, London.

Rhodes, P. (1976). An approach to gynaecology. In *Combined textbook of obstetrics and gynaecology*, (ed. J. Walker, I. McGillivray, and M.C. MacNaughton), pp. 624–9. Churchill Livingstone, Edinburgh.

Speert, H. (1996). *Obstetric and gynaecologic milestones*. Parthenon, London.

Weideger, P. (1978). *Female cycles*. The Women's Press, London.

2 The origins and physiology of menstruation

Steven Campbell and Iain T. Cameron

Menstruation is the physiological process during which healthy adult tissue lining the uterus disintegrates and is expelled from the body. A new surface is formed by rapid healing or regeneration although, intriguingly, scarring does not occur. Menstruation is therefore an unusual event, possibly without parallel in adult mammalian physiology.

Our understanding of human menstruation has been limited by the fact that it has proved difficult to investigate directly. Nevertheless, there have been some observational studies which describe the process in humans and monkeys, and much is known about the events occurring in the endometrium towards the end of the secretory phase of the cycle and early in the proliferative phase following menstruation itself. In addition an increasing amount is now known about the physiological and molecular systems that are likely to be involved.

A silhouette of menstruation

The increase in ovarian progesterone secretion after ovulation and its subsequent fall following regression of the corpus luteum would appear to be the major controlling factors in the events which lead up to menstruation. Progesterone induces a cascade of programmed changes to prepare the endometrium for implantation. In cycles where implantation fails to occur, the corpus luteum involutes, circulating concentrations of progesterone decline, and a second cascade of vascular and stromal changes is then triggered which results in tissue shedding followed by regeneration (Noyes *et al.* 1950; Jansen and Johannisson 1985; Li *et al.* 1988). The implantation cascade might begin with a decline in secretory activity in the glandular epithelium. Whether the epithelium is then reprogrammed to function in implantation or menstruation is not known. Subsequent events primarily involve changes in the stromal compartment of the tissue. In the late luteal phase, permeability of the microvasculature is thought to increase, resulting in stromal oedema, and the arterioles continue to elongate, muscularize, and become coiled. The stromal cells then begin a remarkable process of epithelioid differentiation, commonly known as decidualization, and bone marrow-derived cells invade the tissue. If implantation fails to occur, observations in the monkey suggest that arteriolar vasoconstriction and dilatation are followed by bleeding and tissue shedding in which fibrinolysis and clotting are carefully controlled (Markee 1940). Shortly after the tissue is shed, rapid epithelial regeneration begins by a process similar to wound healing, followed by a period of re-growth of the glands, microvasculature, and stroma. The net effect is that the outer 'functional' layer of the endometrium is lost, leaving behind a thin basal layer from which the tissue is renewed in response to stimulation by oestrogen.

In the description of menstruation that follows an attempt is made to provide an evolutionary answer to the question 'why does menstruation occur in the human?'. The events leading up to and following menstruation are then considered along with a summary of what is known about the process itself. Finally, a description of the molecular control systems that may function during menstruation is provided to promote insight into some of the factors that might play a role in the pathophysiology of dysfunctional menstruation. These factors are considered further in Chapters 3 and 7.

The evolution of menstruation

The ability of the female mammal to expel the products of conception from the genital tract was already present when the ancestors of the egg-laying monotremes appeared in the Jurassic period. As mammalian reproduction evolved in the Cretaceous period with the appearance of marsupials and placentals, the need to deliver live young and their placentas arose. After more than 65 million years of evolution the feto-maternal interface in modern placental mammals varies markedly, ranging from the superficially associated placentomes of the domesticated ungulates (artiodactyls) to the more invasive deciduate type found in humans, higher primates, and other species of mammals including the elephant shrew and the bat. Each of these forms of implantation involves substantial remodelling of the uterus after birth. This process of uterine involution, like menstruation, occurs at a time when the influence of progesterone wanes. Early evolution of the placental mammals would therefore seem to have been accompanied by acquisition of the capacity to involute or remodel the uterus after birth or miscarriage (Clarke 1994). The ability to deliver live young, discharge the lochia through myometrial contraction, and remodel the involuting uterus in the weeks following parturition are therefore more ancient physiological processes than menstruation itself. Tissue remodelling and the coordination of myometrial and endometrial function observed at the time of menstruation may therefore have an evolutionary origin in egg laying, parturition and post-partum events.

Menstruation in mammals

The extent to which menstruation or menstruation-like processes occur throughout the mammalian orders has yet to be investigated exhaustively (Profet 1993; Clarke 1994). To date, menstruation or menstrual-like events have only been observed in humans, non-human primates, the elephant shrew, and species of bat (Dempsey 1939; Macdonald 1971; Graham 1973). Whether menstruation has arisen independently in different mammalian orders by a convergent evolutionary change or has been lost through divergence has not been established. Other mammals, however, undergo a form of bleeding at oestrus (the peri-ovulatory period) or at the end of pseudopregnancy. Even if menstruation arose independently in several lineages, examination of where these animals occur in the mammalian evolutionary tree suggests that the process evolved after the branch point which gave rise to pigs (artiodactyls), horses (perissodactyls), and whales (cetacea).

The existence of menstruation in the human lineage must pre-date the earliest hominid fossils for the phenomenon has been found widely in the primate order. Menstruation has been observed in our nearest evolutionary relatives, chimpanzees, gorillas, orang-utan, and gibbons, as well as in old and new world monkeys (Fig. 2.1). Menstruation with external bleeding does not seem to have been reported in the more primitive prosimian primates. If menstruation evolved indepen-

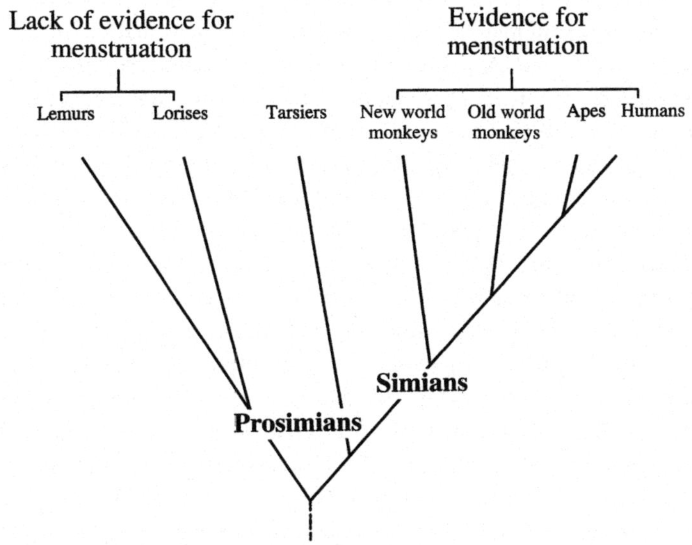

Fig. 2.1 A simplified version of primate evolution showing the species in which menstruation has been demonstrated. Adapted and redrawn from Martin (1990).

dently in primates it is possible that it may have started after the divergence of primitive simians (anthropoids) and prosimians in the Palaeocene epoch around 60 million years ago (Simons 1992). The apparent absence of menstruation in lemuriforms and lorsiforms, and its occurrence in anthropoids, may be related to differences in the mechanism of implantation. Haemochorial placentation, associated with uterine invasion, is found in the menstruating primates whereas the less invasive epitheliochorial form of placentation develops in non-menstruating species (Napier and Napier 1967, 1985; Luckett 1975).

The menstrual cycle in higher primates may be conserved physiologically, for its length shows less variability than does gestation (Napier and Napier 1967). The reproductive cycle in many primate species is approximately four weeks in length. Whether the similarity in periodicity between the menstrual and lunar cycles is coincidental or an ecological factor in reproductive evolution is unknown (see Chapter 1).

Clearly, menstruation of the type observed in humans could not have evolved until the endometrium developed into two distinct layers – the luminal 'functional' layer which is shed and the basal layer which remains and provides the capacity for endometrial regeneration. Macaque endometrium would appear to share this property so it is probably a feature that evolved a considerable time ago (Hill 1939; Padykula *et al.* 1984). Preliminary observations on bovine subjects suggest that there is a gradient of change between the surface epithelium and the myometrium rather than distinct stratified layers (Wylie *et al.* 1995). The evolution of menstruation may therefore have been associated with a change from a more simply organized endometrium to one with distinct stratification.

Why has menstruation been selected for during primate evolution?

The persistence of menstruation for tens of millions of years suggests that either the associated implantation mechanism or menstruation itself confers a significant reproductive advantage. The endometrial cycle and the process of menstruation in most primates has not been described in the same detail as it has in the human. A factor common to humans and chimpanzees is the occurrence of the pre-implantation decidualization reaction in which uterine tissue is pre-programmed to change spontaneously whether implantation occurs or not (Graham 1973, 1981; Gould and Martin 1981; Finn 1987, 1994). Pre-implantation decidualization involves differentiation of the endometrial stromal cells, an influx of bone marrow-derived cells (Loke and King 1995), and a major biochemical and architectural reorganization of stromal extracellular matrix. In women, decidualization commences during both non-conception and conception cycles and continues to develop as pregnancy proceeds. Finn (1994) has argued that it is not the existence of decidualization *per se* that is important because in some species such as the mouse, extensive decidualization is seen after implantation, but menstruation does not occur. He suggests that it is withdrawal of the progestogenic stimulus which triggers the breakdown of endometrial stroma and the loss of superficial parts of the spontaneously decidualized endometrium (Finn and Pope 1984). Furthermore, he has obtained experimental evidence to support this hypothesis by mechanically inducing decidualization in ovariectomized mice primed by exogenous ovarian steroids. Withdrawal of progesterone resulted in menstruation (Finn 1987). This strongly suggests that progesterone-induced decidualization of the endometrium, which begins independently in the human before the embryo implants, creates the appropriate conditions for menstruation to occur after withdrawal of the steroid.

Although the evolutionary advantage of invasive implantation or pre-decidualization is not yet clear it may become so when a better molecular understanding of the implantation mechanism is achieved. As primates evolved and the trophoblast became more highly invasive it may have been necessary for decidualization to start before the embryo had begun to invade the superficial layer of the endometrium so that invasion could be properly contained. This view is consistent with the fact that the lower modern primates, which have not been observed to menstruate, also have a less invasive form of implantation.

Alternatively, menstruation may itself confer specific advantage. Profet (1993) has recently suggested that menstruation has a protective effect by permitting the shedding of pathogens carried into the female body by copulation. Finn (1994) and Clarke (1994) have questioned this argument. Finn (1994) pointed out that menstruation is seen in very few species where internal fertilization occurs. Additionally, Campbell *et al.* (1988, 1993) have argued that menstruation could have the opposite effect and liberate intracellular pathogens such as chlamydia from disintegrating epithelial cells into the lumen of the genital tract. In view of the fact that retrograde menstruation is thought to occur in many women it is hard to envisage menstruation as an efficient cleansing process.

If spontaneous decidualization evolved as a way of containing an invasive trophoblast, it may be that menstruation does itself provide a selective advantage for primates. By evolving as a 'disposable' lining, the functional endometrium may provide a significant selective advantage at relatively minor cost. Increased reproductive success achieved by a rapid regeneration to the pre-pregnancy state would seem to outweigh the burden of losing a few grams of tissue on a regular basis. It should be borne in mind that before the advent of effective contraception and bottle feeding the burden would have been much lighter. For example, women with large families and multiple episodes of lactational amenorrhoea, who in addition had a late menarche and early menopause, would have menstruated less frequently than women of the present day. Although menstruation is therefore likely to assume a greater clinical importance to doctors and may have greater psychological significance to women as time progresses, in evolutionary terms the process may have had less consequence.

A phenomenon that may appear troublesome and superficially wasteful is probably better perceived as the fastest physiological remodelling event so far observed in the adult human body. Within a period of five or six days a spongy glandular tissue of 7–8 mm in thickness is removed and a new epithelial surface is regenerated. Indeed it is difficult to envisage any other mechanism that could achieve such rapid levels of tissue turnover in such a controlled fashion.

Timing of menstruation and the human menstrual cycle

The human menstrual cycle has a modal length of 28 days with ovulation occurring at mid cycle. There is of course a range of cycle lengths in women with a proven history of fertility; cycle length may vary from 21–35 days and still be regarded as normal. Bleeding usually lasts for 3–7 days. The pre-ovulatory phase of the cycle can range from 9 to 23 days and the post-ovulatory phase between 8 and 17 days, determined by the finite lifespan of the corpus luteum (Landgren *et al.* 1980).

Post-ovulatory events leading up to menstruation

Decline in epithelial secretory activity in late luteal phase

The rise in ovarian progesterone secretion following ovulation triggers a very rapid response in the endometrial epithelial cells. Within one day of the luteinizing hormone (LH) surge there are detectable changes on the surface of glandular epithelial cells (Seif *et al.* 1989; Smith *et al.* 1989). Over a period of three days proliferation ceases, a complex series of secretory activities ensues within the glandular epithelial cells, and the glands themselves slowly become more tortuous. Accumulation of glandular secretions within the epithelial cells probably reaches a maximum seven days after the LH surge at the time when implantation is due to occur (Noyes *et al.* 1950; Li *et al.* 1988; Hey *et al.* 1995). Passage of secretions from the gland lumen into the uterine lumen may peak a few days later (Hey *et al.* 1995), four days before the onset of menstruation. Around this time nuclear progesterone receptors become immunohistochemically undetectable in the epithelial cells (Lessey *et al.* 1988; Press *et al.* 1988; Amoso *et al.* 1994). Whether the endometrial glands subsequently play a part in the events surrounding menstruation has yet to be determined, but the fact that they produce vasoactive substances such as endothelins and nitric oxide provides circumstantial evidence for such a role (Cameron *et al.* 1992; Salamonsen *et al.* 1992; Norman and Cameron 1996). Tabibzadeh (1996) has argued that part of the tissue breakdown process involves apoptosis and fragmentation of the endometrial glands due to cell–cell dissociation (dyscohesion), and has suggested that tumour necrosis factor alpha (TNFα) might be involved directly in this process as a local signalling molecule. Our own unpublished histological observations suggest that the amount of apoptosis that occurs at the time of menstruation may vary considerably between different tissue samples.

Changes in the blood vessels

In the week before menstruation, development of the stromal compartment occurs in preparation for the invading embryo. One of the first morphological changes is stromal oedema which begins around day 21. This is probably caused by an increase in permeability of the microvascular endothelium, for experiments with tracer dyes in rodents have demonstrated that the stromal blood vessels become more leaky when decidualization occurs (Psychoyos 1960). One factor that might promote an increase in vascular permeability is vascular endothelial growth factor (VEGF) which is produced by the epithelial cells in increased amounts in the secretory phase of the cycle (Charnock-Jones *et al.* 1993).

Besides changes in the microvasculature there is significant growth and development of the larger blood vessels in the late luteal phase. The endometrial arterioles grow in a spiral fashion from their origin in the myometrium into the endometrium and become muscularized. Regression of endometrial tissue in the days preceding menstruation is thought to increase the number of spirals in these vessels (Markee 1940). Structural changes within the blood vessels during the late secretory phase might contribute to the initiation of bleeding. Ultrastructural studies have demonstrated break-up of the basal lamina in the microvasculature and a reduction in pericyte endothelial cell contact (Roberts *et al.* 1992).

Changes in the stroma

Stromal cell decidualization is one of the next events in the premenstrual, or peri-implantation, sequence. Under the influence of progesterone, the perivascular stromal cells enlarge, form junctional complexes, and deposit basal laminal material, normally found at the basal surface of epithelial cells (Aplin *et al.* 1988). Both collagen type IV (Aplin *et al.* 1995) and laminin (Church *et al.* 1996) are seen in the stroma and increase in amount as pregnancy proceeds. A recent study has shown that withdrawal of progestagen from endometrial stromal cells after two weeks of stimulation *in vitro* resulted in proteinase secretion (Irwin *et al.* 1996; commentary by Liotta 1996). The activity was characteristic of matrix metalloproteinase-2 (MMP-2) although the enzyme was secreted largely in an unactivated higher molecular weight pro-form. Activation of this enzyme, by factors from bone marrow-derived cells, could then lead to stromal extracellular matrix and basement membrane degradation; events which are almost certainly involved in tissue shedding.

In the last three days before the onset of menstruation there is a marked influx of bone marrow-derived cells which continues if pregnancy ensues (Noyes *et al.* 1950; Bulmer 1994; Loke and King 1995). Seventy per cent of these are CD56+ natural killer (NK) cells, 20 per cent CD14+ macrophages, and 10 per cent CD3+ T cells. Whether these cells play a specific role in the process of menstruation has yet to be established. Mast cells, which are present in the endometrial stroma throughout the cycle, degranulate extensively just before and during menstruation (Jeziorska *et al.* 1995, 1996). These cells, which have a different phenotype in the basal and functional layers, release tryptase, an enzyme which can activate precursor forms of the matrix metalloproteinases into the surrounding stroma. In addition, mast cells release histamine, heparin, leukotrienes, cytokines, growth factors, and factors that are chemotactic for eosinophils. Jeziorska *et al.* (1995) have shown that extravascular eosinophils become localized and are activated in the stroma just before menstruation. The eosinophil would also be expected to release proteolytic enzymes such as collagenase and gelatinase and signalling molecules such as platelet activating factor (PAF) and leukotriene C_4.

The onset of bleeding

Menstrual bleeding follows the withdrawal of progesterone from an oestrogen-primed endometrium (Fig. 2.2). The most direct observations of menstruation in the primate were made by Markee (1940) who examined 432 menstrual cycles in 41 macaques over nine years. He transplanted fragments of endometrium into the anterior chamber of the eye so that the tissue could be

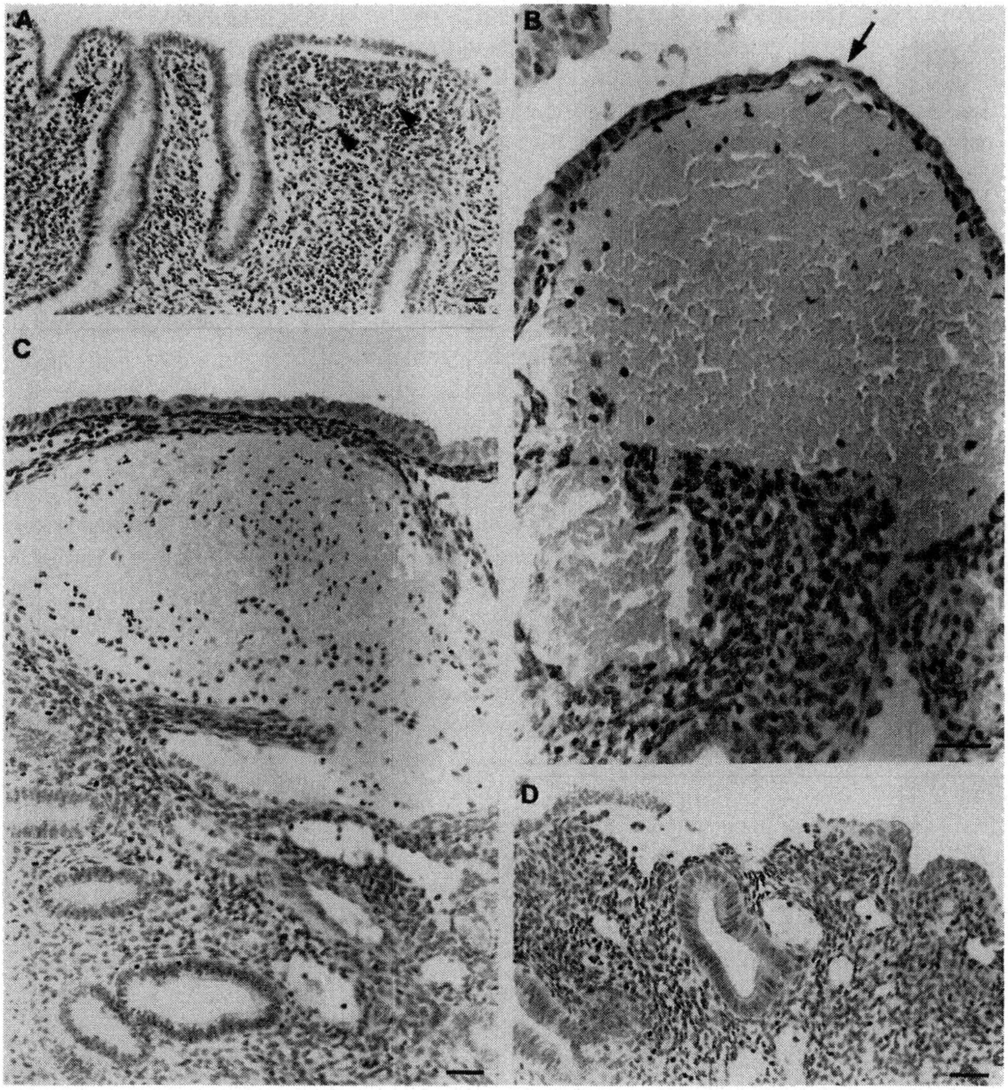

Fig. 2.2 Initiation of menstruation observed in histological sections of human endometria reveals the same features as those observed experimentally by Markee in the macaque. **A:** In this area of an early menstrual phase specimen the surface epithelium has begun to detach from the underlying stroma and the superficial vessels contain fibrinous plugs (arrowheads). **B:** A haemorrhage has occurred in another early menstrual phase specimen. The surface epithelium has become locally detached from the stroma and the underlying space has filled with red blood cells. A local thinning of the surface epithelium (arrow) has occurred and might be the site of an imminent rupture. **C:** A large fibrinous clot has developed in a site very close to that shown in B. **D:** A different pattern of rupture has occurred in this specimen where disruption of the epithelium has happened without the apparent occurrence of haemorrhage. Scale bars = 30 μm.

examined directly under high magnification. The tissue was wedged into the iridal angle and some pieces became externally vascularized within 24 hours. The transplants were observed daily and at the time of menstruation for up to 15 hours each day, when it was possible to see the size and shape of the blood vessels, rupture points, streams of escaping blood, and clots. These experiments provided a unique insight into the process of menstruation. Two to six days before the onset of bleeding the transplants decreased in size, a process that continued even after the last haemorrhage. The reduction in size did not occur simultaneously in each transplant within the same monkey, which suggests that different parts of the uterus may behave in a slightly different fashion in the days before menstruation begins. Both veins and arteries were observed to undergo changes in diameter. Before bleeding was seen the vessels underwent cycles of vasoconstriction and vasodilatation every 60 to 90 seconds. Just prior to menstruation, vasodilatation occurred and the rhythmic contractions ceased over a period of six to nine hours. Vasoconstriction of the spiral but not the straight arterioles took place for a period of four to 24 hours followed, in turn, by vasodilatation. Five patterns of bleeding were then observed:

(1) capillary and arteriolar haemorrhage with formation of haematoma beneath the epithelium;

(2) direct escape of blood with haematoma formation after rupture of arterioles and epithelium;

(3) diapedesis;

(4) venous haemorrhage;

(5) secondary haemorrhage from damaged vessels.

Arteriolar bleeding occurred in spurts but was then controlled by vasoconstriction closer to the basalis. Venous bleeding was also seen which lasted for up to 90 minutes from individual vessels. Markee's experiments suggest that the local modulation of vascular tone is a crucial part of the menstrual process. Vasoconstrictors such as endothelin-1 and prostaglandin $F_{2\alpha}$ ($PGF_{2\alpha}$), and vasodilators such as prostaglandin E_2 (PGE_2), prostacyclin (PGI_2) and nitric oxide would therefore be expected to play a part in these events (see below).

These experiments also showed that endometrium can bleed in isolation from the myometrium. The function of the myometrium may be to contribute to the control of bleeding by constricting the arcuate and radial arteries as they pass towards the endometrium, or to assist with the expulsion of shed tissue. The data pose important questions about the properties and origin of endometrial blood vessels. If the endometrium can become externally vascularized by ocular rather than myometrial arteries, why do they still spiralize and undergo the rhythmic pulsation and subsequent dilatation and constriction thought to be characteristic of uterine arteries? The answer must lie within the endometrium. The function and morphology of the ingrowing arteries must be controlled by the extravascular compartment under the effect of the stromal cells or the stromal cells acting in concert with the epithelium. Markee's observations also raise the possibility that re-growth of new arteries after menstruation may begin in the myometrium.

The study of menstruation in the human has relied on examination of tissue biopsies (Christiaens *et al.* 1980, 1982; van Eijkeren *et al.* 1991). In the study by Christiaens *et al.* (1980), uteri were collected at hysterectomy at precise time periods after the onset of overt bleeding. The uteri were biopsied extensively and examined by light and electron microscopy. Menstrual spotting was associated with small depressed areas of bleeding (1–3 mm diameter) and extravasation of blood was rarely observed histologically. However, the endothelial lining of the blood vessels was damaged at this stage. Between 3.5 and 13 hours after major bleeding, extravasation started in the superficial layers of the endometrium and progressed basally to the deeper layers and pieces of tissue were shed. Vessel endings at the cut edge were filled with fibrin and platelets, and intravascular thrombi were present. In one uterus, after 13 hours of bleeding, most of the functional layer had been shed and the vascular plugs were found at the transition between the functional and basal layers. By late menstruation, vessels ending on the shedding margin were constricted although variable amounts of functional endometrium were left.

Impaired platelet plug formation might be expected in the presence of potent inhibitors of platelet adhesion and aggregation in the endometrium. Prostacyclin, a potent inhibitor of platelet aggregation (Gryglewski *et al.* 1976) is produced by the endometrium and myometrium (Abel and Kelly 1979). Furthermore, recent work has shown that the human endometrium is also a source of nitric oxide (Tseng *et al.* 1996; Telfer *et al.* 1997), a ubiquitous vasodilator and powerful inhibitor of platelet aggregation (Lowenstein and Snyder 1992).

The control of menstrual bleeding

Prostaglandins

Extensive data have accumulated supporting a role for the prostaglandins in the pathogenesis of menorrhagia. Most work has concentrated on direct actions of the prostaglandins on the uterine vasculature. The main endometrial products of the arachidonic acid cascade are prostaglandin E_2 and prostaglandin $F_{2\alpha}$. Endometrial prostaglandin concentrations are low in the proliferative phase and increase in the second half of the cycle (Downie *et al.* 1974). One effect of progesterone is to promote the storage of arachidonic acid which is released as steroid concentrations fall after luteolysis, resulting in prostaglandin formation at the time of menstruation itself. The major prostaglandin in myometrium is prostacyclin.

It has already been suggested that the local production of prostacyclin might contribute to the impaired platelet plug formation seen during menstruation. When the functional endometrium has been shed, prostaglandin E_2 and prostaglandin $F_{2\alpha}$ are thought to control the degree of bleeding from the remaining spiral arteriolar fragments by vasodilatation and vasoconstriction respectively. Indeed, in the endometrium of women with menorrhagia, the balance between prostaglandin E_2 and prostaglandin $F_{2\alpha}$ is tilted in favour of the vasodilator prostaglandin E_2 (Smith *et al.* 1981).

Endothelins

The endothelins are a family of three vasoactive peptides, endothelin-1, endothelin-2 and endothelin-3, which act by binding to two distinct receptor subtypes, ET_A and ET_B (see Cameron and Davenport (1992) for a review). Initially reported as products of vascular endothelium, the endothelins are now known to be released from a variety of epithelial cell types. Endothelin-1, which has been described as the most potent vasoconstrictor yet discovered, is a powerful constrictor of small vessels in the human uterus (Svane *et al.* 1993). Endothelin-like immunoreactivity has been localized to human uterine glandular epithelium (Cameron *et al.* 1992; Salamonsen *et al.* 1992) and was released into the supernatant after endometrial tissue culture (Economos *et al.* 1992). An action for the endothelins in the uterus was further suggested by the demonstration of specific binding sites for iodinated endothelins on myometrium and on endometrial vascular smooth muscle and glandular epithelium. These studies were supported by the demonstration of mRNA for endothelin-1, endothelin-2, and endothelin-3 and the receptors ET_A and ET_B in human endometrium (O'Reilly *et al.* 1992).

Endothelin-1 is thought to mediate vasoconstriction by binding to the ET_A receptor, whereas activation of the ET_B receptor may lead to either vasoconstriction or vasodilatation by the paracrine release of prostacyclin and nitric oxide. Recent studies have demonstrated the presence of ET_A and ET_B receptors in human endometrium throughout the menstrual cycle (Collett *et al.* 1996). ET_A receptor was localized to endometrial stroma. In early secretory phase, ET_B receptors were confined predominantly to glandular epithelial cells within the basalis. By late secretory phase expression of ET_B had spread to the epithelial cells of the 'functional' layer. Subsequently, ET_B receptors were also present in the stroma in menstrual endometrium. The function of ET_B receptors on glandular epithelium is not known but they may play a part in the regenerative process in the early days of the new menstrual cycle.

Platelet activating factor

Platelet activating factor (PAF) is a D-glycerol derivative formed from alkyl-acyl-glycerol-3-phosphocholine by the action of phospholipase A_2 and acetyl transferase. Increasing evidence has shown that PAF may be an important local mediator in the maternal recognition of pregnancy, but it might also play a role in the paracrine control of the uterine vascular bed in the non-pregnant cycle. Platelet activating factor stimulated the release of prostaglandin E_2, but not prostaglandin $F_{2\alpha}$ from separated human endometrial glandular cells from secretory endometrium (Smith and Kelly 1988; Ahmed and Smith 1992). Being a vasoconstrictor, and stimulating platelet aggregation, PAF itself might also make a direct contribution to menstrual haemostasis.

Post-menstrual epithelial regeneration

Despite the repeated nature of menstrual shedding, healing is achieved without the deposition of scar tissue. This suggests a highly controlled response within the stroma and epithelium and well regulated deposition of new extracellular matrix. The surface epithelium (and its underlying basement membrane) is lost after menstruation and is regenerated from the remaining basal portions of the glands (Markee 1940; Ferenczy and Richart 1973; Ludwig *et al.* 1990). Regeneration of the surface epithelium has been examined in histological sections and by transmission and scanning electron microscopy (Ferenczy and Richart 1973; Ferenczy 1976*a*,*b*). The initial stage of healing seems to involve epithelial cell migration and spreading rather than cell proliferation. Cells emerge from the glands in contiguous sheets and re-colonize the surface of the denuded stroma (Fig. 2.3). In

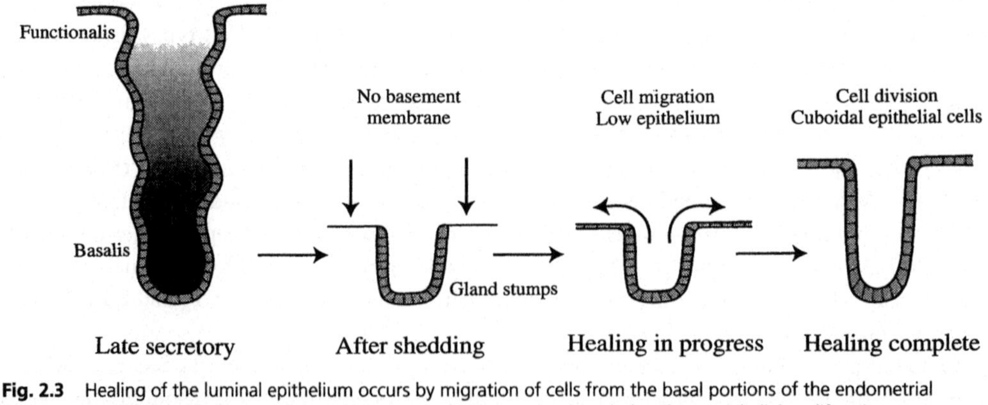

Fig. 2.3 Healing of the luminal epithelium occurs by migration of cells from the basal portions of the endometrial glands. The epithelial cells become flattened and spread out over the denuded surface. Epithelial proliferation commences around the time of epithelial reformation. The cells then become taller. The long axis of the nuclei is re-orientated in an apico-basal direction. This is followed by ciliated cell differentiation. At the same time proliferation within the glandular epithelium results in elongation of the glands.

the course of migration each cell spreads out to occupy a larger area. The newly formed epithelium is therefore thin in cross-section. Cell division restarts around the time of epithelial closure. As a consequence, each epithelial cell has less space to occupy and becomes more cuboidal as the proliferative phase advances. By contrast, cell division within the glandular epithelium leads to an elongation of the glands which are straight tubes at first but become undulatory by the late proliferative phase. Noyes and colleagues (1950) estimated that epithelial cell proliferation was low in the early proliferative phase and increased towards the time of ovulation. The change in glandular morphology could therefore be explained by a difference in the elongation of the glands relative to the stroma.

Angiogenesis

Establishment of a new system of arterioles, capillaries, and venules in the endometrium is critical for re-growth of the tissue. The process involves degradation of the basement membrane around pre-existing blood vessels, endothelial cell migration and proliferation, structural reorganization to form a lumen, and functional maturation. Of the variety of factors known to influence this important process, the fibroblast growth factors (FGFs) and VEGF may play a role in the human endometrium as described in Chapters 3 and 7.

Regeneration of these vessels, especially the capillaries, is more difficult to investigate than the surface epithelium for the latter forms a clearly defined layer. Initial remodelling and closure of the veins and arterioles could occur by a similar combination of cell migration and division as observed in the epithelium. Assessment by colocalization of endothelial cells and proliferative markers suggests that endothelial proliferation is not particularly marked after the end of menstruation. Indeed it is not until the endometrium begins to re-grow that an intricate system of vessels is needed. The way in which new vascular loops develop during each cycle has yet to be fully described. Formation or maintenance of short loops within the basalis after menstruation could provide the basis for the new vascular system. These loops might gradually extend into the functionalis (Fig. 2.4).

Possible roles for oestrogen and polypeptide growth factors in the post-menstrual regeneration of epithelium, stroma, and the vascular system is outlined below.

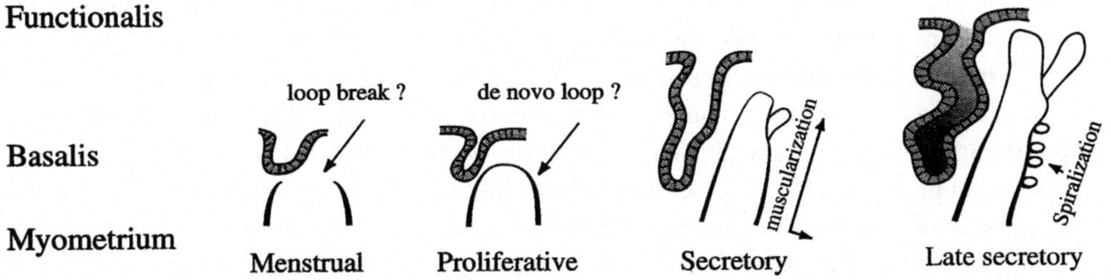

Fig. 2.4 Revascularization after menstruation plays a crucial role in the development of the endometrium and subsequent implantation. It is unclear how new arteriovenous loops develop. It is not known whether broken loops are reinstated by growth or branching from the broken ends of arteries (and veins) or by the extension and elaboration of pre-existing loops which survive within the basalis. Muscularization of the new vessels occurs in a progressive fashion from the basalis towards the luminal surface. The arterioles become spiralized towards the end of the menstrual cycle.

Cytokines

The cytokines comprise a diverse group of proteins which regulate a variety of cellular functions. They are important mediators of immune and inflammatory responses, and of the reparative response to injury. As cytokines influence vasoconstriction, haemostatic platelet-plug formation, mitogenesis, and angiogenesis, they are likely to play a key role in the mechanism of menstruation. Interleukins, tumour necrosis factor alpha (TNFα), and interferons will be outlined here (Tabibzadeh 1994*a*, 1996).

The interleukins may contribute to the control of menstruation by modulating cellular proliferation, inducing the release of other cytokines, and activating stromal T cells. Messenger RNA and protein for interleukin-1α, interleukin-1β, and interleukin receptor antagonist have been demonstrated in human endometrium, and a role for interleukin-1 in the uterus is supported by the detection of binding sites for the cytokine on endometrial epithelial and stromal cells. Other members of the interleukin family found in the uterus include interleukin-6 and interleukin-8 (Critchley *et al.* 1994).

TNFα, or cachectin, has also been detected in endometrium. This peptide exerts a variety of effects including stimulation of the inflammatory response, stimulation and inhibition of growth, and modulation of the immune response. It also has angiogenic and cytotoxic actions (Le and Vilcek 1987), and may be involved in the mechanisms controlling endometrial apoptosis (Tabibzadeh *et al.* 1995).

The interferons, IFNα, IFNβ, and IFNγ, are a family of peptides with antiviral and immunoregulatory activities, which plays an important role in the control of cell growth and differentiation. A potential source of IFNγ in the uterus is the lymphoid aggregates adjacent to the glands of the basal endometrium (Tabibzadeh *et al.* 1988). Interferon γ inhibits proliferation of human endometrial cells *in vitro* and receptors for the cytokine have been demonstrated on human endometrial cells throughout the menstrual cycle (Tabibzadeh *et al.* 1988; Tabibzadeh 1990, 1994*b*).

Growth factors

Transforming growth factors

The transforming growth factors (TGFs) are peptide growth factors with diverse paracrine actions. Although TGFα and TGFβ are similarly named, they represent distinct families of peptides with different structures and actions (De Larco and Todaro 1978; Roberts and Sporn 1988).

Transforming growth factor α binds to the same receptor as epidermal growth factor (EGF) to exert its biological action. In human endometrium, TGFα has been localized to stromal cells in the proliferative phase of the cycle. The distribution was different in the secretory phase, when TGFα-like immunoreactivity was localized to glandular and luminal epithelium, with moderate-to-intense staining around spiral arterioles (Horowitz *et al.* 1993). The presence of TGFα in close proximity to endometrial blood vessels in the luteal phase might suggest a role either in the development of the placental vasculature following implantation, or in the repair process following menstruation.

The TGFβ group, which currently comprises a family of three distinct isoforms, plays a crucial part in the regulation of epithelial homeostasis and epithelial–mesenchymal interactions (Akhurst *et al.* 1992). Of specific relevance to the mechanism of menstruation, TGFβ is expressed after vascular insult and is involved in the repair of damaged epithelium in a variety of human tissues. In addition, it promotes gland formation, and is both chemotactic and angiogenic (Sporn and Roberts 1990).

Epidermal growth factor

Regrowth of the endometrium involves oestrogen-induced cellular proliferation. Increasing evidence indicates that this process is mediated by EGF. This growth factor, first isolated from the submaxillary glands of adult male mice, is a potent stimulator of proliferation in various cell types, including epithelial cells. That EGF can replace the effects of oestradiol on the growth and differentiation of the genital tract in oophorectomized rodents provides compelling evidence for the physiological role of the peptide (Nelson *et al.* 1991).

Insulin-like growth factors and binding proteins

Like EGF, the insulin-like growth factors (IGFs) are widely distributed. They bind to specific binding proteins (IGFBPs), release from which provides a mechanism to control their bioavailability. Animal studies suggested that IGF-1 may increase uterine DNA synthesis *in vitro* (Ghahary *et al.* 1990). In the human, IGFBP-1 (placental protein 12, PP12; see Fay and Grudzinskas (1991) for a review) has been identified as a major secretory product of decidualized endometrium. Whether IGFs are involved in the mechanism of menstruation is not known, but IGFBP-1 mRNA and peptide have been localized to stromal cells in late secretory endometrium (Waites *et al.* 1988; Julkunen *et al.* 1990), suggesting the facilitation of IGF bioavailability at the onset of menstruation.

Conclusion

The precise reason for which menstruation has evolved is unclear, but it seems likely that the process is the inevitable consequence of failed fertilization in species in which implantation involves invasion of extravillous trophoblast into a decidualized endometrium. Although our knowledge of the cellular and molecular processes which control menstruation is incomplete, recent work has described a range of locally derived agents which are likely to govern the onset of menstruation, the degree of menstrual bleeding, and regeneration of the endometrium and its vasculature to prepare for the next cycle. A better understanding of these processes should lead to a more rational approach to the clinical management of disorders of endometrial function.

References

Abel, M.H. and Kelly, R.W. (1979). Differential production of prostaglandins within the human uterus. *Prostaglandins*, **18**, 821–8.

Ahmed, A. and Smith, S.K. (1992). Platelet-activating factor stimulates phosopholipase C activity in human endometrium. *Journal of Cell Physiology*, **152**, 207–14.

Akhurst, R.J., Fitzpatrick, D.R., Fowlis, D.J., Gatherer, D., Millan, F.A., and Slager, H. (1992). The role of TGF-βs in mammalian development and neoplasia. *Molecular Reproduction and Development*, **32**, 127–35.

Amoso, N.A., Crow, J., and Shaw, R.W. (1994). Comparitive immunohistochemical study of oestrogen and progesterone receptors in the Fallopian tube and uterus at different stages of the menstrual cycle and the menopause. *Human Reproduction*, **9**, 1027–37.

Aplin, J.D., Charlton, A.K., and Ayad, S. (1988). An immunohistochemical study of human endometrial extracellular matrix during the menstrual cycle and first trimester decidua. *Cell and Tissue Research*, **253**, 231–40.

Aplin, J.D., Mylona, P., Kielty, C.M., Ball, S., Williams, J.D.L., Church, H.J., and Jones, C.J.P. (1995). Collagen VI and laminin as markers of differentiation of endometrial stroma. In *Molecular and cellular aspects of peri-implantation processes*, pp. 331–51. Springer, New York.

Bulmer, J. (1994). Human endometrial lymphocytes in normal pregnancy and pregnancy loss. *Annals of the New York Academy of Sciences*, **734**, 185–92.

Cameron, I.T. and Davenport, A.P. (1992). Endothelins in reproduction. *Reproductive Medicine Review*, **1**, 99–113.

Cameron, I.T., Davenport, A.P., van Papendorp, C, Barker, P.J., Huskisson, N.S., Gilmour, R.S., *et al.* (1992). Endothelin-like immunoreactivity in human endometrium. *Journal of Reproduction and Fertility*, **95**, 623–8.

Campbell, S. Richmond, S., Haynes, P., Gump, D. Yates, P., and Allen, T.D. (1988). An *in vitro* model of *Chlamydia trachomatis* infection in the regenerative phase of the human endometrial cycle. *Journal of General Microbiology*, **134**, 2077–87.

Campbell S., Yates, P.S., and Richmond, S.J. (1993). *Chlamydia trachomatis* infection of cultured motile cells after uptake of chlamydiae from the substratum. *Journal of General Microbiology*, **139**, 2151–8.

Charnock-Jones, D.S., Sharkey, A.M., Rajput-Williams, J., Burch, D., Schofield, J.P., Fountain, S.A., *et al.* (1993). Identification and localization of alternately spliced mRNAs for vascular endothelial growth factor in human uterus and estrogen regulation in endometrial carcinoma cell lines. *Biology of Reproduction*, **48**, 1120–28.

Christiaens, G.C.M.L., Sixma, J.J., and Haspels, A.A. (1980). Morphology of haemostasis in menstrual endometrium. *British Journal of Obstetrics and Gynaecology*, **87**, 425–39.

Christiaens, G.C.M.L., Sixma, J.J., and Haspels, A.A. (1982). Hemostasis in menstrual endometrium: a review. *Obstetrical and Gynecological Survey*, **37**, 281–303.

Church, H.J., Vicovac, L.M., Williams, J.D.L., Hey, N.A., and Aplin, J.D. (1996). Laminins 2 and 4 are expressed by human decidual cells. *Laboratory Investigation*, **74**, 21–32.

Clarke, J. (1994). The meaning of menstruation in the elimination of abnormal embryos. *Human Reproduction*, **9**, 1204–7.

Collett, G.P., Kohnen, G., Campbell, S., Davenport, A.P., Jeffers, M.D., and Cameron, I.T. (1996). Localization of endothelin receptors in human uterus throughout the menstrual cycle. *Molecular Human Reproduction*, **2**, 439–44.

Critchley, H.O.D., Kelly, R.W., and Kooy, J. (1994). Perivascular location of chemokine interleukin-8 in human endometrium: a preliminary report. *Human Reproduction*, **9**, 1406–9.

De Larco, J.E. and Todaro, G.J. (1978). Growth factors from murine sarcoma virus-transformed cells. *Proceedings of the National Academy of Sciences USA*, **75**, 4001–5.

Dempsey, E.W. (1939). The reproductive cycle of new world monkeys. *American Journal of Anatomy*, **64**, 381–405.

Downie, J., Poyser, N.L., and Wunderlich, M. (1974). Levels of prostaglandins in human endometrium during the normal menstrual cycle. *Journal of Physiology*, **236**, 465–72.

Economos, K., MacDonald, P.C., and Casey, M.L. (1992). Endothelin-1 gene expression and protein biosynthesis in human endometrium: potential modulator of endometrial blood flow. *Journal of Clinical Endocrinology and Metabolism*, **74**, 14–19.

Fay, T.N. and Grudzinskas, J.G. (1991). Human endometrial peptides: a review of their potential role in implantation and placentation. *Human Reproduction*, **6**, 1311–26.

Finn, C.A. (1987). Why do women and some other primates menstruate? *Perspectives in Biology and Medicine*, **30**, 566–73.

Finn, C.A. (1994). The adaptive significance of menstruation. *Human Reproduction*, **9**, 1202–4.

Finn, C.A. and Pope, M. (1984). Vascular and cellular changes in the decidualized endometrium of the ovariectomized mouse following cessation of hormone treatment: a possible model of menstruation. *Journal of Endocrinology*, **100**, 295–300.

Ferenczy, A. (1976*a*). Studies on the cytodynamics of human endometrial regeneration I. Scanning electron microscopy. *American Journal of Obstetrics and Gynecology*, **124**, 64–74.

Ferenczy, A. (1976*b*). Studies on the cytodynamics of human endometrial regeneration II. Transmission electron microscopy and histochemistry. *American Journal of Obstetrics and Gynecology*, **124**, 582–95.

Ferenczy, A. and Richart, R.M. (1973). Scanning and transmission electron microscopy of the human endometrial surface epithelium. *Journal of Clinical and Endocrinology and Metabolism*, **36**, 999–1008.

Ghahary, A., Chakrabarti S., and Murphy, L.J. (1990). Localization of the sites of synthesis and action of insulin-like growth factor-1 in the rat uterus. *Molecular Endocrinology*, **4**, 191–5.

Gould, K.G. and Martin, D.E. (1981). The female genital tract and its secretions. In *Reproductive biology of the great apes* (ed. C.E. Graham), pp. 105–25. Academic Press, New York.

Graham, C.E. (1973). Chimpanzee endometrium and sexual swelling during menstrual cycle or hormone administration. *Folia Primatologica*, **19**, 458–68.

Graham, C.E. (1981). Menstrual cycle of the great apes. In *Reproductive biology of the great apes* (ed. C.E. Graham), pp. 1–43. Academic Press, New York.

Gryglewski, R.J., Bunting, S., Moncada, S., Flower, R.J., and Vane, J.R. (1976). Arterial walls are protected against deposition of platelet thrombi by a substance (prostaglandin x) which they make from prostaglandin endoperoxides. *Prostaglandins*, **12**, 685–713.

Hey, N.A., Li, T.C., Devine, T.L., Graham, R.A., Saravelos, H., and Aplin, J.D. (1995). MUC 1 in secretory phase endometrium: expression in precisely dated biopsies and flushings from normal and recurrent miscarriage patients. *Human Reproduction*, **10**, 2655–62.

Hill, W.C.O. (1939). The menstrual cycle of the toque macaque (*Macaca sinica* L.), with observations on its uterine structure compared with that of other macaques. *Ceylon Journal of Science*, **5**, 21–36.

Horowitz, G.M., Scott, R.T., Drews, M.R., Mavot, D., and Hofmann, G.E. (1993). Immunohistochemical localization of transforming growth factor α in human endometrium, decidua, and trophoblast. *Journal of Clinical Endocrinology and Metabolism* **76**, 786–92.

Irwin, J.C., Kirk, D., Gwatkin, R.B.L., Navare, M., Cannon, P., and Giudice, L.C. (1996). Human endometrial matrix metalloproteinase-2, a putative menstrual proteinase. *Laboratory Investigation*, **97**, 438–47.

Jansen, R.P.S. and Johannisson, E. (1985). Endocrine response in the female. In *Clinical Reproductive Endocrinology*, (ed. R.P. Shearman), pp. 109–64. Churchill-Livingstone, Edinburgh.

Jeziorska, M., Salamonsen, L.A., and Woolley, D.E. (1995). Mast cell and eosinophil distribution and activation in human endometrium throughout the menstrual cycle. *Biology of Reproduction*, **53**, 312–20.

Jeziorska, M., Nagase, H., Salamonsen, L.A., and Woolley D.E. (1996). Immunolocalization of the matrix metalloproteinases gelatinase B and stromelysin 1 in human endometrium throughout the menstrual cycle. *Journal of Reproduction and Fertility*, **107**, 43–51.

Julkunen, M., Koistinen, R., Suikkari, A.M., Seppala, M., and Janne, O.A. (1990). Identification by hybridization histochemistry of human endometrial cells expressing mRNAs encoding a uterine β-lactoglobulin homologue and insulin-like growth factor-binding protein-1. *Molecular Endocrinology*, **4**, 700–7.

Landgren, B.M., Unden, A.L., and Diczfalusy, E. (1980). Hormonal profile of the cycle in 68 normally menstruating women. *Acta Endocrinologica*, **86**, 608–20.

Le, J. and Vilcek, B. (1987). Biology of disease. Tumor necrosis factor and interleukin 1: cytokines with multiple overlapping biological activities. *Laboratory Investigation*, **56**, 234–40.

Lessey, B.A., Killam. A.P., Metzger, D.A., Haney, A.F., Greene, G.L., and McCarty, K.S. (1988). Immunohistochemical analysis of human uterine estrogen and progesterone receptors throughout the menstrual cycle. *Journal of Clinical Laboratory Investigation*, **67**, 334–40.

Li, T.C., Rogers, A.W., Dockery, P., Lenton, E.A., and Cooke, I.D. (1988). A new method of histological dating of human endometrium in the luteal phase. *Fertility and Sterility*, **50**, 52–60.

Liotta, L.A. (1996). Probing the depths of degradation: matrix metalloproteinase-2 and endometrial menstrual breakdown. *Journal of Clinical Investigation*, **97**, 273.

Luckett, W.P. (1975). Ontogeny of the fetal membranes and placenta. In *Phylogeny of the primates* (ed. W.P. Luckett and F.S. Szalay), pp. 157–82. Plenum Press, New York.

Ludwig, H., Metzger, H., and Frauli, M. (1990). Endometrium: tissue remodelling and regeneration. In *Contraception and mechanisms of endometrial bleeding*, (ed. C. d'Arcangues, I.S. Fraser, J.R. Newton, and V. Odlind), pp. 441–66. Cambridge University Press.

Loke, Y.W. and King, A (1995). *Human implantation. Cell biology and immunology*. Cambridge University Press.

Lowenstein, C and Snyder, S.H. (1992). Nitric oxide: a novel biologic messenger. *Cell*, **70**, 705–7.

Markee, J.E. (1940). Menstruation in intraocular endometrial transplants in the rhesus monkey. *Contributions to Embryology*, **28**, 219–308.

Martin, R. (1990). Classification and evolutionary relationships. In *The Cambridge encyclopedia of human evolution* (ed. S. Jones, R. Martin, and D. Pilbeam), pp. 17–23. Cambridge University Press.

Macdonald, G.J. (1971). Reproductive patterns of three species of macaques. *Fertility and Sterility*, **22**, 373–77.

Napier, J.R. and Napier, J.R. (1967). *A handbook of living primates*. Academic Press, London.

Napier, J.R. and Napier, J.R. (1985). *The natural history of the primates*. MIT Press, Cambridge, Massachusetts.

Nelson, K.G., Takahashi, T., Bossert, N.L., Walmer, D.K., and McLachlan, J.A. (1991). Epidermal growth factor replaces estrogen in the stimulation of female genital tract growth and differentiation. *Proceedings of the National Academy of Sciences USA*, **88**, 21–5.

Norman, J.E. and Cameron, I.T. (1996). Nitric oxide in the human uterus. *Reviews of Reproduction*, **1**, 61–8.

Noyes, R.W., Hertig, A.T., and Rock, J. (1950). Dating the endometrial biopsy. *Fertility and Sterility*, **1**, 3–25.

O'Reilly, G., Charnock-Jones, D.S., Davenport, A.P., Cameron, I.T., and Smith, S.K. (1992). Presence of mRNA for endothelin-1, endothelin-2 and endothelin-3 in human endometrium, and a change in the ratio of ET_A and ET_B receptor subtype across the menstrual cycle. *Journal of Clinical Endocrinology and Metabolism*, **75**, 1545–9.

Padykula, H.A., Coles, L.G., McCracken, J.A., King, N.W., Longcope, C., and Kaiserman Abramof, I.R. (1984). A zonal pattern of cell proliferation and differentiation in the rhesus endometrium during the estrogen surge. *Biology of Reproduction*, **31**, 1103–18.

Press, M.F., Udove, J.A., and Greene G.L. (1988). Progesterone receptor distribution in the human endometrium. Analysis using monoclonal antibodies to the human progesterone receptor. *American Journal of Pathology*, **131**, 112–24.

Profet, M. (1993). Menstruation as a defence against pathogens transported by sperm. *The Quarterly Review of Biology*, **68**, 335–86.

Psychoyos, A. (1960). La réaction déciduale est précedée de modification précoces de la perméabilité capillaire de l'uterus. *Comptes Rendus Société Biologique, Paris*, **154**, 1384–7.

Roberts, A.B. and Sporn, M.B. (1988). Transforming growth factor *β*. *Advances in Cancer Research*, **51**, 107–45.

Roberts, D.K., Parmley, T.H., Walker. N.J., and Horbelt, D.V. (1992). Ultrastructure of the microvasculature in the human endometrium throughout the normal menstrual cycle. *American Journal of Obstetrics and Gynecology*, **166**, 1393–406.

Salamonsen, L.A., Butt, A.R., Macpherson, A.M., Rogers, P.A.W., and Findlay, J.K. (1992). Immunolocalization of the vasoconstrictor endothelin in human endometrium during the menstrual cycle and umbilical cord at birth. *American Journal of Obstetrics and Gynecology*, **167**, 163–7.

Seif, M.W., Aplin, J.D. Foden, L.J., and Tindall, V.R. (1989). A novel approach for monitoring the endometrial cycle and detecting ovulation. *American Journal of Obstetrics and Gynecology*, **160**, 357–62.

Simons, E. (1992). The primate fossil record. In *The Cambridge encyclopedia of human evolution* (ed. S. Jones, R. Martin., and D. Pilbeam), pp. 197–208. Cambridge University Press.

Smith, S.K. and Kelly, R.W. (1988). Effect of platelet-activating factor on the release of $PGF_2\alpha$ and PGE_2 by separated cells of human endometrium. *Journal of Reproduction and Fertility*, **82**, 217–76.

Smith, S.K., Abel, M.H., Kelly, R.W., and Baird, D.T. (1981). Prostaglandin synthesis in the endometrium of women with ovular dysfunctional uterine bleeding. *British Journal of Obstetrics and Gynaecology*, **88**, 434–42.

Smith, R.A., Seif, M.W., Rogers, A.W., Li, T.C., Dockery, P., Cooke, I.D., and Aplin, J.D. (1989). The endometrial cycle: the expression of a secretory component correlated with the luteinizing peak. *Human Reproduction*, **4**, 236–42.

Sporn, M.B. and Roberts, A.B. (1990). The transforming growth factor-*β*s: past, present and future. *Annals of the New York Academy of Sciences*, **593**, 1–6.

Svane, D., Larsson, B., Andersson, K.E., and Forman, A. (1993). Endothelin-1: immunocytochemistry, localization of binding sites, and contractile effects in human uteroplacental smooth muscle. *American Journal of Obstetrics and Gynecology*, **168**, 233–41.

Tabibzadeh, S.S. (1990). Evidence of T-cell activation and potential cytokine action in human endometrium. *Journal of Clinical Endocrinology and Metabolism*, **71**, 645–49.

Tabibzadeh, S.S. (1994*a*). Cytokines and hypothalamic–pituitary–ovarian–endometrial axis. *Human Reproduction Update*, **9**, 947–67.

Tabibzadeh, S.S. (1994*b*). Regulatory roles of IFN-gamma in human endometrium. *Annals of the New York Academy of Sciences*, **734**, 1–6.

Tabibzadeh, S.S. (1996). The signals and molecular pathways involved in human menstruation, a unique process of tissue destruction and remodelling. *Molecular Human Reproduction*, **2**, 77–92.

Tabibzadeh, S.S., Satyaswaroop, P.G., and Rao, P.N. (1988). Antiproliferative effect of interferon γ in human endometrial epithelial cells *in vitro*: potential local growth modulatory role in endometrium. *Journal of Clinical Endocrinology and Metabolism*, **67**, 131–8.

Tabibzadeh, S.S., Zupi, E., Babaknia, A., Liu, R., Marconi, D., and Romanini, C. (1995). Site and menstrual cycle-dependent expression of proteins of the tumour necrosis factor (TNF) receptor family, and BCL-2 oncoprotein and phase-specific production of TNFα in human endometrium. *Human Reproduction*, **10**, 277–86.

Telfer, J.F., Irvine, G.A., Kohnen, G., Campbell, S. and Cameron, I.T. (1997). Expression of endothelial and inducible nitric oxide synthase in non-pregnant and decidualized human endometrium. *Molecular Human Reproduction* **3**, 69–75.

Tseng, L., Zhang, J., Peresleni, T.Y., and Goligorsky, M.S. (1996). Cyclic expression of endothelial nitric oxide synthase mRNA in the epithelial glands of human endometrium. *Journal of the Society for Gynecologic Investigation*, **3**, 33–8.

van Eijkeren, M.A., Christiaens, G.C.M.L., Gueze, J.J., Haspels, A.A., and Sixma, J.J. (1991). Morphology of menstrual hemostasis in essential menorrhagia. *Laboratory Investigation*, **64**, 284–94.

Waites, G.T., James, R.F.L., and Bell, S.C. (1988). Immunohistochemical localization of the human endometrial secretory protein pregnancy-associated endometrial α-1-globulin, an insulin-like growth factor binding protein, during the menstrual cycle. *Journal of Clinical Endocrinology and Metabolism*, **67**, 1100–4.

Wylie, A.H.M., Campbell, S. Telfer, J.F., Cameron, I.T., Aughey, E. Robertson, L. and Jeffers, M.D. (1995). Comparison of secretory activity between the bovine and human endometrium. *Journal of Reproduction and Fertility* (Abstract Series), **16**, 60.

3 The endometrial vascular bed

Peter Rogers

Introduction

In searching for a paradigm upon which to base an understanding of the structure and function of the endometrial vascular bed, it is not inappropriate to consider the relative evolutionary histories of both the vascular system and the endometrium. Primitive invertebrate and vertebrate vascular systems first appeared some 500 million years ago. Since that time the vascular system has evolved into a complex organ playing central roles in a number of functions critical to the survival of the organism, including oxygen transport, nutrition, excretion, fluid balance, homeostasis, and immune defence. By contrast, placental mammals and the first primates appeared about 60–70 million years ago, and it is from this time onwards that a functional endometrium has developed.

From this brief evolutionary history it is clear that embryo implantation, placentation, and menstruation are relatively recent events compared to the functioning of the vascular system. On this basis it is possible to conclude that reproductive function, which is orchestrated predominantly by oestrogen and progesterone at the level of the endometrium, has been superimposed on the 'normal' mechanisms that control the vasculature. As a consequence of this, the endometrial vascular bed is constantly responding to the cyclical fluctuations in sex steroids, resulting in repeated alterations in angiogenesis, regression, haemostasis, blood flow, oxygenation, nutrient supply, and tissue fluid balance. From a physiological point of view this is the opposite of what happens in most adult vascular beds, where stability and maintenance of homeostasis are primary functional issues. Despite this, many of the basic mechanisms that control vascular structure and function in the endometrium are similar to those in other vascular beds. The aim of this chapter will be to review the structure and function of the human endometrial vascular bed.

Structure of the endometrial vascular bed

Vascular architecture

The overall architecture of the endometrial vasculature and microvasculature has been well described by numerous workers (Markee 1940; Ramsey 1982; Ferenczy 1987). Blood supply to the endometrium arrives through the radial arteries, which arise from the arcuate arteries within the myometrium. After passing through the myometrial–endometrial junction the radial arteries-split to form the smaller basal arteries that supply the basal portion of the endometrium, and the spiral arterioles which continue up towards the endometrial surface. The spiral arterioles, which supply the functional layer of the endometrium, have a distinctive coiled appearance that becomes more pronounced during the secretory phase of the menstrual cycle. The spiral arterioles are unusual amongst resistance arterioles, in that they lack significant elastin within the internal lamina (Ferenczy 1987). Each spiral arteriole provides blood to a uterine luminal surface area estimated at 4–9 mm^2 (Bartelmez 1933), with little or no overlap between areas. Capillaries branch from the spiral arterioles at all levels supplying the stroma and peri-glandular networks. Just below the endometrial surface the spiral arterioles break up into the prominent sub-epithelial capillary plexus. This plexus drains into a number of venules that pass down through the endometrium, collecting blood from other capillaries on the way. The numerous venules join to form veins which pass out of the endometrium into the myometrium.

The basal portion of the endometrium and its vasculature remains relatively unchanged throughout the menstrual cycle. By contrast, the functional layer of the endometrium is constantly changing in response to circulating sex steroids.

Vascular structure

To a large extent the capillaries, arterioles, and venules of the endometrium are indistinguishable from those of most other tissues in the body. All endometrial vessels are lined by a continuous, single layer of endothelial cells arranged on a vascular basement membrane. The smallest vessels, or capillaries, are usually made up of just these two components, although they can also include pericytes. Pericytes are cells that envelop capillaries, often possessing numerous projections that make contact with several endothelial cells. They are typically a feature of mature rather than growing capillaries, and are normally enveloped in the vascular basement membrane. Pericyte distribution has been studied ultrastructurally in human endometrium (Roberts *et al.* 1992), although the function of these cells is less well understood. A role for pericytes during endometrial preparation for embryo implantation in the rat has been postulated (Lunam and Rogers 1981).

By far the most dominant structural feature of the endometrial vasculature is the spiral arteriole. These specialized arterioles are found only in the endometrium, and play a major role in both placentation and menstruation. Studies using immunohistochemical techniques have shown that endometrial arterioles contain 1–5 layers of vascular smooth muscle cells (Abberton *et al.* 1996). This work also identified a large number of endometrial vessels surrounded by vascular smooth muscle cells that were not spiral arterioles. Although some of these may have been venules, it seems likely that there is also a population of 'straight' arterioles in the functionalis, the existence and function of which have largely been ignored to date.

Microvascular heterogeneity is being recognized increasingly as a key feature of different vascular beds. Thus, in addition to expected differences between arterioles, capillaries, and venules, there are also differences between adjacent vessels of the same class. Examples of this in endometrium include the endothelial expression of intercellular adhesion molecule-1 (ICAM-1), and the basement membrane component heparan sulphate proteoglycan (HSPG) (Tawia *et al.* 1993; Kelly *et al.* 1995). ICAM-1 is found in endometrial arterioles, capillaries, and venules, but unlike platelet endothelial cell adhesion molecule (PECAM or CD31), does not appear in all vessels. HSPG was only demonstrated in approximately 55 per cent of endometrial vessel basement membranes, and also showed no association with any particular vessel type.

The majority of immunohistochemical studies undertaken to date have concluded that endometrial endothelial cells do not contain oestrogen or progesterone receptors (e.g. Critchley *et al.* 1993). However, vascular smooth muscle cells in the endometrium contain both progesterone receptors (Perrot-Applanat *et al.* 1994) and oestrogen receptors (unpublished observation), the latter having also been demonstrated elsewhere in the vasculature (Karas *et al.* 1994). It is thus possible for oestrogen and progesterone to influence the endometrial vasculature in several ways. These include, by paracrine action via the endometrial epithelial and stromal cells, by direct action on vascular smooth muscle cells, by direct non-receptor mediated effects on endothelial cells, and by indirect mechanisms such as overall tissue growth. It has also been reported that endometrial endothelial and vascular smooth muscle cells contain human chorionic gonadotropin/luteinizing hormone receptors (Lei *et al.* 1992), indicating that other reproductive hormones may also have direct actions on the endometrial vasculature.

Structural changes in the endometrial vasculature during the menstrual cycle

In this section a range of different techniques that have been used to investigate endometrial vascular structure across the menstrual cycle will be reviewed.

Histology

Conventional histological dating of endometrial biopsies taken at different stages of the menstrual cycle (Noyes *et al.* 1950) does not place major emphasis on the appearance of the blood vessels. Endothelial proliferation can be seen in conjunction with glandular and stromal proliferation during the proliferative phase of the cycle under the influence of oestrogen, but this is not a major diagnostic feature. The appearance of the endometrial vasculature becomes more important from day 7 post-ovulation onwards, when stromal rather than glandular changes are the main diagnostic features (Ferenczy 1987). From post-ovulation days 8–11 the spiral arterioles become more coiled, appearing as characteristic clusters of multiple vascular profiles in histological sections. From day 9 onwards perivascular predecidual changes start to occur throughout the functionalis, characterized by the conversion of spindle-shaped stromal cells to more ovoid epithelial-like cells. Pre-menstrually (post-ovulation days 11–13) the endometrial stroma is infiltrated by extravasated leucocytes, although the role of the vasculature in this process has not been well studied. During the process of menstruation, the endometrial blood vessels can range from a relatively normal appearance through to a blocked lumen due to endothelial swelling and complete degeneration with ruptured walls and fibrinoid deposits.

In general terms, haematoxylin and eosin stained light microscope sections do not demonstrate the bulk of the endometrial vasculature adequately in biopsy specimens, since most of the smaller vessels collapse during the biopsy procedure. The lack of a visible lumen makes it impossible to differentiate endothelial cells from other stromal cells without the use of ultrastructural or immunohistochemical techniques.

Ultrastructure

There have been several recent ultrastructural studies of the endometrial vasculature during the menstrual cycle (Blackwell and Fraser 1988; Peek *et al.* 1992; Roberts *et al.* 1992). The following description of the endothelial cells, pericytes, and vascular basement membrane during the menstrual cycle is based primarily on the detailed work of Roberts *et al.* (1992).

In the early proliferative phase endothelial cells appear relatively inactive with condensed nuclear chromatin, a small amount of organelle rich cytoplasm, and few microvilli. Pinocytotic vesicles are common on both luminal and basal cell surfaces. Cells presumed to be pericytes are of two appearances, one resembling smooth muscle cells and the second more fibroblast-like. Both types have numerous pinocytotic vesicles and possess cytoplasmic extensions that pass through the basal lamina to make contact with the endothelial cells. The basal lamina or basement membrane surrounding the endometrial capillaries is relatively loose and discontinuous at this time. In the late proliferative phase many endothelial cells and pericytes have enlarged nuclei with diffuse chromatin. Other evidence of increased endothelial cell activation includes more and larger mitochondria, more dilated rough endoplasmic reticulum, increased intermediate and microfilaments, and better developed Weibel–Palade bodies. The capillary basement membrane is thicker and more diffuse than in the early proliferative stages. By the early secretory stage, selected endothelial cells show cytoplasmic growth, with more elaborate Golgi complexes and dilated rough endoplasmic reticulum. Both enlarged and non-enlarged endothelial cells show increased surface blebbing and signs of apparently less active nuclei. Pericytes start to show signs of decidualization with increased size due to more ribosomes, dilated rough endoplasmic reticulum, more elaborate Golgi, and vacuole formation. Pericytes now posses more cell organelles and appear less smooth muscle-like than during the proliferative stage, and the basement membrane becomes more intact and complex. In the midsecretory phase the heterogeneous development of endothelial cells is quite marked, with the larger cells sometimes nearly occluding the capillary lumen. Pericytes are more decidualized and the basement membrane is more developed and elaborate than at any stage of the cycle with many additional laminae enveloping as many as two or three layers of pericytes. In the late secretory/premenstrual phase the endothelial cells appear healthy and in some instances even more hypertrophied than in the midsecretory phase, despite widespread degeneration of other stromal cells. The capillary basement membrane is much more fragmented and there is a marked decrease in the interactions between pericytes and endothelial cells.

Immunohistochemistry and *in situ* hybridization

Immunohistochemical and *in situ* hybridization techniques provide a major avenue for investigating endometrial vascular structure and function during the menstrual cycle. This section has been divided into four broad subject areas – adhesion molecules and integrins, cytokines and growth factors, basement membranes, and vascular smooth muscle cells.

Cellular adhesion molecules play a crucial role in a range of biological processes, including maintenance of tissue integrity, cell–cell and cell–substrate recognition, leucocyte recruitment, and tissue remodelling (Edelman and Crossin 1991). As a dynamic tissue undergoing constant remodelling the endometrium has received considerable recent attention as a model system for investigating adhesion molecules (e.g. Tawia *et al.* 1993; Tabibzadeh *et al.* 1994; Lessey and Castelbaum 1995). ICAM-1 is expressed primarily on endothelial cells throughout the menstrual cycle, with a major increase in immunostaining at the time of menstruation (Tawia *et al.* 1993). ICAM-1 is not expressed by all vessels, although there is no apparent pattern in terms of veins, capillaries, and arterioles as far as the staining is concerned. In contrast to ICAM, PECAM shows strong immunostaining on all blood vessels at all stages of the menstrual cycle. Based on these results, it appears that PECAM is expressed constitutively in the vasculature of human endometrium, and presumably plays some role in maintaining normal vessel integrity.

Interestingly, it does not appear to change at the time of menstruation, when vessel breakdown occurs. In contrast, ICAM-1 expression appears to be increased at the time of menstruation, and presumably plays some role in that process. Neither molecule appears to alter at the time of presumed embryo implantation. Two ligands for ICAM-1 include lymphocyte function-associated antigen-1 (LFA-1) and macrophage antigen-1 (Mac-1). Immunohistochemical studies of the distribution of these ligands in human endometrium (unpublished observations) demonstrate that LFA-1 occurs on cells dispersed throughout the endometrium, both within the stroma and the epithelium, as well as on clusters of cells also spread throughout the endometrium. In contrast Mac-1 only appears on cells scattered throughout the stroma. It was not seen on cells within the epithelium, or on cells clumped together. Both LFA-1 and Mac-1 levels increase around the time of menstruation. However, due to large natural variability between subjects, there were no significant differences in expression of these ligands across the menstrual cycle.

Other adhesion molecules that play a role in the trafficking of white blood cells from the vasculature into the endometrial tissues include vascular cell adhesion molecule 1 (VCAM-1) and E-selectin (Tabibzadeh *et al.* 1994). It has been reported that VCAM-1 is expressed by the endothelial cells in the basalis, but not functionalis, during the proliferative and secretory phases of the cycle. In contrast, E-selectin only appears in the basalis from postovulatory day 3 onwards. Whilst it is clear that these, and other, vascular adhesion molecules play a central part in controlling the recruitment of different white blood cell populations to the endometrium, considerably more work is required before a full understanding of their role in the biology of the endometrium becomes clear.

Integrins are a family of transmembrane glycoproteins that act as receptors for the extracellular matrix. They are heterodimeric complexes made up of α and β subunits, of which there are currently 19 known combinations (Lessey and Castelbaum 1995). There is major interest in the role that integrins may play in determining uterine receptivity for embryo implantation, with particular emphasis on the temporal expression of α_1, α_4, and β_3 integrins by endometrial glandular epithelial cells. To date there has been very little reported work on the role that integrins may play in controlling the endometrial vasculature during the menstrual cycle, despite the fact that they play a key role in controlling vascular integrity (Dejana *et al.* 1993), and more recent reports have identified a key role for $\alpha_V\beta_3$ in regulating angiogenesis (Brooks *et al.* 1994).

Growth factors can be defined as proteins that interact with specific cell membrane receptors to initiate intracellular signalling pathways that result in cell division. Many growth factors are pleiotrophic in action, with the ability to both promote cell differentiation and inhibit mitogenesis in some situations. Cytokines include proteins that modulate a variety of cellular functions, including morphogenesis, chemotaxis, expression of epitopes, and immunoregulatory function. It is becoming increasingly clear that the endometrium expresses a large number of growth factors and cytokines, and that many of these are regulated during the menstrual cycle either directly or indirectly by oestrogen and progesterone (Tabibzadeh and Sun 1992; Giudice 1994). *In vitro* evidence indicates that many growth factors and cytokines can either be produced by, or have actions on, endothelial cells. However, the *in vivo* relevance of *in vitro* experiments should always be questioned critically, especially given the pleiotrophic nature of most of these proteins. Some growth factors and cytokines relevant to specific endometrial vascular functions, such as those known to play a major role in regulating angiogenesis, will be discussed later in this chapter and are also considered in Chapters 2 and 7.

Interleukin-1β has been demonstrated by immunohistochemical methods in endometrial endothelial cells throughout the menstrual cycle, and more strongly in spiral arterioles (Simon *et al.* 1993). There was increased staining in the secretory phase compared to the proliferative phase. Interleukin-1 type 1 receptor was found only in glandular epithelial cells, providing evidence for a mechanism whereby the vasculature can directly modulate epithelial function. Other cytokines expressed by endometrial endothelial cells include interleukin-1α and interleukin-6 (Tabibzadeh and Sun 1992). Transforming growth factor-α shows moderate to intense immunostaining around spiral arterioles during the secretory phase (Horowitz *et al.* 1993), while tumour necrosis factor-α mRNA is found in the vascular smooth muscle cells surrounding spiral arterioles with the protein in smooth muscle and endothelial cells (Philippeaux and Piguet 1993).

Basement membranes play a major role in the structural and functional integrity of blood vessels. Just as endothelial cells can differ in structure, function, and metabolic properties between and within different organs, so too can the composition of the underlying basement membrane. Studies of basement membrane composition in human endometrium reveal that the major components, collagen IV, laminin, and heparan sulphate proteoglycan, are present throughout all stages of the menstrual cycle (Kelly *et al.* 1995). However, whereas the first two of these components appear to be in all vessels, and immunostain with equal intensity throughout the cycle, heparan sulphate proteoglycan is only apparent in approximately 55 per cent of vessels, and its staining intensity is dramatically reduced in menstrual tissue. In addition, breaks and small gaps can be seen in both vascular and glandular basement membrane at the time of menstruation. Thus there is evidence in the endometrium for both vascular basement membrane heterogeneity and regulation during the menstrual cycle.

Vascular smooth muscle cells provide the contractile force around arterioles which enables these vessels to regulate blood flow to the tissues. In a major morphometric study using immunostaining of α-actin to identify vascular smooth muscle cells, it has been shown that total numbers of arterioles per unit volume of endometrium do not alter during the cycle (Abberton *et al.* 1996). In addition, once immunostaining was used to identify arterioles, it became apparent that a significant population of non-spiral, small arterioles was present at all stages of the cycle in human endometrium. The other major findings were that there were no differences in vascular smooth muscle cell α-actin immunostaining between women with and without menorrhagia, but that significant increases in α-actin staining occurred in women showing perimenopausal symptoms. We have also shown using double immunostaining techniques that endometrial vascular smooth muscle cells express oestrogen and progesterone receptors (unpublished observations, see plate 1). The pattern of expression does not seem to alter during the menstrual cycle, and not all vascular smooth muscle cells show positive staining. It has also been suggested that intense staining for progesterone receptors in spiral arteriole smooth muscle cells during pregnancy indicates a key role for progesterone in regulating blood flow to the fetus at this time (Perrot-Applanat *et al.* 1994).

One feature of many of these immunohistochemical and *in situ* hybridization studies is the variability in regional distribution of many proteins in the endometrium. This regional variability, including microvascular heterogeneity within specific regions, makes it critically important that the human endometrium is not considered as a homogeneous tissue when planning research studies or interpreting results.

Hysteroscopy

Hysteroscopy and microhysteroscopy are being used increasingly for diagnostic and operative procedures in gynaecology. Somewhat surprisingly there has been very little published to date on

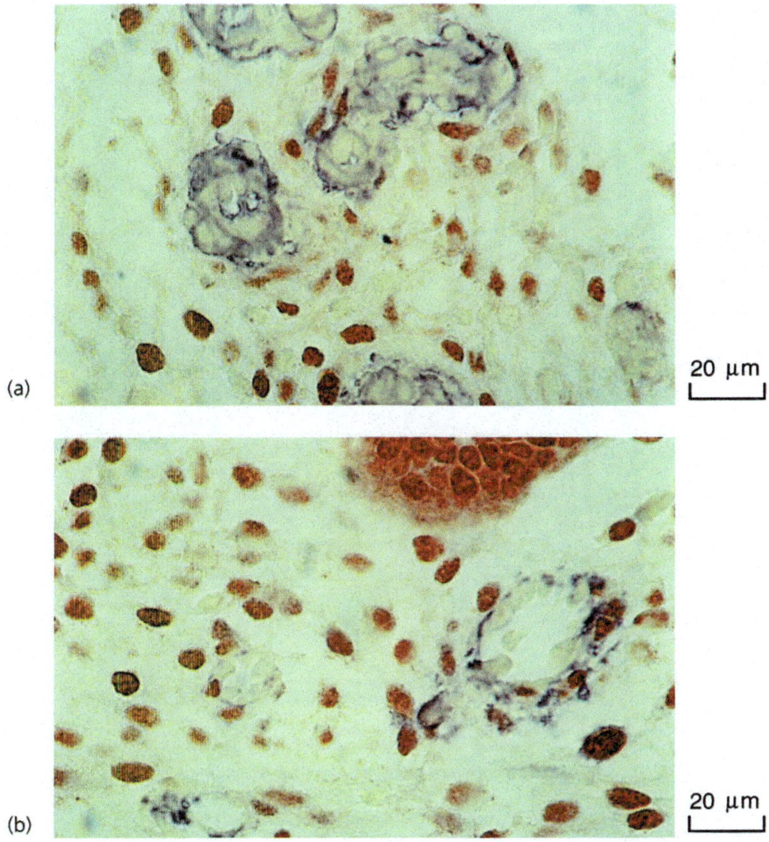

Plate 1 (a) (b) Human secretory phase endometrium with double immunostaining for α-smooth muscle action (blue stain; antibody which selectively marks smooth muscle cells) and progesterone receptor (red stain; antibody which selectively marks the nuclei of cells expressing progesterone receptors). (a) shows several cross-sections of a spiral arteriole. None of the smooth muscle cells of the arteriole show progesterone receptor presence, but other cells closely associated with the spiral arteriole do. By contrast, The vessel in (b) has smooth muscle cells which stain positively for progesterone receptor.

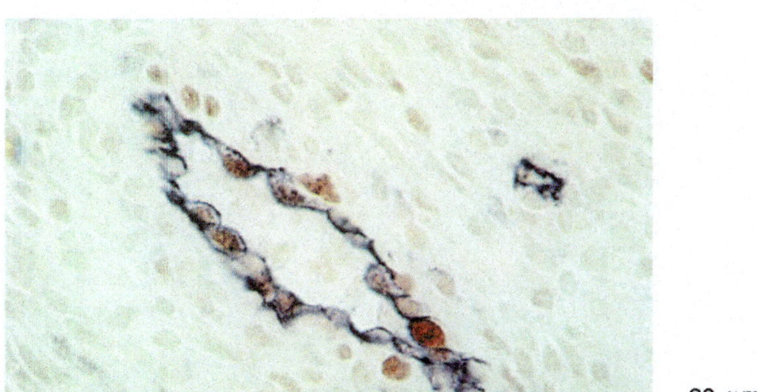

Plate 2 Human secretory phase endometrium with double immunostaining for CD34 (blue stain; antibody which selectively marks endothelial cells) and proliferating cell nuclear antigen (PCNA; red stain; antibody which selectively marks the nuclei of cells in the S phase of the cell cycle). Note several endothelial cells in the vessel wall are positive for PCNA, suggesting that vessel growth is still occurring.

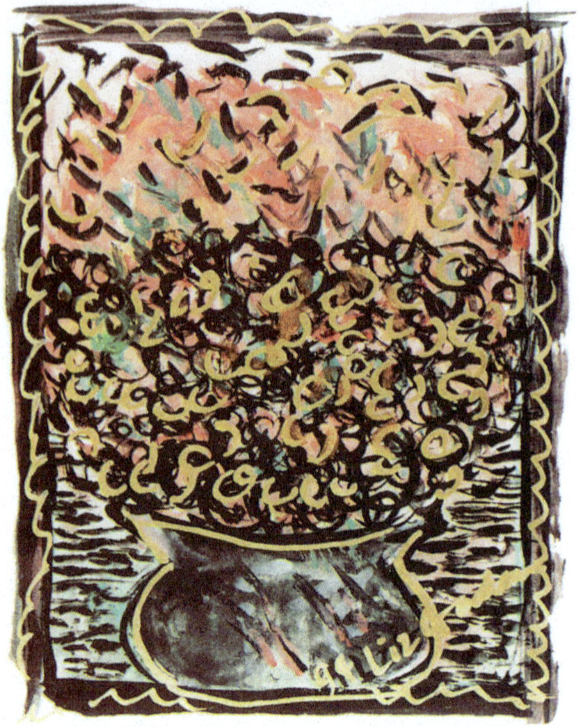

Plate 3 Picture painted before hysterectomy.

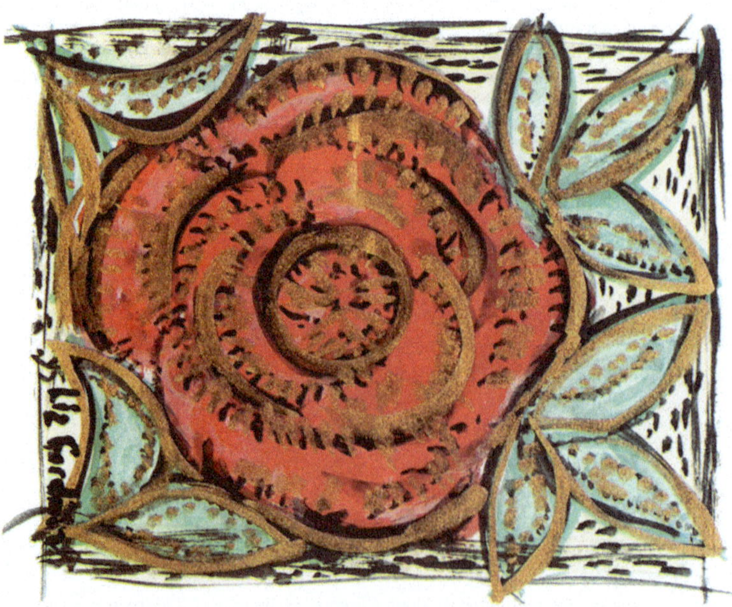

Plate 4 Picture painted after hysterectomy.

endometrial vascular changes during the normal menstrual cycle as visualized with these techniques. The following description is taken from work by van Herendael *et al.* (1987). In the early proliferative phase the main vessels visualized are the basal arterioles running parallel to one another and the endometrial surface. Small coiled arterioles running perpendicular to the surface are seen as interrupted or punctate lines. The late proliferative phase is marked by a rapid growth of the coiled arterioles which become more convoluted and are easily visualized. In the early secretory phase a deeper layer containing the spiral arterioles can be seen under a superficial layer containing a capillary network that spreads around the gland openings. By the late secretory stage, stromal oedema, the decidual response, and glandular secretions combine to reduce or eliminate visualization of the spiral arterioles, so that only the superficial capillary network can be seen. During the premenstrual to menstrual phase small pools of blood collect near the endometrial surface prior to complete endometrial shedding.

Endometrial vascular function during the menstrual cycle

Blood flow

Studies in humans have demonstrated that endometrial blood flow rises during the proliferative phase of the cycle, to reach a peak just before ovulation (reviewed by Fraser and Peek 1992). It has been shown that there is a significant positive correlation between unopposed circulating oestradiol levels and rate of endometrial blood flow. When progesterone levels are elevated, the correlation between oestradiol and blood flow is lost. The method by which oestrogen increases endometrial blood flow is unclear, although a number of mechanisms may be involved. Since endometrial vascular smooth muscle cells contain oestrogen and progesterone receptors, at least some direct effects by these steroids on blood flow seems probable. A number of other vasoactive compounds are under the indirect control of the sex steroids in the uterus. Prostaglandins are readily synthesized in human endometrium and have vasoconstrictive and vasodilatory capabilities. Endothelium derived relaxing factor (EDRF) or nitric oxide will almost certainly play some role at the local level in controlling blood flow, while the potent vasoconstrictor endothelin is also expressed by human endometrium (Economos *et al.* 1992). Other possible vasoactive candidates include leukotrienes, oxytocin, vasopressin, and catecholamines. The myometrium can also act to reduce endometrial blood flow by contracting and thus raising intraluminal pressure.

The recent incorporation of colour Doppler processing in transvaginal transducer/probes has provided a completely new clinical mode for investigating utero-ovarian physiology. There are now a number of reports in the literature showing that an increased uterine artery pulsatility index at the time of embryo transfer may be associated with a reduced implantation rate (Coulam *et al.* 1994; Steer *et al.* 1995). While it appears that colour Doppler assessment of uterine artery flow may have a role to play in determining uterine receptivity for *in vitro* fertilization (IVF), a number of questions about exactly what arterial impedance means at the level of the endometrial microvasculature remain to be answered. For example, the major uterine compartment is the myometrium and not the endometrium, thus it could be assumed that the bulk of blood passing through the uterine artery never reaches the endometrium. It has also been suggested that increased resistance to blood flow, as demonstrated by an increased uterine artery pulsatility index, may represent poor uterine vascularity (Bassil *et al.* 1995). However, since blood flow through a tissue is primarily controlled by contraction and dilation of the resistance arterioles, this may not necessarily be the case. Finally, it is clear that successful implantation can still occur in women with a high pulsatility index, thus raising the fundamental question as to whether uterine artery impedance represents an obligatory marker of uterine receptivity or a related phenomenon. Clearly, further basic and clinical research is required in this emerging area of uterine physiology.

There are two occasions during the normal menstrual cycle when stromal oedema becomes evident; the mid-proliferative and the mid-secretory phases (Noyes *et al.* 1950). Tissue oedema occurs when there is a shift in net fluid flux from the vasculature to the tissues. Fluid flux is governed by relatively simple physical laws, and an increase will occur if blood pressure rises, if the permeability of the vessel wall increases, or if the osmotic pressure of the tissue rises. Although the times of endometrial oedema have been linked to changing levels of sex steroids, and in particular oestrogen, there is little understanding of the exact mechanisms controlling these events, or their physiological purpose.

Angiogenesis

Angiogenesis, or new vessel growth, is usually divided into four main stages (Klagsbrun and D'Amore 1991). These are breakdown of the basement membrane around an existing vessel, migration of endothelial cells towards a stimulus, proliferation of the endothelial cells, and formation of the endothelial cells into a new patent tube or vessel. Other than pathological situations such as wound healing or growth of solid tumours, angiogenesis rarely occurs in the adult. The exception to this is the female reproductive tract, where new blood vessels grow in the ovary and endometrium each cycle.

Between the end of menstruation and ovulation it has been reported that the endometrial vasculature undergoes two different growth phases. The first, which commences during menstruation, is the repair of the vascular bed (Markee 1940). The second is the growth of the vasculature in concert with the rest of the endometrium under the influence of oestrogen during the proliferative phase of the menstrual cycle (Ferenczy *et al.* 1979). In support of these studies Rogers *et al.* (1992) reported two peaks of endothelial cell migratory activity from endometrial explants in culture corresponding to the post-menstrual and mid–late proliferative phases of the cycle. However, a subsequent study (Goodger (Macpherson) and Rogers 1994) demonstrated wide variability in endothelial cell proliferation rates between endometria from the same stages of the menstrual cycle, with no evidence at all for peaks of endothelial cell proliferation either post-menstrually or in the mid–late proliferative phase of the cycle (see plate 2). This result suggests that endothelial cell migration and proliferation are controlled independently during endometrial angiogenesis. If correct, this finding demonstrates that the physiological growth of new blood vessels in the endometrium does not follow the conventionally accepted steps of the angiogenic process exactly. This finding has significant implications for our understanding of how angiogenesis might be controlled in the endometrium, and which angiogenic cytokines may be involved.

That endometrial angiogenesis is a tightly controlled process is demonstrated by the fact that vascular density in the endometrium remains constant throughout the menstrual cycle, despite the large changes in tissue growth and oedema that occur (Rogers *et al.* 1993). However, while many factors known to influence the angiogenic process have been identified in endometrium, the specific mechanisms by which vascular growth is controlled remain unclear. The endometrium and its resident population of macrophages are capable of producing most, if not all, of the major cytokines and factors currently known to play a role in controlling angiogenesis (Giudice 1994; Sunderkotter *et al.* 1994). Publications investigating variations in the expression of some of these factors throughout the menstrual cycle include VEGF (Charnock-Jones *et al.* 1993), fibroblast growth factor (FGF) (Ferriani *et al.* 1993), TGFα (Horowitz *et al.* 1993), IL-1 and IL-6 (Tabibzadeh 1991), EGF (Haining *et al.* 1991), and IL-8 (Critchley *et al.* 1994). However, many of these studies are preliminary in nature and since there is no clear understanding of exactly when or how new blood vessel formation occurs in the endometrium during the menstrual cycle, there is nothing meaningful with which to correlate the reported variations in cytokine expression. In addition, the pleiotrophic nature of most cytokines and the many ways in which their actions are regulated weakens the assumption that they may be involved specifically in endometrial angiogenesis. It is also important to note that endometrial expression of cytokines is usually very varied from subject to subject, and even within the same subject from cycle to cycle. Thus studies involving small groups of women need to be interpreted with caution.

Implantation

In most placental mammals studied to date, a localized increase in endometrial microvascular permeability appears to be one of the first signs of impending implantation. This increase in permeability is seen across a range of implantation modes, in such species as rat (Psychoyos 1960; Rogers *et al.* 1983), guinea-pig (Deanesly 1967), sheep (Boshier 1970), and pig (Keys *et al.* 1986). Despite the ubiquitous nature of this endometrial microvascular response to the implanting embryo, there is still little understanding of either the mechanisms responsible, or the underlying physiological reasons for it. Whether an equivalent increase in vascular permeability occurs in humans is unknown. Oedema is visible around the human implantation site by day 9 post-ovulation (Hertig *et al.* 1956), although this is probably later in the implantation process than that reported above for other mammalian species.

Early trophoblast invasion of the maternal vasculature has been studied in detail in species such as the macaque, the rhesus monkey, and the baboon (Enders 1989; Enders and King 1991). Similar studies have not been performed in the human. Based on the primate work, it appears that the trophoblast migrates rapidly into the endometrium, invading small arterioles, but not veins, directly beneath the implantation site. There is evidence of vascular occlusion, suggesting that trophoblastic lacunae receive their vascular supply by relatively indirect means. During the early stages of invasion, the trophoblast migrates between and along endothelial cells without causing their demise. It is likely that similar processes occur in the human, although this could not be confirmed from the limited historical material available for study.

In normal pregnancy, cytotrophoblast invasion extends through the endometrium to the myometrium. By contrast, women with preeclampsia have abnormally shallow trophoblast invasion. It has recently been shown that pre-eclampsia is associated with abnormal expression of integrins by invasive cytotrophoblasts (Zhou *et al.* 1993). In particular, integrins α_6 and β_4 are expressed far more strongly than normal, while $\alpha_1\beta_1$ is either not upregulated or only weakly expressed by a small proportion of cytotrophoblasts. Thus there is a failure of invasive trophoblast to downregulate adhesion mechanisms, which in turn could lead to the shallow trophoblast invasion that is characteristic of the pre-eclamptic placental bed.

Menstruation

Most of our current understanding of the vascular events during menstruation is still based on the remarkable series of observations using intraocular endometrial transplants in the rhesus monkey published by Markee over 50 years ago (Markee 1940). One to four days prior to the onset of bleeding, venous and arterial stasis occurs, sometimes accompanied by vasodilatation. Four to 24 hours prior to bleeding, vasoconstriction is also seen. About four days prior to menstruation leucocytic infiltration of the endometrium occurs, probably mediated, in part at least, by an upregulation of ICAM-1 adhesion molecule on endothelial cells of some, but not all, endometrial blood vessels (Tawia *et al.* 1993). Menstrual bleeding usually commences from the wall of an arteriole or capillary once a previously constricted spiral arteriole relaxes and blood flow recommences. Approximately 70 per cent of blood is lost in this way. Some blood cells also leave the capillary circulation by diapedesis (approximately 5 per cent of blood loss), as well as by reflux from veins through previously formed breaks in the vasculature (approximately 25 per cent of blood loss). Blood loss from a break in the endometrial vasculature during menstruation normally only lasts for one or two minutes before ceasing due to spiral arteriole vasoconstriction.

One popularly held view based on Markee's observations is that the intense vasoconstriction of the spiral arterioles seen prior to menstruation results in ischaemic necrosis, which in turn leads to tissue shedding once blood flow resumes. While aspects of this may be true, an alternative explanation could be that the recommencement of blood flow after a prolonged stoppage results in ischaemic reperfusion injury (IRI). The tissue damage during IRI results primarily from the generation of highly reactive free radical species as oxygenated blood re-enters the tissue. A similar phenomenon has been described in a number of tissues where blood flow recommences after prolonged stoppage, including heart attacks and surgery. In such instances a significant reduction in tissue damage can be achieved by the use of exogenous free radical scavengers. Similar experiments have yet to be conducted in a menstruating primate.

Throughout the normal menstrual process, the vascular bed shows signs of constant attempts to repair itself. Goodger (Macpherson) and Rogers (1994) demonstrated high levels of endothelial cell proliferation in menstrual endometrium. This agrees with the findings of Charnock-Jones *et al.* (1993), who found high levels of mRNA for VEGF in menstrual endometrium. However, there is also evidence to support the concept that endometrial blood vessels are specifically adapted for the menstrual process. It has been shown that von Willebrand factor levels in endometrial endothelial cells are significantly reduced at the time of menstruation (Au and Rogers 1993). A number of other mechanisms and factors that influence haemostasis and vascular breakdown are also modified during menstruation, including plasminogen activator and plasminogen activator inhibitor type 1 (Gleeson 1994), matrix metalloproteinases (Hampton and Salamonsen 1994), and tissue factor (Lockwood *et al.* 1993). Clinically, it is well established that both prostaglandin synthesis inhibitors and anti-fibrinolytic agents can act to reduce menstrual blood loss in women suffering from menorrhagia (Fraser 1994) thus identifying two further mechanisms that presumably play a central role in controlling menstruation.

Apoptosis, or programmed cell death, plays a key role in the homeostatic maintenance of cell numbers (Schwartzman and Cidlowski 1993). In human endometrium both endothelial cell density and microvascular density remain remarkably constant throughout the menstrual cycle, despite major bursts of tissue growth, large changes in tissue hydration, and highly varied endothelial cell proliferation rates (Rogers *et al.* 1993; Goodger and Rogers 1994). Thus it seems likely that endothelial cell numbers are regulated not only by addition through proliferation but also by removal through apoptosis. Evidence for hormonally regulated mechanisms controlling endometrial apoptosis have been published recently (Gompel *et al.* 1994), using immunohistochemical localization of the protein from the proto-oncogene Bcl-2. Bcl-2, which prolongs cell survival by preventing apoptosis, was expressed primarily in gland cells during the proliferative stage, but disappeared during the secretory phase. Endothelial cells were always Bcl-2 negative, although vascular smooth muscle cells from proliferative-stage small arterioles and secretory-stage spiral arterioles were positive. More recently an immunohistochemical study of Bcl-2 distribution in human endometrium concluded that it was unlikely that Bcl-2 is important in prolonging endometrial cell survival when the luteal phase was prolonged by the use of exogenous human chorionic gonadotrophin (Koh *et al.* 1995). These authors made no comment about Bcl-2 distribution in relation to the endometrial vasculature.

Work in non-endometrial tissues and cells has shown that in addition to Bcl-2, various homologues of Bcl-2 such as Bax and Bak can accelerate apoptosis under certain conditions. It has been suggested that the widespread tissue distribution of Bak mRNA supports the concept that apoptosis is controlled primarily by regulation of molecules such as Bcl-2 (Kiefer *et al.* 1995). Investigation of these mechanisms in the endometrium and its vasculature is still in its infancy, despite the fact that endometrium provides an ideal human model for physiological tissue regression and apoptosis.

Conclusion

In summary it is apparent that the endometrium contains one of the most dynamic and unusual vascular beds in the body. This is perhaps reflected in the large number of endometrial vascular-related disorders that occur in modern day gynaecology. However, despite these clinical problems, the endometrial vasculature provides an important avenue for investigating a wide range of physiological processes in a human model. The constantly changing nature of these blood vessels enables the study of vascular function that is normally only available under pathological circumstances in most other tissues. Thus a more comprehensive understanding of vascular function in endometrium is not only of relevance to many common gynaecological disorders, but may also be of benefit to a wide range of clinical applications in other tissues.

References

Abberton, K.M., Taylor, N.H., Healy, D.L., and Rogers, P.A.W. (1996). Vascular smooth muscle α-actin distribution around endometrial arterioles during the menstrual cycle: increased expression during the perimenopause and lack of correlation with menorrhagia. *Human Reproduction*, **11**, 204–11.

Au, C.L. and Rogers, P.A.W. (1993). Immunohistochemical staining of von Willebrand factor in human endometrium during normal menstrual cycle. *Human Reproduction*, **8**, 17–23.

Bartelmez, G.W. (1933). Histologic studies on the menstruating mucous membrane during menstruation. *Contributions to Embryology*, **142**, 142–57.

Bassil, S., Magritte, J.P., Roth, J., Nisolle, M., Donnez, J., and Gordts, S. (1995). Uterine vascularity during stimulation and its correlation with implantation in in-vitro fertilization. *Human Reproduction*, **10**, 1497–1501.

Blackwell, P.M. and Fraser, I.S. (1988). A morphometric and ultrastructural study of the microvessels of the functional zone of normal human endometrium with some notions on possible secretory functions of the endothelial cells. *Asia-Oceania Journal of Obstetrics and Gynaecology*, **14**, 233–50.

Boshier, D.P. (1970). The pontamine blue reaction in pregnant sheep uteri. *Journal of Reproduction and Fertility*, **22**, 595–6.

Brooks, P.C., Clark, R.A.F., and Cheresh, D.A. (1994). Requirement of vascular integrin $\alpha_V\beta_3$ for angiogenesis. *Science*, **264**, 569–71.

Charnock-Jones, D.S., Sharkey, A.M., Rajput-Williams, J., Burch, D., Schofield, J.P., Fountain, S.A., *et al.* (1993). Identification and localization of alternately spliced mRNAs for vascular endothelial growth factor in human uterus and estrogen regulation in endometrial carcinoma cell lines. *Biology and Reproduction*, **48**, 1120–8.

Critchley, H.O.D., Bailey, D.A., Au, C.L., Affandi, B., and Rogers, P.A.W. (1993). Immunohistochemical sex steroid receptor distribution in endometrium from long-term subdermal levonorgestrel users and during the normal menstrual cycle. *Human Reproduction*, **8**, 1632–9.

Critchley, H.O.D., Kelly, R.W., and Kooy, J. (1994). Perivascular expression of a chemokine interleukin-8 in human endometrium: a preliminary report. *Human Reproduction*, **9**, 1406–9.

Coulam, C.B., Bustillo, M., Soenksen, D.M., and Britten, S. (1994). Ultrasonographic predictors of implantation after assisted reproduction. *Fertility and Sterility*, **62**, 1004–10.

Deansley, R. (1967). The role of the fertilized egg: reactions in the guinea-pig uterus at ovo-implantation and after thread traumatization. *Journal of Reproduction and Fertility*, **14**, 243–8.

Dejana, E., Raiteri, M., Resnati, M., and Lampugnani, M.G. (1993). Endothelial integrins and their role in maintaining the integrity of the vessel wall. *Kidney International*, **43**, 61–5.

Economos, K., MacDonald, P.C., and Casey, M.L. (1992). Endothelin-1 gene expression and protein biosynthesis in human endometrium: potential modulator of endometrial blood flow. *Journal of Clinical Endocrinology and Metabolism*, **74**, 14–19.

Edelman, G.M. and Crossin, K.L. (1991). Cell adhesion molecules: implications for a molecular histology. *Annual Reviews of Biochemistry*, **60**, 155–90.

Enders, A.C. (1989). Trophoblast differentiation during the transition from trophoblastic plate to lacunar stage of implantation in the rhesus monkey and human. *American Journal of Anatomy*, **186**, 85–98.

Enders, A.C. and King, B.F. (1991). Early stages of trophoblastic invasion of the maternal vascular system during implantation in the macaque and baboon. *American Journal of Anatomy*, **192**, 329–46.

Ferenczy, A. (1987). Anatomy and histology of the uterine corpus. In *Blaustein's pathology of the genital tract* (ed. T.G. Kurman), 3rd edn, pp. 257–91. Springer, New York.

Ferenczy, A., Bertrand, G., and Gelfand, M.M. (1979). Proliferation kinetics of human endometrium during the normal menstrual cycle. *American Journal of Obstetrics and Gynecology*, **133**, 859–67.

Ferriani, R.A., Charnock-Jones, D.S., Prentice, A., Thomas, E.J., and Smith, S.K. (1993). Immunohistochemical localisation of acidic and basic FGF in normal human endometrium and endometriosis and the detection of their mRNA by PCR. *Human Reproduction*, **8**, 11–16.

Fraser, I.S. (1994). Menorrhagia – a pragmatic approach to the understanding of causes and the need for investigations. *British Journal of Obstetrics and Gynaecology*, **101**, 3–7.

Fraser, I.S. and Peek, M.J. (1992). Effects of exogenous hormones on endometrial capillaries. In *Steroid hormones and uterine bleeding*, (ed. N.J. Alexander and C. d'Arcangues), pp. 67–79. AAAS Press, Washington.

Giudice, L.C. (1994). Growth factors and growth modulators in human uterine endometrium: their potential relevance to reproductive medicine. *Fertility and Sterility*, **61**, 1–17.

Gleeson, N.C. (1994). Cyclic changes in endometrial tissue plasminogen activator and plasminogen activator inhibitor type 1 in women with normal menstruation and essential menorrhagia. *American Journal of Obstetrics and Gynecology*, **171**, 178–83.

Gompel, A., Sabourin, J.C., Martin, A., Yaneva, H., Audouin, J., Decroix, Y., and Poitout, P. (1994). Bcl-2 expression in normal endometrium during the menstrual cycle. *American Journal of Pathology*, **144**, 1195–202.

Goodger (Macpherson), A.M., and Rogers, P.A.W. (1994). Endometrial endothelial cell proliferation during the menstrual cycle. *Human Reproduction*, **9**, 399–405.

Haining, R.E., Cameron, I.T., van Papendorp, C., Davenport, A.P., Prentice, A., Thomas, E.J., and Smith, S.K. (1991). Epidermal growth factor in human endometrium: proliferative effects in culture and immunocytochemical localization in normal and endometriotic tissues. *Human Reproduction*, **9**, 1200–5.

Hampton, A.L. and Salamonsen, L.A. (1994). Expression of messenger ribonucleic acid encoding matrix metalloproteinases and their tissue inhibitors is related to menstruation. *Journal of Endocrinology*, **141**, R1–R3.

Hertig, A.T., Rock, J., and Adams, E.C. (1956). A description of 34 human ova within the first 17 days of development. *American Journal of Anatomy*, **98**, 435–93.

Horowitz, G.M., Scott, R.T. Jr, Drews, M.R., Navot, D., and Hofmann, G.E. (1993). Immunohistochemical localisation of TGFα in human endometrium, decidua and trophoblast. *Journal of Clinical Endocrinology and Metabolism*, **76**, 786–92.

Karas, R.H., Patterson, B.L., and Mendelsohn, M.E. (1994). Human vascular smooth muscle cells contain functional estrogen receptor. *Circulation*, **89**, 1943–50.

Kelly, F.D., Tawia, S.A., and Rogers, P.A.W. (1995). Immunohistochemical characterization of human endometrial microvascular basement membrane components during the normal menstrual cycle. *Human Reproduction*, **10**, 268–76.

Keys, J.L., King, G.J., and Kennedy, T.G. (1986). Increased uterine vascular permeability at the time of embryonic attachment in the pig. *Biology and Reproduction*, **34**, 405–11.

Kiefer, M.C., Brauer, M.J., Powers, V.C., Wu, J.J., Umansky, S.R., Tomei, L.D., and Barr, P.J. (1995). Modulation of apoptosis by the widely distributed Bcl-2 homologue Bak. *Nature*, **374**, 736–9.

Klagsbrun, M. and D'Amore, P.A. (1991). Regulators of angiogenesis. *Annual Reviews of Physiology*, **53**, 217–39.

Koh, E.A.T., Illingworth, P.J., Duncan, W.C., and Critchley, H.O.D. (1995). Immunolocalization of bcl-2 protein in human endometrium in the menstrual cycle and simulated early pregnancy. *Human Reproduction*, **10**, 1557–62.

Lei, Z.M., Reshef, E., and Rao, Ch. V. (1992). The expression of human chorionic gonadotropin/luteinizing hormone receptors in human endometrial and myometrial blood vessels. *Journal of Clinical Endocrinology and Metabolism*, **75**, 651–9.

Lessey, B.A. and Castelbaum, A.J. (1995). Integrins in the endometrium. *Reproductive Medicine Review*, **4**, 43–58.

Lockwood, C.J., Nemerson, Y., Krikun, G., Hausknecht, V., Markiewicz, L., Alvarez, M., *et al.* (1993). Steroid-modulated stromal cell tissue factor expression: a model for the regulation of endometrial hemostasis and menstruation. *Journal of Clinical Endocrinology and Metabolism*, **77**, 1014–19.

Lunam, C. and Rogers, A.W. (1981). Pericytes in the stroma of the rat uterus. *Journal of Reproduction and Fertility*, **63**, 267–70.

Markee, J.E. (1940). Menstruation in intraocular endometrial transplants in the rhesus monkey. *Contributions to Embryology: Carnegie Institution*, **28**, 219–308.

Noyes, R.W., Hertig, A.T., and Rock, J. (1950). Dating the endometrial biopsy. *Fertility and Sterility*, **1**, 3–25.

Peek, M., Landgren, B.-M., and Johannisson, E. (1992). The endometrial capillaries during the normal menstrual cycle: a morphometric study. *Human Reproduction*, **7**, 906–11.

Perrot-Applanat, M., Deng, M., Fernandez, H., Lelaidier, C., Meduri, G., and Bouchard, P. (1994). Immunohistochemical localization of estradiol and progesterone receptors in human uterus throughout pregnancy: expression in endometrial blood vessels. *Journal of Clinical Endocrinology and Metabolism*, **78**, 216–24.

Philippeaux, M.M. and Piguet, P.F. (1993). Expression of tumor necrosis factor-α and its mRNA in the endometrial mucosa during the menstrual cycle. *American Journal of Pathology*, **143**, 480–6.

Psychoyos, A. (1960). La réaction déciduale est précédée de modifications précoces de la perméabilité capillaire de l'utérus. *Comptes Rendus des Séances de la Socièté Biologie*, **154**, 1384–7.

Ramsey, E.M. (1982). Vascular anatomy. In *Biology of the uterus* (ed. R.M. Wynn), 2nd edn, pp. 59–76. Plenum Press., New York.

Roberts, D.K., Parmley, T.H., Walker, N.J., and Horbelt, D.V. (1992). Ultrastructure of the microvasculature in the human endometrium throughout the normal menstrual cycle. *American Journal of Obstetrics and Gynecology*, **166**, 1391–406.

Rogers, P.A.W., Murphy, C.R., Rogers, A.W., and Gannon, B. (1983). Capillary patency and permeability in the endometrium surrounding the implanting rat blastocyst. *International Journal of Microcirculation: Clinical and Experimental*, **2**, 241–9.

Rogers, P.A.W., Abberton, K.M., and Susil, B. (1992). Endothelial cell migratory signal production by human endometrium during the menstrual cycle. *Human Reproduction*, **7**, 1061–6.

Rogers, P.A.W., Au, C.L., and Affandi, B. (1993). Endometrial microvascular density during the normal menstrual cycle and following exprosure to long-term levonorgestrel. *Human Reproduction*, **8**, 1396–1404.

Schwartzman, R.A. and Cidlowski, J.A. (1993). Apoptosis: the biochemistry and molecular biology of programmed cell death. *Endocrine Reviews*, **14**, 133–51.

Simon, C., Piquette, G.N., Frances, A., and Polan, M.L. (1993). Localization of interleukin-1 type I receptor and interleukin-1β in human endometrium throughout the menstrual cycle. *Journal of Clinical Endocrinology and Metabolism*, **77**, 549–55.

Steer, C.V., Tan, S.L., and Dillon, D. (1995). Vaginal color Doppler assessment of uterine artery impedance correlates with immunohistochemical markers of endometrial receptivity required for the implantation of an embryo. *Fertility and Sterility*, **63**, 101–8.

Sunderkotter, C., Steinbrink, K., Goebeler, M., Bhardwaj, R., and Sorg, C. (1994). Macrophages and angiogenesis. *Journal of Leukocyte Biology*, **55**, 410–22.

Tabibzadeh, S. (1991). Human endometrium: an active site of cytokine production and action. *Endocrine Reviews*, **12**, 272–90.

Tabibzadeh, S. and Sun, X.Z. (1992). Cytokine expression in human endometrium throughout the menstrual cycle. *Human Reproduction*, **7**, 1214–21.

Tabibzadeh, S., Kong, Q.F., and Babaknia, A. (1994). Expression of adhesion molecules in human endometrial vasculature throughout the menstrual cycle. *Journal of Clinical Endocrinology and Metabolism*, **79**, 1024–32.

Tawia, S.A., Beaton, L.A., and Rogers, P.A.W. (1993). Immunolocalization of the cellular adhesion molecules, intercellular adhesion molecule-1 (ICAM-1) and platelet endothelial cell adhesion molecule (PECAM), in human endometrium throughout the menstrual cycle. *Human Reproduction*, **8**, 175–81.

van Herendael, B.J., Stevens, M.J., Flakiewicz-Kula, A., and Hansch, Ch. (1987). Dating of the endometrium by microhysteroscopy. *Gynecological and Obstetrical Investigation*, **24**, 114–18.

Zhou, Y., Damsky, C.H., Chiu, K., Roberts, J.M., and Fisher, S.J. (1993). Preeclampsia is associated with abnormal expression of adhesion molecules by invasive cytotrophoblasts. *Journal of Clinical Investigation*, **91**, 950–60.

4 The practical assessment of endometrial morphology and function

Peter Russell and Ian S. Fraser

Introduction

The central role of the endometrium in reproduction has been increasingly recognized in the past decade as its complexity as an organ has begun to be defined. The endometrium is highly sensitive to changes in hormonal exposure, as are the interactions of its different tissue components. These interactions are regulated by a series of complex molecular changes with a range of effects on morphology and function.

Endometrial histology in health and disease has been extensively described in increasing detail over the past century, but it is only in the past 1–2 decades that the appearances of endometrial surface morphology and aspects of function have begun to be clarified.

The endometrium is now known to have a number of specialized functions, which include:

(1) to produce glandular secretions which permit efficient sperm migration through the uterine cavity;

(2) to produce glandular secretions which nourish sperm and blastocyst;

(3) to permit and to limit implantation of the blastocyst;

(4) to allow placental development and to enhance fetal nourishment;

(5) to participate in the processes leading to the onset of labour;

(6) to undertake a number of immunological surveillance roles, including defence against bacteria and other microbes, and to permit fetal and placental survival and normal growth;

(7) to undergo decidual shedding and remodelling post-partum;

(8) to undergo repeated menstrual shedding and remodelling;

(9) to repeatedly undergo complete surface repair after each menses and pregnancy so that surface scarring and adhesions do not develop;

(10) to remain in an inactive or 'resting' state during childhood, lactation, and post-menopause;

(11) to perform various other complex endocrine and paracrine roles.

Some of these functions are reasonably well defined, but relatively few can be well characterized from a clinical point of view. A variety of different techniques have been developed to gain direct or indirect information about alterations of the endometrium in relation to these specialized functions, whereas the place of others has not yet been defined. It appears that we are on the brink of an explosion of information about the previously mysterious process of embryo implantation.

It is likely that major molecular changes occur on the endometrial surface during the so-called 'window of receptivity' which are not specifically related to changes in classical histology. Tests to characterize these will undoubtedly be developed in the next few years.

Current approaches to endometrial assessment in clinical practice

Diagnostic hysteroscopy

The current 'gold standard' for assessment of the uterine cavity and the endometrial surface is diagnostic hysteroscopy, which is reviewed in detail in Chapters 10 and 11. Attempts at direct visual inspection of the uterine cavity were made as early as the end of the 19th century to try and visualize uterine cancers. These attempts were made using distant light sources reflected by mirrors, and it was not until the development of cold light sources and the rod lens systems in endoscopes in the late 1960s that image clarity was sufficiently good to make hysteroscopy a viable diagnostic technique. More recently, miniature telescopes with narrow rigid or flexible sheaths and remarkably good optics have led to a steadily increasing popularity in routine clinical practice (Gordon and Lewis 1988; Hamou 1991). The technique is so easy and atraumatic that many clinicians now provide this procedure as an outpatient service using minimal local analgesia (Hill *et al.* 1992; Fraser 1993).

Adequate panoramic inspection of the uterine cavity and endometrium requires distention of the cavity with carbon dioxide, normal saline, or a 16–32 per cent dextran solution (Hyskon, Pharmacia). There was a brief vogue for contact hysteroscopy in the late 1970s which gave an interesting view of billowing folds of surface endometrium and vessels but did not allow good assessment of pathology. Optimal use of the modern technique requires some care and a good eye for detail, with systematic assessment and recording of

(1) size and shape of the uterine cavity

(2) contour, colour, and compliance of the endometrial surface

(3) surface vascular distributions and patterns

(4) presence and characteristics of lesions and foreign bodies

(5) appearance and contraction of both tubal ostia

(6) endocervical contour, colour, surface characteristics, and lesions.

Assessment of the size and shape of the uterine cavity and structures within it can be very difficult unless a foreign object of known size (e.g. biopsy forceps) is introduced down an operating sheath. Accurate hysterometry techniques are under development. Pathological lesions which are usually straightforward to identify (but may be more difficult to fully characterize) include submucous and polypoidal intrauterine myomata, endometrial polyps, endometrial adenocarcinoma, septa, adhesions, adherent residual placental or molar tissue, and foreign bodies such as 'lost' intrauterine contraceptive devices or fetal bone fragments. More subtle lesions include superficial endometritis, endometrial fibrosis, moderately severe adenomyosis, endometrial hyperplasias, abnormal vascular patterns and fragility (e.g. with progestogen-only contraceptive use), endometrial stromal oedema, tubal stenosis, and scarring, including poorly healed Caesarean section scars.

Simultaneous use of abdominal or rectal ultrasound guidance may be extremely valuable for the assessment and treatment of occlusive intrauterine adhesions, haematometra, or an intrauterine device embedded in the uterine wall (Fraser *et al.* 1995).

Diagnostic hysteroscopy can be combined with directed biopsy or with semi-directed biopsy or curettage of an abnormal area once the hysteroscope has been removed. The disadvantage of directed biopsy is that the amount of tissue obtained is tiny, and for most clinical purposes a post-hysteroscopic biopsy taken with a larger sampling device from the abnormal region is more satisfactory.

Endometrial biopsy techniques

The aim of these procedures is to provide representative endometrial tissue in good condition for histological or histopathological assessment. This may require careful attention to timing, for example in women with anovulation or infertility, as well as to the choice of technique appropriate for the symptom. Available techniques include the conventional blind curettage, outpatient endometrial biopsy devices, directed hysteroscopic biopsies, semi-directed biopsy or curettage following diagnostic hysteroscopy, and endo-myometrial resection biopsy at operative hysteroscopy.

Diagnostic dilatation and curettage (D&C)

For the whole of this century the 'D&C' has been the commonest gynaecological operation performed in most countries of the world. It has been the mainstay of diagnostic approaches to detect and exclude pathology of the endometrium. In the days when endometrial and endocervical cancer were the most important lesions that a gynaecologist was expected to detect, the D&C served the profession reasonably well. However, over the past 10–15 years there has been an increasingly critical questioning of the effectiveness of this procedure in detecting pathology (Grimes 1982). At the same time, there has been an increasing availability of alternative techniques for imaging the uterus and the uterine cavity in a more definitive manner.

The first major doubts about the value of the D&C came from studies demonstrating a low detection rate for endometrial pathology and calling for care in the determination of indications for this procedure (MacKenzie and Bibby 1978; Grimes 1982; Holst *et al.* 1983). For example, the detection rate for endometrial pathology in younger women and in those with minor intermenstrual and breakthrough bleeding and infertility was extremely low. For many cases, an outpatient endometrial biopsy would give just as high (or low) a likelihood of detection of pathology. Hence, the cost-effectiveness of the thorough 'blind' curettage under general anaesthesia came to be seriously questioned (Grimes 1982; Coulter *et al.* 1993).

Evidence began to accumulate that this 'blind' D&C was a procedure which missed a considerable amount of gross and subtle pathology and the diagnostic hysteroscopy has now become established as the 'gold standard' for assessment of the endometrium (Goldrath and Sherman 1985; Brooks and Serden 1988; Gimpelson and Rappold 1988; Loffer 1989). It is now unquestioned by those who have carried out comparative studies of D&C and hysteroscopy that the D&C alone is greatly inferior in its ability to detect and assess endometrial polyps, intrauterine and submucous myomata, small areas of endometritis or hyperplasia, small cancer, 'lost' IUCDs, uterine septa, intrauterine adhesions, and a range of rare conditions. It should also be mentioned that there is no scientific evidence to support use of a 'therapeutic curettage' for menstrual bleeding disorders such as ovulatory dysfunctional uterine bleeding (Nilsson and Rybo 1971; Haynes *et al.* 1977).

On the other hand, in the absence of access to a hysteroscope, a careful and thorough curettage can usually yield useful information on endometrial pathology such as the endometrial hyperplasias, carcinoma, and extensive endometritis. Endometrial biopsy may also identify these conditions, but the limited sampling achieved by biopsy is only reliable for conditions which uniformly affect the whole endometrial surface.

Effective diagnostic curettage requires limited cervical dilatation to no more than 8 mm, and the use of a small sharp curette to sample systematically all parts of the uterine cavity including the tubal ostial regions. A variety of different techniques are used depending on the type of curette, but the most important message is that the technique should be systematic, thorough, and gentle.

D&C is infrequently associated with complications, but uterine perforation with a cervical dilator or curette occasionally occurs and often cannot be predicted. This rarely causes serious damage, but requires the patient to be kept under observation for a few hours. Healing is usually rapid and complete. This complication is more likely to occur with the post-menopausal or post-partum uterus, even when appropriate care is taken. Other complications include formation of a false passage in the cervix with a dilator, or cervical damage caused by a large dilator resulting in cervical incompetence in the long term. Rarely, post-operative infection or post-operative intrauterine adhesions may occur. These usually occur in very specific situations such as curettage for secondary post-partum haemorrhage and retained products of conception (Asherman 1950).

A variation of the diagnostic D&C which sometimes still provides useful information in the absence of more modern imaging techniques is the fractional curettage. This involves cervical dilatation followed by endocervical curettage (often difficult to judge), followed by endometrial curettage. The two sets of curettings should be sent in separate containers for pathological examination. The theory is that an endocervical adenocarcinoma will be detected in both specimens while an endometrial carcinoma will only be detected in the endometrial curettings.

Most of our knowledge about the histological changes in endometrium in health and disease has come from the billions of D&Cs which have been carried out over the past 100 years, but the time has now been reached when this 'blind' diagnostic technique should only be used when better techniques are unavailable.

Endometrial biopsy

The feasibility of simple outpatient endometrial biopsy or curettage without prior cervical dilatation first became apparent with the design of a narrow metal cannula with a distal side opening bordered by serrated edges (Novak 1935). This device was designed to have a syringe attached to the proximal end to provide suction during removal of the instrument from the uterus. If the device is rotated during removal a lengthy strip of endometrium is sucked into the syringe. The main disadvantage of Novak's curette is that it causes considerable, albeit transient, uterine cramping for many women during removal. Many subsequent devices have been based on similar principles. A popular modern alternative has been the Vabra curette which can provide excellent tissue samples but requires a bulky and non-disposable vacuum source, and also causes substantial cramping (Vuopala 1977). The modern preferred alternative in most centres is Cornier's 'pipelle' (Henig *et al.* 1989) which is a 3.1 mm diameter disposable, semi-rigid plastic tube, with a single distal side opening, and a very close fitting central plunger which provides excellent suction when withdrawn. The whole instrument can be slowly withdrawn and rotated to provide a single continuous endometrial core with excellent characteristics for histological examination. Its semi-rigidity allows for easy insertion in most women, although a cervical tenaculum may be required in many cases. The small size of the device means that cramping is usually less than with other designs.

Numerous alternative approaches to outpatient tissue sampling of the endometrial surface for cytological or histological examination (Kovacs and Burger 1988) which have found favour with some investigators and have generally provided adequate tissue samples include the Gravlee 'jet washer' (Dowling and Gravlee 1964), the Mi–Mark spiral sampler (Milan and Markley 1973), and the 'Gynoscann' surface stripper based on an intrauterine contraceptive device insertion principle (Kovacs *et al.* 1988). None of these have had sufficient advantages to maintain a widespread popularity in view of the simplicity and sampling effectiveness of the pipelle.

Endo-myometrial resection biopsy

Occasionally, there may be a role for a deep (3–5 mm) biopsy collected with a hysteroresectoscope loop to identify adenomyosis or to assess deep lesions of the endometrium (for example, as may sometimes occur with tamoxifen). These biopsies permanently remove a narrow strip of basal endometrium and underlying myometrium which do, however, appear to heal well and the site cannot usually be identified later.

Transvaginal ultrasound scanning

Transvaginal ultrasound scanning is a rapidly developing field which is becoming increasingly useful in the demonstration of fine morphological detail of the pelvic organs (Fleischer and Kepple 1992). One major advantage is the avoidance of the need for a full bladder as with abdominal scanning. The use of a transvaginal probe places the ultrasound transducer close to the structures of interest with minimal thickness of intervening tissue to attenuate the ultrasound waves. This allows use of higher frequency ultrasound waves (3.5–10 MHz) with the consequent demonstration of finer tissue detail. Nevertheless, there are considerable pitfalls to the interpretation of transvaginal images, and this type of ultrasound imaging should only be carried out by those with appropriate training using good quality equipment.

The endometrium can now be depicted in considerable detail using ultrasound scans (Scott 1994). Endometrium has different echogenic characteristics from surrounding myometrium or intraluminal fluid, and these appearances change during the menstrual cycle and in certain pathological states. The endometrium can be demonstrated as a strongly echogenic structure in the central part of the uterus, which appears as a long line in a longitudinal pelvic scan, and as a shorter and rounder linear structure on transverse scanning.

Endometrial thickness is measured ultrasonographically as the double thickness of the two apposed layers, excluding any intracavitary fluid. It is best measured in a longitudinal scan of the uterus. The endometrium is represented by the hyperechoic central signal, and the surrounding hypoechoic region or 'halo' probably represents inner myometrium. Endometrial thickness measurements on transvaginal scanning correlate well with actual endometrial thickness (Fleischer *et al.* 1986) and appear to be important in determining the likelihood of conception in assisted reproduction programmes (Scott 1994). In normal menstrual cycles, endometrial thickness varies from 4–8 mm in the proliferative phase to 7–15 mm in the secretory phase. These measurements may be substantially greater in women on ovulation induction programmes. Endometrial volume has also been calculated, varying from 1.6 ± 0.4 ml (mean ± SD) in the mid to late proliferative phase of the cycle to 3.4 ± 0.8 ml in the secretory phase (Fleischer *et al.* 1988).

The nature of the endometrial echo also changes during the cycle (Fig. 4.1) from a thin echogenic interface during menses to a thicker, evenly echoic line in the early to mid-proliferative phase. In the periovulatory period the endometrium appears multilayered with a hypoechoic layer within the inner endometrium, a hyperechoic luminal line, and hyperechoic outer endometrial regions. The hypoechoic region probably represents the appearance of tissue oedema in the upper layers of the endometrium. The greater echogenicity of endometrium during the secretory phase is probably a reflection of the greater density of secretory material in glands.

Abnormalities of endometrial appearance and thickness may be apparent in a number of pathological conditions (Fig. 4.2). These abnormalities may be further clarified or enhanced by developments such as colour flow or duplex Doppler, or by the instillation of saline solution (Nanini *et al.* 1981; Parsons and Lense 1993) or instillation of specially developed, novel hyperechoic media into the uterine cavity to delineate the shape of surface structures such as endometrial

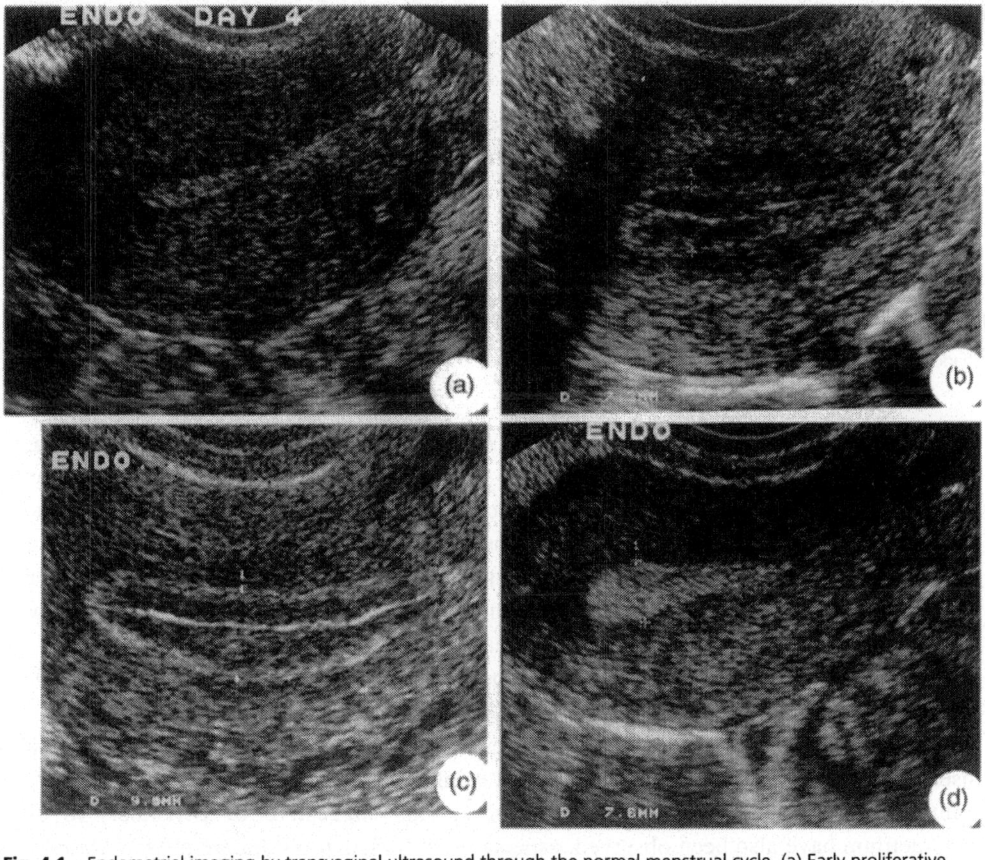

Fig. 4.1 Endometrial imaging by transvaginal ultrasound through the normal menstrual cycle. (a) Early proliferative phase (day 4) – thin homogeneous endometrial echo. (b) Pre-ovulatory phase (day 13) – thicker endometrium demonstrating the 'triple line sign' (see text). (c) Pre-ovulatory phase (day 13) – demonstrating the endometrium at higher magnification. (d) Mid to late secretory phase (four days before menstruation) – thick, homogeneous endometrial echo. (Images courtesy of Dr Philippa Ramsay.)

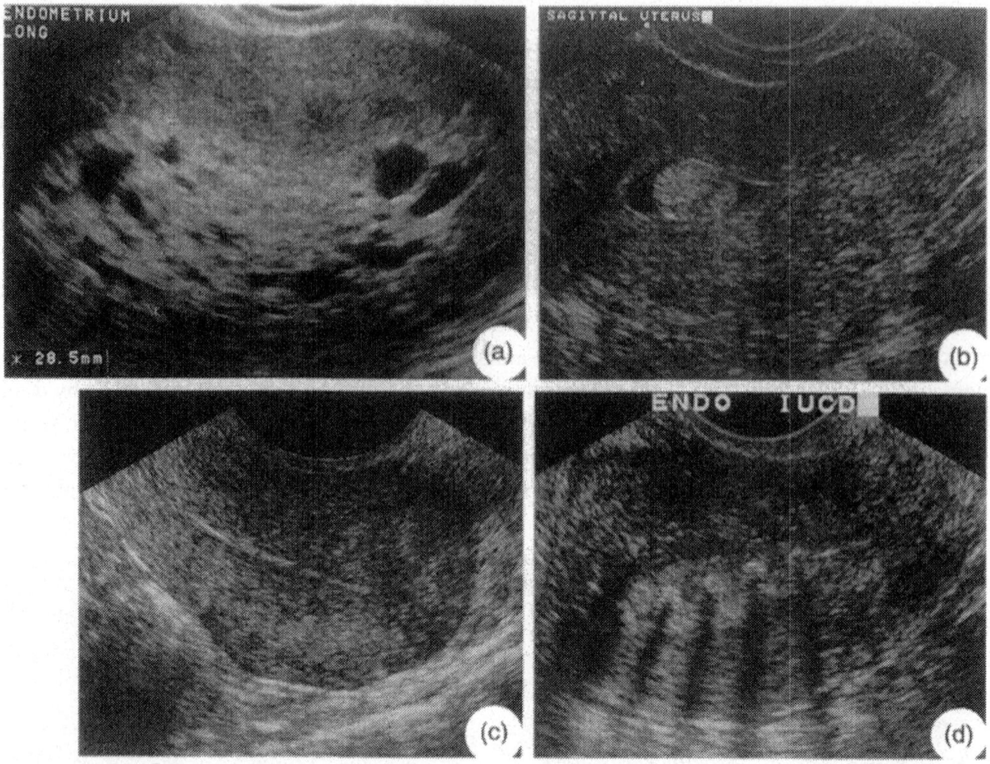

Fig. 4.2 Endometrial imaging by transvaginal ultrasound of four uterine abnormalities. (a) Simple (cystic) endometrial hyperplasia, demonstrating a thick brightly echogenic endometrium containing multiple irregular cystic spaces. (b) Well circumscribed, brightly echogenic endometrial polyp surrounded by echolucent free fluid, probably blood. (c) Very thin, regular pseudosecretory endometrium due to combined oral contraceptive use. (d) Lippes loop IUCD surrounded by secretory endometrium. The loops of the IUCD are seen in cross-section as five bright echogenic foci causing posterior shadowing. (Images courtesy of Dr Philippa Ramsay.)

polyps, submucous myomas or cancer, or the shape of the tubal lumen (Balen 1994; Campbell *et al.* 1994). Colour flow and duplex Doppler may be helpful in demonstrating prominent low resistance (diastolic) blood flow in cases of endometrial carcinoma. The uterine arterial pulsatility index of pulsed Doppler varies across the menstrual cycle and further refinement of these techniques may provide useful information on changes in blood flow with changes in uterine function. Ultrasound assessment with an intrauterine probe may also provide additional information about certain types of endometrial or myometrial lesions (Kikuchi *et al.* 1995).

Uterine size and the changing size and shape of the uterine cavity can now be measured by transvaginal scanning in a way which was not previously possible by other techniques. This should replace the rather crude direct measurements which were originally carried out prior to insertion of intrauterine contraceptive devices using such ingenious ideas as the Hasson 'wing sound' (Hasson 1980, 1985). Uterine contractions suggestive of peristalsis involving endometrium have also been observed, especially in the late proliferative phase (Abramowicz and Archer 1990). Three-dimensional ultrasound assessments of endometrial and myometrial pathology might also become feasible in routine practice in the near future (Steiner *et al.* 1994).

Pathological conditions affecting the endometrium in which specific abnormalities of ultrasonographic appearance, thickness, or Doppler impedance may be demonstrated include endometrial polyps, submucous or intracavity myomas, synechiae (adhesions), septa, intracavity fluid, luteal phase defects, inflammatory conditions, intramyometrial cystic collections of fluid (including haematometra), diffuse and focal adenomyosis, endometrial hyperplasia, carcinoma, and abnormalities of early pregnancy.

In untreated post-menopausal women, endometrial thickness varies between 2 and 8 mm, but increases in women on hormone replacement therapy (up to 10 mm). A steadily increasing body of evidence indicates that endometrial thickness measurements may be useful in excluding endometrial hyperplasia and carcinoma in post-menopausal women (see Chapter 21). Most investigations have indicated that a thickness of 5 mm or less is a strong reassurance against the presence of hyperplasia or adenocarcinoma (Granberg *et al.* 1991; Varner *et al.* 1991), although rare exceptions have been reported (Dijkhuizen *et al.* 1996).

Morphology of the normal endometrium

Accurate interpretation is best achieved when the biopsy sample or curettings are taken from the body or fundus region of the uterus and fixed immediately in either formalin/acetic acid/alcohol (FAA) or 10 per cent buffered formalin. FAA is preferred because it better preserves cytological characteristics (equivalent to Bouin's fixative) and causes lysis of red blood cells, thus facilitating tissue handling, whereas formalin results in comparatively poor cellular details. The specimen should be wiped from the curette on to gauze and immersed in the fixative. It should then be processed between soft foam pads, to prevent loss during processing.

Endometrial dating is a somewhat subjective process and, depending upon the precise stage of the cycle, a discrepancy of ± 1 day in relation to the calendar day of ovulation or menstruation is acceptable for experienced histopathologists. In less experienced hands and at some stages of the cycle, this discrepancy may be greater (Gibson *et al.* 1991). In our institution, dating is related to a stylized 28 day cycle, with the first day of bleeding designated day 1, and ovulation occurring at the conclusion of the 14th day. The original descriptions of endometrial dating were provided by Noyes *et al.* (1950), with more precise morphometric criteria being described by Li *et al.* (1988). The degree of precision of these techniques has been questioned (Arthur and Khan 1996).

Proliferative phase

In the proliferative phase, changes are not distinctive enough to allow accurate dating, but they do follow a sequential pattern. Under the influence of oestradiol, the endometrium shows proliferation of glandular, stromal, and vascular endothelial cells, producing a measurable thickening of the uterine mucosa. This proliferative response is non-uniform, being more prominent in the superficial two-thirds of the functional layer ('functionalis') of the body and fundus than in the deeper third and basalis, or than the endometrium of the isthmic and cornual regions. Nuclear DNA synthesis and mitotic activity are high, correlating with high levels of nucleolar organizer regions (NORs) on chromosomes 13–15, 21, and 22 (Wilkinson *et al.* 1990). The straight tubular glands of the early proliferative phase (Fig. 4.3) become larger, more tortuous and more crowded during mid and late proliferative phases. This proliferative process begins to subside by the 11–14th day.

At an ultrastructural level, oestradiol is responsible for production of ultrastructural organelles in glandular, stromal, and vascular endothelial cells (such as free and bound ribosomes, adenosine

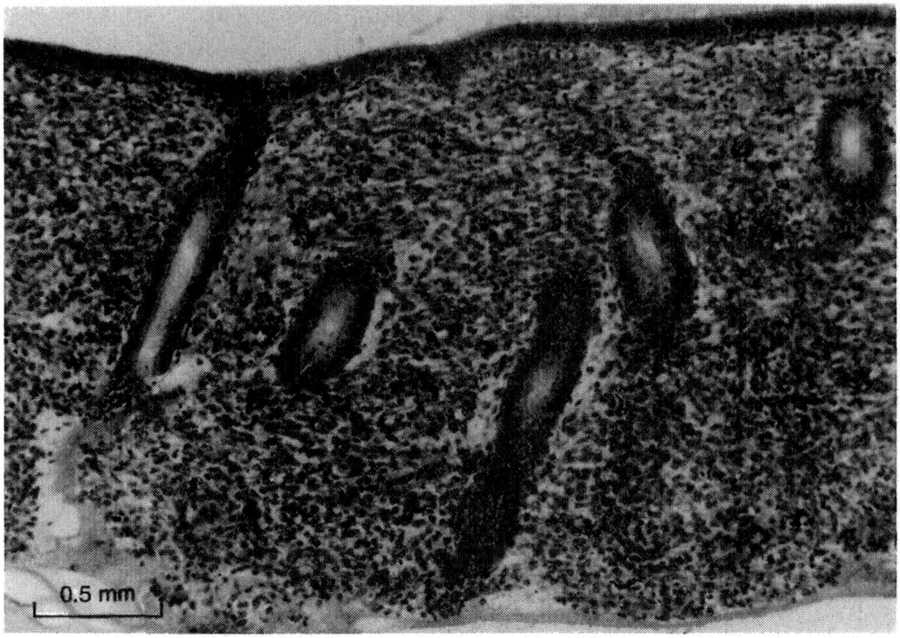

Fig. 4.3 Early proliferative endometrium. Straight tubular glands of uniform size are regularly distributed in hypercellular, slightly oedematous stroma. Glandular epithelial cells have basophilic cytoplasm, sharp luminal borders, and mitoses. Stromal cells have inapparent cytoplasm. H and E; × 35.

triphosphate (ATP)-rich mitochondria, and Golgi and primary lysosomes (Ferenczy *et al.* 1979)) which are responsible for a protein matrix, energy, and synthesis and storage of enzymes, respectively. The surface and glandular cells acquire numerous cilia and microvilli, the latter being cytoplasmic extensions to increase overall cell surface and thus enhance excretory, secretory, and absorptive functions.

Secretory phase

In the postovulatory or secretory phase, under the influence of progesterone, the oestradiol-primed endometrium undergoes rapid architectural and cellular changes, sufficiently distinct to permit accurate dating (Hendrickson and Kempson 1980). During the first 24–36 hours after ovulation (i.e. the 15th day of a 'normal' 28-day cycle, or the first day post-ovulation), the endometrium is not distinguishable from that seen in the late proliferative phase. On the 16th day (2nd day postovulation) of the cycle, small discrete glycogen-containing vacuoles appear between the nuclei and basal lamina of the glands in the functional layer. In all other respects the glands remain indistinguishable from those of the late proliferative phase. Glandular cells are still tall columnar, with amphophilic luminal cytoplasm and mitoses. It is important to note that similar changes may be produced by oestrogens alone in the absence of ovulation, and it is suggested that presumptive evidence of ovulation be predicated on finding well developed subnuclear vacuoles in > 50 per cent of cells in > 50 per cent of glands in the curettage material; this is usually well exceeded by the 17th day (third day postovulation) of the cycle (Fig. 4.4). Using electron microscopy ovulation is characterized by the appearance of giant mitochondria within the glandular epithelial cells and the so-called nucleolar channel system (seen as early as the

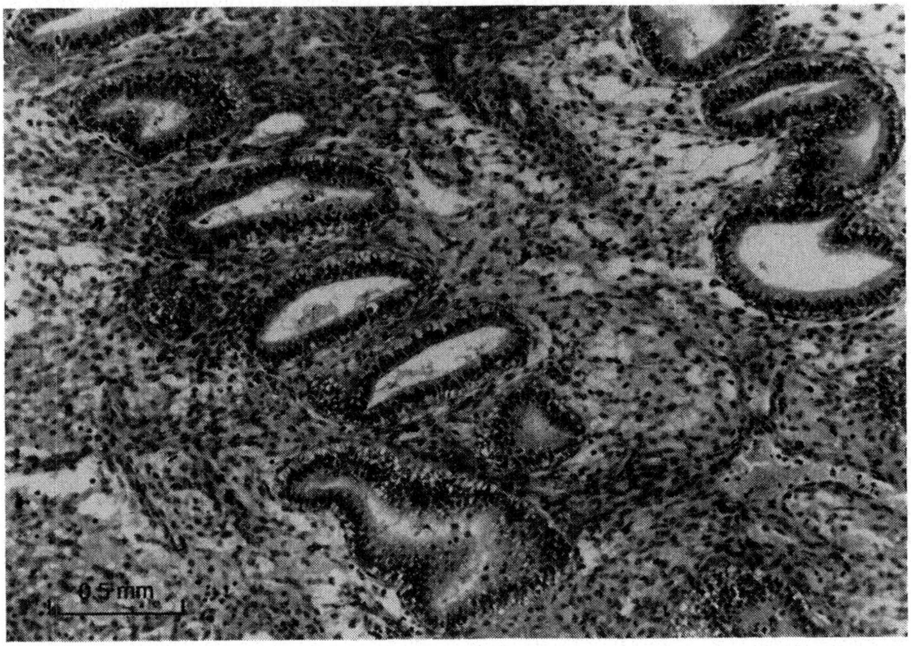

Fig. 4.4 Early secretory phase endometrium, corresponding to the third post-ovulatory day. Glands are slightly dilated. Glandular epithelial cells show widespread basal vacuolation, but still exhibit sharp luminal borders and mitoses. H and E; × 35.

15th day of the cycle) formed by helical infolding of nuclear membranes into the nuclear or nucleolar substances (More *et al.* 1974).

On the 18th day (four day post-ovulation), supranuclear vacuolation is also seen. On the 19th and 20th days (fifth and sixth days post-ovulation), apical glycoprotein-rich and mucopolysaccharide-rich cytoplasmic fragments are expelled into the glandular lumen by protrusion and eventual detachment (Wilkinson *et al.* 1990) with consequent loss of vacuolization of the supranuclear cytoplasm. The peak of glandular secretions is intended to coincide with the usual time of blastocyst implantation on the 21st day (seventh day post-ovulation). Nuclear DNA synthesis and mitotic activity cease in glandular epithelial cells by the 19th day, under the influence of progesterone, which antagonizes the proliferative activity of oestradiol by interfering with the recycling or replenishment of cytoplasmic oestradiol-receptors (Katzenellenbogen 1980), and by inducing the 17 β-hydroxysteroid dehydrogenase enzyme involved in the interconversion of oestradiol and oestrone (Song and Fraser 1995). Progesterone prevents these cells from entering the premitotic (G_1 and S) phases of the cell cycle.

From the 20th day (sixth day postovulation), stromal changes take pre-eminence in endometrial dating. These changes are stromal oedema (days 20–23, maximal on the 22nd day in response to a mid-luteal peak of serum oestradiol and probably mediated by prostaglandins and mast cell secretory products), coiling of spiral arterioles (days 22–25), and pseudo-decidualization of the stroma (23rd through 28th days). The mid-luteal peak of oestradiol may play a role in priming the endometrium for blastocyst implantation. Prostaglandin E_2 and other growth factors promote vascular endothelial mitotic activity. Endothelial proliferation leads to coiling of the endometrial arterioles, producing vascular clusters in the upper functionalis. Stromal pseudo-decidualization begins around spiral arterioles and capillaries of the functionalis. Simultaneously, glands form intraluminal epithelial projections ('ferning'). Periarteriolar pseudo-decidualization (Fig. 4.5(a)) is more obvious on the 24th day (tenth day post-ovulation) due to the conversion of non-descript stromal cells into large polyhedral epithelial-like cells with enlarged nuclei and abundant cytoplasm, by processes of both hypertrophy and hyperplasia (mitosis). Progesterone receptors remain stable without great fluctuation in these cells throughout the secretory phase and indicate a probable role for progesterone in their cytoplasmic differentiation (Bergeron *et al.* 1988; Song and Fraser 1995). Histochemically, pseudo-decidual cells contain glycogen and Periodic Acid Schiff (PAS)-positive mucins. They often stain immunohistochemically with vimentin and desmin but not with cytokeratins or epithelial membrane antigen. Ultrastructurally, they have intercellular gap-junction nexuses, composed of hexagonal microtubules forming an open-channel system between adjacent cells to facilitate the passage of electrolytes and molecules and play a role in cell contact inhibition (Lawn *et al.* 1971; Wilkinson *et al.* 1990).

Confluent pseudo-decidual change of stromal cells under the endometrial surface epithelium occurs by the 25th day (11th day post-ovulation), producing the 'compacta'. This process extends on the following two days (12th and 13th days post-ovulation), and the glands demonstrate coiling and ferning. The endometrial stroma exhibits large numbers of endometrial granulocytes, the so-called metrial cells or 'K' cells (see below).

Menstrual phase

Menstruation is a process which normally lasts 3–5 days, during which time the endometrium rapidly fragments and degenerates, with most of the surface shedding occurring within the first 24–48 hours (Ludwig *et al.* 1990). The actual extent of tissue desquamation is still controversial, and probably varies considerably from one woman to another. Tissue fragmentation and necrosis are succeeded by tissue regeneration. The functionalis, on the 28th day through to the second day of the following cycle (Fig. 4.6), is typified by fissures and degenerate, pseudo-decidual cells which rapidly lose their eosinophilic cytoplasm and produce small rounded cellular aggregates of crowded naked nuclei, admixed with fragments of glands as well as acute and chronic (lymphoid) inflammatory cells. Lysosomal and other proteinase autodigestion destroys glandular and stromal cells and also vascular endothelium. Vascular injury promotes platelet deposition within the vascular lumen and is followed by multiple foci of ischaemic necrosis. On the second to fourth days of the new cycle, the functionalis gradually separates from the underlying basalis, commencing in the fundus and extending towards the isthmus (Ludwig and Metzger 1976; Lindeman 1979). Reparative re-epithelialization occurs by extension of the residual basal glandular epithelium over the denuded surface. The peripheral regions of the endometrial cavity, such as the isthmus and peritubal ostium remain more or less intact during menstruation, and also contribute to the re-epithelialization which is complete by the fifth day of the new cycle, heralding the cessation of bleeding. The ability of endometrial epithelial cells to migrate and heal wounds rapidly, as well as electron microscopic data, do not support the view that new endometrial surface and glandular epithelium are regenerated directly from persistent, secretory spongiosa (Flowers and Wilborn 1978) or stromal cells (Baggish *et al.* 1967). The latter may contribute to endometrial repair indirectly, by their positive influence on growth factors (Taketani and Masahiko 1991) or by providing cellular support to the migrating surface epithelial cells. Mechanisms of menstrual breakdown are reviewed more fully in Chapter 2.

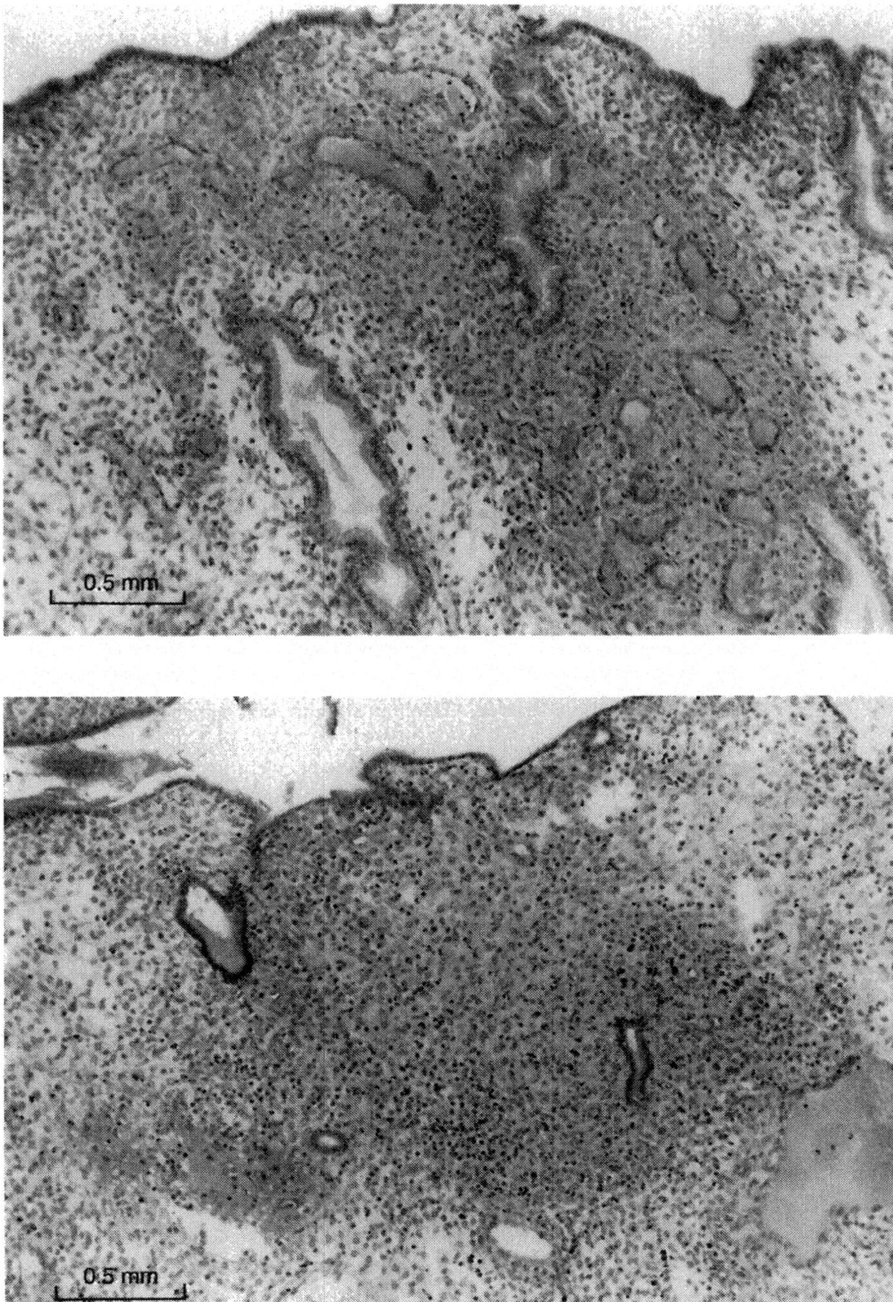

(a)

(b)

Fig. 4.5 (a) Late secretory endometrium, corresponding to the tenth post-ovulatory day. Superficial spiral arterioles are cuffed by a distinct zone of stromal pseudo-decidual change. Glands are large, tortuous, and distended by secretory product. H and E; × 50. (b) Contrast with endometrium associated with combination oral contraceptive therapy and corresponding to approximately the 11th day of continuous exposure to the progestational component. The small size and sparse distribution of the glands is due to concurrent inhibition of the proliferative effect of oestrogen by the progestogen. H and E; × 35.

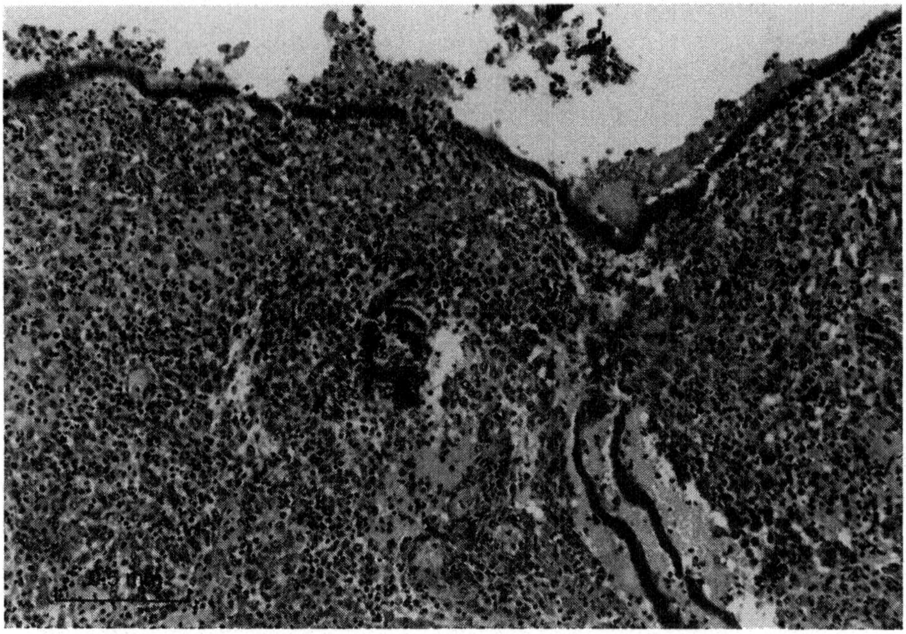

Fig. 4.6 Early menstrual endometrium. Fragmentation has commenced, with formation of blood lakes, rounding up of stromal cells, and infiltration by neutrophil polymorphs. Residual eosinophilic cytoplasm is still present in many stromal cells of the superficial compacta as evidence of adequate luteal effect in the secretory phase. H and E; × 35.

Gestational endometrium

In the event of pregnancy, the endometrium between the 22nd and 28th days of the cycle exhibits so-called 'gestational hypersecretory' change, characterized by glandular epithelial cell changes (cellular enlargement, ferning, re-emergence of vacuolation, nuclear variability) and luminal secretions, stromal oedema and vascular congestion, and extension of the pseudo-decidual reaction. These early events are exaggerated forms of those seen in the non-pregnant secretory endometrium. While not in themselves diagnostic of pregnancy, they are strongly suggestive (this should be noted in the pathologist's report) and a rigorous search should be undertaken in the curettage material to identify trophoblast, or linear fibrin deposition, which represents the placental site. In the absence of trophoblast or fibrin, changes indistinguishable from gestational endometrium may also be found in association with bilateral corpora lutea or a persistent corpus luteum cyst (Hendrickson and Kempson 1980).

The gestational endometrium becomes more distinctive by the fourth week of pregnancy (menstrual dating). Glands show more pronounced luminal ferning. Exaggeration of the nuclear changes gives rise to the so-called Arias-Stella reaction, typified by pavement-like clear cells with large hyperchromatic angulated nuclei. Nuclear enlargement in the Arias-Stella reaction is due to nuclear polypoidy. The Arias-Stella reaction may also be seen in the glandular epithelium of the cervix, the Fallopian tube, or in endometriosis (Silverberg and Arias-Stella 1972).

The pseudo-decidualized stromal cells are transformed into larger epithelioid cells and constitute the decidua vera. Such cells are most obvious in the upper one-third of the endometrium where they give rise to the compacta layer. Electron microscopically, these decidual cells are richer in organelles, including intermediate filaments, cigar-shaped mitochondria, and granular endoplasmic reticulum, than their non-gestational counterparts (Lawn *et al.* 1971; Wilkinson *et al.* 1990), and are connected by nexuses between cytoplasmic filipodial projections. Similar ultrastructural changes are present in response to exogenous progestogen therapy (Song and Fraser 1995).

Spiral arterioles are larger in calibre and thicker walled than they are in the non-pregnant state. Some show acute atherosis, with concentric intimal proliferation of myofibroblasts and foamy cells, apparently in response to trophoblastic invasion of endometrial vessels.

Inactive and atrophic endometrium

Peri-menopausal and post-menopausal endometrium which is architecturally similar to that seen in early proliferative phase but without features of active proliferation or secretion is termed 'inactive'. The glands tend to be oriented parallel to the surface epithelium rather than vertically, and the lining epithelial cells are low columnar to cuboidal with pseudostratified amitotic nuclei. The stroma is dense and uniformly hypercellular.

Atrophic endometrium is typified by a thin mucosa (< 0.5 mm), with reduced numbers of small glands and a reduced volume of stroma. The glandular and surface epithelia are low and cuboidal and devoid of cilia and mitotic activity. The stroma often appears collagenized, similar to that of the isthmus or lower uterine segment in younger women. Atrophic endometrium frequently has cystically dilated glands. These are also lined by flattened atrophic epithelium which readily distinguishes them from those seen in simple (cystic) hyperplasia. This appearance is often referred to as cystic atrophy, and is thought to reflect low level oestrogenic response of otherwise atrophic endometrial epithelium.

Vascular anatomy

The endometrium has a rich vascular supply derived from the radial arteries of the underlying myometrium. These penetrate the endometrium at regular intervals as the basal arteries, which in turn give off horizontal and vertical branches, the former supplying the basal layer and the latter the overlying functionalis. The arterioles in the functionalis are referred to as *spiral arterioles*. Their superficial arborization and connections with the epithelial precapillary system, as well as extreme tortuosity during the menstrual cycle, are a function of the ovarian steroid hormones. Histologically, endometrial arteries do not exhibit a subendothelial elastica, except in their basal portion. Endometrial vascular arborization is best seen immunohistochemically by staining for factor VIII-related antigen, CD34 or *Ulex europaeus* (Song *et al.* 1995). Veins and lymphatics are in close proximity to the endometrial arterioles and glands, respectively. Lymphatics appear to be uncommon in the endometrium, but are somewhat more easily identified in the basal layer (Blackwell and Fraser 1981).

Inflammatory cell elements in the normal endometrium

The human endometrium contains significant numbers of inflammatory cells, predominantly T lymphocytes and histiocytes, with minor populations of B lymphocytes, Langerhans cells, natural killer cells, endometrial granulated lymphocytes, and polymorphonuclear leukocytes. Immunocompetent plasma cells are normally absent. Perivascular lymphoid aggregates resembling follicles may be present in the endometrial stroma, particularly during the proliferative phase. They are not thought to play a significant role, if any, in the local secretory immune system. Indeed, endometrial glands do not synthesize immunoproteins (Rebello *et al.* 1975). In the secretory phase, there is a marked increase in the presence of scattered single T lymphocytes in the stroma. Endometrium contains moderate numbers of mast cells, located chiefly in the basalis and easily identified in H and E stained sections of FAA-fixed tissues by their brightly eosinophilic cytoplasm, or by Giemsa stains in formalin-fixed tissues. Their number is stable throughout the cycle (they are activated in the late secretory phase), but drops with age, particularly post-menopausally. Polymorphonuclear leukocytes are seen normally only in menstrual phase, after the onset of tissue breakdown.

In the late secretory phase, endometrial granulated lymphocytes, the so-called metrial cells or 'K' cells, become prominent. These cells resemble eosinophils with coarse, brightly eosinophilic cytoplasmic granules, but have a single, kidney-shaped hyperchromatic nucleus. They were formerly thought to be of endometrial stromal origin and to contain relaxin in the granules; more recently they have been shown to be members of the large granular lymphocyte series (Bulmer *et al.* 1987), staining positively for the leukocyte and cell surface antigens designated by the following abbreviations: LCA, CD2, OKT10 (CD38), UCHL1 (CD45RO), and Leu-19 (CD56) and negatively for Leu-7 (CD57), CD3, CD4, CD5, CD7, CD16, and HLA-DR (Song and Fraser 1995). Because of their gradual numeric increase during the secretory phase and their maximum concentration during early pregnancy, it is thought that they are under the control of progesterone and that they may play a role in implantation and placentation.

Endometrial-morphology in hyperplasia and carcinoma

Endometrial hyperplasias, and the closely related processes of metaplasia, are a mixed group of abnormal structural proliferations and cellular changes, some of which precede endometrial carcinoma. Hyperplasia is characterized by a proliferation of irregularly sized, shaped, and distributed glands with an increase in the ratio of glands/stroma when compared to normal proliferative phase endometrium. It is most commonly found in response to excess oestrogenic stimulation (Fig. 4.7). Metaplasias (cytoplasmic changes such as 'eosinophilic', squamous, tubal or 'ciliated cell', 'secretory/clear cell', and mucinous), may be seen separately but are frequently superimposed upon hyperplasia or, indeed, carcinoma.

Endometrial hyperplasia is divided histologically into two broad categories, simple (formerly cystic) and complex (formerly adenomatous). Simple hyperplasia exhibits crowded, abnormally shaped glands with luminal dilatation and glandular buds, but separated by easily identifiable stroma. Nuclei are predominantly elongate, vertically oriented, and often pseudostratified. Mitoses are always present but may be quite variable. Complex hyperplasia differs from simple hyperplasia partly in degree, showing more closely crowded glands with loss of the intervening stroma, but also the presence of luminal buds or infoldings of the epithelium, with bridging causing complex or multiple lumens, or abnormal branching of the glands giving rise to complicated external contours. True epithelial stratification may be seen, and mitoses are again present but variable. The stroma is usually inconspicuous but, in about 25 per cent of cases, is distinguished by the presence of large lipid-laden foamy stromal cells with small pyknotic nuclei (Fechner *et al.* 1979).

Each of the subcategories of hyperplasia is further divided into those *without* or *with* cellular (nuclear) atypia. In practise, simple hyperplasia with atypia is uncommonly encountered, with many cases of apparent atypia being due to one of the metaplasias. The significance of cellular atypia is based on elegant long-term follow-up studies (Ferenczy and Gelfand 1989; Kurman *et al.* 1985; Baak *et al.* 1992) which showed that progression to carcinoma occurred in less than

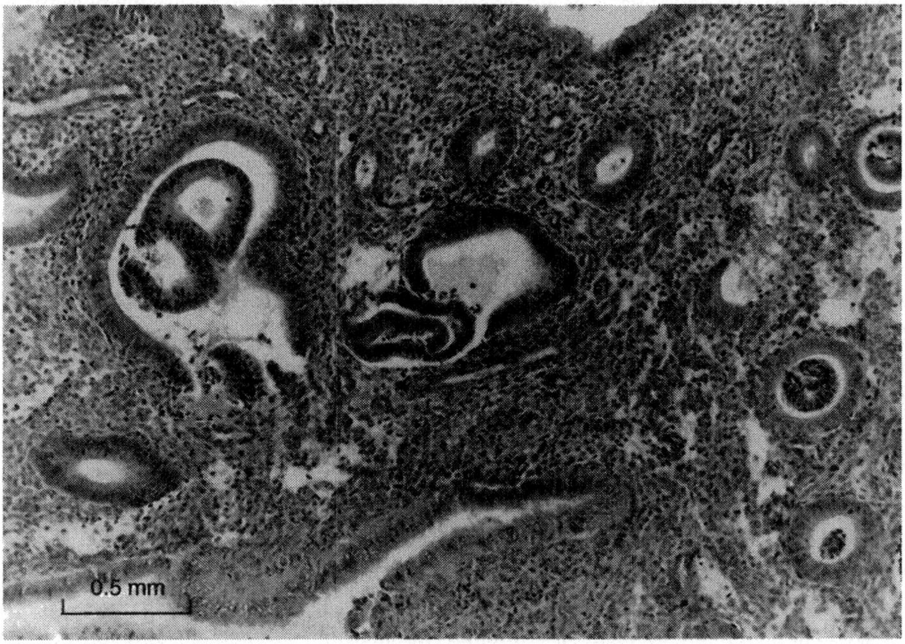

Fig. 4.7 Anovulatory or disordered proliferative endometrium is the first recognizable pattern of unopposed oestrogen stimulation and is characterized by irregular size and distribution of proliferative type glands. Tubal metaplasia (bottom) is often observed. Continued exposure to oestrogens causes progression of these changes to hyperplasia. H and E; × 35.

2 per cent of cases of endometrial hyperplasia without atypia but in 23 per cent of cases with atypia.

As may reasonably be inferred from the above discussion, the spectrum of endometrial hyperplasias includes gradational changes from one to the other. The distinction between complex hyperplasias with atypia and well differentiated endometrial carcinoma and all of its 'metaplastic' variants is also one of interpretation of subtle changes and quantitation of these changes. The simplest distinction is made in the presence of a host stromal response to invading carcinoma manifest as altered or fibroblastic ('desmoplastic') stroma separating disorderly and irregular glands. In the now quite widely accepted schema of Kurman and Norris (Kurman and Norris 1982; Norris *et al.* 1983), the independent presence of a 'confluent glandular pattern' characterized by crowded, complex, or cribriform glands, not separated by stroma, or an 'extensive papillary pattern' are each regarded as diagnostic of carcinoma. These latter features should occupy fields of at least 2 mm dimension in the sections of curettage material if a useful prediction of well differentiated carcinoma in the residual (uterine) endometrium is to be made. The term 'adenocarcinoma-*in-situ*' should be avoided. Moderately and poorly differentiated carcinomas do not require sophisticated diagnostic parameters for their identification.

Specialized functions of the endometrium

There has been considerable progress in the past decade to develop and apply research techniques which clarify the complex endocrine, molecular, and physiological changes occurring in human endometrium in relation to implantation, pregnancy, menstruation, and a variety of pathological conditions (Findlay 1994; Metzger 1995). As it has become clear that the endometrium is a highly complex and specialized tissue, attempts have been made to assess the possible clinical relevance of changes in these functions. Most tests remain in the realms of laboratory and clinical research, but undoubtedly some will have major implications for clinical medicine. Features that are likely to have future relevance include the biochemical changes associated with implantation, changes in endocrine function of the endometrium, and local blood flow and vascular fragility. Accurate measurements of the size and shape of the uterine cavity and pathological structures may also become important.

At the present time, there is an explosion of information on changes in the molecular and cellular biology of the endometrium through the menstrual cycle and pregnancy with gradually increasing understanding of some of the changes which occur in certain pathological conditions (Findlay 1994; Metzger 1995). These interactions are likely to become more clinically relevant within the next decade and clinicians will need to become familiar with the different migratory leukocytes, hormones (for example prolactin and the renin–angiotensin system), growth factors, cytokines, prostaglandins, endothelins, matrix metalloproteinases, lysosomal enzymes, and numerous other protein secretions.

Conclusions

The main approach to the assessment of human endometrium still entails some form of curettage followed by the application of classical histology. This provides valuable, if somewhat crude, information about function and the presence of certain pathologies. Macroscopic imaging of the endometrium can be provided by increasingly sophisticated vaginal ultrasound techniques, but the ‘gold standard’ for detection and exclusion of endometrial pathology is accepted to be diagnostic hysteroscopy with directed biopsy. These approaches provide little information about function, although there is likely to be an explosion of clinically relevant information on this aspect as modern sophisticated methods of assessment of molecular interaction and physiological function are refined.

References

Abramowicz, J.S. and Archer, D.F. (1990). Uterine endometrial peristalsis – a transvaginal ultrasound study. *Fertility and Sterility*, **54**, 451–7.

Arthur, I.D. and Khan, S.M. (1996). The application of standard and morphometric dating criteria for luteal phase endometrial specimens collected by outpatient sampling. *British Journal of Obstetrics and Gynaecology*, **103**, 473–4.

Asherman, J.G. (1950). Traumatic intrauterine adhesions. *Journal of Obstetrics and Gynaecology of the British Commonwealth*, **57**, 892–6.

Baak, J.P.A., Wise-Brekelmans, E.C.M., Fleege, J.C., van der Putten, H.W.H.M., and Bezemer P.D. (1992). Assessment of the risk of endometrial cancer in hyperplasia, by means of morphological and morphometric features. *Pathology Research and Practice*, **188**, 856–9.

Baggish, M.S., Pauerstein, C.J., and Woodruff, J.D. (1967). Role of stroma in regeneration of endometrial epithelium. *American Journal of Obstetrics and Gynecology*, **99**, 453–9.

Balen, F. (1994). Ultrasound contrast agents. *Clinical Radiology*, **49**, 77–82.

Bergeron, C., Ferenczy, A., Toft, D.O., Schneider, W., and Shyamala, G. (1988). Immunocytochemical study of progesterone receptors in the human endometrium during the menstrual cycle. *Laboratory Investigation*, **59**, 862–9.

Blackwell, P. and Fraser, I.S. (1981). Superficial lymphatics in the functional zone of the normal human endometrium. *Microvascular Research*, **21**, 142–52.

Brooks, P.G. and Serden, S.P. (1988). Hysteroscopic findings after unsuccessful dilatation and curettage for abnormal bleeding. *American Journal of Obstetrics and Gynecology*, **158**, 1354–7.

Bulmer, J.N., Hollings, D., and Ritson, A. (1987). Immunocytochemical evidence that endometrial stromal granulocytes are granulated lymphocytes. *Journal of Pathology*, **153**, 281–8.

Campbell, S., Bourne, T.H., Tan, S.L., and Collins, W.P. (1994). Hysterosalpingo contrast sonography (Hy Co Sy) and its future role within the investigation of infertility in Europe. *Ultrasound in Obstetrics and Gynecology*, **4**, 245–53.

Coulter, A., Klassen, A., Mackenzie, I.Z., and McPherson, K. (1993). Diagnostic dilatation and curettage: is it used appropriately? *British Medical Journal*, **306**, 236–9.

Dijkhuizen, E.P.H.L.J., Brolman, H.A.M., Potters, A.E., Bongers, M.Y., and Heintz, A.P.M. (1996). The accuracy of transvaginal ultrasonography in the diagnosis of endometrial abnormalities. *Obstetrics and Gynecology*, **87**, 345–9.

Dowling, E.A. and Gravlee, L.C. (1964). Endometrial cancer diagnosis. A new technique using a jet washer. *Alabama Journal of Medical Science*, **1**, 412–16.

Fechner, R.E., Bossart, M.I., and Spjut, H.J. (1979). Ultrastructure of endometrial stromal foam cells. *American Journal of Clinical Pathology*, **72**, 628–33.

Ferenczy, A. and Gelfand, M. (1989). The biologic significance of cytologic atypia in progesterone-treated endometrial hyperplasia. *American Journal of Obstetrics and Gynecology*, **160**, 126–31.

Ferenczy, A. Bertrand, G., and Gelfand, M.M. (1979). Proliferation kinetics of human endometrium during the normal menstrual cycle. *American Journal of Obstetrics and Gynecology*, **133**, 859–67.

Findlay, J.K. (ed.) (1994). *Molecular biology of the female reproductive system*. Academic Press, San Diego.

Fleischer, A.C. and Kepple, D.M. (1992). Benign conditions of the uterus, cervix and endometrium. In *Transvaginal ultrasound*, (ed. D.A. Nyberg, L.M. Hill, M. Böhm-Velez, and E.B. Mendelson), pp. 21–14, Mosby Year Book, St Louis

Fleischer, A.C., Kalemeris, G.C., and Machin, J.E. (1986). Sonographic depiction of normal and abnormal endometrium with histopathologic correlation. *Journal of Ultrasound Medicine*, **5**, 445–52.

Fleischer, A.C., Mendelson, E.B., and Böhm-Velez, M. (1988). Transvaginal and transabdominal sonography of the endometrium. *Seminars in Ultrasound*, **9**, 81–96.

Flowers, C.E. Jr and Wilborn, W.H. (1978). New observations on the physiology of menstruation. *Obstetrics and Gynecology*, **51**, 14–16.

Fraser, I.S. (1993). Personal techniques and results for outpatient diagnostic hysteroscopy. *Gynaecological Endoscopy*, **2**, 29–33.

Fraser, I.S., Song, J.Y., Jansen, R.P.S., Ramsay, P., and Boogert, T. (1995). Hysteroscopic lysis of intrauterine adhesions under ultrasound guidance. *Gynaecological Endoscopy*, **4**, 35–40.

Gibson, M., Badger, G.J., and Byrne, F. (1991). Error in histologic dating of secretory endometrium: variance component analysis. *Fertility and Sterility*, **56**, 242–7.

Gimpelson, R. and Rappold, H. (1988). A comparative study between panoramic hysteroscopy with directed biopsies and dilatation and curettage. A review of 276 cases. *American Journal of Obstetrics and Gynecology*, **158**, 489–92.

Goldrath, M.H. and Sherman, A.I. (1985). Office hysteroscopy and suction curettage: can we eliminate the hospital diagnostic dilatation and curettage? *American Journal of Obstetrics and Gynecology*, **152**, 220–9.

Gordon, A.G. and Lewis, B.V. (1988). *Gynaecological endoscopy*. Chapman and Hall, London.

Granberg, S., Wikland, M., and Karlsson, B. (1991). Endometrial thickness as measured by endovaginal ultrasonography for identifying endometrial abnormality. *American Journal of Obstetrics and Gynecology*, **164**, 47–55.

Grimes, D.A. (1982). Diagnostic dilatation and curettage: a reappraisal. *American Journal of Obstetrics and Gynecology*, **142**, 1–6.

Hamou, J. (1991). *Hysteroscopy and microcolpohysteroscopy: text and atlas*. Appleton and Lange, Norwalk, Connecticut.

Hasson, H.M. (1980). Uterine geometry and IUD performance. In *Medicated intrauterine devices, physiological and clinical aspects*, (ed. E.S.E. Hafez and W.A.A. Van Os), pp. 11–12. Martinus Nijhoff, Amsterdam.

Hasson, H.M. (1985). Clinical studies of the wing sound II metrology device. In *Intrauterine contraception: recent advances and future prospects*, (ed. G.I. Zatuchni), pp. 126–41. Harper and Row, Philadelphia.

Haynes, P.J., Hodgson, H., Anderson, A.B.M., and Turnbull, A.C. (1977). Measurement of menstrual blood loss in patients complaining of menorrhagia. *British Journal of Obstetrics and Gynaecology*, **84**, 763–9.

Hendrickson, M.R. and Kempson, R.L. (1980). Surgical pathology of the uterine corpus. In *Major problems in pathology* (ed. J.L. Bennington), Vol. 12, pp. 36–98. W.B. Saunders, Philadephia.

Henig, I., Chan, P., and Tredway, D.R. (1989). Evaluation of the pipelle curette for endometrial biopsy. *Journal of Reproductive Medicine*, **34**, 786–9.

Hill, N.C.W., Broadbent, J.A.M., and Magos, A.L. (1992). The role of outpatient hysteroscopy. *Contemporary Reviews in Obstetrics and Gynaecology*, **4**, 209–14.

Holst, J., Koskella, O., and Von Schoultz, B. (1983). Endometrial findings following curettage in 2018 women according to age and indications. *Annales Chirurgia et Gynecologia*, **72**: 274–7.

Katzenellenbogen, B.S. (1980). Dynamics of steroid hormone receptor action. *Annual Review of Physiology*, **42**, 17–32.

Kikuchi, A., Okai, T., Kobayashi, K., Sakai, M., Ryo, E., and Taketani, Y. (1995). Intrauterine ultrasonography with a high frequency probe: preliminary report. *Obstetrics and Gynecology* **85**, 457–61.

Kovacs, G.T. and Burger, H.G. (1988). Endometrial sampling for women on perimenopausal hormone replacement therapy. *Maturitas*, **10**, 259–62.

Kovacs, G.T., Burger, H.G., Hailes, J., and Medley, G. (1988). A new method of endometrial sampling – the Gynoscann: a comparison with Vabra curettage. *Medical Journal of Australia*, **148**, 498–503.

Kurman, R.J. and Norris, H.J. (1982). Evaluation of criteria for distinguishing atypical endometrial hyperplasia from well differentiated carcinoma. *Cancer*, **49**, 2547–59.

Kurman, R.J., Kaminski, P.F., and Norris, H.J. (1985). The behavior of endometrial hyperplasia. A long-term study of 'untreated' hyperplasia in 170 patients. *Cancer*, **56**, 403–12.

Lawn, A.M., Wilson, E.W., and Finn, C.A. (1971). The ultrastructure of human decidual and predecidual cells. *Journal of Reproduction and Fertility*, **26**, 85–93.

Li, T.C., Rogerts, A.W., Dockery, P., Lenton, E.A., and Cooke, I.D. (1988). A new method of histological dating of human endometrium in the luteal phase. *Fertility and Sterility*, **49**, 52–60.

Lindeman, H.J. (1979). Hysteroscopic data during menstruation. In *The biology of the fluids of the female genital tract*, (ed. F.K. Beller and G.F.B. Schumacher) pp. 225–9. Elsevier–North Holland, Amsterdam.

Loffer, F.D. (1989). Hysteroscopy with selective endometrial sampling compared with dilatation and curettage for abnormal uterine bleeding: the value of a negative hysteroscopic view. *Obstetrics and Gynecology*, **73**, 16–20.

Ludwig, H. and Metzger, H. (1976). The re-epithelization of endometrium after menstrual desquamation. *Archiv für Gynakology*, **221**, 51–60.

Ludwig, H., Metzger, H., and Frauli, M. (1990). Endometrium: tissue remodelling and regeneration. In *Contraception and mechanisms of endometrial bleeding*, (ed. C. D'Arcangues, I.S. Fraser, J.R. Newton, and V. Odlind), pp. 441–61. Cambridge University Press.

Mackenzie, I.Z. and Bibby, J.G. (1978). A critical assessment of dilatation and curettage in 1029 women. *Lancet*, **ii**, 556–8.

Metzger, D.A. (ed.) (1995). The endometrium. *Infertility and reproductive medicine of North America*, Vol. 6, pp. 263–459. W.B. Saunders, Philadelphia.

Milan, A.R. and Markley, R.L. (1973). Endometrial cytology by a new technique. *Obstetrics and Gynecology* **42**, 469–75.

More, I.A.R., Armstrong, E.M., McSeveney, D., and Chatfield, W.R. (1974). The morphogenesis and fate of the nucleolar channel system in the human endometrial glandular cells. *Journal of Ultrastructural Research*, **47**, 74–82.

Nanini, R., Chelo, E., Branconi, F., Tantini, C., and Scarselli, G.F. (1981). Dynamic echohysteroscopy: a new diagnostic technique in the study of female infertility. *Acta Europaeus Fertilitas*, **12**, 165–71.

Nilsson, L. and Rybo, G. (1971). Treatment of menorrhagia. *American Journal of Obstetrics and Gynecology*, **110**, 713–20.

Norris, H.J., Tavassoli, F.A., and Kurman, R.J. (1983). Endometrial hyperplasia and carcinoma. Diagnostic considerations. *American Journal of Surgical Pathology*, **7**, 839–46.

Novak, E. (1935). A suction-curettage apparatus for endometrial biopsy. *Journal of the American Medical Association*, **104**, 1947–8.

Noyes, R.W., Hertig, A.T., and Rock, J. (1950). Dating the endometrial biopsy. *Fertility and Sterility*, **1**, 3–25.

Parsons, A.K. and Lense, J.J. (1993). Sonohysterography for endometrial abnormalities. *Journal of Clinical Ultrasound*, **21**, 87–97.

Rebello, R., Green, F.H.Y., and Fox, H. (1975). A study of the secretory immune system of the female genital tract. *British Journal of Obstetrics and Gynaecology*, **82**, 812–20.

Scott, R.T. (1994). Ultrasonographic evaluation of the endometrium during ovulation induction. In *Imaging in infertility and reproductive endocrinology* (ed. R. Jaffe, R.A. Pierson, and J.S. Abramowicz), pp. 53–61. Lippincott, Philadelphia.

Silverberg, S.G. and Arias-Stella, J. (1972). Arias-Stella phenomenon in spontaneous and therapeutic abortion. *American Journal of Obstetrics and Gynecology*, **112**, 777–82.

Song, J.Y. and Fraser, I.S. (1995). Effects of progestogens on human endometrium. *Obstetric and Gynecologic Survey*, **50**, 385–94.

Song, J.Y., Markham, R., Russell, P., Wong, T., Young, L., and Fraser, I.S. (1995). The effect of high-dose medium- and long-term progestogen exposure on endometrial vessels. *Human Reproduction*, **10**, 797–800.

Steiner, H., Staudach, A., Spitzer, D., and Schaffer, H.I. (1994). Three-dimensional ultrasound in obstetrics and gynaecology: techniques, possibilities and limitations. *Human Reproduction*, **9**, 1773–8.

Taketani, Y. and Masahiko, M. (1991). Evidence for direct regulation of epidermal growth factor receptors by steroid hormones in human endometrial cells. *Human Reproduction*, **6**, 1365–9.

Varner, R.E., Sparks, J.M., and Cameron, C.D. (1991). Transvaginal sonography of the endometrium in postmenopausal women. *Obstetrics and Gynecology*, **78**, 195–203.

Vuopala, S. (1977). Diagnostic accuracy and clinical applicability of cytological and histological methods for investigating endometrial carcinoma. *Acta Obstetrica et Gynecologica Scandinavica*, **70** (Suppl.), 1–72.

Wilkinson, N., Buckley, C.H., Chawner, L., and Fox, H. (1990). Nucleolar organiser regions in normal, hyperplastic and neoplastic endometrium. *International Journal of Gynecological Pathology*, **9**, 55–9.

5 Menstruation, surgery, and women

Ann M. Voda, Phyllis Kernoff Mansfield, and Jan L. Root

> And did we find regularity in the menstrual cycle? Anything but! Variation so clearly characterized every history that we wondered how the word regular had come to be applied; not only that, but so firmly entrenched. As biometricians, we were prone to define a term like regular in a strictly mathematical sense, as straight lines of circled onset dates, which never appeared on the cards as we studied them individually, and in great numbers each new year. Surely, if we were persistent enough in assembling data, we could convince those who were apt to regard the menstrual cycle as 'regular' as the superlative of falsehood. (from Alan E. Treloar's diary ~1930s)

Introduction

Two significant maturational events associated with a woman's reproductive system are menarche and menopause, the onset and closure of menstrual bleeding. Between these two reproductive landmarks, on average every 23 to 38 days, for an estimated 30 to 40 years, a woman's body prepares for the implantation of a conceptus in the uterus. If implantation does not occur, the uterine endometrium is shed over a period of four to seven days via a process that becomes very familiar to women – menstruation. Until recently, knowledge of the menstrual cycle was generated either through myth and folklore, or research based upon the biomedical, quantitative research paradigm. Each has had its own unique impact on how the menstrual cycle is viewed today, and is discussed briefly in the sections that follow.

Myth and folklore

According to writers of *The curse, a cultural history of menstruation*, in the beginning, menstrual blood inspired fear and wonder in humans. Both men and women realized that menstrual blood set woman apart from man in a mysterious, magical way. Menstrual blood flowed, but women were not disabled from such blood loss, nor did they die. Only the creation of a new life could alter an almost predictable pattern of bleeding (Delaney *et al.* 1988). Many 19th century peoples regarded menstrual blood with extreme respect, even fear, constructing taboos to protect themselves from impurity, illness, or death. In our own not-too-distant past, the fear of menstrual blood caused women to be burned at the stake for incidents that happened in their communities coincident with menstrual bleeds. Menstruating women, in traditional Chinese culture, were perceived as not clean. To eliminate contamination, they were forbidden to enter temples, to have sex, to swim, and even forbidden to hang laundry over other people's clothing, especially a man's (Cornacchia 1995).

Fortunately, most peoples who live in westernized societies today no longer believe that a menstruating woman's blood is responsible for either societal or individual problems, and except for a few societies on which we have current information (Beyene 1989; duToit 1990), a menstruating woman is no longer viewed as possessing supernatural power, someone who can curse a village, spoil meat, sour milk, etc. Yet, Grahn (1993) perpetuates the mythical connection between the menstrual and the lunar cycles, for example:

> Humans have a fundamental and unique tool of external–internal measurement in the synchronization of the menstrual cycle and the lunar cycle. ... Only the human cycle, at 29½ days, coincides with the cycle of the moon.

The message here is that menstruation is normal as long as it is periodic and regular, that is coinciding with the lunar interval of 28–29 days (Grahn 1993). If a woman does not conceive, the expectation is that menstruation will occur with amazing regularity (Grahn 1993). Drawing upon material from history, folklore, and myth, Grahn also advances an hypothesis in which she argues that menstrual blood has been the centre of all creativity on the planet since the creation of the universe. Why, she questions, when images of blood surround us daily in human societies – wounds, death, birthing, TV violence – does menstrual blood, the only non-traumatic source of blood, remain hidden?

> ...this is the most hidden blood, the one so rarely spoken of and almost never seen, except privately by women, who shut themselves in a little room too quickly and in many cases disgustedly change their pads and tampons, wrapping the bloodied cotton so it won't be seen by others, wrinkling their faces at the odor, flushing or hiding the evidence away. ... menstrual blood, like water, just flows. Its fountain existed long before knives or flint; menstruation is the original source of blood.

Biomedical, quantitative approach to research

On the one hand, utilizing the quantitative paradigm has served effectively to increase knowledge about the physiology and hormonal mechanisms which regulate the menstrual cycle. On the other hand, however, the method has created several problems. First, it has promoted a dichotomization of menstrual experiences as either regular/normal or irregular/pathological; second, researchers utilizing the method have ignored the significance of an individual's experience in understanding the totality of the menstrual experience; and third, knowledge generated has not explored the impact that values, language, and cultural expectations could have upon research outcomes (Root 1992).

Most studies of menstrual cycle function have been based upon the misconception that healthy, normal menstrual function is characterized by one pattern: regularity. Predicating research based upon such an assumption forces menstrual experiences into a dichotomy – either the menstrual cycle conforms to the established norm, or it does not. In other words, menstrual experiences need to be as regular and predictable as the lunar cycle to be normal. If they are not, they are irregular and abnormal (Root 1992). Words such as 'failure,' 'pathological', and 'dysfunctional' are commonly used to describe variations from the normal 28 day cycle pattern. Exclusive reliance on an illness or failure model prevents any possibility of understanding the menstrual cycle from a normal perspective. A focus on problems or differences in the phenomenon of menstruation itself, whether within or among women, has not been without consequences to health for menstruating women.

As such, the material in this chapter is organized as follows: first, an overview of menstruation as a normal biologic process in the lives of women is presented; second, a review of the factors that have influenced the contemporary views of menstruation as disease is offered; third, menstruation as a periodic, irregular event is discussed. The chapter concludes with a discussion of reproductive surgeries, the impact on women's health and quality of life, and suggestions for clinicians.

Menstruation as a normal, biological process

By definition, menstruation is a natural, healthy process of cleansing the uterus. Technically, it is only one phase of the menstrual cycle: the periodic shedding of the uterine endometrium in a process referred to as a sterile inflammatory reaction (Shaw and Roche 1985). Approximately once a month for 30 to 35 years of reproductive life, the menstrual cycle repeats itself. During a span of 26–30 days during prime reproductive years (ages 20–39), all menstrual cycle activities are coordinated to promote changes in the endometrium, ovulation, and implantation of a fertilized egg. As such, almost one-half of a woman's life is spent in a body that is in a constant, regulated state of change as a result of cyclic fluctuations in a variety of hormones. Within the parameters of a 'monthly' cycle, from the time of sexual maturation the human female prepares for a possible pregnancy. If hormone synthesis is not maintained, endometrial tissue (which had proliferated during the follicular phase of the cycle, and was transformed into a secretory glandular structure during the luteal phase) regresses at a rate which is parallel to a decrease in blood levels of the sex hormones (Shaw and Roche 1985). During the regressive phase, the endometrium is characterized by increased signs of cell injury, cell depletion, and signs of intracellular resorption and reorganization. It is injury to blood vessels via kinking and vasoconstriction that causes red blood cells to suffuse (moisten) the endometrium, causing menstruation.

The endometrium has been observed to shed in layers. Knowing this led Profet (1993) to hypothesize that menstruation, instead of being a sign of failed fertility, is a sterile, inflammatory reaction, which functions not only to cleanse the uterus, but to protect it against pathogens carried into the body via sperm, thus protecting fertility. Profet's theory has been challenged by researchers who counter that menstruation, rather than ridding the uterus of bacteria, is more likely to be the time of greatest bacterial contamination, because open areas are created by constriction and dilation of arterioles, with subsequent elimination of necrotic tissue (Toufexis 1993).

A fact not widely known by women is that in prime reproductive years, most endometrial build-up is resorbed. Menstruation, by definition, then, is more accurately referred to as 'menstrual discharge', which, according to Shaw and Roche (1985), is a combination of cellular debris, fluid, and blood. An estimate of around 26 ml has been postulated as the normal volume of loss of menstrual discharge for healthy women who have a preponderance of ovulatory cycles (Shaw 1973). No research-based data are available to indicate with any confidence whether the resorptive process changes in perimenopausal women as they make the transition to menopause.

Menstruation as disease

Certain misconceptions about the menstrual cycle persist. For example, reproductive endocrinologists agree that the menstrual cycle is not simply switched on at menarche and off at menopause; hormonal and bodily changes precede the first menstruation as well as the last (Hafez 1980; Buckler and Anderson 1994; Longcope 1994). Yet, when the onset of menstrual bleeds becomes unpredictable, or the interval between bleeds increases or decreases, and/or the quality of the bleed changes from light to heavy (as in perimenopause), with the passing of clots, these changes are viewed as abnormal, and diagnosed as dysfunctional, needing to be fixed. In this context, Profet (1993) suggests that routinely regarding irregular bleeding as an endocrine problem to be stopped with hormone therapy could be counterproductive to menstrual health.

The view of the menstrual cycle as problematic persists because much of past menstrual cycle research has been predicated upon the misconception that the menstrual cycle is highly regular, and thus, predictable. In reality, the menstrual cycle is more accurately characterized by irregularity (Treloar *et al.* 1967; Vollman 1977). Except for the longitudinal studies of Treloar *et al.* on menstrual cycle interval, what characterizes the normal pattern of menstruation in women across the life span is, by and large, unknown (Rodrigues *et al.* 1976; Machin *et al.* 1987; Belsey and Farley 1988).

Other views of the menstrual cycle are that it is a burden, a cross to bear, a shameful event to be hidden away, or a sign of a failed pregnancy (Grahn 1993; Root 1992; Martin 1988; Profet 1993). Since the sources of this information arose out of society itself (Root 1992), it is not surprising to find that the uterus itself is considered to be the source of many problems, and is conceptualized as a disposable, rather than an essential, organ – one that cramps, bleeds, carries babies, and gets cancer (Laurence and Weinhouse 1994). If a woman does not conceive, the expectation is that menstruation will occur. If a woman's primary role in society is viewed as responsibility for reproduction of the species, menstruation is a failed pregnancy.

Conceptualizing menstruation as a burden, disease, or a failure, according to Martin (1988), serves to maintain and justify the subordinate status of women in society, as well as promoting and sustaining a theory of the defective woman. Although current medical texts explicitly acknowledge menstruation and the menstrual cycle as natural, non-pathological events, Martin suggests that the assumption that menstruation is intrinsically pathological continues to be widespread, and is articulated via a metaphor congruent with the ideology of contemporary westernized society, a metaphor of failed production. Martin believes that if understanding the menstrual cycle is conceptually organized around production, for example the 'production' of a new human, then menstruation can only represent failure (a failed pregnancy).

This culturally accepted view of menstruation as inherently pathological was demonstrated by Martin (1988), who discovered after examining the most widely used obstetrical texts, published between 1700 and the 1980s, that prior to 1800 male and female functions were viewed as analogous. Discussions in the texts emphasized the similarities rather than the differences between the sexes in physiology and function. Menstruation was characterized as a process essentially analogous to sweating in men – the primary purpose of the latter was to rid men of harmful bodily wastes. Menstruation was viewed as a way to fulfil the same purpose in women. Martin argued that the social disruptions brought about by the industrial and scientific revolutions forced society to create new ways of understanding the relationships between men and women. Hence, a new understanding of the physiological processes connected with reproduction centred on the differences between the sexes rather than the similarities. Functions previously acknowledged as valued female functions were now denigrated. Nineteenth-century writers medicalized the menstrual cycle, stressing the debilitating and pathological nature of menstruation (Martin 1988), whereas 20th century writers transformed menstrual distress into pre-menstrual syndrome (PMS), a disorder that is reported to disrupt or even destroy lives (Lever and Brush 1981; Keye 1988;

Voda 1997). PMS, by definition, is the cyclic occurrence of symptoms of sufficient severity to interfere with some aspect of life, which appear with a consistent and predictable relationship to menses (Keye 1988).

Related to PMS, Root (1992) offers some instructive insights. First, she examined the word 'syndrome,' asking: what is a syndrome? By definition, a syndrome is a number of symptoms occurring together, which characterize a specific disease state (Webster 1983). By virtue of this definition, PMS is a disease. Next, Root examined the commonly accepted definition of disease, which is a particular destructive process in the body which may interrupt or impair any or all of the natural and normal functioning (Webster 1983). One menstrual cycle researcher attributes 150 different signs and symptoms to PMS (Moos 1968). This means, literally, that there could be 150 ways for a woman to be diseased and have normal function impaired.

The PMS model has been effective in providing a framework from which to discuss certain problematic aspects of the menstrual cycle. On the one hand, it is useful for women in that it formally legitimizes problematic aspects of the menstrual cycle that previously were denied (Keye 1988). On the other hand, however, to label as problematic any normal change associated with the menstrual cycle increases the risk of being diagnosed with PMS and being diseased (Root 1992; Voda 1997).

Root (1992) concluded her probe into PMS asking: if a premenstrual change is problematic for a woman, does this need to imply that the problem is an indication of something abnormal? If so, the PMS model of women as diseased is essentially flawed – it operates from an implicit assumption that a woman's condition when she is not menstruating or about to menstruate is her normal condition. In other words, women who are not premenstrual or menstruating are assumed to be in a state like men are all the time, for example, in a balanced, physiologically steady state. Women, however, do not exist day-to-day in a physiologically steady state, any more than men do. During menstrual life, they are always in one phase or another of the menstrual cycle. Change, then, not steadiness, is the norm. As such, to be a cycling woman means change, and change is normal. To apply the PMS model to all menstruating women who experience normal premenstrual changes, implicitly labels them as diseased (Voda 1997).

The bottom-line paradigm here is that biological explanations for human actions – PMS, menopause, and so on – tend to focus on women, not men – women's hormones, their menstruations, and, at menopause, their lack of female hormones (Hedricks 1992). Lange (1983), a feminist critic, hypothesizes that the view of menstruating women as diseased, unbalanced, inherently weak and/or inferior, has its roots deeply embedded in Aristotelian ideology. In a critique of *The biology or reproduction*, Lange suggests that Aristotle's theory of 'concoction' (which is based upon the ability of the male to produce semen, and not menstrual blood), established as dogma early on the view that the male of the species is more valuable than the female. Menstrual blood does not contain sperm; semen does. Sperm is necessary for impregnation and is *the* vital fluid for creating a new human. Based upon differences in reproductive ability, females, because they could not concoct semen, were viewed as weak and inferior when compared to males. The female reproductive functions of gestation and birthing were also described as animalistic, since these same processes were also observed to occur in the females of lower animals (no matter that the males of lower species also impregnated females).

Lander (1988), another feminist critic, like Profet, questioned the physiological necessity of menstruation in human females. Unlike Profet, however, Lander theorized that in humans it is an evolutionary anomaly. In other words, the menstrual cycle as women now experience it will at some future time become obsolete; reproduction will occur without the necessity of a monthly menstrual discharge. Lander suggests that women's physiology has had little time to adapt to the change from oestrus (in lower animals) to menstruation in humans. She speculates that modern-day woman's genes are the genes of a woman in hunter/gatherer societies, a woman who was always pregnant and never menstruated. In her attempt to explain why women menstruate and men do not, Lander implicitly uses man as the standard – men do not menstruate, women do. As such, menstruation in women is viewed as an evolutionary artifact – in time, women will evolve to as high a level as man, and they will not menstruate. Obliteration of the genotype for menstruation is viewed as the ultimate goal to eliminate that event. Lander's theory, albeit unintentional, is similar to Aristotle's theory about women as imperfect, because reproductive function in women differs from that in men. Implicit in Lander's argument, then, is the idea that menstruation is abnormal. The message here is that even feminists can fall prey to westernized societies' view of menstruation as abnormal, and needing to be fixed.

Small wonder, then, that Root (1992), in her study of menstruation, found that on average, women reported nothing positive about menstruation. A perception of the 'natural' defectiveness of menstruating women and the justification for that perception is now institutionalized in western societies. Implicit in the institutional view of menstruation is the assumption that women are responsible for maintaining the public code of conduct around menstruation, so as to keep it extremely private. Women are expected to control the presence of menstrual blood and keep it strictly confined to the private sphere. The assumed regularity/predictability of menstruation, both when it occurs and what it will be like, and the social construction of menstruation as a shameful, secretive event, are foundational for justifying the expectation that a woman's menstrual condition never inadvertently be made public (Root 1992).

Menstruation as a periodic and bloody event

Much of the past menstrual cycle research has been predicated upon an unsubstantiated belief that the menstrual cycle is highly regular, and thus, predictable. In reality, the menstrual cycle is more accurately characterized by irregularity (Treloar *et al.* 1967; Vollman 1977).

Once menarche has occurred, as previously mentioned, an almost universal assumption is that menstrual bleeds will issue forth in a regular manner, that is, about every 28 days, and that a girl, now turned woman, is fertile once maturation commences. This assumption is based upon the belief that at menarche, the female reproductive system is mature, when in fact it is not. The normal postmenarcheal menstrual cycle pattern, as reported by Treloar *et al.* (1967), is characterized first by irregularities in onset of bleeds. Vollman (1977) documented that a high percentage of these menstruations were anovulatory. According to Treloar *et al.*, a woman does not reach reproductive system maturity until her 20s, when, during the interval between ages 20 and 39, the menstrual cycle pattern repeats itself with some regularity. This statement, however, is not meant to imply that the menstrual cycle repeats itself in a regular manner. On the contrary, according to Treloar (1935; Treloar *et al.* 1967), the term 'regularity,' as applied to the menstrual cycle, is totally in appropriate. It is a vague term and should not be taken to mean 'without variation.'

In 1967, the 'classic' menstrual cycle paper by Treloar *et al.* was published, in which analyses of menstrual intervals over a 30 year period were reported. The subjects were women who had enrolled in the 'menstruation reproductive history (MRH) program' in the 1930s. A detailed description of the program is found elsewhere (Voda *et al.* 1991). Unfortunately, the data reported in the 1967 article have been overlooked or disregarded by many authors of medical, nursing, and other related texts, since the misconception that the menstrual cycle is a regular, temporal event, that is, one that occurs every 28 days, persists. That this belief has been institutionalized is demonstrated by the regimen established for reproductive-age women who take oral contraceptives. Women take a birth control pill each day for 21 days, then stop for 7 days in order to induce a menstrual bleed (Parke-Davis 1995). This kind of regimen reinforces the idea that the menstrual cycle interval is regular and 28 days in duration.

Treloar and colleagues (1967) found anything *but* regularity in the menstrual cycle! As the following summary indicates, variation, rather than regularity, characterized every menstrual history examined.

Menstrual periodicity

From the mid-1930s to 1961, 2702 participants in the MRH program had recorded 25 825 person-years of menstrual histories. Analyses of these data generated the following findings.

1. For approximately seven years post-menarche, variability in the menstrual interval was the norm, decreasing gradually, until about age 20, at which time a period of relative stability prevailed.
2. From ages 21 to 39, inclusive, menstrual intervals were observed to be the most stable, but were still characterized by variability more than regularity.
3. From age 41 onward, which marks the transition to menopause, wide variability in menstrual cycle intervals is the norm rather than the exception.

The variability in menstrual interval duration as reported by Treloar *et al.* (1967) is shown in Fig. 5.1, which is a graph of data from the original article, based upon the analyses of 25 825 person-years of data.

The data in the graph are categorized in three zones: 'menstrual year', 'chronological age', and 'premenopausal year'. At menarche, shown on the graph as the beginning of menstrual year zero, on average, 5 per cent of the menstrual intervals were observed to be 18.3 days or less, 25 per cent were 24.6 days, 50 per cent were 29.1 days, and proceeding up to the 95th per cent frequency distribution, one finds that 5 per cent of menstrual intervals were estimated at 83.1 days or longer. The range in duration between menstrual bleeds at menarche, time zero, then, is substantial – from 18.3 days at the lower end to 83.1 days at the upper end.

The data in the graph also document the wide range of variability in menstrual onsets throughout menstrual life. If one follows the horizontal line of the graph from menstrual year zero and menarche, to menstrual year 2, and moves upward along this line, all values for menstrual interval duration decreased substantially from year zero, albeit still exhibiting variability. As one moves to the right on the graph, duration of menstrual interval decreases until about menstrual year 7, when, generally speaking, the menstrual interval durations approximate the recorded patterns for women at chronological age 20. An examination of the chronological age zone indicates that women can expect to experience about 20 years of relative regularity of menstruation onset and duration between menstrual intervals. Moving along the graph to the right to zone 3, premenopausal year, the data suggest that the transition to menopause occurs more slowly in terms of time to reach the end point, and durations between bleeds reach more extremes than those in the post-menarchal years. What is gleaned from the data in this zone is that as women make the transition from zone 2 to zone 3, they enter a period in which the duration between menstrual

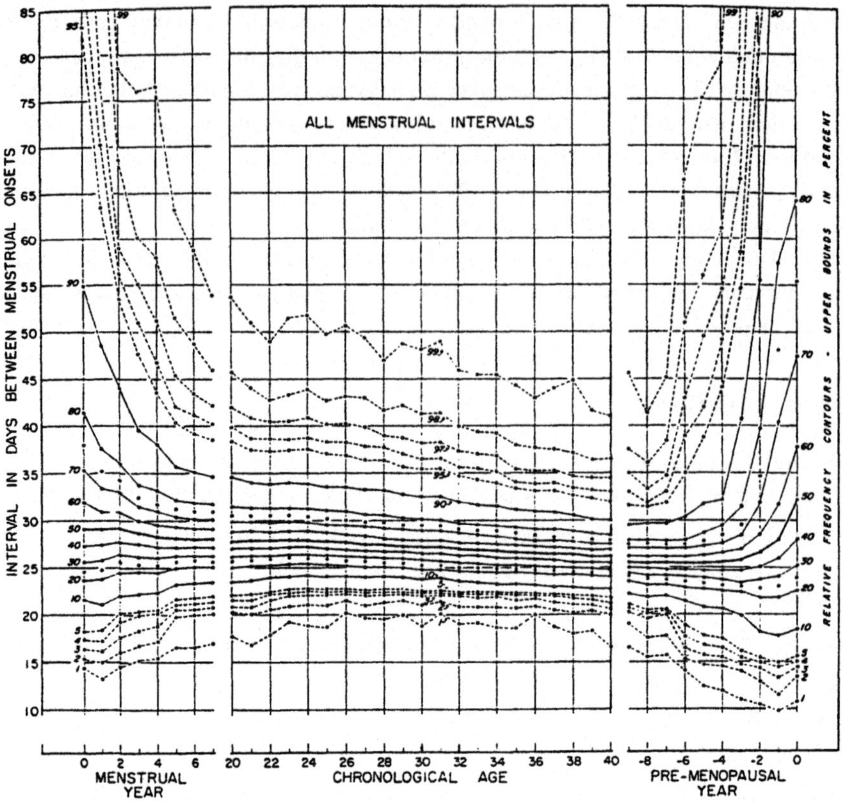

Fig. 5.1 The variability in menstrual interval (from Treloar *et al.* 1967, with permission).

bleeds is characterized by much more variability than that found in either zone 1 or zone 2. Treloar and colleagues concluded from this observation that increasing variability in menstrual interval, with long durations between bleeds, pre-menopausally, could be considered normal.

Factors that contribute to the variability in menstrual interval among women and within individual women are not known with any certainty. Clearly, one's genotype, health status, as well as stress level, have the potential to affect menstruation onset. One stressor well known to health care workers is the trauma associated with surgery. It is not unusual for postoperative women patients to state that they have just had their period start, even though it was not due for another week. Root (1992) performed an extensive review of the menstrual cycle literature to identify whether life events as stressors could alter the menstrual cycle pattern. What she found was that most menstrual studies relied upon alterations in menstrual cycle duration to support that stress affects a woman's cycle. Only two studies demonstrated a clear association between hormonal and/or anatomical effects and stress. In one instance, a physician in London during the Second World War examined the endometrial tissue of amenorrhoeic women who had been close to bomb explosions. The pathology report on these women was that endometrial development had been arrested (Loeser 1941). In the other situation, frequent blood hormone assays were done on two women admitted to hospital to evaluate the effect of hospitalization on the menstrual cycle. In both women, hormone levels indicated that ovulation was delayed until the women were released from hospital (Peyser *et al.* 1973). Root concluded that the linear causality model, upon which most of the life-event studies were based, was probably an inappropriate assumption.

Menstrual bleeding

As reported by Treloar *et al.* (1967), between ages 20 and 40, the duration between menstrual cycle intervals shows a characteristic length and variability that remains stable until the transition to menopause. Prior to menopause (see zone 3 in Fig. 5.1), changes in duration of menstrual interval begin (Treloar *et al.* 1967), as well as changes in bleeding (Voda and Mansfield 1994). The mean blood loss in menstrual discharge at this time may exceed 80 ml per menstruation, which is the clinical definition of menorrhagia (Hallberg *et al.* 1966; Powell 1991).

Approximately 80 per cent of women may expect to experience irregular bleeding as they go through the menopause (Seltzer *et al.* 1990). The high frequency of this change in bleeding pattern has important consequences for perimenopausal women. In the absence of normative guidelines to assess bleeding, menopausal women, particularly, are at risk for both physical and emotional disruption as the pattern of bleeding changes. Women view the bleeding change as loss of control of an important bodily function (Patterson and Hale 1985); this loss of control becomes a source of anxiety in that the change in pattern is perceived as a sign of 'illness', that 'something is wrong', and as such, becomes a vitally important emotional health issue for women (Berken 1986; Root 1992; Mansfield and Jorgensen 1992).

A change in bleeding pattern is also a concern to physicians, because of its potential to be a precursor of a more serious condition. Gambrell (1992) suggests that the most frequent problem encountered by physicians who treat primarily women is related to vaginal bleeding, with the complaints being highest in perimenopausal women. In the absence of normative guidelines to evaluate whether such bleeding is normal or abnormal, Gambrell and others (Jutras and Cowan 1990) recommend that each peri- and post-menopausal woman who complains of heavy bleeding undergo a thorough evaluation. By thorough is meant a pap smear, biopsy of cervical lesions, bimanual examination to detect whether there is uterine enlargement or masses, and cervical and uterine curettage.

Assessment of the volume of menstrual blood loss is considered to be the most important single parameter of the menstrual history (Rankin *et al.* 1962; Shaw 1973; Greenberg 1981; Fraser *et al.* 1984). Yet, only a handful of studies have been conducted which document how menstruation changes as women make the transition to menopause. Even the Treloar MRH study (Voda *et al.* 1991) did not collect menstrual blood volume data. Data from several cross-sectional studies suggest that the volume of menstrual discharge changes from light to moderate, to very heavy with clotting, as the journey to menopause progresses (Neugarten *et al.* 1963; Root 1992; Mansfield and Boyer 1990; Voda and Mansfield 1994).

Studies of menstrual blood loss on women of various ages suggest that older women lose more menstrual blood than younger women (Hallberg *et al.*1966; Rybo *et al.* 1985; Sporrong *et al.* 1992). Menorrhagia, generally, is viewed as a sign of an underlying gynaecological problem, or at least, as a sign that pathology needs to be ruled out. However, actual cases of menorrhagia are difficult to identify or objectively diagnose without the collection of used vaginal tampons or napkins. The Fraser *et al.* (1981) study of drug treatments for menorrhagia included only participants with a convincing history of menorrhagia. Study participants reported passing clots, and having to use multiple menstrual products simultaneously, which were inadequate to control menstrual flow. When blood loss was measured, only 30 of 69 women actually had a measured blood loss of 80 ml or more, and 20 per cent had a measured blood loss of 35 ml or less. Based on these findings, the authors raised serious concerns about the diagnosis of menorrhagia as it is made in routine clinical practice, and on which decisions are made to employ a variety of diagnostic methods and treatments, including hysterectomy.

According to Fraser *et al.* (1985), most clinicians are unaware of the extent of errors in a woman's perception of volume of menstrual discharge when they present with a complaint of heavy bleeding. A study done in the United Kingdom found that 53 per cent of the women of various ages who complained of heavy menstrual bleeding did indeed have a loss that repeatedly measured more than 80 ml. The remainder, 47 per cent, had variable amounts of blood loss, from mild to moderate, which suggests that women take into account other factors when estimating losses (Haynes *et al.* 1977). More recently, work done using objective methods to measure the volume of blood lost and then correlating the measured loss with a subjective scale, also documents that wide variability in bleeding exists among women (Fraser *et al.* 1981, 1984, 1985; Voda and Mansfield 1994).

Seltzer and colleagues (1990) reviewed the medical records of 500 perimenopausal women, categorizing bleeding patterns as follows: abrupt onset of amenorrhoea was found in 12 per cent of the women; 37 per cent reported oligomenorrhoea and/or hypomenorrhoea; and 18 per cent (91 of 500) were heavy bleeders. The latter group was comprised of women with menorrhagia (defined as bleeding for an excessive length of time), hypermenorrhoea (defined as excessive amounts of bleeding), and metrorrhagia, or irregular bleeding between cycles. When the researchers combined the 91 heavy bleeders into one group, they discovered that one-third of these women did indeed have gynaecological problems. However, only the women who also bled between cycles (metrorrhagia) were diagnosed with malignancies. Even so, the researchers concluded that any woman with a complaint of heavy bleeding should seek immediate medical attention.

In the absence of a reliable and valid rating scale to assess the quality of menstrual bleeding in pre-, peri-, and postmenopausal women, clinicians, by and large, formulate diagnoses and treat women based upon a woman's self-report that the pattern of bleeding and/or menstrual cycle onset has changed. As the number of women in the perimenopause increases – for example, in 1990 approximately one-third of all women in the USA were age 50 or older, and by the year 2000, estimates indicate that more than 719 million women over age 45 will inhabit the planet – gynaecologists and primary care physicians will encounter more and more mid-life women with the chief complaint of a change in the menstrual bleeding pattern. In the US, it is estimated that almost two-thirds of women consult a gynaecologist for primary care (Hegerfeld 1994). As such, the ability to assess accurately the volume of blood loss is a critical aspect of the menstrual history. Gambrell (1992) recommends that clinicians carefully concentrate on the characteristics of the bleeding, the duration and frequency of flow, as well as any previous episodes of abnormal bleeding.

Until recently, no valid way to estimate the volume of blood loss has been available to clinicians. As indicated above, a heavy menstrual bleed is defined clinically as more than 80 ml of blood loss per menstruation. This is a fine definition of heavy bleeding if one is a researcher, but useless to a clinician with a busy practice. To measure the blood loss accurately, menstrual products would need to be collected, blood extracted from the products, and then measurement of the haemoglobin concentration of the blood portion of the menstrual discharge would have to be made (Fraser 1992). The process is very time consuming and appropriately belongs in a research laboratory.

Mansfield created a six-point bleeding scale, which subsequently was modified as the Mansfield, Voda, Jorgensen bleeding scale (MVJBS), for use by women to rate the volume of menstrual discharge. The tool has been used in two studies; it has demonstrated face and content validity, and recently established criterion validity (Voda and Mansfield 1994; Barre *et al.* 1995).

In the first study (Voda and Mansfield 1994), the researchers studied a non-clinical sample of 505 premenopausal women – participants of the Treloar MRH program – ages 35 to 55, who used the MVJBS to prospectively rate the volume of menstrual discharge and clotting, using a three-point scale. They found that the quality of bleeding changed as women aged; 69.5 per cent of the sample documented a change in the menstrual bleeding pattern over a period of one year. The heaviest ratings of blood flow and passing of clots were found on day two of the bleeding interval. By day six, bleeding and clotting had stopped for most women. The highest mean ratings for bleeding and clotting respectively on day two were 3.8 (using the six-point scale) and 1.6 (using the three-point scale). Women 45 and older reported more change in menstrual interval and heavier bleeding than younger participants.

The second study two was carried out to establish MVJBS validity. A subset of 40 participants in study number one were invited simultaneously to collect all menstrual products over three menstrual cycles and to rate the quality of the bleeding using the MVJBS. The actual weights of menstrual discharge captured on menstrual products were compared with the ratings of menstrual discharge made by participants using the six-point MVJBS. The procedure used to collect menstrual products is described elsewhere (Barre *et al.* 1995). The prospective data collection technique is a particular strength of the MVJBS, as it involves immediate, rather than retrospective, rating of menstrual discharge, and it is naturalistic, that is, it does not require women to change or modify the timing of when menstrual products are changed (Barre *et al.* 1995). Thirty-two women completed the study. Results indicate that women are better able to discriminate menstrual discharge loss in the upper ranges of the scale (moderate, heavy, very heavy bleeding with gushing) than in the lower range. What this means is that the women in this study were very accurate when rating menstrual discharge at the high end of the scale. When the discharge was low or small, women were less accurate. Since the most serious gynaecological problems found by Seltzer *et al.* (1990) were in those women who were heavy bleeders with metrorrhagia, the researchers believe that the MVJBS can be used in research and clinical settings accurately to identify a heavy bleeder who is at risk for pathology. Further work needs to be done to establish whether the scale is valid for women throughout menstrual life.

There is some urgency connected to this task, as misconceptions about the menstrual cycle continue to be the norm rather than the exception. Recently, even a women's health newsletter reported: 'Studies demonstrate that women generally have four or five years of "abnormal" bleeding prior to the onset of menopause' (Reynolds 1995). Rather than characterizing the bleeding as different from that of pre-menopausal, reproductive years, this woman-oriented publication described bleeding changes as abnormal. From a clinical diagnostic perspective, Hawkins *et al.* (1995) define abnormal vaginal bleeding as 'any variation from a woman's usual menstrual pattern'.

Gynaecological surgery and women

In the 1960s, self-report of excessive menstrual blood loss by women was the symptom that was most commonly treated by hysterectomy (Rankin *et al.* 1962). In the 1980s, Fraser observed that large numbers of hysterectomies were being performed on Australian women who reported having heavy bleeding, even though the complaint could not be confirmed subjectively or objectively.

Gynaecology, as a specialty, has been criticized for years for the high rates of hysterectomy, primarily when no abnormality is detected by pathologic study. Jutras and Cowan (1990) believe that most hysterectomies are performed for clear-cut indications, to include the public's fear that unusual or irregular vaginal bleeding represents a potential serious medical problem. Cancer phobia by the public, they argue, is problematic, and physicians who provide health care for women will at some time encounter a patient seeking a surgeon who will take out her uterus.

Hysterectomy is one of the most common surgeries performed on US women. In 1980, 649 000 US women had hysterectomies. The rate increased in 1985 to 670 000, and then decreased to 528 000 in 1988 and 541 000 in 1989 (Chapin and Pereles 1992). It is an invasive procedure with a high risk of complications. The hospital stay time for the procedure can range from two to four days. Recovery from the procedure can take from four to six weeks. Coffey, President of the US Hysterectomy Educational Resources Foundation (HERS), claims that the impact that hysterectomy has on a woman's life, or the effect that it has on family and friends, is neither indicated in the medical literature, nor are physicians aware of it (Coffey 1993).

Some hysterectomies are performed to correct dysfunctional uterine bleeding, uterine fibroids, or endometriosis (Garcia and Cutler 1983; Cutler 1988; Coffey 1993). Five per cent of reported hysterectomies are done to treat cancer of the uterus (Boring *et al.* 1991). Still other hysterectomies are prescribed medically for no other reason than a woman's reproductive life being over and the uterus having no value (Cutler 1988). The median age of a woman undergoing hysterectomy in the US is 40.9 years, with the greatest number of procedures being performed on women between the ages of 30 and 49 (National Center for Health Statistics 1987). In 1984, between 20 and 30 per cent of all hysterectomies performed in the US were combined with oophorectomy (Elixhauser *et al.* 1993). Until the recent US NIH Consensus Statement (National Institutes of Health 1994) on ovarian cancer, screening, treatment, and follow-up, a standard of practice recommended by US gynaecological surgeons was to perform prophylactic oophorectomy in women undergoing hysterectomy for benign disease in order to protect against ovarian cancer. Prophylactic oophorectomy does indeed lower the risk of ovarian cancer in both pre- and postmenopausal women. It is now believed, however, that a greater risk to those oophorectomized women may result, that is, a significant reduction in life expectancy due to heart disease and osteoporosis, if women are non-compliant regarding oestrogen replacement (Averette and Nguyen 1994).

No research-based data are available to verify that the rate of ovarian cancer in women increases if ovaries are retained when hysterectomy is performed. Data available are appallingly unreliable. According to Utian (1990), occurrence rates of ovarian cancer in women who have ovaries retained are estimated to range from 1 in 500 to 1 in 5000. These data are inadequate to support the need to perform prophylactic oophorectomy unless certain risk factors are present. For example, a woman with one first-degree relative with ovarian cancer has a 5 per cent lifetime risk of ovarian cancer developing, and is not considered at high enough risk for prophylactic oophorectomy, whereas the risk of ovarian cancer developing in women from families with hereditary ovarian cancer syndromes is considered to be sufficiently high to warrant surgery (Averette and Nguyen 1994). The American Cancer Society estimates that 26 700 new cases of ovarian cancer will occur in the US in 1996, and more than 55 per cent will die of the disease (Parker *et al.* 1996).

Removal of a woman's ovaries, by definition, is castration. The term castration implies an inability to produce hormones from human gonads due to surgery or other treatments, such as radiation or chemotherapy. No matter how castration is accomplished, it poses serious metabolic consequences for women and men. Young, premenopausal women have little choice for a healthy quality of life unless they replace the estrogen that has been prematurely eliminated from the body. These women cannot synthesize estradiol, and have a diminished capacity to synthesize androgens and weaker estrogens. Castrated women are truly 'oestrogen deficient;' they absolutely require hormone replacement. Several feminist colleagues object to the use of the word castration when referring to women, suggesting that it is a term for the surgical removal of a male's testicles (Voda 1997). Surgical removal of the ovaries, is, by definition, oophorectomy; surgical removal of the testicles is orchidectomy. Removal of the gonads in either sex is, by definition, castration.

Far too many US women in the past were made oestrogen-deficient through hysterectomy with oophorectomy, and experienced both oestrogen- and non-oestrogen-related symptoms. Hysterectomy eliminates the source of any bleeding problem; it also increases the risk of developing chronic conditions, and may significantly alter sexual arousal and responsiveness (Cutler 1988). A recent article in the *New England Journal of Medicine* suggested that a good many US physicians are not sure about what is an appropriate indicator to perform hysterectomy. The authors of the article concluded that there is insufficient information on conditions that lead to hysterectomy, as well as outcomes of the procedure; that alternatives to hysterectomy are not always considered; and that the kind of treatment a woman wants is not necessarily taken into consideration (Carlson *et al.* 1993).

Physicians have long assumed that hysterectomy with ovarian conservation would not affect the menopausal transition, and it should not initiate the common menopausal complaints, such as hot flushes, night sweats, and vaginal dryness, as does hysterectomy with bilateral oophorectomy. The research of Oldenhave and colleagues (1993) suggests that this assumption is not correct. When the researchers compared women who had undergone hysterectomy with ovarian conservation (one or both ovaries), with a sample of women who did not have surgery, the women with ovarian conservation reported moderate to severe vasomotor complaints more often than non-hysterectomized women. A similar finding was reported with the symptom of vaginal dryness. The findings of Oldenhave and co-workers are not isolated results. A review of the literature reported by the International Health Foundation (1993) found that an increased incidence of the typical signs of ovarian failure occurred in a substantial number of premenopausal, hysterectomized women, which resulted in an early age onset of menopause.

One explanation for why hysterectomized women experience symptoms may be interference with ovarian blood supply. Normally, blood is carried to the ovaries by the ovarian artery and the ovarian branches of the uterine artery. During hysterectomy there is a possibility that the uterine artery branches may be ligated and removed with the uterus. Evidence that this is so is provided from studies on hysterectomized women with ovarian conservation who had lower plasma levels of estrogen and progesterone, and higher gonadotrophin levels than age-matched controls (International Health Foundation 1993).

Other explanations for symptoms suggest interference with uterine blood supply and nerves. According to Coffey (1993), a US women's health activist, if blood vessels and/or nerves to the uterus happen to be cut during surgery, sensation to the vagina, clitoris, and nipples may be lost. If ligaments happen to be cut, the pelvis may broaden and widen. Inability to engage in sexual intercourse for some women following hysterectomy may be due to the formation of scar tissue. If adequate pelvic support has not been maintained, abdominal organs can drift down into the area previously occupied by the uterus, displacing other organs. Women who report having problems post-hysterectomy, or no longer having sexual feelings, have in the past been told that these problems are in their heads, when in fact, excision of ligaments, lymph nodes, and other structures, can destroy blood vessels that contribute to engorgement during sexual arousal (Williamson 1992). This is not to say that all women who have hysterectomy suffer or are not satisfied with the outcome. Indeed, with new surgical techniques, pre-and post-hysterectomy support groups, and hormonal interventions when necessary, many women are satisfied. The problem that remains, according to West and Dranov (1994), is the inability to predict which women will be unequivocally helped, and which will experience disabling side-effects. Many hysterectomized women in the Tremin Trust program (the 1930s and 1960s cohorts) report satisfaction post-hysterectomy (Voda 1997). Of course, the 1930 cohort of women are now in their 70s, and positive responses may be due to poor recall. However, the women in their 40s and early 50s appear to resonate a similar level of satisfaction.

Cohen and colleagues (1994) recently examined the concerns expressed by 55 US women during convalescence after hysterectomy. The data were gathered as part of a study of early hospital discharge and home follow-up after hysterectomy for an eight-week period. A review of the diaries of these women generated 727 comments/concerns related to the surgery. These were subsequently characterized as three themes: concerns about physical convalescence (ranging from pain, activities of daily living, incision, urinary problems, etc.); concerns related to social interaction (ranging from emotional aspects, family concerns, professional support, finances, etc.); and concerns about the changes that were expected after hysterectomy, such as body image, hot flushes, sexuality, partner attitude, ageing, etc.

The uterus, for some women, is proof that they are female. If a woman's gender identity is based on her uterus, then a woman will have problems post-hysterectomy and her femininity must be redefined in new terms. According to Williamson (1992), some women, following hysterectomy, may not understand that they will no longer menstruate; others believe that they will no longer be able to reach orgasm; still others believe that the uterus is the primary organ of excretion to rid the body of impurities. Women are known to grieve over the loss of menstrual rhythmicity (Williamson 1992). The monthly onset of menstrual cycle bleeds, the rhythmic changes, are viewed as a friend, a long-time companion, a rhythm of life and predictability, and a symbol of unity with other women. For these women, the menstrual cycle represents life itself, humanity's link with generations past, present, and future (Voda 1997). From this perspective, there are a good many women who do not view the uterus as a disposable organ. This woman-centered view of menstruation is diametrically opposed to that of some clinicians, who, according to feminists, view the uterus as a useless, bleeding, cancer-prone, disposable organ (Laurence and Weinhouse 1994). Stanley West, a US gynaecologist, criticizes the American way of hysterectomy and what it does to women, suggesting that it says more about physicians than it does about disease. According to West, it is the outdated attitude physicians harbour about women patients that has created the problem (West and Dranov 1994). The bad news is that these attitudes have their roots deeply embedded in biased and/or myth-laden assumptions about women. The good news is that most of these are fixable.

For a start, Martin (1991) recommends removing the metaphorical lens through which medicine views women–menstruation as failed production, and menopause as loss of central (hormonal) organization and control. According to Martin, the onset of menstrual flow, when viewed as failure to produce (a baby), is like an idle factory, unused inventory. Words used in medical descriptions of menstruation (and which I have cited in this chapter as well) tend to emphasize waste and debris, and illustrations in texts describing the menstrual phases characterize menstruation as a bomb which has exploded – a graphic picture of destruction and disorganization.

There are, of course, differing non-medical views of menstruation that are just as problematic. As discussed previously, Lander (1988) implicitly advanced an hypothesis of menstruation in women as abnormal. Men don't menstruate, so why should women? Lander believes that women are still in the process of evolving, developing. At some time in the future, there will be no need for menstruation, as women will have evolved to a higher level of development. In contrast, Profet (1993) views menstruation as a very important mechanism to protect against pathogen-initiated infections. Profet believes that all female animals menstruate – that ridding pathogens through the process was adaptive for survival.

Whether or not human females and males have evolved to the highest degree of biological efficiency, and whether menstruation cleanses the body of pathogens is academic. For now, males and females are genetically programmed to play different biological roles with respect to reproduction. In this respect, biology is destiny for both men and women. This statement is not to be construed to mean that the authors are biological reductionists. It is a fact that women ovulate, gestate, and menstruate, and males impregnate – normal biological functions which will not be replaced in the near, or even distant, future. Concealment of ovulation and intrauterine gestation are biological processes that were selected to ensure survival of the human species. As such, unless a hormonal method of birth control is being used, a woman's body during reproductive years periodically prepares at the organ and system level for the possibility of conception and the implantation of a fertilized ovum. That is a biological fact! If a woman chooses not to conceive, menstruation ensues, and as menstruation commences, the follicular phase of the menstrual cycle has begun anew. For some women, the cyclic phenomenon continues over a period of thirty plus years until the genetically preprogrammed time arrives – menstruation ceases, and menopause occurs.

Perhaps an appropriate closure for this chapter is to offer suggestions as to how readers might begin to reconceptualize reproductive/biological events in a woman's life, all of which have their beginning and their end in the menstrual cycle.

Suggestions

First, as suggested by Martin (1991), reread the gynaecological texts in current use, asking the following questions.

- Are there hidden meanings in the biological discourse presented as it relates to the role of women in reproduction, the function of vaginal bleeding, and woman's status and health needs at menopause?
- Is a change in menstruation viewed as a normal or abnormal process?
- Is the menstrual cycle perceived as a source of pain, suffering, and disease, or a mechanism for the production of a new human?
- Is the menstruation onset described as a regular, clock-like event, as predictable as the lunar cycle? Or is it understood to be a complex function that is expressed in a variety of temporal patterns, whether within or among women?

- There is no biological counterpart to a woman's uterus in men. How do texts describe the function of a woman's uterus at menopause? A useless, bleeding organ, a potential source of disease, or a valuable organ that contributes to the quality of post-menopausal life?
- Are ovaries described as hidden sources of disease at menopause, needing to be surgically removed when a hysterectomy is done? There are biological counterparts to a woman's gonads in men, the testicles. Do texts in which male reproductive diseases are discussed suggest widespread castration of mid-life men to prevent certain disease(s)?

Then, examine current texts or articles that outline treatment protocols and/or standards of practice as the basis for surgical intervention or hormonal or drug treatment of menstruating women. Seek to identify whether these publications are based upon the outcomes of 'good' science, or a science where methods of procedure of 'doing' science become the means to an end, that is, a source of data to justify intervention.

Conclusion

Almost all women will experience changes in the perceived regularity of menstrual cycle onset, and/or in the quality of bleeding pattern. These changes are sometimes viewed as abnormal or dysfunctional, leading to clinical intervention. Menstruation is expected to be regular; it is not. Women are expected to coexist with men in a physiologically steady state; they do not, nor do men! As such, women live precariously, along a line of fault. On one side of the fault is the institutionalized view of menstruation, the socially constructed view women have accepted as truth, a view, in large part, that supports dysfunction, disease, and intervention. On the other side of the line is woman's perception of actual every-day menstrual experience, a view of menstruation as normal, yet not always considered in the methods of traditional biomedical science. Fortunately, the line of fault has begun to heave, quake, and shake: interventions and manipulations of the menstrual cycle have decreased, and women's voices are defining women's experiences.

References

Averette, H.E. and Nguyen, H.N. (1994). The role of prophylactic oophorectomy in cancer prevention. *Gynecologic Oncology*, **55**, S38–41.

Barre, D., Voda, A.M., and Mansfield, P.K. (1995). Validating a paper and pencil measure of menstrual blood loss. Society for Menstrual Cycle Research Conference, Montreal, Canada, June 2–4, 1995.

Belsey, E.M. and Farley, T.M.M. (1988). The analysis of menstrual bleeding patterns: a review. *Contraception*, **38**, 129–55.

Berken, C. (1986). In behalf of women over 40: understanding the importance of the menopause. *Social Work*, Sept/Oct, 378–84.

Beyene, Y. (1989). *From menarche to menopause*. Suny, New York.

Boring, C.C., Squires, T.S., and Tong, T. (1991). Cancer statistics 1991. *CA – A Cancer Journal for Clinicians*, **41**, 19–36.

Buckler, H.M. and Anderson, D.C. (1994). The perimenopausal state and incipient ovarian failure. In *Treatment of the postmenopausal woman: basic and clinical aspects*, (ed. R. Lobo), pp. 11–24. Roman Press, New York.

Carlson, K.J., Nichols, D.H., and Schiff, I. (1993). Indications for hysterectomy. *New England Journal of Medicine*, **328**, 856–60.

Chapin, J.L. and Pereles, S.A. (1992). Women's access to the health care system. In *The women's health data book, a profile of women's health in the United States* (ed. J.A. Horton). The Jacobs Institute of Women's Health, Washington, DC.

Coffey, N.W. (1993). An introduction to hysterectomy, the operation and its lifelong consequences. *HERS Newsletter*, **V**, 2–4.

Cohen, S.M., Hollingsworth, A., Rubin, M., Graff, B., Thomas, J., Morgan, M., *et al.* (1994). Issues of convalescence after hysterectomy. In *Proceedings, Society for Menstrual Cycle Research: Mind Body Rhythmicity: A Menstrual Cycle Perspective*, pp. 213–15. Hamilton & Cross, Seattle, WA,

Cornacchia, C. (1995). Across the divide. *The Gazette*, June 12.

Cutler, W.B. (1988). *Hysterectomy before and after*. Harper and Row, New York.

Delaney, J., Lupton, M.J., and Toth, E. (1988). *The curse: a cultural history of menstruation.* University of Illinois Press, Urbana, IL.

duToit, B.M. (1990). *Aging and menopause among South African women.* Suny, New York.

Elixhauser, A., Andrews, R.M., and Fox, S. (1993). *Clinical classifications for health policy research: discharge statistics by principal diagnosis and procedure.* Providers studies research note 17, August 1993. United States Department of Health and Human Services, PHS, AHCPR, Publication #93–0043.

Fraser, I.S. (1992). Personal communication.

Fraser, I.S., Pearse, C., Sherman, R.P., Elliott, P.M., McIlveen, J., and Markham, R. (1981). Efficacy of mefenamic acid in patients with complaint of menorrhagia. *Obstetrics and Gynecology*, **58**, 543–51.

Fraser, I.S., McCarron, G., and Markham, R. (1984). A preliminary study of factors influencing perception of menstrual blood volume. *American Journal of Obstetrics and Gynecology*, **149**, 788–93.

Fraser, I.S., McCarron, G., Markham, R., and Resta, T. (1985). Blood and total fluid content of menstrual discharge. *Obstetrics and Gynecology*, **65**, 194–8.

Gambrell, R.D. (1992). Abnormal vaginal bleeding: routes of investigation. *Menopause Management*, 28–31.

Garcia, R. and Cutler, V. (1983). *Menopause: a guide for women and the men who love them.* Norton, New York.

Grahn, J. (1993). *Blood, bread and roses: how menstruation created the world.* Beacon Press, Boston, MA.

Hafez, E.S.E. (1980). *Human reproduction: conception and contraception* (2nd edn). Harper and Row, Hagerstown, MD.

Hallberg, L., Hogdahl, A.M., Nilsson, L., and Rybo, G. (1966). Menstrual blood loss–a population study. *Acta Obstetrica Gynecologica Scandinavica*, **45**, 320–351.

Hawkins, J.W., Roberto-Nichols, D.M., and Havey, J.L.S. (1995). *Protocols for nurse practitioners in gynecologic settings.* Tiresias Press, New York.

Haynes, P.T., Hodgson, H., Anderson, A.B.M., and Turnbull, A.C. (1977). Measurements of menstrual blood loss in patients complaining of menorrhagia. *British Journal of Obstetrics and Gynaecology*, **84**, 763–8.

Hedricks, C. (1992). Menopause has no part in the year of the woman. *The Society for Menstrual Cycle Research Newsletter*, **9**, 3.

Hegerfeld, C.K. (1994). Publisher's notes. *Women's Health Connections*, II:3, Aug/Sept.

Oddens, B.J. (1993). Hysterectomy with ovarian conservation suspected to lead to an earlier climacteric. *International Health Foundation Newsletter*, 1993–1. Brussels.

Jutras, M.L. and Cowan, B.D. (1990). Abnormal bleeding in the climacteric. *Obstetrics and Gynecology Clinics of North America*, **17**, 409–25.

Keye, W.R. (1988). *The premenstrual syndrome*. W.B. Saunders, Philadelphia.

Lander, L. (1988). *Images of bleeding: menstruation as ideology*. Orlando Press, New York.

Lange, L. (1983). Woman is not a rational animal: on Aristotle's biology of reproduction. In *Discovering reality* (ed. S. Harding and M.B. Hintikka), pp. 1–15 D. Reidel Dordrecht, The Netherlands.

Laurence, L. and Weinhouse, B. (1994). *Outrageous practices*. Ballantine Books, New York.

Lever, J. and Brush, M.G. (1981). *Premenstrual tension*. McGraw Hill, New York.

Loeser, A.A. (1941). Effect of emotional shock on hormone release and endometrial development. *Lancet*, **i**, 518–19.

Longcope, C. (1994). The endocrinology of menopause. In *Treatment of the postmenopausal woman* (ed. R. Lobo), pp. 47–56. Roman Press, New York.

Machin, D., D'Arcangues, C., Busca, B., Farley, T.M.M., and Pinol, A. (1987). Vaginal bleeding patterns – the problem and an example data set. *Applied Stochastic Models and Data Analysis*, **3**, 27–35.

Mansfield, P.K. and Boyer, B. (1990). The experience, concerns, and health care needs of women in menopausal transition. *Annals of the New York Academy of Sciences*, **592**, 448–9.

Mansfield, P.K. and Jorgensen, C.M. (1992). Menstrual pattern changes in middle-aged women. In *Menstrual health research* (ed. A. Dan and L. Lewis). University of Illinois Press.

Martin, E. (1988). Medical metaphors of women's bodies: menstruation and menopause. *International Journal of Health Services*, **18**, 237–54.

Martin, E. (1991). Metaphors of bleeding in women. *NAACOG's Clinical Issues in Perinatal and Womens Health Nursing: Bleeding in Women* (ed. D.W. Perlis), pp. 83–8. J.B. Lippincott, Philadelphia.

Martin 1991 and Powell 1991 are from the some volume namely: *NAACOG's Clinical Issues in Perinatal and Woman's Health Nursing: Bleeding in women* (ed. D.W. Perlis), pp. x–xx. J.B. Lippincott, Philadelphia.

Moos, R.H. (1968). The development of a menstrual distress questionnaire. *Psychosomatic Medicine*, **30**, 853–67.

National Center for Health Statistics (1987). *Hysterectomies in the United States 1965–84*. Vital Health Statistics, PHS, Centers for Disease Control DHSS Publication #PHS88–1753, Washington, D.C.

National Institutes of Health (1994). NIH Consensus statement. *Ovarian cancer: screening, treatment, and follow up*. Vol. 12 (April), pp. 5–7. NIH,

Neugarten, B.L., Wood, V., Kraines, R.J., and Loomis, B. (1963). Women's attitudes towards the menopause. *Vita Humana*, **6**, 140–51.

Oldenhave, A., Jaszmann, L.J.B., Everaerd, W., and Haspels, A.A. (1993). *American Journal of Obstetrics and Gynecology*, **168**, 765–71.

Parke-Davis (1995). Loestrin product description. *Menopause mangement*.

Parker, S., Tong, L.T., Bolden, S., and Wingo, P.A. (1996). Cancer Statistics, 1996. *CA – A Journal for Clinicions*, **46**, 5–27.

Patterson, E.T. and Hale, E.S. (1985). Making sure: integrating menstrual care practices into activities of daily living. *Advances in Nursing Science*, **4**, 18–31.

Peyser, M.R., Ayalon, D., Harrell, A., Toaff, R., and Cordova, T. (1973). Stress induced delay of ovulation. *Obstetrics and Gynecology*, **42**, 667–71.

Powell, L.L. (1991). Evaluation of abnormal genital bleeding. In *NAACOG's Clinical Issues in Perinatal and Women's Health Nursing: Bleeding in Women* (ed. D.W. Perlis), pp. 328–38. J.B. Lippincott, Philadelphia.

Profet, M. (1993). Menstruation as a defense against pathogens transported by sperm. *The Quarterly Review of Biology*, **68**, 335–81.

Rankin, G.L.S., Veall, N., Huntsman, R.G., and Liodell, J. (1962). Measurement with ^{51}Cr of red-cell loss in menorrhagia. *Lancet*, **i**, 567–9.

Reynolds, T. (1995). Midlife health: a guide for the 40-something woman. *National women's health report*, Vol. 17. National Women's Health Center, Washington, DC.

Rodrigues, G., Faundes-Latham, A., and Atkinson, L. (1976). An approach to the analysis of menstrual patterns in the critical evaluation of contraceptives. *Studies in Family Planning*, **7**, 42–51.

Root, J.L. (1992). Women's perceptions of the experience of menstruation. Unpublished D. Phil. thesis. University of Utah College of Health.

Rybo, G., Lemar, J., and Tibblin, E. (1985). Epidemiology of menstrual blood loss. In *Mechanism of menstrual bleeding* (ed. D.T. Baird and E.A. Michie), pp. 181–93. Serono Symposia Publications, Raven Press, New York.

Seltzer, V.L., Beryamen, F., and Deutsch, S. (1990). Perimenopausal bleeding patterns and pathologic findings. *Journal of the American Medical Women's Association*, **45**, 132–4.

Shaw, S.T. Jr (1973). Quantitation of menstrual blood loss. *Postgraduate Medicine*, **53**, 204–8.

Shaw, S.T. Jr and Roche, P.C. (1985). The endometrial cycle: aspects of hemostatis. In *Mechanism of menstrual bleeding* (ed. D.T. Baird and E.A. Michie). Serono Symposia Publications and Raven Press, New York.

Sporrong, T., Rybo, G., Mattson, L.A., Vilbergson, G., and Crona, N. (1992). An objective and subjective assessment of uterine blood loss in post-menopausal women on hormone replacement therapy. *British Journal of Obstetrics and Gynaecology*, **99**, 399–401.

Toufexis, A. (1993). A woman's best defense? *Time*, October 4 (1993), pp. 72–3.

Treloar, A.E. (1935). Unpublished diary.

Treloar, A.E., Boynton, R.E., Behn, B.G., and Brown, B.W. (1967). Variation of the human menstrual cycle through reproductive life. *International Journal of Fertility*, **12**, 77–113.

Utian, W.H. (1990). The menopause in perspective: from potions to patches. *Annals of the New York Academy of Sciences*, **592**, 1–7.

Voda, A.M. (1997). *Menopause Me and You, the sound of women pausing*. Haworth Press, New York.

Voda, A.M. and Mansfield, P.K. (1994). Menstrual bleeding patterns in premenopausal women. In *Proceedings, Society for Menstrual Cycle Research: Mind Body Rhythmicity: A Menstrual Cycle Perspective*, pp. 1–11. Hamilton and Cross, Seattle, W.A.

Voda, A.M., Morgan, J.M., Root, J.L., and Smith, K.R. (1991). The Tremin Trust research program (5–19). In *Menstruation health and illness* (ed. N. Woods and D. Taylor). Hemisphere Press, New York.

Vollman, R.F. (1977). *The menstrual cycle*. W.B. Saunders, Philadelphia.

Webster's third new international dictionary (1983). Unabridged. Merriam-Webster, Springfield, MA.

West, S. and Dranov, P. (1994). *The hysterectomy hoax*. Doubleday, New York.

Williamson, M.L. (1992). Sexual adjustment after hysterectomy. *Journal of Obstetric. Gynecologic and Neonatal Nursing*, **21**, 42–7.

11 Menorrhagia

6 Definition and epidemiology of menorrhagia

Angela Coulter

Definition and historical background

Menorrhagia is 'excessive' menstrual blood loss or, in lay terms, heavy periods. The widely accepted clinical definition is a blood loss of 80 ml or more per period. This cut-off point was derived from a community study of menstrual blood loss conducted in Gothenberg, Sweden, in the 1960s, in which 80 ml represented the 90th centile of the distribution (Hallberg *et al.* 1966). These researchers found that the incidence of anaemia was significantly increased in women with blood losses over 60 ml and they recommended that a blood loss greater than 80 ml should be regarded as pathological. However, this apparently clear-cut definition masks a tangle of scientific debate and clinical uncertainty.

Menorrhagia is one of a number of menstrual problems that are quite commonly experienced. Others include dysmenorrhoea (painful periods), premenstrual syndrome (a combination of symptoms including depression, anxiety, tiredness, irritability, bloatedness, breast tenderness, and headache), metrorrhagia (irregular or prolonged periods), polymenorrhoea (frequent periods), oligomenorrhoea (infrequent and scanty periods), epimenorrhoea (inter-menstrual bleeding), and amenorrhoea (absent menstrual periods). Despite the fact that many of these problems are extremely common, they have been categorized as 'menstrual abnormalities' and allocated greek-derived clinical labels. They are an increasingly frequent cause of general practice consultation and specialist referral (Coulter *et al.* 1988) and considerable health service resources are devoted to their management. The increasing incidence of complaints about menstrual problems is probably related to the fact that women in the second half of the 20th century experience many more menstrual cycles than their ancestors did (Rees and Turnbull 1989). Frequent pregnancies, followed by two to three years of lactational amenorrhoea, meant that prior to the widespread adoption of effective methods of contraception a woman would experience only 30 to 40 menstrual periods during her entire reproductive life, as compared to today's average of about 400 menstrual cycles. Yet menorrhagia is not a new problem. There are references to excessive menstrual bleeding in the writings of Pliny (AD 23–79) and Galen (AD 129–199) (Wilbush 1988). Several historical texts link this problem to the menopause. At the end of the 17th century, Thomas Sydenham studied the problem and its treatment:

> But as to the Flux … [that] … comes most commonly a little before the Time the Courses are about to leave them, viz. about the Age of Forty-five if they flow early, but about Fifty if they come somewhat later; from these as it is said, a little before they quite go away (like a Candle burnt to the Socket which gives the greatest light, just as it is about to go out) they flow

> impetuously, and subject the poor Women almost continually to Hysterick Fits, by reason of the quantity of Blood which is continually evacuated...
>
> Let eight Ounces of Blood taken from the Arm, the next Morning give the common purging Potion, which must be repeated every third day for twice and every Night at Bedtime through the whole Course; let her take an Anodyne made with one Ounce of Diacodium.
>
> *(Sydenham 1701, quoted in Greer 1992)*

In the 18th century Astruc, physician to Louis XV of France, described the problem in similar terms:

> The climacteric does not necessarily require treatment. Though variable, as cessation approaches 'in general women begin to be irregular'. 'In some women the menses cease without accident ... [yet] in others the cessation brings on very strong hysteric fits. In some there happen floodings that are long, obstinate and dangerous. In others a fluor albus ... difficult of cure, is left.'
>
> *(Astruc 1762, quoted in Wilbush 1988)*

Various theories about the aetiology of menorrhagia were proposed by these early writers and a variety of treatments recommended. In the 19th century a British physician named Tilt surveyed 500 women, 138 of whom complained of 'flooding'. He estimated that the problem afflicted around 30 per cent of all women in the years preceding the menopause (Tilt 1851) – a figure which, as we shall see, is remarkably similar to current estimates of the prevalence of perceived heavy periods.

Aetiology of menorrhagia

The debate about what causes the problem continues to this day. It is generally accepted that the aetiology is multifactorial, although the precise biological mechanisms are still the subject of much doubt and conjecture. Broadly, current understanding of the factors causing menorrhagia can be grouped into four: pathological causes, including fibroids and other endometrial abnormalities, systemic disorders, and hormonal disturbances; iatrogenic causes, including various methods of contraception; psychological causes; and other causes, including genetic and behavioural factors.

Pathological causes

Fibroids

Uterine fibroids, or leiomyomata, are smooth muscle tumours which develop in the myometrium or wall of the uterus. They are very common; it has been estimated that between 20 and 25 per cent of women over the age of 30 have fibroids (West and Lumsden 1989; Vollenhoven *et al.* 1990). Fibroids occur in the reproductive years and reduce in size after the menopause. Their aetiology is unclear, but is thought to be hormonally related. The risk of fibroids is highest in nulliparous women and reduces with increasing parity. Non-smokers have a higher relative risk of fibroids than smokers. The risk is reduced in oral contraceptive users and increased among those who are obese (Ross *et al.* 1986; Parazzini *et al.* 1988). It has been suggested that fibroids and gall stones may share a common aetiology (Misciagna *et al.* 1987).

A leading article in the *British Medical Journal* (Baird and West 1988) asserted that fibroids give rise to 'menstrual problems, iron deficiency anaemia, pelvic discomfort, infertility and miscarriage', but in fact there is dispute about nearly all of these claims. Although it seems likely that large fibroids cause pain and discomfort, small fibroids are often asymptomatic. They are rarely associated with cancer: estimates of the proportion of malignancies found in fibroids removed at hysterectomy suggest that the incidence is between 0.1 and 0.7 per cent (Liebsohn *et al.* 1990).

Fibroids are commonly assumed to be a cause of menorrhagia, but the association is not well documented, with only a few small case series in the literature. Rybo (1982) studied 215 women with objectively measured menorrhagia and found that the prevalence of fibroids increased with higher levels of blood loss, but only 49 (23 per cent) of the women had fibroids. Fraser and colleagues (1986) reported the surgical removal of fibroids in four women who had a mean menstrual blood loss before treatment of 304 ml. After treatment there was a dramatic reduction in mean loss to 52 ml. The same investigators performed hysteroscopic investigations on a selected group of 139 patients complaining of menorrhagia and measured their menstrual blood loss (Fraser 1990). The blood loss in 47 of the women was found to be well within the normal range (i.e. less than 60 ml). Only three of these women (6 per cent) had fibroids, whereas fibroids were present in 12 (20 per cent) of the 59 women with moderately heavy loss (60–120 ml) and 12 (36 per cent) of the 33 women with losses greater than 120 ml.

There is dispute about the mechanisms by which uterine fibroids might cause increased blood loss (West and Lumsden 1989; Vollenhoven *et al.* 1990). They may be linked to increased vascularity of the uterus or they may be associated with abnormal ovarian function which might affect blood loss, although this theory has been challenged (see below). It is possible that they cause increased prostaglandin production which could lead to menorrhagia. Alternatively, increased blood loss may be the result of an increase in the uterine cavity surface area due to fibroids, but again this is disputed (Chimbira *et al.* 1980*a*). Although fibroids are often recorded as the discharge diagnosis in women undergoing hysterectomy following a complaint of menorrhagia, it seems likely that they are often incidental to the excess bleeding rather than its cause.

Endometriosis and adenomyosis

Other abnormalities of uterine tissue, including endometriosis (endometrial tissue outside the uterine cavity) and adenomyosis (endometrial glands and stroma deep within the myometrium) are also sometimes thought to be a cause of menorrhagia, although they may be a consequence of heavy bleeding rather than the cause (Kennedy 1993). Estimates of the prevalence of these conditions vary widely and cannot be established definitively (Azziz 1989; Thomas 1993). The most common symptoms of endometriosis are pelvic pain and dyspareunia (pain during intercourse), but this condition is sometimes suspected in women who present with increased blood loss (Stephenson and Campbell 1960; Sensky and Liu 1980). Fraser *et al.* (1986) measured blood loss in five women with adenomyosis and eleven with endometriosis. Three of those with adenomyosis and four with endometriosis had menorrhagia. However, Mahmood and colleagues (1991) studied 1200 women undergoing laparoscopy or abdominal hysterectomy for sterilization, infertility, chronic pelvic pain, or dysfunctional uterine bleeding. Two hundred and one (17 per cent) of the patients were diagnosed as having endometriosis. Those with endometriosis were significantly more likely to complain of dysmenorrhoea, dyspareunia, and irregular periods, but they were no more likely to report heavy bleeding than those without obvious pelvic abnormalities.

Other endometrial abnormalities

Rybo (1982) studied 213 women with objectively measured menorrhagia and found endometrial polyps in only eight (4 per cent) women and endometrial hyperplasia in five (2 per cent).

He concluded that both types of endometrial pathology were uncommon causes of menorrhagia.

Systemic disorders

A number of bleeding disorders are associated with a higher risk of menorrhagia. These include thrombocytopaenia, thrombocytopathy, Fanconi's anaemia, and Von Willebrand's disease (Claessens and Cowell 1981; Fraser *et al.* 1986). Blood loss measurements in small series of women with these diseases have confirmed that the majority suffer from menorrhagia (Makarainen and Ylikorkala 1986; van Eijkeren *et al.* 1990). Other diseases which have been implicated in the aetiology of menorrhagia include various thyroid disorders including myxoedema (van Eijkeren *et al.* 1989; Wilansky and Greisman 1989).

It is sometimes suggested that menorrhagia may be an indication of the presence of serious pathology such as endometrial cancer or pelvic inflammatory disease, although there is little evidence to support this. The possibility of endometrial cancer is the ostensible reason why so many women presenting with menorrhagia are referred for dilatation and curettage (D&C), but in fact this is almost certainly unnecessary in women under the age of 40 years (Coulter *et al.* 1993) and those with this disease are more likely to present with blood-stained vaginal discharge, or intermenstrual or post-coital bleeding (Rees 1993).

Most women treated for menorrhagia have no organic pathology and it is likely that in about 80 per cent of cases the disorder is the result of local endometrial factors (Cameron and Smith 1992). It used to be believed that hormonal disturbance, in particular anovulation, was the underlying cause of otherwise unexplained menorrhagia. While this may be the cause of menstrual problems in adolescent girls (Coupey and Ahlstrom 1989), or perimenopausal women (Mishell *et al.* 1984), it does not appear to be a satisfactory explanation in the vast majority of cases (Boyd 1986).

Currently favoured theories stress the importance of biochemical factors. There is dispute about the role of increased fibrinolytic activity (Cole and Clarkson 1972; Bonnar *et al.* 1976; Rybo 1982). However, studies of the physiology of menstruation have isolated prostaglandins as possibly implicated in the pathogenesis of menorrhagia and dysmenorrhoea. An imbalance in the different types of prostaglandins could be important. Recently a number of investigators have postulated that excess production of the type of uterine prostaglandins which act as vasodilators may lead to increased blood loss (Smith *et al.* 1981; Hagenfeldt 1987; Adelantado *et al.* 1988; Cameron 1989; Rees 1989; van Eijkeren *et al.* 1989).

Iatrogenic causes

Intrauterine contraceptive devices (IUCDs)

The most important iatrogenic causes of menorrhagia are those associated with methods of contraception. IUCDs have been shown to increase blood loss in a large number of studies (Hefnawi *et al.* 1973; Israel *et al.* 1974; Malmqvist *et al.* 1974; Liedholm *et al.* 1975; Larsson *et al.* 1975; Guillebaud *et al.* 1976; Rybo 1978, Andrade *et al.* 1979; Shaw *et al.* 1980; Tauber *et al.* 1981; Pedron *et al.* 1982; Gao Ji *et al.* 1986; Toppozada 1987; Andrade and Orchard 1987). The underlying mechanisms causing this effect remain unclear. Indeed, there is still uncertainty about the origins of the contraceptive effect of these devices. Studies which have measured menstrual blood loss before and after insertion of the Lippes loop have shown that it leads to a lasting and significant increase of between 20 and 40 ml per period, a doubling of the average loss. The increase associated with copper IUCDs is less, approximately 50 per cent above pre-insertion levels, but the reason for this difference between the devices is not at all clear.

On the other hand, progestagen-releasing devices reduce the volume of bleeding by between 40 and 90 per cent (Nilsson 1977; Gallegos *et al.* 1977; Bergqvist and Rybo 1983; Luukkainen *et al.* 1990; Andersson and Rybo 1990). For this reason this type of IUD has been advocated as a cure for menorrhagia, although inter-menstrual bleeding is common in the first few months after insertion.

Sterilization

There has long been concern that female sterilization may result in an increased likelihood of menstrual disturbances (Rioux 1977). It has been hypothesized that interfering with the Fallopian tubes may cause reduced oestrogen excretion and thus lead to menstrual problems (Cattanach and Milne 1988). Although many studies have been carried out to investigate this possibility, the question poses complex methodological problems.

Some investigators have studied self-reported menstrual change, for the most part finding little difference between sterilized and non-sterilized women (Brown *et al.* 1988; Rulin *et al.* 1989). Only one study included objective assessment of blood loss measurement (Kasonde and Bonnar 1976). Menstrual blood loss was measured for three months before and for six to 12 months after tubal ligation in 25 women and no significant effects were found. Most of the large studies of the menstrual consequences of sterilization have used hospital admissions as the main outcome variable. Vessey *et al.* (1983) found an increase in hospital referrals and admissions for menstrual disorders among women who had undergone tubal ligation, although they were not more likely to undergo hysterectomy than a comparison group of women whose husbands had undergone vasectomy. Cohen (1987) found an increased risk of hysterectomy among women who underwent tubal ligation at a young age (under 30), but no elevated risk for women aged 30 and over. A large Danish study using routine data on hospital admissions found that sterilized women were three times more likely to undergo hysterectomy than women who had not been sterilized, but the authors felt that this difference could be attributed to prior bleeding disorders and prior contraceptive use (Kjer and Knudsen 1990). Shy *et al.* (1992) found that sterilized women were twice as likely to be hospitalized for menstrual disorders as a general population sample of non-sterilized women and this risk was especially marked among women sterilized before their 30th birthday, who had a six-fold elevated risk.

Interpreting this apparent association between prior sterilization and hospitalization for menstrual disorders is problematic. It is possible that there is a biological mechanism by which sterilization interferes with the supply of blood to the ovaries resulting in hormonal dysfunction and menstrual problems. On the other hand, it is also possible that women who have opted for sterilization are those who have a preference for surgical intervention and they may therefore be more willing to undergo gynaecological surgery than those who have used other contraceptive methods. Equally plausible is the suggestion that the permanent loss of fertility represented by tubal ligation removes a barrier when considering treatment options for menorrhagia, so these patients' doctors may be more likely to recommend hysterectomy than they would to women who have retained their fertility.

Oral contraception

Use of oral contraception appears to reduce blood loss (Mishell 1982). In a community sample only 5 per cent of oral contraceptive users reported heavy periods compared to 16 per cent of those using IUCDs, 13 per cent of those who had been sterilized, and 11 per cent of those using other methods of contraception or none (Brown *et al.* 1988). The most important evidence comes from another British community survey which included objective measurement of blood loss (Cole *et al.* 1971). These investigators found that the mean loss for the 23 oral contraceptive users in the study was 12.7 ml, compared to 56.3 ml among the 25 IUD users and 37.9 ml for the remaining 280 women.

Since oral contraceptive users experience lighter menstrual periods, a change from this method of contraception may be an important cause of perceived increased blood loss leading to consultation and consequent diagnosis of menorrhagia. Every woman has only her own previous experience of menstruation as a guide to normality and since oral contraceptives are frequently used from the late teenage years onwards, many women may be ignorant of their own 'normal' bleeding pattern until they cease using this method of contraception.

Psychological causes

Since the ancient Greeks, writers have blamed the uterus for abnormal behaviour and mental instability (Chodoff 1982). Plato's theory of the 'wandering womb' and ideas about 'hysterical disturbance' caused by diseased genital organs continued to exert an influence on medical thought in the 18th and 19th centuries and their influence can still be detected today. Nowadays the tendency is to assume that causality operates in the opposite direction, i.e. that menstrual disorders are caused by psychological disturbance rather than the other way around. So, for example, Blaikley writing in the *Lancet* in 1949 argued that psychogenic factors were 'a far commoner cause of menorrhagia than some of the others which are fully described', and in 1950 an American gynaecologist asserted that 'functional uterine bleeding is frequently psychological in origin' (Rogers 1950). Dutton, a Canadian gynaecologist, claimed that 'psychological disturbances are the principal cause of functional uterine bleeding during the prime reproductive years' (Dutton 1965). He studied 155 women who presented with heavy menstrual bleeding in whom no organic cause was identified. Psychological disturbance was identified in 83 per cent of these patients, compared to a prevalence of 33 per cent in a comparison group whose bleeding disorders were attributed to fibroids, prolapse, cervicitis, or endometriosis. Dutton concluded that the anxiety experienced by his patients must be a cause rather than a consequence of their bleeding problems.

Lennane and Lennane (1973) published an influential article in the *New England Journal of Medicine* criticizing gynaecologists' propensity to assume psychogenic origins for the problems afflicting their female patients. Pointing to the lack of a sound scientific basis for these beliefs, they argued that the tendency to blame patients' neuroses for conditions for which the doctors could find no physical basis amounted to sexual prejudice and was damaging to patients. However, many studies of women presenting at gynaecological outpatient clinics for bleeding problems have indicated that the prevalence of psychiatric morbidity is higher than would be expected in a general population (Sainsbury 1960; Ballinger 1977; Gath *et al.* 1982; Greenberg 1983; Byrne 1984; Ryan *et al.* 1989).

A community study in Oxford demonstrated an association between perceived heavy bleeding and psychiatric morbidity as measured by the 'present state examination' and the 'general health questionnaire', although the relationship with these symptoms was not as strong as it was with dysmenorrhoea and premenstrual syndrome (Gath *et al.* 1987). The authors suggested that psychiatric treatment rather than treatment aimed at ameliorating the gynaecological symptoms may be more appropriate in some cases. Others have suggested that hysterectomies are often performed unnecessarily on women whose underlying problem is psychiatric rather than physical (Waldemar *et al.* 1987). On the other hand, a number of prospective studies of women undergoing hysterectomy have shown a reduction in rates of psychiatric morbidity after the operation, suggesting that the operation may ameliorate psychological problems as well as physical ones (Oates and Gath 1989).

There are several possible explanations for this apparent association between complaints of menorrhagia and psychiatric symptoms. It is entirely plausible that the stress and social discomfort of heavy bleeding in itself could cause anxiety or depression. Alternatively another factor, such as hormonal imbalance, might cause both depression and bleeding disorders. The perception of menstrual change could be a symptom of depression; or it could present a convenient physical trigger for consultation for an underlying psychological problem, possibly unrecognized by the general practitioner or gynaecologist. Final resolution of this puzzle will require large-scale population-based prospective studies incorporating menstrual blood loss measurement, subjective and objective assessments of menstrual problems, standardized psychiatric assessment, and clinical investigation. Currently there are no such studies in the published literature.

Other possible causes

There are few publications on the descriptive epidemiology of menorrhagia. There is no evidence that age influences menstrual blood loss. Rybo found similar median values in blood loss measurements among women aged 15, 23, 30, 40, and 45 (Rybo 1982). However, the oldest age group (mostly perimenopausal women) had the highest mean loss in population studies (Hallberg *et al.* 1966; Cole *et al.* 1971). Rybo and Hallberg's (1966) study of twins suggested a genetic link. There was a significant correlation between the menstrual losses of sisters in monozygotic pairs but no correlation between dizygotic twins. The same investigators also found that blood loss was related to parity, although the difference was statistically significant only in the younger age groups (Rybo and Hallberg 1966). The relationship between numbers of children and heavier menstrual loss has been found in some other studies (Barer and Fowler 1936; Cole *et al.* 1971; Khatri and Gupta 1978; Hefnawi *et al.* 1980*a*), though not all (Elwood *et al.* 1968). Hysterectomy for dysfunctional uterine bleeding is positively associated with parity (Vessey *et al.* 1992). There is also evidence of an increased risk of menorrhagia associated with smoking (Sloss and Frerichs 1983; Brown *et al.* 1988). Other suggested associated factors include diet and body mass index (van Eijkeren *et al.* 1989). One study, which looked at the effect of iron supplementation on reported blood loss among women complaining of menorrhagia, suggested that chronic iron deficiency might be a cause as well as a consequence of menorrhagia (Taymor *et al.* 1964).

In Britain working class women have been found to be more likely to report menstrual problems (Blaxter 1987) and they are more likely to consult their GPs for these problems (Royal College of General Practitioners 1990). Having consulted for menorrhagia, women who have not received higher education are more likely to indicate a preference for surgical rather than medical treatment (Coulter *et al.* 1994). This may explain the higher rate of hysterectomy experienced by working class women or women with lower educational status observed in at least three studies

(Coulter and McPherson 1986; Vessey *et al.* 1992; Kuh and Stirling 1995). Whether these patterns represent greater morbidity among working class women, perhaps related to their greater propensity to smoke, or cultural differences which make them more likely to opt for treatment, is very hard to determine.

Prevalence of heavy bleeding

Before one can attempt to assess needs for treatment for menorrhagia, it is necessary to determine the prevalence of the condition in the female population. The clinical definition involves objective measurement of menstrual blood loss to estimate the proportion with losses greater than 80 ml, or 60 ml if the lower threshold is preferred. However, as we have seen these thresholds were chosen for statistical rather than clinical reasons. Iron deficiency is not an inevitable consequence of heavy blood loss and anyway it can be treated by iron supplementation or dietary change. Since objective measurement is not carried out in normal clinical practice and since women's perceptions of heavy loss are the key determinants of consultation rates and subsequent treatment, an estimate of subjectively assessed heavy loss is also an essential prerequisite for assessing the likely demand for medical intervention.

Objective measurement

The development of techniques for measuring menstrual blood loss was prompted by the quest to establish the precise relationship between menstrual loss and iron-deficiency anaemia. This became particularly important following the widespread uptake of IUCDs for contraception, especially in developing countries where dietary deficiencies accompanied by increased menstrual blood loss meant that many women using these devices were at risk of developing anaemia. Early studies used a variety of measurement techniques, including weight measurements and radio isotopic methods, which had the drawback of being unreliable or laborious and expensive (Barer and Fowler 1936; Baldwin *et al.* 1961; Price *et al.* 1964; Hytten *et al.* 1964; Jacobs and Butler 1965). In 1964 Hallberg and Nilsson developed the alkaline haematin method in which blood was extracted from tampons and towels soaked in a sodium hydroxide solution and examined spectrophotometrically (Hallberg and Nilsson 1964). Using this method Hallberg and colleagues conducted the first population study of the distribution of menstrual blood loss (Hallberg *et al.* 1966). The results are summarized in Table 6.1, where they are compared with the only other randomly selected population study which measured blood loss objectively (Cole *et al.* 1971).

It can be seen that these studies were in fairly close agreement in that the mean loss was around 40 ml, with a median of 30 ml, and that 90 per cent of the female population had losses of less than 80 ml, with 20 per cent losing 60 ml or more. These estimates are broadly in line with other studies measuring blood loss in selected populations, mostly prior to insertion of intrauterine devices. Mean menstrual blood loss in these studies ranged from 24 ml to 45 ml (Gao Ji *et al.* 1987; Andrade and Orchard 1987). The largest study so far was conducted by Hefnawi and colleagues (1980*a*, *b*) who measured blood loss in 774 family planning clinic attenders in Cairo, none of whom were using oral contraceptives or intrauterine devices. They used the atomic absorption technique for iron determination and calculated a mean menstrual blood loss in their population of 25.6 ml, with a range from 1.2 to 146.7 ml. The studies by Hallberg *et al.* (1966)

Table 6.1 Population studies of measured menstrual blood loss

Study	Hallberg *et al.* 1966	Cole *et al.* 1971
Country	Sweden	England
MBL method	Alkaline haematin	Atomic absorption
No. of subjects	476	348
Age range	15–50	17–44
Selection:	Random	Random
Mean loss (ml)	43.4 ± 2.3	37.5 ± 3.3
Median loss (ml)	30.0	27.6
Range	10.4–83.9*	0.1–280
Loss > 80 ml	11.0%	9.5%
Loss > 60 ml	19.0%	20.7%

* 10th and 90th percentile.

and Cole *et al.* (1971) differed in the proportion of the total population found to have low haemoglobin levels. In Gothenberg, 29 per cent of the study population had haemoglobin levels below 12 g/100 ml, whereas the proportion in Cole's Northumbrian study was 15 per cent. This may be because iron supplementation was more common in the British sample. There was a correlation between menstrual loss and haemoglobin levels in both studies, but Cole *et al.* (1972) discovered that the association was as strong in low menstrual losses as at high levels. On this basis they argued that the association between menstrual loss and haematological indices was not likely to be due to iron depletion.

Differences in mean menstrual blood volume in the various studies may be due to population differences or to different methods of measuring blood loss. The alkaline haematin method is currently the most popular method of measurement. It appears to be accurate as long as it is based on more than one measurement (due to within-subject variation, it is necessary to take at least two measurements), although a number of authors have recommended modifications (Shaw *et al.* 1972; Shaw 1977; Newton *et al.* 1977; van Eijkeren *et al.* 1986; Vasilenko *et al.* 1988). The test measures haemoglobin in the fluid discharge, on the assumption that this gives a reliable estimate of total loss. However, this assumption has been challenged by Fraser and colleagues (1985) who studied total fluid loss and blood loss in 28 women. The mean measured blood loss was 30.6 ± 6.1 ml, but the total fluid loss was 74.4 ± 10.3 ml, indicating that most of the fluid volume of the menstrual discharge may be derived from sources other than blood. If the main aim of diagnosis is to detect the risk of iron-deficiency anaemia, it is probably more important to have an accurate measurement of blood loss than other fluids, but if true, Fraser's finding may help to explain the discrepancies between patients' subjective impressions of blood loss and objective measurements (see below).

Subjective assessment

In the Swedish study (Hallberg *et al.* 1966), women were asked to describe their blood loss in one of three categories – light, medium, or heavy. Fifty one (11 per cent) out of 474 women considered their loss light, 274 (58 per cent) said it was medium, and 149 (31 per cent) said it was heavy. When compared to objectively measured loss, there appeared to be considerable discrepancies in the assessments. So, for example, 26 per cent of those with losses well within the normal range (below 60 ml) wrongly considered their loss to be heavy and 40 per cent of those with heavy losses (over 80 ml) considered theirs moderate or light. Similar discrepancies between subjective and objective assessments have been found in a number of studies. Haynes *et al.* (1977) measured blood losses in 66 women complaining of heavy periods and found that 24 per cent had losses below 80 ml. Chimbira and colleagues (1980*b*) found no correlation between measured menstrual blood loss and the subjective assessments of 92 women, neither was there a relationship between numbers of days of bleeding or numbers of pads and tampons used. Fraser and colleagues measured blood loss in 69 women with a convincing complaint of menorrhagia and found that only 38 per cent had losses over 80 ml, although 59 per cent would qualify with an upper limit of normal of 60 ml (Fraser *et al.* 1984).

In everyday practice, clinical assessment relies on questions about the 'heaviness' of loss, the numbers of pads and tampons used, the number of days bleeding, soiling of clothes, bedding, and furniture and whether or not clots are passed. In most of the studies the majority of women in each broad grouping were reasonably accurate in their assessments, but for a significant number of individuals their assessments were wildly different from the objective measurements. This would suggest that the usual methods of diagnosis are unreliable guides to blood loss in individuals. As has already been argued, this is probably due to the fact that women do not have a 'gold standard' against which to assess their own menstrual loss. An additional problem arises from the varying absorbency rates of different brands of pads and tampons, which together with differences in tolerance of soaked sanitary materials make these indicators particularly unreliable (Grimes 1979). Recently a pictorial chart has been developed which proved to be reasonably accurate as an indicator of loss in a clinical trial in which subjects all used the same brand of pads and tampons (Higham *et al.* 1990). However, it would seem to have limited use in clinical practice unless patients could be persuaded to use a standard type of sanitary material.

The important factor determining consultation rates for heavy bleeding is, of course, subjective perception rather than objectively verified menorrhagia. For some reason social scientists, who might be expected to be interested in women's subjective experiences, have virtually ignored menorrhagia. There is a large literature on menstrual problems in social science publications, but the studies have been almost exclusively concerned with the pre-menstrual syndrome. Where menorrhagia is mentioned (e.g. Golub 1992; Scambler and Scambler 1993), it is only as part of a general discussion about menstrual problems and no estimates of prevalence have been attempted. A recent population survey conducted by a market research organization carried out face-to-face home interviews with a nationally representative quota sample of 1069 women aged 16–45 years to determine the prevalence of menstrual problems (Corrado 1990). Three hundred and thirty-one women, 31 per cent of the sample, reported that they had experienced heavy periods. Twenty-eight per cent of these said they had always had heavy periods, 17 per cent said they developed following a pregnancy, and 6 per cent attributed them to use of IUCDs. More than a third (36 per cent) of the 541 women who reported heavy or painful periods within the four months prior to the survey had consulted a general practitioner for this problem.

It is interesting to compare the prevalence of heavy periods reported in this modern British survey with Hallberg's findings from Gothenberg in the 1960s and with those reported by Tilt in 1851. In all of these studies just under a third of the women surveyed have complained of heavy menstrual loss. This complaint would appear to be neither culturally nor temporally specific!

References

Adelantado, J., Rees, M., Bernal, A.L., and Turnbull, A. (1988). Increased uterine prostaglandin E receptors in menorrhagic women. *British Journal of Obstetrics and Gynaecology*, **95**, 162–5.

Andersson, J.K. and Rybo, G. (1990). Levonorgestrel-releasing intrauterine device in the treatment of menorrhagia. *British Journal of Obstetrics and Gynaecology*, **97**, 690–4.

Andrade, A. and Orchard, E.P. (1987). Quantitative studies on menstrual blood loss in IUD users. *Contraception*, **36**, 129–44.

Andrade, A., de Souza, J.P., Rowe, P., and Shaw, S. (1979). Effect of prior pregnancy and combined oral contraceptives on baseline menstrual blood loss and bleeding response to intrauterine devices. *Contraception*, **20**, 19–27.

Azziz, R. (1989). Adenomyosis: current perspectives. *Obstetrics and Gynecology Clinics of North America*, **16**, 221–35.

Baird, D.T. and West, C.P. (1988). Medical management of fibroids. *British Medical Journal*, **296**, 1684–5.

Baldwin, R., Whalley, P., and Pritchard, J. (1961). Measurements of menstrual blood loss. *American Journal of Obstetrics and Gynecology*, **81**, 739–42.

Ballinger, C.B. (1977). Psychiatric morbidity and the menopause: survey of a gynaecological outpatient clinic. *British Journal of Psychiatry*, **131**, 83–9.

Barer, A. and Fowler, W. (1936). The blood loss during normal menstruation. *American Journal of Obstetrics and Gynecology*, **31**, 979–86.

Bergqvist, A. and Rybo, G. (1983). Treatment of menorrhagia with intrauterine release of progesterone. *British Journal of Obstetrics and Gynaecology*, **90**, 255–8.

Blaikley, J.B. (1949). Menorrhagia of emotional origin. *Lancet*, **ii**, 691–4.

Blaxter, M. (1987). Health and social class. Evidence on inequality in health from a national survey. *Lancet*, **ii**, 30–3.

Bonnar, J., Kasonde, K., Haddon, M., Hassanein, M.K., and Allington, M.J. (1976). Fibrinolytic activity *in utero* and bleeding complications with intrauterine contraceptive devices. *British Journal of Obstetrics and Gynaecology*, **83**, 160–4.

Boyd, M. (1986). Dysfunctional uterine bleeding. *The Canadian Journal of Surgery*, **29**, 305–7.

Brown, S., Vessey, M., and Stratton, I. (1988). The influence of method of contraception and cigarette smoking on menstrual patterns. *British Journal of Obstetrics and Gynaecology*, **95**, 905–10.

Byrne, P. (1984). Psychiatric morbidity in a gynaecology clinic: an epidemiological survey. *British Journal of Psychiatry*, **144**, 28–34.

Cameron, I.T. (1989). Dysfunctional uterine bleeding. *Baillière's Clinical Obstetrics and Gynaecology*, **3**, 315–27.

Cameron, I.T. and Smith, S.K. (1992). Menorrhagia. In *Haemostasis and thrombosis in obstetrics and gynaecology* (ed. I. Greer, A. Turpie and C. Forbes), pp. 77–93. Associated Books, London.

Cattanach, J.F. and Milne, B.J. (1988). Post-tubal sterilisation problems correlated with ovarian steroidogenesis. *Contraception*, **38**, 541–50.

Chimbira, T., Anderson, A., Naish, C., Cope, E., and Turnbull, A. (1980*a*). Reduction of menstrual blood loss by danazol in unexplained menorrhagia: lack of effect of placebo. *British Journal of Obstetrics and Gynaecology*, **87**, 1152–8.

Chimbira, T., Anderson, A., and Turnbull, A. (1980b). Relation between measured menstrual blood loss and patient's subjective assessment of loss, duration of bleeding, number of sanitary towels used, uterine weight and endometrial surface area. *British Journal of Obstetrics and Gynaecology*, **87**, 603–9.

Chodoff, P. (1982). Hysteria and women. *American Journal of Psychiatry*, **139**, 545–51.

Claessens, E. and Cowell, C. (1981). Dysfunctional uterine bleeding in the adolescent. *Pediatric Clinics of North America*, **28**, 369–78.

Cohen, M.M. (1987). Long-term risk of hysterectomy after tubal sterilization. *American Journal of Epidemiology*, **125**, 410–19.

Cole, S. and Clarkson, A. (1972). Menstrual blood loss and fibrin degradation products. *British Medical Journal*, **1**, 78–9.

Cole, S., Billewicz, W., and Thomson, A. (1971). Sources of variation in menstrual blood loss. *Journal of Obstetrics and Gynaecology of the British Commonwealth*, **78**, 933–9.

Cole, S., Thomson, A., Billewicz, W., and Black, A. (1972). Haematological characteristics and menstrual blood losses. *Journal of Obstetrics and Gynaecology of the British Commonwealth*, **79**, 994–1001.

Corrado, M. (1990). *Women's health in 1990*. Research study conducted on behalf of Parke-Davies Research Laboratories. MORI (Market Opinion and Research International).

Coulterm, A. and McPherson, K. (1986). The hysterectomy debate. *Quarterly Journal of Social Affairs*, **2**, 379–96.

Coulter, A., McPherson, K., and Vessey, M. (1988). Do British women undergo too many or too few hysterectomies? *Social Science and Medicine*, **27**, 987–94.

Coulter, A., Klassen, A., MacKenzie, I., and McPherson, K. (1993). Diagnostic dilatation and curettage: is it used appropriately? *British Medical Journal*, **306**, 236–9.

Coulter, A., Peto, V., and Doll, H. (1994). Patients' preferences and general practitioners' decisions in the treatment of menstrual disorders. *Family Practice*, **11**, 67–74.

Coupey, S. and Ahlstrom, P. (1989). Common menstrual disorders. *Adolescent Gynecology*, **36**, 551–71.

Dutton, W.A. (1965). Psychological factors in 155 patients with functional uterine bleeding. *Canadian Medical Association Journal*, **92**, 398–405.

Elwood, P., Rees, G., and Thomas, J. (1968). Community study of menstrual iron loss and its association with iron deficiency anaemia. *British Journal of Preventive and Social Medicine*, **22**, 127–131.

Fraser, I.S. (1990). Hysteroscopy and laparoscopy in women with menorrhagia. *American Journal of Obstetrics and Gynecology*, **162**, 1264–9.

Fraser, I.S., McCarron, G., and Markham, R. (1984). A preliminary study of factors influencing perception of menstrual blood loss volume. *American Journal of Obstetrics and Gynecology*, **149**, 788–93.

Fraser, I.S., McCarron, G., Markham, R., and Resta, T. (1985). Blood and total fluid content of menstrual discharge. *Obstetrics and Gynaecology*, **65**, 194–8.

Fraser, I.S., McCarron, G., Markham, R., Resta, T., and Watts, A. (1986). Measured menstrual blood loss in women with menorrhagia associated with pelvic disease or coagulation disorder. *Obstetrics and Gynecology*, **68**, 630–3.

Gallegos, A., Aznar, R., Merino, G., and Guizer, E. (1977). Intrauterine devices and menstrual blood loss: a comparative study of eight devices during the first six months of use. *Contraception*, **17**, 153–61.

Gao Ji, Zeng Su, Sun Boling, Wu Shangchun, Dong Jing, Cong Jie, *et al.* (1986). Menstrual blood loss, hemoglobin and ferritin concentration of Beijing women wearing steel ring, VCu 200, and TCu 220c IUCDs. *Contraception*, **34**, 559–71.

Gao Ji, Zeng Su, Sun Boling, Fan Huimin, and Han Lihui. (1987). Menstrual blood loss and haematologic indices in healthy Chinese women. *Journal of Reproductive Medicine*, **22**, 822–6.

Gath, D., Cooper, P., and Day, A. (1982). Hysterectomy and psychiatric disorder: 1. Levels of psychiatric morbidity before and after hysterectomy. *British Journal of Psychiatry*, **140**, 335–50.

Gath, D., Osborn, M., Bungay, G., Iles, S., Day, A., Bond, A., and Passingham, C. (1987). Psychiatric disorder and gynaecological symptoms in middle aged women: a community survey. *British Medical Journal*, **294**, 213–18.

Golub, S. (1992). *Periods: from menarche to menopause*, Sage, London.

Greenberg, M. (1983). The meaning of menorrhagia: an investigation into the association between the complaint of menorrhagia and depression. *Journal of Psychosomatic Research*, **27**, 209–14.

Greer, G. (1992). *The change*. Penguin London.

Grimes, D. (1979). Estimating vaginal blood loss. *Journal of Reproductive Medicine*, **22**, 190–2.

Guillebaud, J., Bonnar, J., Morehead, J., and Matthews, A. (1976). Menstrual blood-loss with intrauterine devices. *Lancet*, **i**, 387–90.

Hagenfeldt, K. (1987). The role of prostaglandins and allied substances in uterine haemostasis. *Contraception*, **36**, 23–35.

Hallberg, L. and Nilsson, L. (1964). Determination of menstrual blood loss. *Scandinavian Journal of Clinical and Laboratory Investigation*, **16**, 244–8.

Hallberg, L., Hogdahl, A.M., Nilsson, L., and Rybo, G. (1966). Menstrual blood loss – a population study. *Acta Obstetrica et Gynecologica Scandinavica*, **45**, 320–51.

Haynes, P., Hodgson, H., Anderson, A., and Turnbull, A. (1977). Measurement of menstrual blood loss in patients complaining of menorrhagia. *British Journal of Obstetrics and Gynaecology*, **84**, 763–8.

Hefnawi, F., Askalani, H., and Zaki, K. (1973). Menstrual blood loss with copper intrauterine devices. *Contraception*, **9**, 133–9.

Hefnawi, F., El-Zayat, A., and Yacout, M. (1980*b*). Physiologic studies of menstrual blood loss I. Range and consistence of menstrual blood loss in and iron requirements of menstruating Egyptian women. *International Journal of Gynaecology and Obstetrics*, **17**, 343–8.

Hefnawi, F., El-Zayat, A., and Yacout, M. (1980*a*). Physiologic studies of menstrual blood loss II. Physiologic variables affecting the magnitude of menstrual blood loss. *International Journal of Gynaecology and Obstetrics*, **17**, 348–52.

Higham, J., O'Brien, P., and Shaw, R. (1990). Assessment of menstrual blood loss using a pictorial chart. *British Journal of Obstetrics and Gynaecology*, **97**, 734–9.

Hytten, F., Cheyne, G., and Klopper, A. (1964). Iron loss at menstruation. *Journal of Obstetrics and Gynaecology of the British Commonwealth*, **71**, 255–9.

Israel, R., Shaw, S., and Martin, M. (1974). Comparative quantitation of menstrual blood loss with the Lippes Loop, Dalkon Shield, and Copper T intrauterine devices. *Contraception*, **10**, 63–71.

Jacobs, A. and Butler, E.B. (1965). Menstrual blood-loss in iron-deficiency anaemia. *Lancet*, **ii**, 407–9.

Kasonde, J. and Bonnar, J. (1976). Effect of sterilisation on menstrual blood loss. *British Journal of Obstetrics and Gynaecology*, **83**, 572–5.

Kennedy, S. (1993). Endometriosis. In *Women's problems in general practice* (ed. A. McPherson). Oxford University Press.

Khatri, R. and Gupta, A. (1978). Effect of childbirth on menstrual pattern. *Indian Journal of Medical Research*, **67**, 66–72.

Kjer, J.J. and Knudsen, L. (1990). Hysterectomy subsequent to laparoscopic sterilisation. *European Journal of Obstetrics and Gynecology and Reproductive Biology*, **35**, 63–8.

Kuh, D. and Stirling, S. (1995). Socioeconomic variation in hospital care for diseases of the female genital system and breast in a national cohort aged 15–43. *British Medical Journal*, **311**, 840–3.

Larsson, B., Hamberger, L., and Rybo, G. (1975). Influence of copper intrauterine contraceptive devices (Cu-7-IUD) on the menstrual blood-loss. *Acta Obstetrica et Gynecologica Scandinavica*, **54**, 315–18.

Liebsohn, S., d'Ablaing, G., Mishell, D.R., and Schlaerth, J.B. (1990). Leiomyosarcoma in a series of hysterectomies performed for presumed uterine leiomyomas. *American Journal of Obstetrics and Gynaecology*, **162**, 968–76.

Lennane, K.J. and Lennane, R.J. (1973). Alleged psychogenic disorders in women – a possible manifestation of sexual prejudice. *The New England Journal of Medicine*, **288**, 288–92.

Liedholm, P., Rybo, G., Sjoberg, N., and Solvell, L. (1975). Copper IUD – influence on menstrual blood loss and iron deficiency. *Contraception*, **12**, 317–25.

Luukkainen, T., Lahteenmaki, P., and Toivonen, J. (1990). Levonorgestrel-releasing intrauterine device. *Annals of Medicine*, **22**, 85–90.

Mahmood, T.A., Templeton, A.A., Thomson, L., and Fraser, C. (1991). Menstrual symptoms in women with pelvic endometriosis. *British Journal of Obstetrics and Gynaecology*, **98**, 558–63.

Makarainen, L. and Ylikorkala, O. (1986). Primary and myoma-associated menorrhagia: role of prostaglandins and effect of ibuprofen. *British Journal of Obstetrics and Gynaecology*, **93**, 974–8.

Malmqvist, R., Petersohn, L. and Bengtsson, L. (1974). Menstrual bleeding with copper-covered intrauterine contraceptive devices. *Contraception*, **9**, 627–33.

Misciagna, G., Mangini, V., Messa, C., Argese, V., Lacatena, M., Trentadue, R., and Giorgio, I. (1987). Gallstones and uterine fibroids. *Surgery, Gynecology and Obstetrics*, **165**, 429–34.

Mishell, D.R. (1982). Noncontraceptive health benefits of oral steroidal contraceptives. *American Journal of Obstetrics and Gynaecology*, **142**, 809–16.

Mishell, D., Fisher, H., Haynes, P., Seegar-Jones, G., and Smith, R. (1984). Menorrhagia: a symposium. *Journal of Reproductive Medicine*, **29**, 763–82.

Newton, J., Barnard, G., and Collins, W. (1977). A rapid method for measuring menstrual blood loss using automatic extraction. *Contraception*, **16**, 269–82.

Nilsson, C.G. (1977). Comparative quantitation of menstrual blood loss with a d-norgestrel-releasing IUD and a Nova-T-Copper device. *Contraception*, **15**, 379–87.

Oates, M. and Gath, D. (1989). Psychological aspects of gynaecological surgery. *Bailliere's Clinical Obstetrics and Gynaecology*, **3**, 729–49.

Parazzini, F., La Vecchia, C., Negri, E., Cecchetti, G., and Fedele, L. (1988). Epidemiologic characteristics of women with uterine fibroids: a case–control study. *Obstetrics and Gynecology*, **72**, 853–7.

Pedron, N., Gallegos, A., Lozano, M., and Aznar, R. (1982). Menstrual blood loss estimates in women using Copper 7 and Multiload-250 intrauterine devices. *Contraception*, **26**, 475–83.

Price, D., Forsyth, E., Cohn, S., and Cronkite, E. (1964). The study of menstrual and other blood loss, and consequent iron deficiency by Fe59 whole-body counting. *The Canadian Medical Association Journal*, **90**, 51–4.

Rees, M. (1989). Heavy, painful periods. *Baillière's Clinical Obstetrics and Gynaecology*, **3**, 341–56.

Rees, M. (1993). Menstrual problems. In *Women's problems in general practice* (ed. A. Mcpherson). Oxford University Press.

Rees, M. and Turnbull, A.C. (1989). Menstrual disorders – an overview. *Baillière's Clinical Obstetrics and Gynaecology*, **3**, 217–26.

Rioux, J.E. (1977). Late complications of female sterilisation: a review of the literature and a proposal for further research. *Journal of Reproductive Medicine*, **19**, 329–40.

Rogers, F.S. (1950). Emotional factors in gynecology. *American Journal of Obstetrics and Gynecology*, **52**, 321–7.

Ross, R.K., Pike, M.C., Vessey, M.P., Bull, D., Yeates, D., and Casagrande, J.T. (1986). Risk factors for uterine fibroids: reduced risk associated with oral contraceptives. *British Medical Journal*, **293**, 359–63.

Royal College of General Practitioners, Office of Population Censuses and Surveys, Department of Health. (1990). *1981–1982 Morbidity statistics from general practice. Third national study: socio-economic analyses*, Series MB5. HMSO, London.

Rulin, M., Davidson, A., Philliber, S., Graves, W., and Cushman, L. (1989). Changes in menstrual symptoms among sterilised and comparison women: a prospective study. *Obstetrics and Gynecology*, **74**, 149–54.

Ryan, M., Dennerstein, L., and Pepperell, R. (1989). Psychological aspects of hysterectomy. *British Journal of Psychiatry*, **154**, 516–22.

Rybo, G. (1978). The IUD and endometerial bleeding. *The Journal of Reproductive Medicine*, **20**, 175–82.

Rybo, G. (1982). Variations of menstrual blood loss. *Research and Clinical Forums*, **4**, 81–9.

Rybo, G. and Hallberg, L. (1966). Influence of heredity and environment on normal menstrual blood loss. *Acta Obstetrica et Gynecologica Scandinavica*, **45**, 389–410.

Sainsbury, P. (1960). Psychosomatic disorders and neurosis in outpatients attending a general hospital. *Journal of Psychosomatic Research*, **4**, 261–73.

Scambler, A. and Scambler, G. (1993). *Menstrual disorders*, Tavistock/Routledge, London.

Sensky, T.E. and Liu, D.T. (1980). Endometriosis: associations with menorrhagia, infertility and oral contraceptives. *International Journal of Gynaecology and Obstetrics*, **17**, 573–6.

Shaw, S. (1977). On quantifying menstrual blood loss. *Contraception*, **16**, 283–5.

Shaw, S., Aaronson, D., and Moyer, D. (1972). Quantitation of menstrual blood loss – further evaluation of the alkaline hematin method. *Contraception*, **5**, 497–513.

Shaw, S., Andrade, A., de Souza, J.P., Macaulay, L., and Rowe, P. (1980). Quantitative menstrual and intermenstrual blood loss in women using Lippes Loop and Copper T intrauterine devices. *Contraception*, **21**, 343–52.

Shy, K., Stergachis, A., Grothaus, L., Wagner, E., Hecht, J., and Anderson, G. (1992). Tubal sterilization and risk of subsequent hospital admission for menstrual disorders. *American Journal of Obstetrics and Gynecology*, **166**, 1698–706.

Sloss, E. and Frerichs, R. (1983). Smoking and menstrual disorders. *International Journal of Epidemiology*, **12**, 107–9.

Smith, S.K., Abel, M., Kelly, R., and Baird, D. (1981). A role for prostacyclin (PGI2) in excessive menstrual bleeding. *Lancet*, **i**, 522–4.

Stephenson, C.S. and Campbell, C.G. (1960). The symptoms, physical findings and clinical diagnosis of pelvic endometriosis. *Clinics in Obstetrics and Gynecology*, **3**, 441–55.

Tauber, P., Kloppel, A., Goodpasture, J., Burns, J., Ludwig, H., and Zaneveld, L. (1981). Reduced menstrual blood loss by release of an antifibrinolytic agent from intrauterine contraceptive devices. *American Journal of Obstetrics and Gynecology*, **140**, 322–8.

Taymor, M., Sturgis, S., and Yahia, C. (1964). The etiological role of chronic iron deficiency in production of menorrhagia. *Journal of the American Medical Association*, **187**, 323–7.

Thomas, E.J. (1993). Endometriosis. *British Medical Journal*, **306**, 158–9.

Tilt, E.J. (1851). *On the preservation of the health of women at the critical periods of life*. London. Churchill, (Quoted in Wilbush 1988.) London.

Toppozada, M. (1987). Treatment of increased menstrual blood loss in IUD users. *Contraception*, **36**, 145–57.

van Eijkeren, M., Scholten, P., Christiaens, G., Alsbach, G., and Haspels, A. (1986). The alkaline hematin method for measuring menstrual blood loss – a modification and its clinical use in menorrhagia. *European Journal of Obstetrics and Gynecology and Reproductive Biology*, **22**, 345–51.

van Eijkeren, M., Christiaens, G., Sixma, J., and Haspels, A. (1989). Menorrhagia: a review. *Obsterical and Gynaecological Survey*, **44**, 421–9.

van Eijkeren, M., Christiaens, G., Haspels, A., and Sixma, J. (1990). Measured menstrual blood loss in women with a bleeding disorder or using oral anticoagulant therapy. *American Journal of Obstetrics and Gynaecology*, **162**, 1261–3.

Vasilenko, P., Kraicer, P., Kaplan, R., deMasi, A., and Freed, N. (1988). A new and simple method of measuring menstrual blood loss. *Journal of Reproductive Medicine*, **33**, 293–7.

Vessey, M., Huggins, G., Lawless, M., McPherson, K., and Yeates, D. (1983). Tubal sterilisation: findings in a large prospective study. *British Journal of Obstetrics and Gynaecology*, **90**, 203–9.

Vessey, M., Villard-Mackintosh, L., McPherson, K., Coulter, A., and Yeates, D. (1992). The epidemiology of hysterectomy: findings in a large cohort study. *British Journal of Obstetrics and Gynaecology*, **99**, 402–7.

Vollenhoven, B.J., Lawrence, A.S., and Healy, D.L. (1990). Uterine fibroids: a clinical review. *British Journal of Obstetrics and Gynaecology*, **97**, 285–98.

Waldemar, G., Werdelin, L., and Boysen, G. (1987). Neurologic symptoms and hysterectomy: a retrospective survey of the prevalence of hysterectomy in neurologic patients. *Obstetrics and Gynecology*, **70**, 559–63.

West, C.P. and Lumsden, M.A. (1989). Fibroids and menorrhagia. *Bailliere's Clinical Obstetrics and Gynaecology*, **3**, 357–74.

Wilansky, D.L. and Greisman, B. (1989). Early hypothyroidism in patients with menorrhagia. *American Journal of Obstetrics and Gynecology*, **160**, 673–7.

Wilbush, J. (1988). Menorrhagia and menopause: a historical review. *Maturitas*, **10**, 5–26.

7 The pathophysiology of menorrhagia

Stephen K. Smith

Introduction

Menorrhagia is the subjective complaint of heavy periods. Its cause in the vast majority of cases is unknown. As one of the commonest referrals for gynaecological consultation (Bradlow *et al.* 1992) this statement may appear surprising. Yet when one considers the burden of proof needed to identify the cause of such a complex disease and when one views the highly pragmatic means used in the past to deal with the problem it is perhaps less surprising. However, a new urgency to this conundrum is now with us. Regular menstruation is the consequence of the use of widespread fertility regulation and thus in the past has only been a problem of the developed world, about 20 per cent of the total population of women of reproductive age. However, with the spread of effective fertility regulation worldwide and the global reduction of family size, the rest of the world's population will for the first time experience regular menstruation.

The present treatments employed in the developed world for this problem, being mostly surgical, are either not safely available in the developing world or provide too large a burden on health care costs. If this is the case, then many millions of women will have their quality of life severely depleted. Additionally, major changes are occurring in the status of women and the demand from them for better control of the problem will surely increase. So where to begin?

A definition of menorrhagia

Strictly speaking, menorrhagia is the regular loss of a menstrual fluid volume which exceeds the upper two standard deviations of the corrected mean blood loss of the population. Population based studies to define this level are only available for Swedish and British women (Hallberg *et al.* 1966; Cole *et al.* 1971).

There are no such studies for Oriental or African women. In clinical practice 31 per cent of British women describe their blood loss as heavy (Corrado 1990), but 40 per cent of women with proven heavy periods do not think their loss is excessive. Studies into the pathophysiology of the condition must therefore be guarded in the absence of measured menstrual blood loss. Furthermore great care must be used in assessing associative data which in the past have been used erroneously for evidence.

This is particularly so in a speciality which is predominantly surgical where surgeons need to persuade both themselves and their patients of the supremacy of their skills over the disease.

Hormones and menorrhagia

In the past, confusion arose from the misunderstanding that most women with the problem had anovulatory cycles and were in the early post-menarchal or late perimenopausal years. There have never been any reliable data to refute or substantiate this claim. Now it is clear that only about 10 per cent of women complaining of heavy periods are anovulatory (Cameron *et al.* 1990) but there are few data to describe the median and range of blood loss in women who bleed as a consequence of anovulatory cycles. This is not to deny that some women bleed very heavily after such a cycle but why this occurs on some occasions but not others is not known. The standard explanation is that there is a build up of endometrium under the proliferating influence of oestrogen which is not antagonized by progesterone. This can only be true for the epithelial cells which may eventually show cystic glandular hyperplasia. This is not an explanation for the increased menstrual loss. Steroids, as will be discussed, undoubtedly regulate many of the putative factors involved in menstrual bleeding but it is not clear which are the critical agents which induce and then regulate menstrual loss.

Menstruation

Any explanation of menorrhagia must start with an understanding of the normal process of menstruation, defined as the initiation of uterine bleeding consequent upon the systemic withdrawal of the ovarian steroids, oestradiol-17β and progesterone. As bleeding in these circumstances is predictable, it raises an important conceptual issue. Is heavy menstrual bleeding a disease or does it just reflect the upper range of normal loss? Certainly, as will be discussed, defined disease such as the presence of a large necrotic fibroid in the uterine cavity may cause heavy bleeding, but is menorrhagia a disease and does it reflect aberrant regulation of menstrual loss in women whose loss is within the normal range? Whilst a combination of mechanisms must initiate and regulate menstrual bleeding, three distinct mechanisms are suggested to control menstrual loss.

The vascular theory

The most celebrated explanation for both the initiation and regulation of menstrual loss is the vascular theory of Markee (1940). Oestrogen or progesterone withdrawal results in vasoconstriction of the spiral arterioles. The period of vasoconstriction lasts between 4 and 24 hours and is followed by vasodilatation and the flow of blood into the distal endometrium. There is no direct evidence to suggest that abnormalities of constriction contribute to excessive menstrual loss in women. Only associative and indirect evidence are available. In view of the presumed importance of this process, agents which regulate vascular tone have been studied extensively.

Prostaglandins

The consistent observation that non-steroidal anti-inflammatory drugs reduce menstrual blood loss by approximately 30 per cent in women with essential menorrhagia (Guillebaud *et al.* 1978; Fraser *et al.* 1981; Rybo *et al.* 1981; Hall *et al.* 1987; Cameron *et al.* 1990) and those with an IUCD *in situ* (Davies *et al.* 1981; Makarainen and Ylikorkala 1986) raised the prospect that prostaglandins (PGs), weak vasoregulatory agents, were involved in the process. Smith *et al.*

(1981*a*, *b*) showed a change in the ratio of PGs away from constricting $PGF_{2\alpha}$ to the neutral PGE_2. Reducing overall PG levels was assumed to reduce the effects of $PGF_{2\alpha}$. Non-steroidal anti-inflammatory drugs block PG production by antagonizing cyclo-oxygenase activity. It is presumed that the effect comes from inhibiting PGs which favour dilatation against those favouring constriction. There is no direct experimental evidence to substantiate this view and little has been added to this subject over the past 15 years!

Endothelins

Endothelins are widely recognized as potent constrictors of the vasculature. Cameron *et al.* (1993) demonstrated that the endometrium is a rich source of endothelin-1, and that endothelin A and B receptors are expressed in human endometrium (O'Reilly *et al.* 1993). Abnormalities of endothelin expression or of the receptors at the time of menses may thus be expected to result in altered vascular tone and increased menstrual loss. No studies have yet directly linked disturbances of endothelin/endothelin receptor expression to excessive menstrual loss, though reduced immunostaining for endothelin was demonstrated in the endometrium of women using the depot progestagen Norplant® (Marsh *et al.* 1995).

Nitric oxide

The recent identification of endothelium-derived relaxing factor as nitric oxide has raised the prospect of this agent being involved in menorrhagia. Nitric oxide synthase immunoreactivity and *in situ* hybridization demonstrated its expression in the endometrium but an association with abnormal bleeding has not yet been shown (Telfer *et al.* 1995, 1997). Similarly, agents altering nitric oxide generation have yet to be shown to alter menstrual blood loss.

Haemostasis

The process of haemostasis in the endometrium is not like that found in other parts of the body and more closely reflects fetal wound healing. This must be true otherwise the monthly repair of the endometrium would produce scar tissue with fibrosis similar to that seen with Asherman's syndrome. A key feature of haemostasis in the uterus is the changed nature of menstrual blood. It is assumed that coagulation occurs in the distal endometrium. This seems so because platelets found in the endometrial cavity are deactivated and do not respond to collagen as would normally be expected (Rees *et al.* 1984*a*). Fibrinolysis is mediated by plasmin which is prepared by proteolytic cleavage of plasminogen by urokinase-type and tissue-type plasminogen activators (uPA and tPA respectively) (Dano *et al.* 1985). In turn, these activators are controlled by inhibitors, Plasminogen Activator Inhibitor (PAI 1) and PAI 2 (Loskutoff *et al.* 1989; Kruithof 1990) which are expressed in endometrium (Casslen *et al.* 1995; Schatz *et al.* 1995). The endometrium is a rich source of tPA and uPA suggesting that coagulation occurs but is rapidly reversed by profound fibrinolysis. Menstrual endometrium is characterized by the absence of platelet fibrin clots in the lumen and broken surfaces of ruptured blood vessels (Christiaens *et al.* 1980). Normally the exposure of platelets to collagen and other extracellular matrices induces the clotting process with the deposition of fibrin/platelet plugs. These are only found in the endometrium on the first day of heavy bleeding. After that time they are absent.

The explanation for this finding is that menstrual loss is controlled by vasoconstriction in the basal part of the endometrium, thus obviating the need for coagulation. Two pieces of evidence further suggest the importance of this mechanism for the control of menstrual bleeding even if it is not similar to coagulation elsewhere in the body. Firstly, certain individuals with systemic bleeding disorders do have measured excessive menstrual blood loss (Fraser *et al.* 1986). Secondly, increased fibrinolytic activity has been shown in the endometrium of women with increased menstrual loss (Gleeson *et al.* 1993), and finally tranexamic acid, an inhibitor of fibrinolysis, reduces menstrual loss by about 50 per cent (Andersch *et al.* 1988; Gleeson *et al.* 1994; Preston *et al.* 1995).

Tissue growth and remodelling

Endometrium

More recently, the importance of growth factors and cytokines to the development of the endometrium has been appreciated (Smith and Haining 1991; Smith 1994*a*, *b*; Tabibzadeh 1991, 1994). Similarly, tissue remodelling is also dependent on the integrity of the extracellular matrix (ECM). The endometrium demonstrates the most profound hormone-dependent tissue remodelling in the body and these two factors are likely to be important in the process of menstruation. They will be described in this section because although there is as yet no direct evidence linking them to menorrhagia, it is likely that disorders of this system could be responsible for menorrhagia.

The most active proliferation occurs at the time of menstruation and begins on the second day of bleeding. This involves proliferation of the basal glands which, by the end of about the fifth day, has resulted in the complete re-epithelialization of the uterine surface. Although oestradiol has always been considered the proliferating agent, levels of this hormone are very low at this time. Perhaps the best known growth factor regulating epithelial proliferation is epidermal growth factor (EGF).EGF is expressed in human epithelial cells throughout the menstrual cycle (Haining *et al.* 1991*a*, *b*) and stimulates endometrial epithelial cell proliferation (Haining *et al.* 1991*b*; Zhang *et al.* 1995). Expression of EGF and its receptor EGF-R is induced by oestradiol. The assumption must be that there is sufficient EGF in the residual glands to stimulate growth in the circumstances of the menstruating endometrium. Once oestradiol secretion increases in the proliferative phase, then the hormone probably mediates its action by genomic mechanisms. Certainly EGF can mimic the proliferative effects of oestradiol on the endometrium in transgenic mice lacking the oestradiol receptor (Ignar Trowbridge *et al.* 1992, 1993). Clearly a large number of growth factors, including the insulin-like growth factors (IGFs) and their binding proteins, are expressed in endometrium and EGF, IGF, and fibroblast growth factors (FGFs) all promote cellular proliferation (Smith 1994*a*, *b*; Tabibzadeh 1994). However, there is no evidence to date which indicates that altered wound healing is a factor in the aetiology of menorrhagia.

Vasculature

As bleeding arises from blood vessels an additional explanation of heavy bleeding is impaired repair of the damaged blood vessels of the endometrium. It was calculated that about 70 per cent of the volume of menstrual loss arises from the spiral arterioles. Most bleeding occurs in the first three days of the period (Haynes *et al.* 1977). Impaired repair may contribute to the excessive loss. Repair of the vasculature must occur within two to three days of the onset of bleeding. As might be expected, this remarkable regenerative process depends on high levels of angiogenic growth factors. Apart from the endometrium and the ovary, endothelial cell turnover in the adult animal is usually very slow.

An increasing number of angiogenic growth factors are now recognized (Risau 1990; Smith 1994*b*). The most well known are the family of fibroblast growth factors. Immunoreactive FGF 1 and 2 is present in epithelial cells of the endometrium throughout the cycle. Other studies indicate that the FGF 2 protein is stimulated in endometrium by oestradiol and suppressed by progesterone (Presta 1988). The issues concerning FGFs relate to the precise mechanism of their biological regulation. Firstly, they do not contain a secretory signal sequence and should not be secreted from the epithelial cells. However, FGFs could be released with the extensive tissue destruction and cell death that arises at menstruation. Most likely, they are then deposited on heparan sulphate proteoglycans of the extracellular matrix (ECM) and released following enzymatic degradation of the matrix. However, immunohistochemical staining does not support this view as there is little immunoreactivity for FGFs in the ECM. This does not mean that FGFs are not released acutely at menses. Surprisingly, FGF immunoreactivity is elevated in post-menopausal endometrium compared to that of pre-menopausal tissue.

Vascular endothelial growth factor (VEGF) is a multiple spliced heterodimeric growth factor with significant angiogenic activity (Gospodarowicz *et al.* 1989; Ferrara and Henzel 1989; Connolly *et al.* 1989; Tischer *et al.* 1991). Unlike FGF, the coding sequence contains a secretory signal domain resulting in the ability of cells to release the protein. The splicing removes various exons, one of which contains the heparin binding domain. This results in the secretion of different splice variants which vary in their cellular localization. The higher molecular weight proteins 206, 189, and 165 bind heparin and are present, like FGF, in the ECM and attached to proteoglycans on the cell surface. The 145 variant may be preferentially expressed in malignant tissue whilst the 121 type does not bind heparin. VEGF is expressed by a variety of cells in the endometrium (Charnock-Jones *et al.* 1993). It is expressed throughout the menstrual cycle by the glandular epithelium. In addition, it is secreted by macrophages which constitute about 8 per cent of the endometrial cell types. It also appears to be expressed by the large decidual cells found clustered around spiral arterioles in the latter part of the luteal phase of the cycle (Sharkey *et al.* 1996). Unlike the FGFs, levels of mRNA encoding the protein are increased in the presence of progesterone and are highest in secretory endometrium (Sharkey, personal communication). This steroidal regulation, however, is two orders of magnitude lower than the regulation exerted by hypoxia. Levels of VEGF mRNA are greatest in glandular epithelium at the time of menses (Charnock-Jones *et al.* 1993). VEGF expression is upregulated by hypoxia and the assumption is that the intense vasoconstriction which precedes menstruation induces distal hypoxia and increased expression of VEGF. This would be appropriate as rapid angiogenesis will be needed once the functional layer is lost. No studies have yet demonstrated reduced VEGF synthesis in the endometrium of women with menorrhagia. Other cytokines are almost certainly involved in this complex interplay between vascular control and tissue remodelling. Tumour necrosis factor (TNF)α released by macrophages around the spiral arterioles is responsible for changes in vascular tone, and Critchley *et al.* (1995) have also shown increased immunoreactive interleukin 8 around spiral arterioles.

The endometrium is a rich source of cytokines, many of the functions of which are pleiotrophic, and new means of identifying the key agents are going to be needed before the central pathways can be defined and then applied to the clinical situation.

Matrix

An alternative hypothesis to that of spiral arteriolar constriction is that of enhanced matrix degradation. The extracellular matrix promotes the structural integrity of tissue. The matrix components include collagens, fibronectin, laminin, gelatins, entactins, hyaluronic acid, and proteoglycans. Cellular expression of the heterodimeric integrins in endometrium provides the link between the ECM and individual cells of the endometrium (Hynes 1987; Ruoslahti *et al.* 1991; Lessey *et al.* 1992, 1994). Degradation of the matrix is regulated by the matrix metalloproteinases (MMPs). Three broad groups of enzymes have been described which include collagenases, gelatinases, and stromelysins (Tabibzadeh and Babaknia 1995). Endometrial stroma is known to express MMP-1, MMP-2 (type IV collagenase), MMP-3 (stromelysin-1), and MMP-10. The epithelium expresses MMP-7 (matrilysin). This expression is controlled by progesterone (Osteen *et al.* 1994; Schatz *et al.* 1994). Interestingly, epithelial expression of MMP-7 is suppressed by transforming growth factor (TGFβ_2) synthesized in the stromal compartment which is further regulated by progesterone. Removal of progesterone would be expected to withdraw the suppressive action and release metalloproteinase activity. This should result in degradation of the matrix and breakdown of the endometrium.

However, this is almost certainly too simple an explanation. Tissue inhibitors of metalloproteinase activity, TIMP-1 and -2, are expressed in human endometrium (Rodgers *et al.* 1992; Hampton and Salamonsen 1994). It is suggested that TGFβ also regulates degradative enzyme expression by inducing TIMP-1 expression in the endometrium (Graham *et al.* 1992). There is clearly a complex regulatory mechanism which keeps degradation under control. There are no published studies as yet which tie any of these compounds to disorders of menstruation.

Potentially, disorders of matrix arrangement would be expected to be more important for premenstrual bleeding, though if menorrhagia does arise from deranged tissue remodelling it could conceivably be relevant.

Uterine fibroids

There is a consistent view that uterine fibroids cause excessive menstrual blood loss. Over 30 per cent of uteri removed for menorrhagia have fibroids (Carlson *et al.* 1993). However, there is no evidence that in general fibroids cause heavy periods, except in rare cases. The problem with the data as they stand is that most women who have a hysterectomy for heavy periods do not have heavy periods and the underlying incidence of fibroids is very high. There is a poor correlation between uterine cavity volume and measured menstrual blood loss, and a poor clinical correlation between fibroid size and subjective menorrhagia (Rees *et al.* 1984*b*). However, there is a greater consensus with respect to intrauterine or submucosal fibroids. But again great caution must be applied in assessing associative data. Indeed the only way forward at present is individual case studies which are of limited scientific value. None the less, we recently completed a study in two women which emphasizes the point. Both patients had measured menstrual blood loss in excess of 1 litre. One patient had a pedunculated 5 × 5 cm intra-cavity fibroid. Removal of the fibroid returned the patient's periods to normal. In the second case multiple small submucosal fibroids (>17) were present, hysteroscopic excision of which, again resulted in normal periods. Fraser *et al.* (1986) reported on four cases of leiomyomata treated by myomectomy in which the measured mean menstrual blood loss declined from 304 ml to a mean of 52 ml.

Uterine polyps

There is little evidence to link intrauterine polyps with menorrhagia. Here again the problem is one of definition and reporting. Most gynaecologists do not see enough cases with measured menstrual blood loss to undertake such studies and the underlying incidence of the finding is unknown.

Considerations on the pathophysiology of menstruation

It is fair to say that the precise cause of excessive menstrual bleeding arising from the withdrawal of oestradiol-17β and/or progesterone remains unknown. Several tantalizing features point to putative explanations. Firstly, disturbances in prostaglandin release are consistently found in women with proven heavy periods with or without an intrauterine contraceptive device *in situ* (Smith *et al.* 1981*a*; Rees *et al.* 1984*c*; Ylikorkala and Vinnikka 1983) and inhibitors of PG synthesis reduce menstrual blood loss. Secondly, abnormalities of coagulation are found in the endometrium and again inhibitors of fibrinolysis produce, on average, a 50 per cent reduction of menstrual blood loss (Preston *et al.* 1995). More recent studies identifying the complex interplay between cells and the extracellular matrix and the determination that steroids, through growth factors, can regulate this relationship point to a further mechanism. Tissue degradation arising from progesterone withdrawal would clearly be consistent with the observed changes of menstruation. As yet no pathological changes in this system have been found. However, new agents which interfere with tissue remodelling may be of therapeutic benefit in the future. Similarly, progestogens delivered to the uterine cavity seem to provide a highly effective treatment for menorrhagia probably acting via a range of mechanisms including inhibition of proliferation and regulation of tissue degradation. Gene transfer to the endometrium may provide an additional means of delivering genes to the uterus without the concomitant systemic side-effects associated with current medication (Charnock-Jones *et al.* 1997).

All of these new strategies will be needed to provide women with the type of choice they will want to make in order to redress the biological imbalance of menstrual function arising from the widespread desire to restrict family size.

References

Andersch, B., Milson, I., and Rybo, G. (1988). An objective evaluation of flurbiprofen and tranexamic acid in the treatment of idiopathic menorrhagia. *Acta Obstetrica Gynecologica Scandinavica*, **67**, 645–8.

Bradlow, J., Coulter, A., and Brooks, P. (1992). *Patterns of referral.* Oxford Health Services Research Unit.

Cameron, I.T., Haining, R., Lumsden, M.A., Thomas, V.R., and Smith, S.K. (1990). The effects of mefenamic acid and norethisterone on measured menstrual blood loss. *Obstetrics and Gynecology*, **76**, 85–8.

Cameron, I.T., Plumpton, C., Champeney, R., van Papendorp, C.L., Ashby, M.J., and Davenport, A.P. (1993). Identification of endothelin-1, endothelin-2 and endothelin-3 in human endometrium. *Journal of Reproduction and Fertility*, **98**, 251–5.

Carlson, K.J., Nichols, D.H., and Schiff, I. (1993). Indications for hysterectomy. *New England Journal of Medicine*, **328**, 856–60.

Casslen, B., Nordengren, J., Gustavsson, B., Nilbert, M., and Lund, L.R. (1995). Progesterone stimulates degradation of urokinase plasminogen activator (u-PA) in endometrial stromal cells by increasing its inhibitor and surface expression of the u-PA receptor. *Journal of Clinical Endocrinology and Metabolism*, **80**, 2776–84.

Charnock-Jones, D.S., Sharkey, A.M., Rajput-Williams, J., Burch, D., Schofield, J.P., Fountain, S.A., *et al.* (1993). Identification and localization of alternatively spliced mRNAs for vascular endothelial growth factor in human uterus and oestrogen regulation in endometrial carcinoma cell lines. *Biology of Reproduction*, **48**, 1120–8.

Charnock-Jones, D.S., Sharkey, A.M., Jaggers, D.C., Jin Yoo, H., Heap, R.B., and Smith, S.K. (1997). In-vivo gene transfer to the uterine endometrium. *Human Reproduction*, **12**, 17–20.

Christiaens, G.C.M.L., Sixma, J.J., and Haspels, A.A. (1980). Morphology of haemostasis in menstrual endometrium. *British Journal of Obstetrics and Gynaecology*, **87**, 425–39.

Cole, S., Billewicz, W., and Thomson, A. (1971). Sources of variation in menstrual blood loss. *Journal of Obstetrics and Gynaecology of the British Commonwealth*, **78**, 933–9.

Connolly, D.T., Heuvelman, D., Nelson, R., Olander, J.V., Eppley, B.L., Delfino, V.J., *et al.* (1989). Tumor vascular permeability factor stimulates endothelial cell growth and angiogenesis. *Journal of Clinical Investigation*, **84**, 1470–8.

Corrado, M. (1990). *Women's health in 1990*. Research study conducted on behalf of Parke-Davies Research Laboratories. MORT (Market Opinion and Research International).

Critchley, H.O.D., Susil, B., Kooy, J., Mamers, P.M., Healy, D.L., and Rogers, P.A.W. (1995). Endometrial histology and vascular appearance following endometrial ablation. *Gynaecological Endoscopy*, **4**, 27–33.

Dano, K., Andreasen, P.A., Grondahl-Hansen, J., Kristensen, P., Nielsen, L.S., and Skriver, J. (1985). Plasminogen activators, tissue degradation and cancer. *Advances in Cancer Research*, **44**, 139–266.

Davies, A.J., Anderson, A.B.M., and Turnbull, A.C. (1981). Reduction by naproxen of excessive menstrual bleeding in women using intrauterine devices. *Obstetrics and Gynecology*, **57**, 74–8.

Ferrara, N. and Henzel, W.J. (1989). Pituitary follicular cells secrete a novel heparin binding growth factor specific for vascular endothelial cells. *Biochemical and Biophysical Research Communications*, **161**, 851–8.

Fraser, I.S., Pearse, C., Shearman, R.P., Elliott, P.M. McIlveen, J., and Markham, R. (1981). Efficacy of mefenamic acid in patients with a complaint of menorrhagia. *Obstetrics and Gynecology*, **58**, 543–51.

Fraser, I.S., McCarron, G., and Markham, R. (1986). Measured menstrual blood loss in women with menorrhagia associated with pelvic disease or coagulation disorder. *Obstetrics and Gynecology*, **68**, 630–3.

Gleeson, N., Devitt, M., Sheppard, B.L., and Bonnar, J. (1993). Endometrial fibrinolytic enzymes in women with normal menstruation and dysfunctional uterine bleeding. *British Journal of Obstetrics and Gynaecology*, **100**, 768–71.

Gleeson, N.C., Buggy, F., Sheppard, B.L., and Bonnar, J. (1994). The effect of tranexamic acid on measured menstrual loss and endometrial fibrinolytic enzymes in dysfunctional uterine bleeding. *Acta Obstetricia et Gynecologica Scandinavica*, **73**, 274–7.

Gospodarowicz, D., Abraham, J.A., and Schilling, J. (1989). Isolation and characterisation of a vascular endothelial cell mitogen produced by pituitary-derived folliculo stellate cells. *Proceedings of the National Academy of Sciences USA*, **86**, 7311–15.

Graham, C.H., Lysiak, J.J., McCrae, K.R., and Lala, P.D. (1992). Localization of transforming growth factor-beta at the human fetal–maternal interface: role in trophoblast growth and differentiation. *Biology of Reproduction*, **46**, 561–72.

Grimes, D.A. (1994). Shifting indications for hysterectomy: nature, nurture, or neither? *Lancet*, **344**, 1652–3.

Guillebaud, J., Anderson, A.B.M., and Turnbull, A.C. (1978). Reduction by mefenamic acid of increased menstrual blood loss associated with intrauterine contraception. *British Journal of Obstetrics and Gynaecology*, **85**, 53–62.

Haining, R.E.B., Schofield, J.P., Jones, D.S.C., Rajput-Williams, J., and Smith, S.K. (1991a). The identification of mRNA for EGF and TGFα present in low copy number in human endometrium and decidua using RT-PCR. *Journal of Molecular Endocrinology*, **6**, 207–14.

Haining, R.E.B., Cameron, I.T., van Papendorp, C., Davenport, A.P., Prentice, A., Thomas, E.J., and Smith, S.K. (1991*b*). Epidermal growth factor in human endometrium: proliferative effects in culture and immunocytochemical localization in normal and endometriotic tissue. *Human Reproduction*, **6**, 1200–5.

Hall, P. Maclachlan, N., Thorn, N., Nudd, M.W.E., Taylor, C.G., and Garrioch, D.B. (1987). Control of menorrhagia by the cyclo-oxygenase inhibitors naproxen sodium and mefenamic acid. *British Journal of Obstetrics and Gynaecology*, **94**, 554–8.

Hallberg, L., Hogdahl, A.M., Nilsson, L., and Rybo, G. (1966). Menstrual blood loss – a population study. *Acta Obstetrica Gynecologica Scandinavica*, **45**, 320–51.

Hampton, A.L. and Salamonsen, L.A. (1994). Expression of messenger ribonucleic acid encoding matrix metalloproteinases and their tissue inhibitors is related to menstruation. *Journal of Endocrinology*, **141**, R1–3.

Haynes, P., Hodgson, H., Anderson, A., and Turnbull, A. (1977). Measurement of menstrual blood loss in patients complaining of menorrhagia. *British Journal of Obstetrics and Gynaecology*, **84**, 763–8.

Hynes, R.O. (1987). Integrins: a family of cell surface receptors. *Cell*, **48**, 549–54.

Ignar Trowbridge, D.M., Nelson, K.G., Bidwell, M.C., Curtis, S.W., Washburn, T.F., McLachlan, J.A., and Korach, K.S. (1992). Coupling of dual signaling pathways: epidermal growth factor action involves the estrogen receptor. *Proceedings of the National Academy of Sciences USA*, **89**, 4658–62.

Ignar Trowbridge, D.M., Teng, C.T., Ross, K.A., Parker, M.G., Korach, K.S., and McLachlan, J.A. (1993). Peptide growth factors elicit estrogen receptor-dependent transcriptional activation of an estrogen-responsive element. *Molecular Endocrinology*, **7**, 992–8.

Kruithof, E.K.O. (1990). Plasminogen activator inhibitor type 2: biochemical and biological aspects. In *Protease inhibitors* (ed. A. Takada, M.M. Sumama, and D. Collen), pp. 15–22. Elsevier, Amsterdam.

Lessey, B.A., Damjanovich, L., Coutfaris, C., Castelbaum, A., Albelda, S.M., and Buck, C.A. (1992). Integrin adhesion molecules in the human endometrium. Correlation with the normal and abnormal menstrual cycle. *Journal of Clinical Investigation*, **90**, 188–95.

Lessey, B.A., Castelbaum, A.J., Buck, C.A., Lei, Y., Yowell, C.W., and Sun, J. (1994). Further characterization of endometrial integrins during the menstrual cycle and in pregnancy. *Fertility and Sterility*, **62**, 497–506.

Loskutoff, D.J., Sawdey, M., and Mimuro, J. (1989). Type 1 plasminogen activator. *Progress in Hemostasis and Thrombosis*, **9**, 87–115.

Makarainen, L. and Ylikorkala, O. (1986). Ibuprofen prevents IUCD-induced increases in menstrual blood loss. *British Journal of Obstetrics and Gynaecology*, **93**, 285–8.

Markee, J.E. (1940). Menstruation in intraocular endometrial transplants in the rhesus monkey. *Contributions to Embryology, Carnegie Institute*, **28**, 219–308.

Marsh, M.M., Butt, A.R., Riley, S.C., Rogers, P.A.W., Susil, B, Affandi, B.A., *et al.* (1995). Immunolocalization of endothelin and neutral endopeptidase in the endometrium of users of subdermally implanted levonorgestrel (Norplant®). *Human Reproduction*, **10**, 2584–9.

O'Reilly, G., Charnock-Jones, D.S., Davenport, A.P., Cameron, I.T., and Smith. S.K. (1992). Presence of messenger ribonucleic acid for endothelin-1, endothelin-2, and endothelin-3 in human endometrium and a change in the ratio of ETA and ETB receptor subtype across the menstrual cycle. *Journal of Clinical Endocrinology and Metabolism*, **75**, 1545–9.

Osteen, K.G., Rodgers, W.H., Gaire, M., Hargrove, J.T., Gorstein, F., and Matrisian, L.M. (1994). Stromal–epithelial interaction mediates steroidal regulation of metalloproteinase expression in human endometrium. *Proceedings of the National Academy of Sciences USA*, **91**, 10129–33.

Presta, M. (1988). Sex hormones modulate the synthesis of basic fibroblast growth factor in human endometrial adenocarcinoma cells: implications for the neovascularization of normal and neoplastic endometrium. *Journal of Cellular Physiology*, **137**, 593–7.

Preston, J.T., Cameron, I.T., Adams, E.J., and Smith, S.K. (1995). Comparative study of tranexamic acid and norethisterone in the treatment of ovulatory menorrhagia. *British Journal of Obstetrics and Gynaecology*, **102**, 401–6.

Rees, M.C.P., Demers, L.M., Anderson, A.B.M., and Turnbull, A.C. (1984*a*). A functional study of platelets in menstrual fluid. *British Journal of Obstetrics and Gynaecology*, **91**, 667–73.

Rees, M.C.P., Dunnill, M.S., Anderson, A.B.M., and Turnbull, A.C. (1984*b*). Quantitative uterine histology during the menstrual cycle in relation to measured menstrual blood loss. *British Journal of Obstetrics and Gynaecology*, **91**, 662–6.

Rees, M.C.P., Anderson, A.B.M., Demers, L.M., and Turnbull, A.C. (1984*c*). Endometrial and myometrial prostaglandin release during the menstrual cycle in relation to menstrual blood loss. *Journal of Clinical Endocrinology and Metabolism*, **58**, 813–18.

Risau, W. (1990). Angiogenic growth factors. *Progress in Growth Factor Research*, **2**, 71–9.

Rodgers, W.H., Osteen, K.G., Matrisian, L.M., Navbre, M., Guidice, L.C., and Gorstein, F. (1992). Expression and localization of matrilysin, a matrix metalloproteinase in human endometrium during the reproductive cycle. *American Journal of Obstetrics and Gynecology*, **168**, 253–60.

Rouslahti, E. and Yamaguchi, Y. (1991). Proteoglycans as modulators of growth factor activities. *Cell*, **64**, 867–9.

Ruoslahti, E. (1991). Integrins. *Journal of Clinical Investigation*, **87**, 1–5.

Rybo, G., Nilsson, S., Sikstrom, B., and Nygren, K.G. (1981). Naproxen in menorrhagia. *Lancet*, **i**, 608–9.

Schatz, F., Papp, C., Toth Pal, E., and Lockwood, C.J. (1994). Ovarian steroid-modulated stromelysin-1 expression in human endometrial stromal and decidual cells. *Journal of Clinical Endocrinology and Metabolism*, **78**, 1467–72.

Schatz, F., Aigner, S., Papp, C., Toth Pal, E., Hausknecht, V., and Lockwood, C.J. (1995). Plasminogen activator activity during decidualization of human endometrial stromal cells is regulated by plasminogen activator inhibitor 1. *Journal of Clinical Endocrinology and Metabolism*, **80**, 2504–10.

Smith, S.K. (1994*a*). Growth factors in the human endometrium. *Human Reproduction*, **9**, 936–46.

Smith, S.K. (1994*b*). Angiogenic growth factor expression in human pregnancy. In *Early fetal growth and development* (ed. R.H.T. Ward, S.K. Smith, and D. Donnai), pp. 183–96. Royal College of Obstetricians and Gynaecologists.

Smith, S.K. and Haining, R.E.B. (1991). The investigation and management of excessive menstrual bleeding. In *Recent advances in obstetrics and gynaecology*, Vol. 17, (ed. J. Bonnar), pp. 171–89. Churchill Livingstone, Edinburgh.

Smith, S.K., Abel, M.H., Kelly, R.W., and Baird, D.T. (1981*a*). Prostaglandin synthesis in the endometrium of women with ovular dysfunctional uterine bleeding. *British Journal of Obstetrics and Gynaecology*, **88**, 434–42.

Smith, S.K., Abel, M.H., Kelly, R.W., and Baird, D.T. (1981*b*). A role for prostacyclin (PG12) in excessive menstrual bleeding. *Lancet*, **i**, 522–4.

Tabibzadeh, S. (1991). Human endometrium; an active site of cytokine production and action. *Endocrine Reviews*, **12**, 272–90.

Tabibzadeh, S. (1994). Cytokines and the hypothalamic–pituitary–ovarian–endometrial axis. *Human Reproduction*, **9**, 947–67.

Tabibzadeh, S. and Babaknia, A. (1995). The signals and molecular pathways involved in implantation, a symbiotic interaction between blastocyst and endometrium involving adhesion and tissue invasion. *Molecular Human Reproduction*, **1**, 1579–602.

Telfer, J.F., Lyall, F., Norman, J.E., and Cameron, I.T. (1995). Identification of nitric oxide synthase in human uterus. *Human Reproduction*, **10**, 19–23.

Telfer, J.F., Irvine, G.A., Kohnen, G., Campbell, S., and Cameron, I.T. (1997). Expression of endothelial and inducible nitric oxide synthase in non-pregnant and decidualized human endometrium. *Molecular Human Reproduction* **3**, 69–75.

Tischer, E., Mitchell, R., Hartman, T., Silva, M., Gospodarovicz, D., Fiddes, J.C., and Abraham, J.A. (1991). The human gene for vascular endothelial growth factor. *Journal of Biological Chemistry*, **266**, 11947–54.

Ylikorkala, O. and Vinnikka, L. (1983). Comparison between antifibrinolytic and antiprostaglandin treatment in the reduction of increased menstrual blood loss in women with intrauterine contraceptive devices. *British Journal of Obstetrics and Gynaecology*, **90**, 78–83.

Zhang, L., Rees, M.C.P., and Bicknell, R. (1995). The isolation and long term culture of normal human endometrial epithelium and stroma. *Journal of Cell Science*, **108**, 323–31.

8 Menstrual problems in adolescence

D. Keith Edmonds

Introduction

During adolescence, girls become preoccupied with the physical and emotional changes which occur over a number of years, and which translate the girl into a fully sexually and reproductively competent adult female. These changes are also associated with changes in emotional and intellectual status, which identify the adult female as different from the adult male. The outward changes of breast growth, pubic hair and axillary hair growth, and the attainment of full adult height usually precede the outward manifestation of maturity, i.e. the menarche. For many girls their first menstrual period is truly the sign of adulthood and psychologically extremely important to achieve. However, it is also associated with times of stress and the absolute wish to be normal. Thus, changes that occur which are abnormal may have a very serious impact on psychological well-being. Being normal as an adolescent and accepted as a normal member of that peer group is extremely important. In differentiating the range of normality from true abnormality, an understanding of the onset and control of puberty is essential, as in many cases, misinformation leads these adolescent teenagers to states of anxiety which can be well avoided, and a deep knowledge and understanding of the adolescent will make management effective and help her to achieve normal adulthood. In fact, in some cases, poor management of menstrual problems at the time of adolescence may leave her with a life-long menstrual phobia which may be used in later life as a prop against adversity.

The neuroendocrinology of puberty

The outward physical changes of puberty are a result of the production of oestradiol-17β from the ovary. The ovary is capable of producing oestradiol in response to FSH stimulation at any time during fetal life or infancy (Kaplan *et al.* 1976; Lee 1988). The oocytes are incorporated into the ovary in very early embryonic life at around five to six weeks gestation, and from 20 weeks gestation onwards have the potential to produce oestradiol in normal quantities. It is the lack of FSH secretion during childhood that leaves the female infant without oestradiol. The pituitary gland itself is capable of producing FSH throughout life if the appropriate stimulus is applied, (i.e. gonadotrophin releasing hormone, GnRH), and, in fact the hypothalamus itself is capable of producing and secreting ample amounts of GnRH to maintain full function of the pituitary also (Yen 1991). Thus, the control of the onset of puberty must begin when the hypothalamus receives its stimulus to release GnRH and this stimulus has to come from a higher central level in the brain.

The neuroendocrine system consists of three strata – the pituitary gland, the arcuate nucleus of the medial basal hypothalamus, and the higher cortical centres. The arcuate nucleus controls GnRH release with intermittent bursts of secretion into the hypothalamo-pituitary circulation. The pulse generator is probably within the GnRH-secreting neurones, and neurotransmitters from higher centres in the CNS may either stimulate or inhibit the release of GnRH. A number of hypotheses are currently being explored to try to explain this control mechanism. Modulators which have been suggested to play a role are noradrenaline, dopamine, central opiates, neuropeptide Y, glutamate, aspartate, and other neuroactive amino acids (Lee 1988; Gore *et al.* 1993; Prasad *et al.* 1993; Brann 1995). It seems that the control of GnRH release involves activation of the *N*-methyl-D-aspartate receptor in the hypothalamus and it is possible that, in conjunction with epidermal growth factor (EGF) receptors which seem also to be activated at the time of puberty, this is the way in which the control of GnRH secretion is modulated (Bourguignon *et al.* 1992; Brann 1995). Recently work from Ma *et al.* (1994) has suggested that the gene encoding for transforming growth factor α is activated at this time and thus there is now scientific evidence to suggest that the onset of puberty is genetically controlled and it would seem at the present time this is likely to be a gene which activates both the *N*-methyl-D-aspartate and EGF receptors. This activation of the receptor would explain why the downregulated state of childhood has been previously unexplained, i.e. that the hypothalamus and pituitary seem to be insensitive to the oestradiol feedback mechanisms that they become so sensitive to in adult life. Thus, in childhood the activation of these genes changes the sensitivity back to normal, similar to the fetal state in which there was no suppression. One may further postulate that outside central influences such as weight loss or exercise may well influence the receptor gene, thereby either delaying the onset of puberty or, in the post-pubertal female, inducing secondary amenorrhoea through exactly the same mechanism of switching off the gene and thus inactivating the receptor.

The normal onset of puberty

Pulsatile release of gonadotrophins, in response to central pulsatile release of GnRH, begins around eight or nine years of age and is first detected during the sleep period. Eventually these episodic releases of FSH and LH increase throughout the nocturnal period and extend into pulsations which can be detected throughout the 24 hour day. The amplitude of these pulses, which is initially quite high during the nocturnal period, falls and eventually the adult pattern of gonadotrophin pulses is manifest with inherent ovarian response and oestradiol production. GnRH pulses occur, on average, every 60 to 90 minutes in the follicular and early luteal phases of the menstrual cycle; and from the middle to late luteal phases, the frequency diminishes to every 180 minutes (Boyer *et al.* 1974). Before the onset of menstruation, the initiation of a new menstrual cycle begins with late luteal phase increases in FSH secretion, which initiates the next recruitment of follicles for the ensuing cycle.

The timing of the onset of puberty has been changing over the past 100 years, and there is no doubt that in those countries which have improved their socioeconomic status the onset of puberty has occurred at an increasingly early age. In 1905 the mean age of menarche in the United Kingdom was 15 years (Kennedy 1933), but by 1980 the mean age of the onset of puberty was 12.6 years with a range of 10 to 16 years (Wyshak 1983). The attainment of significant body weight seems to be closely related with the initiation of puberty and conversely the failure to attain adequate body fat (e.g. anorexia nervosa of childhood) is closely associated with a delay in the onset of puberty. It would seem therefore that the maturation process which leads to the activation of the gene involved in GnRH secretion is influenced by ideal environmental factors for reproduction and that failure to attain these criteria prevents the gene from being switched on, thereby avoiding pregnancy in an undesirably underweight female. It may be that the modulator of this process is production of central β endorphins as part of the control mechanism (Quigley *et al.* 1980). Other than socioeconomic conditions, chronic disease may also influence the age of onset of puberty, particularly central disabilities. It is interesting to note that the mean ages of menarche in children with neural tube defects, epilepsy, and cerebral palsy are all earlier than the mean for the normal population (Edmonds 1989). However, puberty may be delayed in these children because chronic illness restricts their ability to achieve normal weight gain.

The secondary sexual characteristic changes of puberty are manifest in a cascade of events which usually follows a typical pattern. Breast and pubic hair development usually begin together and this is followed by a growth spurt and then the onset of menarche; axillary hair growth tends to be the last of the secondary sexual characteristics to appear. The secondary sexual characteristics are classified into five stages as reported by Tanner (1962). This classification should be used when clinical assessment of puberty is being made.

Menstrual patterns in adolescence

The majority of early menstrual cycles are irregular and anovulatory. This is hardly surprising when, with our understanding of the neuroendocrine control of the onset of puberty, the process is a gradual one leading to the eventual adult pattern of GnRH secretion. This evolution takes on average 10 years from age 7 to 17, and menarche will therefore occur at a somewhat random time during this 10 year period, when endometrial growth is sufficient to induce a menstrual loss. Thus, the pattern of GnRH secretion and subsequent pulsatile release of FSH will give widely ranging levels of oestradiol in the circulation, and as a result of this, widely different endometrial responses. The failure to achieve the adult pulsatile pattern of cyclicity immediately is completely normal, and therefore irregular anovulatory cycles in the initial years of puberty are inevitable. In the study by Apter and Vikho (1987) the pattern of early cycles was studied using progesterone concentrations as an indicator of ovulation. Studies prior to this used basal body temperature charts as a means of detecting ovulation and these are notoriously unreliable, although the studies by Vollman (1977) and Dewhurst *et al.* (1971) found similar results. Apter and Vikho (1987) showed that 85 per cent of cycles in the first post-menarchal year are anovulatory, and during the ensuing nine years post-menarchally, the fully ovulatory cycle is achieved in 100 per cent of cases, reflecting hypothalamo-pituitary ovarian maturation. Anovulatory cycles are notoriously irregular and therefore, any adolescent female presenting with irregular cycles in which there is no concern about heavy menstrual loss need only be reassured, if her development is otherwise normal. In the vast majority of cases maturation over the ensuing years will bring regular menstrual cycles associated with normal fertility.

Menstrual abnormalities in adolescence

As we have seen, the problems of menstrual disorder in the adolescent are aberrations of hypothalamic control in the vast majority of cases. The normal menstrual flow that a woman can expect is on average around 30 ml per cycle with an upper limit of 80 ml per cycle (Hallberg *et al.* 1966). Bleeding that occurs at less than 21 days or with greater than seven days duration may be considered abnormal, but not infrequently cycle length may be prolonged and when menstruation occurs it can be very heavy. These cycles are almost entirely anovulatory and are seen at the extremes of reproductive life, in adolescence and in the perimenopausal woman. Adolescents presenting with disorders of menstruation must be very carefully evaluated. It is more common for the mothers of adolescent girls to recount the menstrual difficulties rather than the girl herself, and it is this maternal anxiety that often brings girls to the gynaecologist. Very often, if interviewed separately, girls will declare a much less anxious attitude towards their periods than their mothers are expressing. This form of imprinting of menstrual abnormalities is a very difficult one to overcome, and mothers who have perceived menstrual problems themselves may imprint the fear of the menstrual period on to their daughters. When these children are investigated, they are found to have completely normal menstrual loss, but their fear and anxiety may give them a false impression of their periods. Thus, great care must be taken in truly evaluating the menstrual loss patterns of adolescents.

It is important to exclude an organic cause for the disorder, and therefore anovulatory bleeding is a diagnosis of exclusion. Rarely, teenagers may have carcinomas of the vagina or cervix, or occasionally granulosa cell tumours of the ovary leading to oestrogen production and heavy menstrual loss. They may also have polycystic ovarian disease, and this may well be the basis of the anovulatory state. However, great care has to be taken in diagnosing this condition, as ultrasonically, the ovaries may well have a polycystic appearance in adolescents, but this is more likely to be the multi-cystic ovary and until a detailed endocrine evaluation has been performed to support the ultrasound changes in the ovary, then the diagnosis must be made with great caution. Rarely some children may have coagulation disorders. In the much quoted paper of Claessens and Cowell (1981), it was suggested that 19 per cent of teenagers presenting with abnormal uterine bleeding might have a primary coagulation disorder. However, this has been questioned as not the experience that most gynaecologists have had, and in a recent study by Falcone *et al.* (1994), a 10 year review of the primary diagnosis of dysfunctional bleeding in three paediatric hospitals in Montreal revealed bleeding disorders in only two of 61 patients. One of these had immune thrombocytopenic purpura and the other had acute promyelocytic leukaemia. The diagnosis of a coagulation disorder must always be borne in mind, but the diagnosis would seem to be quite rare.

In evaluating the diagnosis of bleeding disorders in adolescents, the best screening test is a full blood count. It is then possible to make a clinically objective assessment of the severity of the bleeding, and thereafter to use this in management. Girls who truly seem to be bleeding very heavily may rarely have normal values of haemoglobin, but their ferritin concentrations may be reduced, indicating iron deficiency without anaemia. Therefore, the additional measurement of plasma ferritin may be justified in some cases. However, the majority of cases may be classified on haemoglobin alone. The full blood count allows assessment of platelets, thereby excluding idiopathic thrombocytopenia if necessary. In approaching the treatment, therefore, one can divide patients into three groups – those with haemoglobin concentrations greater than 12 g per 100 ml, those with between 10 and 12 g, and those with less than 10 g per 100 ml.

Normal haemoglobin concentration

In this group of patients the most important treatment is reassurance. Here, menstrual dysfunction is probably not associated with excessive menstrual loss and, although this may be inconvenient, it is not a health hazard. In the vast majority of cases, by simple explanation and reassurance that the cycle will in fact establish a normal pattern, no further treatment will be necessary. It is important to follow these adolescents up at six-monthly intervals until their cycle is established so that they have the support that they need to achieve the normality they expect.

Mild to moderate anaemia

In those children whose haemoglobin concentrations lie between 10 and 12 g/100 ml, again reassurance and explanation is required. Iron supplements may be useful in alleviating any tiredness due to mild anaemia and these should be encouraged. The use of endocrine therapy needs to be discussed with the adolescent and her parents and may be used in one of a number of ways. She may either use oral progestogens or the combined oral contraceptive pill. Both these approaches may be entirely successful in controlling menstrual loss due to anvoluatory bleeding and neither interferes with the maturation process necessary at the level of the hypothalamus to establish the normal menstrual cycle. Thus, short term usage of either of these preparations is usually sufficient to control the menstrual loss difficulties until the mature menstrual cycle is established. Again, patients must be re-evaluated at regular intervals to ensure that the control of their periods is adequate and that their anaemia, albeit mild, is resolving. It is usually recommended that therapy is stopped after a year to evaluate the natural cycle maturation process, and this is repeated six monthly thereafter until cycle control is gained.

Severe anaemia

In those girls with severe anaemia, there are two circumstances which need to be considered: when they are not actively bleeding and when they are acutely bleeding. In the former, again an explanation is necessary but the oral contraceptive pill is by far the best therapy. Progestogens are usually inadequate and the dose of contraceptive pill needs to be adjusted to the individual. However, in the vast majority of cases, this is sufficient to control the bleeding and again, similar management to those in the mildly anaemic group is thereafter followed. In the acutely bleeding group, blood transfusion must be considered on admission, and transfusion performed if necessary. Intravenous conjugated oestrogen may be administered (15 to 25 mg, 6 to 12 hourly) until bleeding is controlled. In the process of the dysfunctional bleed, lack of endometrial growth causes the problem of arterial bleeding, and therefore a rise in oestrogen is mandatory to promote endometrial cell growth and arterial occlusion. Once control of the bleeding has been gained in this manner, cyclical oestrogens and progestogens can be administered in the form of the oral contraceptive pill. Only extremely rarely is dilatation and curettage indicated, and in these circumstances it would be when a diagnosis of a uterine pathology is suspected, e.g. a sarcoma, where a uterine biopsy will be necessary to make the diagnosis. As the vast majority of these girls will have a normal uterus on ultrasound, and imaging of the endometrium will not reveal an abnormality, curettage is really an unnecessary investigation as no abnormality will be detected. In rare circumstances where intravenous oestrogen is not effective or the oral contaceptive pill is not controlling the cycle, the use of GnRH analogues can be considered and this will create a hypo-oestrogenic state, thereby stopping the bleeding. The administration of ‘add-back’ therapy in the form of HRT can then be considered in order to provide oestrogen and to calculate the dose of oral hormone therapy that will be required to control the cycle.

The recent development of the levonorgestrel impregnated IUCD may well bring a new alternative to the treatment of this condition (see Chapter 13). Its use in adults has suggested that amenorrhoea will result in 90 per cent of patients. However, the adolescent uterus may not be receptive to this type of intrauterine device in its current form, but in the future there may well be a device of a suitable design available, to enable local control of periods without the side-effect profiles of progestogens given orally, and also without interference in the maturation process or in the ovulation process itself.

Menstrual disorders and mental subnormality

In adolescents with severe mental retardation the management of the menstrual cycle is extremely difficult for the parents or carers. Not only do they have the difficulty of managing the hygiene associated with menstrual loss in girls who have no ability to recognize the onset of bleeding, but also the menstrual cycle brings behavioural abnormalities in these patients, particularly with control of their medication with regard to seizures. This in itself presents an extremely difficult problem and great discussion has to occur in order to explore all avenues of treatment. If amenorrhoea is a necessary aim then depot progestogens are, without doubt, the best form of therapy. This may be either as Depo-Provera® or Norplant®. In chosing either of these, management is determined by following up the girls to make sure they are amenorrhoeic. All carers must be warned that breakthrough bleeding is not uncommon and occasionally this may result in continuous bleeding. In terms of alternatives, if the oral contraceptive pill is chosen, then the other medication that these patients are taking must be taken into account when choosing the dose of oral contraceptive pill. Many of them are on anti-epileptic therapy and this demands a higher dose of oestrogen in order to gain efficacy. Continuous use of the oral contraceptive pill can be useful in these circumstances, and may in itself create amenorrhoea which is a satisfactory way of controlling the situation. The suggestion that endometrial resection could be used in these circumstances seems unlikely to be successful. Whilst it may be attractive theoretically, the chances of regeneration of the endometrium in very young girls may be high. In those patients in whom control of menstrual loss is medically impossible then a surgical approach with hysterectomy has to be considered. This may require discussion with social workers, psychiatrists, and other health care workers involved in the case before a decision can be taken, but with informed consent and the appropriate counselling these decisions sometimes have to be made.

Menstrual problems in the adolescent and environmental factors

A number of environmental factors may affect menstruation during adolescence. These have become increasingly apparent during recent years, and highlight the need to observe other factors apart from normal aberrations when considering the girl who presents with oligomenorrhoea.

Adolescents often suffer from body image aberration. The fashion design industry has epitomized the ideal female as being tall and thin. Women's clothes' designers illustrate modern fashion through models who fit this image. Teenage girls, therefore, understandably are influenced by these images and may well try to achieve some degree of imitation through dieting. This type of dieting may be harmless, but in severe cases may lead to anorexia nervosa. In those girls who diet without reducing their body fat below 17 per cent there is really little impact on the menstrual cycle, but those who continue to lose body weight and become amenorrhoeic may well induce the hypo-oestrogenic state with its end results of decreased bone density. The attainment of peak bone density is crucial for normal skeletal structure and strength. Herzog *et al.* (1993) demonstrated that failure to achieve peak bone density during teenage years may result in long-term problems of osteoporosis at a relatively young age. It is a misconception that teenagers who are amenorrhoeic are not at risk of osteoporosis and it is therefore essential that the post-menarchal teenage girl who becomes amenorrhoeic, particularly in association with decreased weight, is closely followed and prescribed supplementation with either calcium or oral oestrogen in order to achieve normal bone mass (Bonjour 1991; Lloyd *et al.* 1993).

For many years it has been believed that athletes have a delayed onset of menarche, and this delayed onset of menarche has been investigated and proven to be a truism (Morgan and London 1993). However, it has always been assumed that it is the exercise which induces the delay, and in those athletes who train particularly hard, alterations in their cortisol and central changes which may influence gonadotrophin release are the explanation for the delay (Loucks 1989). However, in a recent study by Baxter-Jones *et al.* (1994), longitudinal studies of gymnasts, swimmers, and tennis players have demonstrated that there is an intrinsic delay within the normal range of athletes, which is almost certainly merely a reflection of the selection of girls who wish to indulge in sport, as opposed to those girls who do not. Thus some form of sport-specific selection has occurred and the late maturation is, in many ways, an advantage for the athlete which selects her to follow her sporting prowess. It is unlikely that stress has any influence over the menstrual cycle during adolescent years, unless it is associated with weight loss. There are no studies which have demonstrated a stress-related response in terms of changed menstrual cycle control, and it is much more likely that the stress and pubertal menstrual cycle irregularity are associated and not 'cause-and-effect'.

Dysmenorrhoea in adolescence

Dysmenorrhoea or painful menstruation is extremely common in teenage girls and 75 per cent of all teenagers probably have some degree of dysmenorrhoea. In some 15 per cent this limits their daily activity at the time of their pelvic pain. Dysmenorrhoea may manifest itself in two ways in adolescents. Without doubt the vast majority present with primary dysmenorrhoea or dysmenorrhoea in association with normal pelvic organs. Only a small percentage of teenagers will have a pathological cause for dysmenorrhoea or secondary dysmenorrhoea (see Chapters 22 and 23).

In a study by Andersch and Milsom (1982) 50 per cent of their patient population reported that at some time during their adolescent years they had missed time from either school or work as a result of dysmenorrhoea. However, only a third of these had ever sought the help of a gynaecologist or doctor.

The aetiology of dysmenorrhoea is due to myometrial stimulation, in many cases secondary to endometrial prostaglandin production, and teenage girls have been found to produce excessive amounts of prostaglandin, thereby inducing their symptom complex (Lundstrom 1986). Primary dysmenorrhoea usually begins with the onset of menstruation and lasts between 24 and 72 hours. The pain is typically crampy and spasmodic, usually in the lower abdomen or supra-pubically and may well radiate down the inner parts of the thigh. If the pain begins several days prior to the onset of menstruation it is more likely that this is a secondary dysmenorrhoea problem, secondary to an organic cause.

Table 8.1 Prostaglandin synthetase inhibitors

Type I	
Salicylic acid esters	Aspirin, diflunisal
Acetic acids	Diclofenac, indomethacin
Propionic acids	Ketoprofen, ibuprofen, naproxen
Fenamic acids	Mefenamic acid
Type II	
Pyrozolones	Phenylbutazone
Oxicans	Piroxicam

Secondary dysmenorrhoea may be due to pelvic inflammatory disease, congenital abnormalities of the genital tract, endometriosis, or ovarian cysts. In any patient, adolescent or otherwise, with secondary dysmenorrhoea problems which are persisting, a laparoscopic assessment of the pelvis is mandatory if a diagnosis is to be made and an appropriate treatment instituted.

The treatment of primary dysmenorrhoea revolves around two modalities, either the use of non-steroidal anti-inflammatory drugs or the oral contraceptive pill. Both of these are suitable for use in the adolescent and non-steroidal anti-inflammatory drugs are probably the commonest used medication in teenage years. They are prostaglandin synthetase inhibitors, and are extremely effective in controlling the pain of dysmenorrhoea. There are a number of non-steroidal anti-inflammatory drugs available, and they fall into two types – carboxylic acid derivatives and inolic acid derivatives (Table 8.1). Control of dysmenorrhoea can be achieved in well over 90 per cent of adolescent females using these drugs. In those in whom they are not effective, the oral contraceptive pill is extremely effective, because it induces endometrial atrophy and reduces endometrial prostaglandin production. In any girl in whom non-steroidal anti-inflammatory drugs and oral contraceptive pills have failed to control dysmenorrhoea, it is crucial to rule out organic or psychological causes for her manifestation of pelvic pain. However, other strategies for dealing with the pain can also be entertained. In a study by Helms (1987), acupuncture was found to be successful in 90 per cent of cases when it was applied for the treatment of primary dysmenorrhoea. Further alternatives in terms of strategies for reducing intrauterine pressure are the use of the calcium channel blockers (such as nifedipine), though there are a number of side-effects associated with these agents which do not make them the drugs of first choice at the present time.

References

Andersch, B. and Milsom, I. (1982). An epidemiologic study of young women with dysmenorrhoea. *American Journal of Obstetrics and Gynecology*, **144**, 155–60.

Apter, D. and Vikho, R. (1977). Serum pregnenelone, progesterone, 17-hydroxyprogesterone, testosterone, and di-hydrotestosterone during female puberty. *Journal of Clinical Endocrinology and Metabolism*, **45**, 1039–45.

Baxter-Jones, A.D., Helms, P., Baines-Preece, J., and Preece, M. (1994). Menarche in intensively trained gymnasts, swimmers and tennis players. *Annals of Human Biology*, **21**, 407–15.

Bonjour, J.P. (1991). Critical years and stages of puberty for spinal and femoral bone mass accumulation during adolescence. *Journal of Clinical Endocrinology and Metabolism*, **73**, 555–63.

Bourguignon, J.P., Gerard, A., Alvarez-Gonzalez, M.L., Fawe, L., and Franchimont, P. (1992). Gonadal independent developmental changes in activation of *N*-methyl-D-aspartate receptors involved in gonadotropin releasing hormone secretion. *Neuroendocrinology*, **55**, 634–41.

Brann, D.W. (1995). Glutamate: a major-excitatory transmitter in neuroendocrine regulation. *Neuroendocrinology*, **61**, 213–25.

Claessens, E.A. and Cowell, C.A. (1981). Acute adolescent menorrhagia. *American Journal of Obstetrics and Gynecology*, **139**, 277–82.

Dewhurst, C.J., Cowell, C.A., and Barrier, L.C. (1971). The regularity of early menstrual cycles. *Journal of Obstetrics and Gynaecology of the British Commonwealth*, **78**, 1093–5.

Edmonds, D.R. (1989). Menstrual changes in adolescence. *Baillière's Clinical Obstetrics and Gynaecology*, **3**, 329–39.

Falcone, T., Desjardins, C., Bourque, J., Granger, L., Hemmings, R., and Quiros, E. (1994). Dysfunctional uterine bleeding in adolescents. *Journal of Reproductive Medicine*, **39**, 761–4.

Gore, A.C., Mitshushima, D., and Terasawa, E. (1993). A possible role for neuropeptide Y in the control of the onset of puberty in female rhesus monkeys. *Neuroendocrinology*, **58**, 23–34.

Hallberg, L., Hogdahl, A.M., Nilsson, L., and Rybo, G. (1966). Menstrual blood loss – a population study. *Acta Obstetrica et Gynecologica Scandinavica*, **45**, 244–8.

Helms, J.M. (1987). Acupuncture for the management of primary dysmenorrhoea. *Obstetrics and Gynecology*, **69**, 51–6.

Herzog, W., Minne, H., Deter, C., Hirdig, G., Schellberg, D., Wustru, C. *et al.* (1993). Outcome of bone mineral density in anorexia nervosa patients 11.7 years after first admission. *Journal of Bone Mineral Research*, **8**, 597–605.

Kaplan, S.L., Grumbach, M.M., and Aubert, M.L. (1976). The ontogenesis of pituitary hormones and hypothalamic factors in the human fetus. *Recent Progress in Hormone Research*, **32**, 161–70.

Kennedy, W. (1933). The menarche and the menstrual type. *Journal of Obstetrics and Gynaecology of the British Empire*, **40**, 792–5.

Lee, P.A. (1988). The neuroendocrinology of puberty. *Seminars in Reproductive Medicine*, **6**, 13–20.

Lloyd, T., Andon, M.B., Rolling, N., Martel, J.R., Landis, J.R., Demers, L.M. *et al.* (1993). Calcium supplementation and bone mineral density in adolescent girls. *Journal of the American Medical Association*, **270**, 841–4.

Loucks, A.B. (1989). Alterations in the hypothalamo–pituitary–adrenal axis in athletic women. *Journal of Clinical Endocrinology and Metabolism*, **68**, 402–11.

Lundstrom, V. (1986). The uterus. In *Prostaglandins and their inhibitors in clinical obstetrics and gynecology* (ed. N. Bygdeman, G.S. Berger, and L.G. Reith), pp. 59–82. MTP Press, Lancaster.

Ma, Y.J., Costa, H.E., and Ojeda, S.R. (1994). Developmental expression of the genes encoding transforming growth factor alpha and its receptor in the hypothalamus of the female rhesus macaque. *Neuroendocrinology*, **60**, 346–59.

Morgan, A. and London, S. (1993). Effects of excessive exercise and weight loss on adolescent menstrual cyclicity. *Adolescent and Pediatric Gynecology*, **6**, 63–70.

Prasad, B., Conover, C.D., Barker, D.K., Rabii, J., and Advis, J.P. (1993). Feed restriction in prepubertal lambs: effect on puberty, LHRH, neuropeptide Y, and Beta-endorphin release from the postero-lateral median eminence. *Neuroendocrinology*, **57**, 1171–81.

Quigley, M.E., Sheehan, K.L., Csaper, K.F., and Yen, S.S.C. (1980). Evidence of increased dopaminergic and opioid activity in patients with hypothalamic hypogonadotropic amenorrhoea. *Journal of Clinical Endocrinology and Metabolism*, **50**, 949–54.

Tanner, J.M. (1962). *Growth and adolescence*. Blackwell, Oxford.

Vollman, R.F. (1977). *The menstrual cycle*. W.B. Saunders, Philadelphia.

Wyshak, G. (1983). Secular changes in age at menarche. *Annals of Human Biology*, **10**, 75–83.

Yen, S.S.C. (1991). The hypothalamic control of pituitary hormone secretion. In *Reproductive endocrinology* (3rd edn), (ed. S.S.C. Yen and R.B. Jaffe), pp. 132–58. W.B. Saunders, Philadelphia.

9 Menstrual dysfunction secondary to medical disease

Jenny Higham

Introduction

Menstruation, being the end result of a complex endocrine pathway, is susceptible to a wide variety of influences. Disruption of menstruation can be provoked by both systemic and local disease. This chapter concerns the precipitation of the common problem of excessive menstrual bleeding by ill-health. It should be remembered that only a very small proportion of menorrhagia cases can be attributed correctly to systemic disease. For these few, however, the correct diagnosis may result in successful curative therapy, rather than disappointing palliative medication or unnecessary surgery.

Despite frequent mention in standard textbooks as to the association of menorrhagia with disease, there is a paucity of objective data on the subject. The estimation of menstrual blood loss on the basis of a patient's history is notoriously unreliable (Chimbira *et al.* 1980; Fraser *et al.* 1984). There is no reason, however, to suspect that women who have a medical problem should be any more accurate in the assessment of their menstrual loss in comparison with women in general. The complaint of excessively heavy loss may not be a loss of more than 80 ml per cycle but to that individual is an increase in menstrual flow in comparison to that previously experienced.

The stage of the menstrual cycle is also acknowledged to influence medical disease. Conditions such as epilepsy, migraine, asthma, myasthenia gravis, and diabetes mellitus are often noted to have cycle-dependent fluctuations. The severity and manifestation of symptoms almost always has premenstrual and menstrual exacerbations. Arguably, emotional factors such as pre-menstrual dysphoria may affect a woman's disease perception, but there are a range of confirmatory observations and measurements which give credence to a cyclical phenomenon (Magos and Studd 1985).

Potential precipitants of menorrhagia

The diseases most commonly considered in association with the precipitation of menorrhagia are listed in Table 9.1 and discussed below.

Endocrine disease

Thyroid dysfunction

Thyroid disorders are the most common endocrinological abnormality associated with menstrual disturbance. Hypothyroidism is noted in most texts as being a potent cause of menorrha-

Table 9.1 Medical diseases thought to be associated with menorrhagia

Endocrine disease	Thyroid dysfunction Pituitary/adrenal gland abnormalities
Haematological disease	Coagulation defects Platelet abnormalities Sickle cell disease
Autoimmune disease	Systemic lupus erythematosus
Hepatic, renal and cardiac disease	Liver disease Renal disease Cardiac disease
Metabolic disease	Gaucher's disease
Other causes	Infection Psychological disturbance Altitude Arteriovenous malformations Pregnancy related Tubal occlusion

gia and one which is amenable to treatment. What published data exist to support this assertion?

Scott and Mussey (1964) questioned 50 hypothyroid women and found that abnormal menstrual patterns were present in 56 per cent. Amongst these, menorrhagia was the most common complaint. One woman whose loss was measured was found to be losing 135 ml per period. Another study which detailed the menstrual bleeding pattern of women with thyroid disease found that 17 of 18 patients with thyrotoxicosis had oligo- or amenorrhoea. Of those with myxoedema, 8 out of 10 had ovulatory failure, with only two experiencing normal ovulation and menses (Goldsmith *et al.* 1952). Changes in the FSH/LH ratio in such patients have been implicated in the mechanism of this ovulatory failure (Akande 1975).

A study of 15 women found to have 'mild' hypothyroidism stated that their complaint of menorrhagia disappeared after administration of corrected doses of thyroxine. However, blood loss was not measured (Wilansky and Greisman 1989). Objective menstrual blood loss measurement prior to and during correction of hypothyroidism to the euthyroid state gives additional support to the causal association between this condition and menorrhagia. A dramatic, although possibly only temporary, reduction of losses in excess of 400 ml to within the normal range was noted during this time (Higham and Shaw 1992).

A further interesting aspect of the association between hypothyroidism and menorrhagia is the development of an acquired form of von Willebrand's disease in untreated hypothyroidism (Smith *et al.* 1987; Blesing *et al.* 1990). The haemostatic defects were noted to revert back to normal when thyroxine supplementation was instituted and the patients were returned to the euthyroid state.

Pituitary/adrenal gland abnormalities

Three studies have documented the pituitary and ovarian hormone levels in otherwise normal women with objectively proven menorrhagia compared with normal controls (Haynes *et al.* 1979;

Cameron 1989; Eldred and Thomas 1994). None of the authors were able to establish a relationship between either the ovarian or pituitary hormone levels and the variation in menstrual blood loss between the two groups. That is not to say, however, that pituitary disease could not produce menorrhagia. It should be noted that at the extremes of reproductive life, namely in the peri-menarche and towards the menopause, the incidence of anovulation increases (Treloar *et al.* 1967).

Hyperprolactinaemia, hypopituitarism, adrenal insufficiency, and acromegaly most commonly result in oligo- or amenorrhoea. Cushing's disease is reputed to be associated with a variety of menstrual cycle disorders including menorrhagia. There is little evidence to support this assertion, though menstrual abnormalities were reported to be corrected following bilateral adrenalectomy (Smals *et al.* 1977). The mechanism by which elevated glucocorticoids might cause menorrhagia is uncertain, though the hyperandrogenaemia might lead to oligomenorrhoea with subsequent anovulatory dysfunctional uterine bleeding.

Haematological disease

Coagulation disorders

A definite association between abnormal menstruation and systemic bleeding disorders has been reported (Table 9.2) (Bonnar *et al.* 1983). Quick (1966) described a variety of inherited blood coagulation disorders which resulted in subjective menorrhagia. Many women, therefore, suffering with these conditions, will present for treatment of their menorrhagia at some time during their reproductive life. 'Simple' operative procedures such a dilatation and curettage can provoke torrential bleeding, requiring blood transfusion, cryoprecipitate, and uterine packing (Greer *et al.* 1992). In the past, coagulopathy and resultant menorrhagia or post-partum haemorrhage was responsible for a number of deaths.

Fraser *et al.* (1986) made objective blood loss measurements in 15 women with various coagulation disorders, demonstrating that some had menorrhagia of the most dramatic kind, with monthly losses of between 750 and 1000 ml. This was not always the case, however; one woman on warfarin had a blood loss of 59.1 ml.

van Eijkeren *et al.* (1990) set out to verify these findings. The mean menstrual blood loss in six women with a congenital or acquired bleeding disorder was 219 ml (range 60 to 568 ml), with

Table 9.2 Haemostatic blood disorders presenting with abnormal menstrual bleeding

Coagulation abnormalities	Von Willebrand's disease Factor IX deficiency Haemophilia A carriers Prothrombin Factors V, VII, X
Platelet defects	Thrombocytopenia Glanzmann's thrombasthenia Bernard–Soulier syndrome Aplastic anaemia Leukaemia

five of the six women having objective menorrhagia (blood loss greater than 80 ml). Despite Fraser's case, anticoagulation therapy has acquired the reputation for increasing menstrual blood loss. van Eijkeren and colleagues also measured the menstrual blood loss of 11 women on anticoagulants. The average blood loss was 98 ml with almost half of the women having menorrhagia. There was no correlation between anticoagulant state and blood loss. The authors concluded that their evidence supported the association between both bleeding disorders and oral anticoagulation and increased menstrual loss. The incidence of haemorrhagic diatheses is not thought to be increased in adult women with menorrhagia. However, adolescent menorrhagia may have a coagulation disorder as an underlying cause (see Chapter 8). Claessens and Cowell (1981) studied 59 young girls whose menorrhagia had precipitated an acute hospital admission and in whom no obvious gynaecological pathology was found. 29 per cent had a coagulation disorder.

Platelet disorders

Haemorrhagic diatheses due to platelet dysfunction are a heterogeneous and poorly understood group of conditions. Platelets have a vital role in promoting haemostasis and it is not surprising therefore that a substantial reduction in platelet numbers or defects in their ability to function correctly could precipitate excessive menstrual bleeding (Table 9.2). The onset of menstrual bleeding at the menarche may be the first time an inherited platelet defect becomes apparent.

There have been a number of case reports describing the association between rare hereditary disorders such as Bernard–Soulier syndrome and other forms of platelet dysfunction and menorrhagia (Cartwright *et al.* 1994) which have been treated successfully with exogenous ovarian steroids (Sharma *et al.* 1991).

Reduction in platelet numbers (thrombocytopenia) can result from other disturbances of platelet production and distribution or from excessive platelet destruction. Poor production can result from a failure of the bone marrow function secondary to damage, malignant replacement, or deficiency states. Additionally, there are the rare congenital hereditary thrombocytopenias.

Immune destruction of platelets due to either idiopathic thrombocytopenic purpura or systemic autoimmune disorders is the most common cause of reduced platelet count in women of reproductive age. Objective blood loss measurement in five women with thrombocytopenia demonstrated substantial menorrhagia. In broad terms, the degree of menorrhagia was proportional to the severety of thrombocytopenia (Fraser *et al.* 1986).

Sickle cell disease

A preliminary study of women with this condition suggested that they experienced shorter menstrual cycles than control women. In addition their periods were longer and heavier and were associated with a greater incidence of dysmenorrhoea (Samuels-Reid and Scott 1985).

Autoimmune disease

Systemic lupus erythematosus

Systemic lupus erythematosus (SLE) is a disease of unknown aetiology in which organ systems are involved in an inflammatory process. There is a production of antibodies which react with nuclear, cytoplasmic, and cell membrane antigens. The syndrome usually runs a variable course, with disease activity greatest in the interval between ovulation and menstruation. Menstrual abnormalities are common in female sufferers, especially during active disease phases. An increase in menstrual loss is particularly associated with antibodies to clotting factors or with SLE associated thrombocytopenia. Serological screening for this condition has been advocated in cases where either the history is suspicious or there is unsatisfactory response to the standard menorrhagia treatments (Fraser 1994).

Hepatic, renal, and cardiac disease

Liver disease

Hepatic impairment can produce a wide variety of menstrual disturbances from amenorrhoea to protracted profuse flow. Of those women with end-stage disease prior to transplantation, almost 50 per cent had at least one year of amenorrhoea. Laifer and Guido (1995) support the premise that such menstrual dysfunction is corrected following successful transplantation. The immunosuppressive medication required following transplantation is not thought to have a detrimental effect on menstrual loss. This is supported by a study of women immunosuppressed by the human immunodeficiency virus which found no association between either symptomatic and asymptomatic immunosuppressed women or their respective CD4 lymphocyte counts and the quantity of menstrual loss (Shah *et al.* 1994).

Stellon and Williams (1986) studied the gynaecological intervention in women before their liver disease was diagnosed. Those with a subsequent diagnosis of primary biliary cirrhosis had significantly more dilatation and curettage and hysterectomy operations performed, when compared with matched patients with chronic active hepatitis or alcoholic liver disease. The main indication for hysterectomy was menorrhagia. A study of female patients with primary biliary cirrhosis found an abnormal relationship between the sex steroids and sex hormone binding globulin (Wilkinson *et al.* 1983).

Impairment of hepatic metabolism restricts the therapeutic options available to treat menstrual problems. In terms of contraception, barrier methods and subsequent sterilization appear to be the safest option. However, surgery may also present an increased risk of haemorrhage if there is impairment of clotting ability.

Renal disease

A review of women with renal disease referred to the gynaecology clinic found that by far the most common reason for this was menorrhagia (59 per cent); only 5 per cent of women referred considered their cycle normal in both interval and flow (Cochrane and Regan, personal communication). Menorrhagia is a frequent complaint amongst renal patients, which if left unchecked may necessitate blood transfusion. This in turn may limit the possibility of a woman having a successful renal transplant because of the development of atypical antibodies. Excessive blood loss is therefore to be avoided, especially in those being dialysed and awaiting transplantation. Non-steroidal anti-inflammatory drugs are contraindicated and several other therapeutic modalities have limited efficacy. High dose medroxyprogesterone acetate has been found to be useful in such patients (Cochrane and Regan, personal communication).

Following successful renal transplantation and the restoration of normal renal function, it is often assumed that endocrine function will also revert to normal with a resultant improvement in menstrual problems. In the experience of Cochrane and Regan, this was not the case and subjective complaints of menorrhagia persisted. Similarly, a study of women with chronic renal failure found that all patients with end-stage renal disease had amenorrhoea. An assessment of the pituitary–ovarian axis was made in those women with renal disease who were still menstruating, prior to and after the commencement of therapy to improve renal function. Following the initiation of the therapy there was no significant alteration in hormonal profiles or menstrual pattern. The authors suggested that factors apart from hormonal imbalance were responsible for the menstrual disturbances noted in patients with chronic renal failure (Otieno *et al.* 1993).

Cardiac disease

The effect of congenital heart disease on menstruation has been studied (Canobbio *et al.* 1995). Ninety eight women were divided into two groups depending on whether they had acyanotic or cyanotic disease and asked to completed a questionnaire concerning their menstrual pattern. The results were compared with those of matched controls. The only significant differences between the groups were of a slightly later menarche and increased incidence of breakthrough bleeding in women with congenital heart disease. Overall, menstrual patterns, including the subjective quantity of flow, were similar to those in the general population.

Metabolic disease

Gaucher's disease

Gaucher's disease is a lipid storage disease in which deficient glucocerebrosidase enzyme activity causes widespread glucocerebroside accumulation. Like SLE, it is a multisystem disease. When 53 women were interviewed, examined, and investigated, heavy menstrual bleeding was found to be a major problem which responded well to therapy with low-dose oral contraceptives (Granovsky-Grisaru *et al.* 1995). Again, blood loss was not measured objectively.

Other causes

Infectious disease

Though acute pelvic infection can cause irregular menstrual bleeding, infection is an uncommon cause of chronic menorrhagia. Amenorrhoea is a more typical menstrual response to serious infection.

Psychological influences

Psychosomatic and psychiatric influences on the menstrual cycle and menstrual symptoms are considered in detail in Chapters 26 and 27.

Frank's 1945 review of the literature about uterine bleeding due to extragenital disturbance noted that 'worry, fright, fatigue, nervous shock, sexual excesses, and perversions' could influence menstrual bleeding. A case of menorrhagia apparently arising to protect a patient from her desire for extramarital relationships is reported.

Overall, women who subjectively considered their menstrual loss to be heavy were more likely to experience negative mood changes with a period (Snowden and Christian 1983). A study of the incidence of psychiatric symptoms in women with gynaecological symptoms found a significant association between psychiatric morbidity and complaints of flooding, passing clots, and subjectively very heavy periods (Gath *et al.* 1987). The association of menstrual function with depression has also been explored (Greenberg 1983). In general, however, indices of subjectively excessive menstruation do not appear strongly related to mental state. This was surprising perhaps, as menorrhagia may have been expected to induce emotional distress.

Arteriovenous malformations

Uterine arteriovenous malformations (AVM) are rare causes of massive uterine bleeding. The condition can be either congenital or acquired secondary to uterine trauma (Ghosh 1986; Fleming *et al.* 1989). Alternatively, AVMs may arise as a result of gestational trophoblastic disease (Vogelzang *et al.* 1991). Techniques such as Doppler flow ultrasound and pelvic angiography are increasing the ability to make this rare diagnosis, for which selective vessel embolization offers a successful method of treatment (Manolitsas *et al.* 1994). Curettage may precipitate life-threatening haemorrhage and is therefore contraindicated when AVM is suspected.

Pregnancy related

Although not a disease, the seasoned clinician should not forget the potential role of pregnancy and its complications on matters gynaecological. Molar change and retained products of conception (the latter often accompanied by infection) are particularly important causes of profuse uterine bleeding which can occasionally present as menorrhagia.

Tubal occlusion

Tubal occlusion has been postulated as a precipitant of menorrhagia and hence could be an iatrogenic 'disease' (Muldoon 1972). Kasonde and Bonnar (1976) were not able to support this hypothesis, finding no significant difference in the objective menstrual blood loss measurement in 25 women prior to and then 6 and 12 months following the excision and ligation of a small portion of Fallopian tube. A further study, which included four different methods of tubal occlusion, found no significant changes in objectively quantified menstrual blood loss up to a year following the procedure (Sahwi *et al.* 1989). It is more likely that the perceived increase in menstrual blood loss following surgical sterilization is related to discontinuation of oestrogen/progestagen contraceptive preparations and the consequent loss of their beneficial effect on menstrual bleeding. Additionally, it is possible that the higher than average incidence of hysterectomy in sterilized women might be a reflection of a group who prefer surgical treatment as a therapeutic option.

Altitude

Although not subjected to a rigorous controlled trial, an increase in altitude is said to augment menstrual loss. It is reported that waitresses in the Swiss Alps had to descend from the high altitude of a resort on the Jungfraujoch to lower levels on account of the development of severe menorrhagia (Frank 1945)!

Conclusion

A number of diseases are potentially responsible for disturbances of menstrual function. Systemic disease is an unusual cause of menstrual disorders. However, the possibility of a non-gynaecological disorder should be borne in mind, particularly in women with significant findings on history taking or if there is an unexpected response to standard management. It should not be forgotten that as 30 per cent of women will experience at least subjective menorrhagia at some stage of their reproductive life, menstrual dysfunction may coexist with underlying medical disease by chance.

References

Akande, E.O. (1975). Plasma concentration of gonadotrophins, oestrogen and progesterone in hypothyroid women. *European Journal of Obstetrics and Gynaecology*, **82**, 552–6.

Blesing, N.E., Hambley, H., and McDonald, G.A. (1990). Acquired von Willebrand's disease and hypothyroidism: report of a case presenting with menorrhagia. *Postgraduate Medical Journal*, **66**, 474–6.

Bonnar, J., Sheppard, B.L., and Dockeray, C.J. (1983). The haemostatic system and dysfunctional uterine bleeding. *Research and Clinical Forums*, **5**, 27–36.

Cameron, I.T. (1989). Dysfunctional uterine bleeding. *Baillière's Clinical Obstetrics and Gynaecology*, **3**, 315–27.

Canobbio, M.M., Rapkin, A.J., Perloff, J.K., Lin, A., and Child, J.S. (1995). Menstrual patterns in women with congenital heart disease. *Paediatric Cardiology*, **16**, 12–15.

Cartwright, I.J., Hampton, K.K., Macneil, S., Colvin, B.T., and Preston, F.E. (1994). A haemorrhagic platelet disorder associated with altered stimulus-response coupling and abnormal membrane phospholipid composition. *British Journal of Haematology*, **88**, 129–36.

Chimbira, T.H., Anderson, A.B., and Turnbull, A.C. (1980). Relation between measured menstrual blood loss and patient's subjective assessment of loss, duration of bleeding, number of sanitary towels used, uterine weight and endometrial surface area. *British Journal of Obstetrics and Gynaecology*, **87**, 603–9.

Claessens, E.A. and Cowell, C.A. (1981). Acute adolescent menorrhagia. *American Journal of Obstetrics and Gynecology*, **139**, 277–80.

Eldred, J.M. and Thomas, E.J. (1994). Pituitary and ovarian hormone levels in unexplained menorrhagia. *Obstetrics and Gynecology*, **84**, 775–8.

Fleming, H., Ostor, A.G., Pickel, H., and Fortune, D.W. (1989). Arteriovenous malformations of the uterus. *Obstetrics and Gynecology*, **73**, 209–14.

Frank, I.L. (1945). Uterine bleeding and extragenital disturbances. *American Journal of Medical Science*, **210**, 787–98.

Fraser, I.S. (1994). Menorrhagia – a pragmatic approach to the understanding of causes and the need for investigations. *British Journal of Obstetrics and Gynaecology*, **101**, 3–7.

Fraser, I.S., McCarron, G., and Markham, R. (1984). A preliminary study of factors influencing perception of menstrual blood loss volume. *American Journal of Obstetrics and Gynecology*, **149**, 788–93.

Fraser, I.S., McCarron, G., Markham, R., Resta, T., and Watts, A. (1986). Measured menstrual blood loss in women with menorrhagia associated with pelvic disease or coagulation disorder. *Obstetrics and Gynecology*, **68**, 630–3.

Gath, D., Osborn, M., Bungay, G., Iles, S., Day, A., Bond, A., and Passingham, C. (1987). Psychiatric disorder and gynaecological symptoms in middle aged women: a community survey. *British Medical Journal*, **294**, 213–18.

Ghosh, T.K. (1986). Arteriovenous malformation of the uterus and pelvis. *Obstetrics and Gynecology*, **68**, 40S–43S.

Goldsmith, R.E., Sturgis, S.H., Lerman, J., and Stanbury, J.B. (1952). The menstrual pattern in thyroid disease. *Journal of Clinical Endocrinology and Metabolism*, **12**, 846–55.

Granovsky-Grisaru, S., Aboulafia, Y., Diamant, Y.Z., Horowitz, M., Abrahamov, A., and Zimran, A. (1995). Gynecologic and obstetric aspects of Gaucher's disease: a survey of 53 patients. *American Journal of Obstetrics and Gynecology*, **172**, 1284–90.

Greenberg, M. (1983). The meaning of menorrhagia: an investigation into the association between the complaint of menorrhagia and depression. *Journal of Psychosomatic Research*, **27**, 209–14.

Greer, I.A., Lowe, G.D.O., Walker, J.J., and Forbes, C.D. (1992). Congenital coagulopathies in obstetrics and gynaecology. In *Haemostasis and thrombosis in obstetrics and gynaecology* (ed. I.A. Greer, A.G.G. Turpie, and C.D. Forbes), pp. 459–85, Chapman & Hall Medical, London.

Haynes, P.J., Anderson, A.B., and Turnbull, A.C. (1979). Patterns of menstrual blood loss in menorrhagia. *Research and Clinical Forums*, **1**, 73–8.

Higham, J.M. and Shaw, R.W. (1992). The effect of thyroxine replacement on menstrual blood loss in a hypothyroid patient. *British Journal of Obstetrics and Gynaecology*, **99**, 695–6.

Kasonde, J.M. and Bonnar, J. (1976). Effect of sterilization on menstrual blood loss. *British Journal of Obstetrics and Gynaecology*, **83**, 572–5.

Laifer, S.A. and Guido, R.S. (1995). Reproductive function and outcome of pregnancy after liver transplantation in women. *Mayo Clinics Proceedings*, **70**, 388–94.

Magos, A. and Studd, J. (1985). Effects of the menstrual cycle on medical disorders. *British Journal of Hospital Medicine*, **33**, 68–77.

Manolitsas, T., Hurley, V., and Gilford, E. (1994). Uterine arteriovenous malformation – a rare cause of uterine haemorrhage. *Australia and New Zealand Journal of Obstetrics and Gynaecology*, **34**, 197–9.

Muldoon, M.J. (1972). Gynaecological illness after sterilization. *British Medical Journal*, **274**, 84–5.

Otieno, M.R., McLigeyo, S.O., Kigondu, C.S., and Rogo, K.O. (1993). Menstrual disorders in patients with chronic renal failure. *East African Medical Journal*, **70**, 6–9.

Quick, A.J. (1966). Menstruation in hereditary bleeding disorders. *Obstetrics and Gynecology*, **28**, 37–48.

Sahwi, S., Toppozada, M., Kamel, M., Anwar, M.Y., and Ismail, A.A. (1989). Changes in menstrual blood loss after four methods of female tubal sterilization. *Contraception*, **40**, 387–98.

Samuels-Reid, J. and Scott, R.B. (1985). Characteristics of menstruation in sickle cell disease. *Fertility and Sterility*, **43**, 139–41.

Scott, J.C. and Mussey, E. (1964). Menstrual patterns of myxedema. *American Journal of Obstetrics and Gynecology*, **90**, 161–5.

Shah, P.N., Smith, J.R., Wells, C., Barton, S.E., Kitchen, V.S., and Steer, P.J. (1994). Menstrual symptoms in women infected by the human immunodeficiency virus. *Obstetrics and Gynecology*, **83**, 397–400.

Sharma, J.B., Buckshee, K., and Sharma, S. (1991). Puberty menorrhagia due to Bernard Soulier syndrome and its successful treatment by 'Ovral' hormone tablets. *Australian and New Zealand Journal of Obstetrics and Gynaecology*, **31**, 369–70.

Smals, A.G.H., Kloppenborg, P.W.C., and Benraad, T.J. (1977). Plasma testosterone profiles in Cushing's syndrome. *Journal of Clinical Endocrinology and Metabolism*, **45**, 240–5.

Smith, S.R., Auger, M.J., MacCallum, P.K., Rodgers, M., Taberner, D.A., Thornton, J.G., Parapia, L.A., and Minford, A.M.B. (1987). Hypothyroidism and von Willebrand's disease. *Lancet*, **i**, 1314–15.

Snowden, R. and Christian, B. (1983). *Patterns and perception of menstruation*. Croom Helm/ St Martin's Press, London.

Stellon, A.J. and Williams, R. (1986). Increased incidence of menstrual abnormalities and hysterectomy preceding primary biliary cirrhosis. *British Medical Journal*, **293**, 297–8.

Treloar, A.E., Boynton, R.E., Behn, B.G., and Brown, B.W. (1967). Variation of the human menstrual cycle through reproductive life. *International Journal of Fertility*, **12**, 77–126.

van Eijkeren, M.A., Christiaens, G.C.M.L., Haspels, A.A., and Sixma, J.J. (1990). Measured menstrual blood loss in women with a bleeding disorder or using oral anticoagulant therapy. *American Journal of Obstetrics and Gynecology*, **162**, 1261–3.

Vogelzang, R.L., Nemcek, A.A., Skrtic, Z., Gorrell, J., and Lurain, J.R. (1991). Uterine arteriovenous malformations: primary treatment with therapeutic embolization. *Journal of Vascular Interventionist Radiology*, **2**, 517–22.

Wilansky, D.L. and Greisman, B. (1989). Early hypothyroidism in patients with menorrhagia. *American Journal of Obstetrics and Gynecology*, **160**, 673–7.

Wilkinson, M.I., Iqbal, M.J., Johnson, P.J., and Williams, R. (1983). Abnormal relationship between sex steriods and SHBG in primary cirrhosis. *Gut*, **24**, A490.

10 Menorrhagia: clinical investigation

Hilary O.D. Critchley

Introduction

Disorders of menstruation are the commonest indication for women to seek medical attention. Up to 20 per cent of healthy menstruating women report an excessively heavy monthly blood loss (Jacobs and Butler 1965; Hallberg *et al.* 1966; van Eijkeren *et al.* 1989). Menstruation itself has been defined as the 'shedding of the superficial layers of the endometrium following the withdrawal of ovarian steroids. The process is associated with a variable degree of blood loss and usually lasts for up to six days' (Cameron *et al.* 1996). The increase in dissatisfaction with menstrual aberrations may be a reflection of the fact that women experience more menstrual cycles than they did at the turn of the century. The average woman nowadays experiences in the order of 400 menstrual cycles during her reproductive years, in contrast to the 40 or so cycles she would have been exposed to over 50 years ago (Short 1984; Rees and Turnbull 1989). The increased numbers of menstrual cycles are due to the fewer pregnancies and reduced lactation periods chosen by women in the latter half of this century.

In the United Kingdom over 70 000 women undergo hysterectomy each year and despite the emergence of hysteroscopic methods of treatment the figures for both types of surgical treatment are increasing (Bridgman 1994; Coulter 1994). It is now estimated that almost 20 per cent of women in the UK will have had a hysterectomy by the age of 55 years (Vessey *et al.* 1992). In contrast, hysterectomy rates in Norway are half those of Britain and the lifetime risk of having a hysterectomy in the USA (based on 1975 data) was 62 per cent (Teo 1991). Furthermore, the management cost to the general practitioner and hospital services has been estimated as between £250 and £500 million per annum in the United Kingdom (Smith and Haining 1994). Fifty per cent of women, however, have no systemic or pelvic pathology and have normal ovulatory cycles (Haynes *et al.* 1979; Chimbira *et al.* 1980) despite complaints of menstrual dysfunction. A woman's decision to seek treatment is unlikely to be unifactorial and may be influenced by cultural issues, perception of her doctor's attitudes to menstrual complaints, and, importantly, her expectations about treatment (Warner 1995).

Clinical evaluation

Adequate clinical investigation of women complaining of menorrhagia requires a detailed gynaecological history establishing the perception and tolerance of menstrual blood loss and its impact upon quality of life (specifically disturbance of social, occupational, and sexual activities) (Table 10.1). Changes in contraceptive habit may result in an altered perception of menstrual bleeding.

Table 10.1 The clinical evaluation of menorrhagia: Important features of clinical evaluation

History (A prospective approach may be more accurate)	
• duration and heaviness of flow	
• sudden change more likely to be pathological	
• own perception of monthly blood loss	
• social/occupational/sexual disturbance	
• concern about underlying disease	
• symptoms of iron deficiency anaemia	
• exacerbation of underlying depression (poor tolerance)	
• current contraception	
• menstrual tolerance after sterilization	
Investigation	
Examination	Bimanual pelvic examination
	Cervical smear if due
Full blood count	
Selected patients	Ferritin, TSH, coagulation screen

There is no evidence for increased blood loss following sterilization (Kasonde and Bonnar 1975), although women using oral contraception prior to sterilization may have been accustomed to a lighter monthly blood loss (Cole *et al.* 1971). It is important to differentiate 'ovular' and 'anovular' cycles. Eighty per cent of women with three consecutive regular periods have ovulatory cycles. Normal cycle length may range from 21 to 35 days. If anovular cycles are suspected, serial progesterone measurement in serum or urine may be useful. There is no abnormality of hypothalamic–pituitary–ovarian function in women with excess menstrual blood loss who have regular cycles. Anovulation will be more common at both ends of the spectrum of reproductive life, i.e. in adolescence and in the perimenopausal years. Obesity may lead to anovulatory cycles and aberrant menses. In such cases, weight reduction alone should improve the pattern of menstrual loss. The woman may be excessively concerned about serious underlying disease such as cancer. The history should elicit endocrine (e.g. thyroid) disorder or coagulopathy, if present, (e.g. von Willebrand's disease, thrombocytopenic purpura). Chronic liver and renal disease will also result in disordered menstruation. Besides general examination to seek signs of anaemia and underlying medical or endocrine disease, clinical examination should include a bimanual examination to detect abnormalities in the pelvis. A cervical smear should be performed if required.

Further appropriate investigations as indicated should be undertaken. In most cases a full blood count should be conducted and serum ferritin measured if descriptions of blood loss indicate very heavy loss. Even among women with monthly measured blood loss less than 80 ml, 13 per cent are anaemic and half have ferritin concentrations below 'normal'.

Thyroid disease and coagulation disorders should be excluded when suspected on history and examination by measuring thyroid-stimulating hormone (TSH) concentrations and a coagulation screen. However, these tests are not indicated as routine first line investigations. Fibroids may be detected during a pelvic examination and subsequently confirmed with pelvic ultrasound if desired. Occasionally a diagnostic laparoscopy will be indicated, for example, if endometriosis is suspected. All too often, however, the history and examination are unremarkable.

Assessment of menstrual blood loss

The classic population study of Hallberg and colleagues (1966) showed measured menstrual blood loss to have a skewed distribution with a mean loss of 35 ml and a 90th percentile of 80 ml. It is appropriate to define what is meant by excessive monthly menstrual blood loss, and the upper limit of normal has been defined as 60–80 ml (Cameron 1989). Certainly, if menstrual blood loss exceeds 50–60 ml in a woman taking an average western diet, negative iron balance will result (Rybo 1966). Objective measurement of menstrual blood loss can be determined easily using the alkaline haematin method (Hallberg and Nilsson 1964) but this may be unrealistic in practice in busy clinical settings. This method requires menstrual pads to be soaked in 5 per cent sodium hydroxide. Haemoglobin is converted to alkaline haematin and blood loss may be calculated by comparing the optical density of an aliquot of the alkaline haematin solution (at 540 nm) with the optical density of a known volume of venous blood similarly processed.

However, very few women undergoing surgical intervention for 'heavy periods' have had their menstrual blood loss measured. No standard clinical assessment of menorrhagia exists. Subjective descriptions of menstrual blood loss may be unreliable as only 38 per cent of women who complain of menorrhagia had average monthly blood losses greater than 80 ml per period (Fraser *et al.* 1984). It is notable that in over half of referrals for 'menorrhagia' the women do not even report their periods as 'very heavy' and hence in these situations excessive loss is unlikely (Warner 1994).

The actual volume of blood loss may not in fact be a good indicator of the menstrual experience. Menstrual fluid consists of both blood and non-blood fluid. Indeed, fluid volume ranges from 1.9–9 times that of blood volume (Fraser *et al.* 1985). However, women with heavy menstrual blood loss also describe a heavy fluid loss. The variability between individuals is great (Fraser *et al.* 1985). Recently there has been reconsideration of a semi-quantitative method to allow visual assessment of menstrual blood loss (Higham *et al.* 1990; Janssen *et al.* 1995). This study measured objective menstrual blood loss by the alkaline haematin method and also required women to keep semi-objective assessment of the volume based on a pictorial chart, which recorded the amount of and degree to which their sanitary wear was soiled. A score was calculated for each bleeding episode and a cut-off point was chosen above which menorrhagia was likely and below which a diagnosis of menorrhagia was unlikely.

Evaluation of the uterine cavity

A wide array of methods is available for evaluating the uterine cavity:

- dilatation and curettage (D&C)
- hysteroscopy plus endometrial sampling
- ultrasound evaluation of uterine architecture and endometrial thickness
- endometrial sampling (pipelle, Gynocheck, Vabra aspiration).

The main indication for assessing the uterine cavity is to exclude sinister intrauterine pathology which is seen most often in older women (over 45 years of age) with anovulatory cycles (Lewis 1993).

Dilatation and curettage

Dilatation and curettage (D&C) has been the 'gold standard of uterine evaluation' for many years (Fig. 10.1). Seven women per 1000 still undergo dilatation and curettage each year in the United Kingdom (Coulter *et al.* 1993). Indeed, dilatation and curettage procedures are six times more common in Britain than in the USA (Coulter *et al.* 1993; Fig. 10.2). However, the procedure is rarely indicated in women under 40 years. In young women under 40 years who complain of heavy but regular menses a D&C is unlikely to reveal significant pelvic disease (Mackenzie and Bibby 1978; Grimes 1982; Royal College of Obstetricians and Gynaecologists 1994). Over 15 years ago, in 1978, Mackenzie and Bibby questioned the diagnostic value of a D&C. Three to four thousand D&Cs would have to be performed to detect one endometrial cancer in women under 35 years (Vessey *et al.* 1979). Yet even in 1994 the numbers of women undergoing this procedure are still increasing!

In 1982, Grimes reappraised the role of diagnostic dilatation and curettage and based a comparison of two techniques on data derived over twenty years. Table 10.2 (derived from the publication by Grimes in 1982) identifies salient features of his comparison between a diagnostic 'D&C' and endometrial sampling by Vabra aspiration (VA).

Although a 'D&C' is a relatively safe procedure, it is associated with a higher risk of complications than Vabra aspiration, for example perforation or infection. Both methods of endometrial sampling appear to provide adequate samples for histological analysis. However, Grimes (1982) pointed out that the sensitivity and specificity of a D&C are unknown and that endometrial lesions may be undetected in up to 10 cases per 100.

It was most interesting that a study performed prior to hysterectomy, evaluating the completeness with which samples of endometrium were obtained at D&C, revealed that only half of the

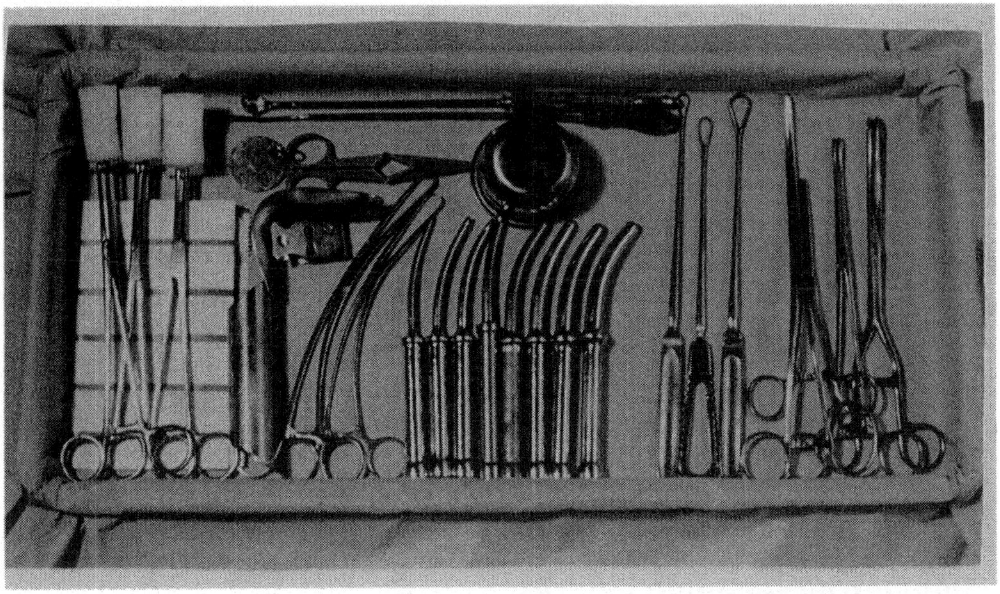

Fig. 10.1 A standard instrument tray for dilatation and curettage (D&C) – the previous 'gold standard of uterine evaluation'.

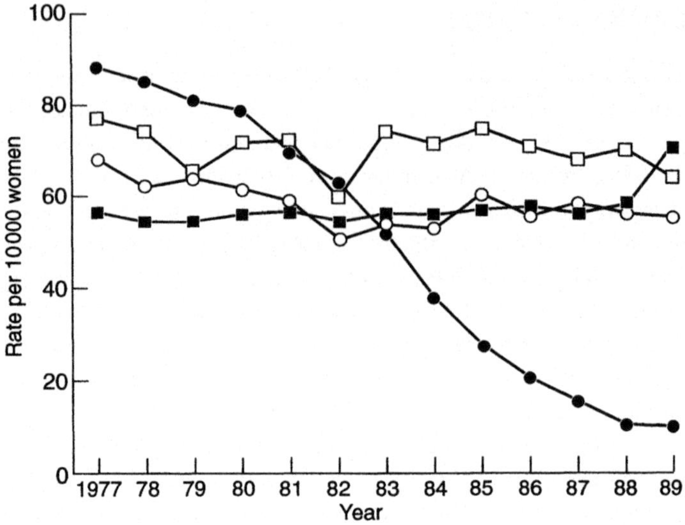

Fig. 10.2 D&C rates between 1977 and 1990. Trends over time in rates of dilatation and curettage in England and Wales ■ (data for Wales before 1982 only), Oxford region ○, Scotland □, and United States ●. Rates have remained stable in the UK. In contrast, in the USA rates have markedly declined. Reproduced with permission from Coulter *et al.* (1993).

Table 10.2 Comparison of diagnostic D&C and Vabra aspiration (VA) (adapted from Grimes 1982)

Characteristic	D&C (*n* = 13 598)	VA (*n* = 5851)
Safety		
Infection rate*	3–5	0–4
Perforation rate*	6–13	0–4
Adequacy of specimen†	0.77–0.94	0.85–0.99
Diagnostic accuracy		
Adenocarcinoma	Unknown	0.96
Polyps	Unknown	0.80

* Per 1000 procedures.
† Number of procedures providing samples adequate for histological diagnosis/total number of procedures.

cavity was sampled (Stock and Kambour 1975). At least 5 per cent of cases of endometrial carcinoma may be missed by dilatation and curettage alone (Schild and Kutta 1992), and evidence is accumulating to suggest that hysteroscopy combined with endometrial sampling may be superior to dilatation and curettage in the accurate diagnosis of pathology.

Endometrial sampling devices

A number of endometrial sampling devices are now available. Novak (1935) pioneered endometrial sampling techniques in an outpatient setting. In the 1970s the Vabra curette was introduced.

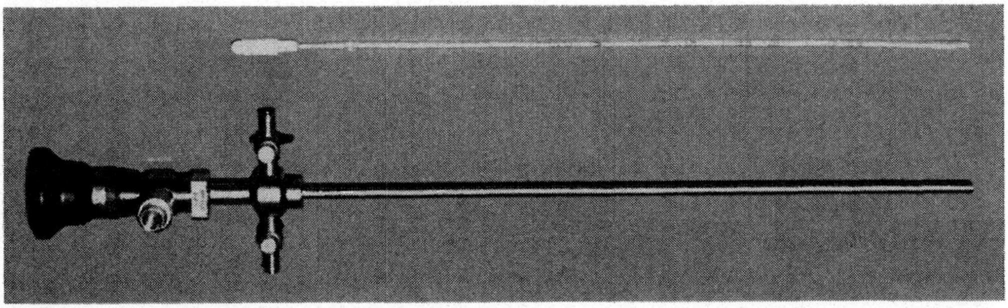

Fig. 10.3 Endometrial sampling device – pipelle sampler (upper); rigid hysteroscope for outpatient or in-patient use (lower).

The more recently introduced pipelle sampler (Fig. 10.3) is simpler to use and patients experience less discomfort (Kaunitz *et al.* 1988). However, the pipelle device does sample less endometrial area than the Vabra sampler (4 per cent versus 40 per cent; Rodriguez *et al.* 1993) but amounts of tissue sampled are adequate for diagnosis as long as the appropriate area of tissue has been biopsied. All blind sampling procedures may miss submucous fibroids and polyps. There is a reservation that endometrial sampling alone may not in fact collect a representative specimen of endometrial tissue. This has led to the introduction of hysteroscopic evaluation of the uterine cavity to complement endometrial biopsy. Table 10.3 summarizes the advantages and disadvantages of D&C versus endometrial sampling conducted by a pipelle or Vabra aspirator. As yet, no randomized controlled trial has been conducted to compare outpatient endometrial sampling and D&C.

Hysteroscopy

Hysteroscopy is an increasingly popular alternative/adjunct to dilatation and curettage. Hysteroscopes (Fig. 10.3, 10.4) are now manufactured with a sufficiently narrow diameter (i.e. 4 mm) to permit use in an outpatient setting without need for anaesthesia, since in appropriately selected women cervical dilatation is unnecessary (Taylor and Hamou 1983; Mencaglia *et al.*

Table 10.3 'D&C' versus endometrial sampling

Procedure	Disadvantages	Advantages
D&C	May miss 10% of lesions Less than half of the cavity curetted Requires anaesthesia Risks trauma (1.7% complication rate)	Detects endometritis
Endometrial sampling (Pipelle or VA)	Pipelle samples 4.2% surface area vs. 41.6% by VA	96% agreement with pathology No anaesthesia required

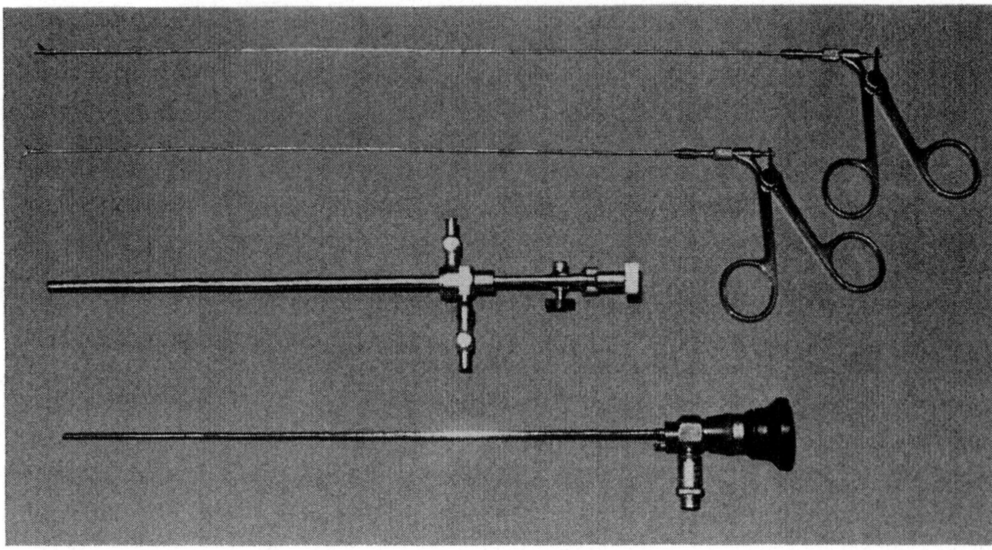

Fig. 10.4 Hysteroscope for use in an outpatient or in-patient setting. In this model it is possible to introduce a small biopsy forceps or scissors along the sheath of the hysteroscope.

1987). Careful selection of patients and adequate counselling of women with regard to their expectations of the procedure are essential. A history of cervical surgery such as a previous cone biopsy or a Manchester repair, with the possibility of subsequent cervical stenosis, may result in difficulty in passing the hysteroscope through the internal cervical os. The possibility of vagal stimulation and 'cervical shock' should be remembered and appropriate resuscitative measures should be available. Recently Gillespie and Nichols (1994) reported that in an unselected group of patients outpatient hysteroscopy was well tolerated in 80 per cent of subjects (irrespective of diagnostic indicator and without local analgesia). Two-thirds of patients were shown to have a normal or atrophic endometrium (Table 10.4).

Table 10.4 Outpatient hysteroscopy: indications and diagnoses (above); diagnosis made in 160 outpatient examinations (below) (reproduced with permission from Gillespie and Nichols 1994)

Menorrhagia	58	(29%)
Irregular bleeding	32	(16%)
Irregular bleeding with HRT	45	(22.5%)
Post-menopausal vaginal bleeding	46	(23%)
Other	19	(9.5%)
Total	**200**	
Normal endometrium	57	(36%)
Atrophic endometrium	48	(30%)
Fibroids	37	(23%)
Endometrial polyp	8	(5%)
Adhesions	8	(5%)
Malignancy	2	(1%)
Total	**160**	

Some sources consider endometrial biopsy unnecessary in the presence of normal hysteroscopic appearances (Mencaglia *et al.* 1987; Loffer 1989). However, caution is required as the recognition of normality with hysteroscopic visualization of the cavity has a considerable 'learning curve'. Furthermore it should be remembered that different distension media produce different appearances. It is probably safest to recommend endometrial sampling at the time of hysteroscopic evaluation – for example, Fig. 10.5(a) illustrates an endocervical polyp viewed with gas distension (carbon dioxide) whilst Fig. 10.5(b) shows the same polyp seen after fluid distension.

The uterine distension media used for hysteroscopy are either a low flow (≤ 100 ml per minute) and low pressure (≤ 100 mm of mercury) of carbon dioxide gas or fluid (dextran 70, 1.5 per cent glycine, or sorbitol). Carbon dioxide gas is particularly convenient in the outpatient setting. It has been recommended (Lewis 1990) that a hysteroscopy is best performed in the postmenstrual or proliferative phase of the cycle. At this time the endometrium is thin. Blood within the cavity inhibits a clear view and thus hysteroscopy is best avoided during menstruation. The contraindications to hysteroscopy include active pelvic inflammatory disease and pregnancy.

The Royal College of Obstetricians and Gynaecologists' (1994) guidelines recommend hysteroscopy with endometrial sampling as the method of choice for investigation of heavy regular bleeding which has failed to improve with medical management, and intermenstrual bleeding in

(a)

(b)

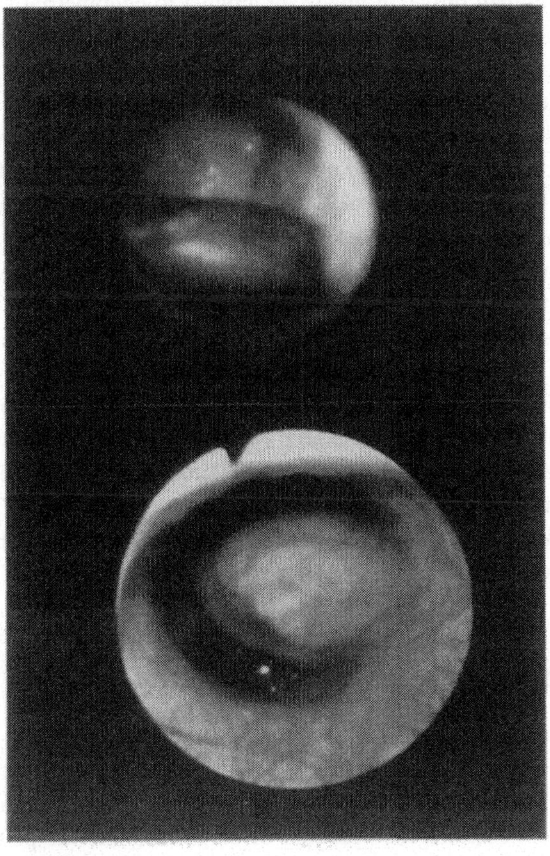

Fig. 10.5 (a) Endocervical polyp viewed with gas distention medium (carbon dioxide). **(b)** The same endocervical polyp viewed after fluid distension of the uterine cavity.

women under 40 years of age. Recent commentaries (Lewis 1990, 1993; Gillespie and Nichols 1994) have gone further in suggesting that outpatient hysteroscopy and endometrial sampling should largely replace dilatation and curettage under general anaesthetic for the investigation and diagnosis of endometrial abnormalities at all ages. Diagnosis may still have to await the pathology report just as it does with tissue samples collected at the time of curettage under anaesthetic (Gillespie and Nichols 1994). Hysteroscopy itself has been compared with the previously popular procedure of curettage (Gimpelson and Rappold 1988). The former was equally efficacious with regard to the provision of information in 79 per cent of cases. Panoramic hysteroscopy was superior in 18 per cent of cases; whereas curettage was found to be superior in only 3 per cent of procedures. One of the important and consistent findings in this report was the detection by hysteroscopy of endometrial polyps and submucous fibroids in women who have been subjected to multiple 'negative' curettage procedures. Furthermore, intrauterine synechiae may be detected with hysteroscopy but remain obscure with biopsy or curettage alone. Hence these authors (Gimpelson and Rappold 1988) argue strongly that hysteroscopy is the investigation of choice for evaluation of intrauterine pathology.

Ultrasound

Ultrasound evaluation may prove an important adjunct to endometrial sampling for the clinical investigation of menorrhagia, permitting evaluation of uterine architecture and the measurement of endometrial thickness. In appropriately selected patients, transvaginal ultrasound, with better resolution (since the distance between the ultrasound probe and the reproductive organs is reduced compared to abdominal ultrasound), is increasing in popularity. The former allows assessment of fibroids and polyps if the resolution is good. Endometrial thickness has limited, if any, relevance to the pre-menopausal woman although, of course, it is of value in post-menopausal patients. There is a good correlation between ultrasound evaluation of endometrial thickness (by convention, double thickness) and measurement of the endometrium from hysterectomy specimens (Andolf and Jorgensen 1988). An accuracy to within 1 mm has been reported. Endometrial thickness does increase in the normal secretory phase of the menstrual cycle. Studies have demonstrated that in post-menopausal women an ultrasound measured endometrial thickness of ≤ 5 mm over the whole uterine cavity excluded the likelihood of endometrial cancer in subjects who presented with post-menopausal bleeding (Nasri and Coast 1989; Goldstein *et al.* 1990). Subsequent data, however, have exposed a small (6 per cent) incidence of endometrial cancer where the endometrium measured < 5 mm (Dorum *et al.* 1993). This would suggest that such ultrasound measurement should be complemented with endometrial sampling, such as with a pipelle sampling device.

Concluding remarks

In women with clinical symptoms, ultrasound evaluation is unlikely to be sensitive enough to confidently exclude neoplastic pathology and more detailed evaluation of the uterine cavity is required, i.e. a hysteroscopy with endometrial sampling. Indeed, hysteroscopic examination has been cited as the most cost-effective method of diagnosing uterine pathology in older women (Effective Health Care Bulletin 1995).

A clinical dilemma remains with respect to younger women complaining of menorrhagia as to whether detailed endometrial evaluation is warranted. The recent guidelines from the Royal College of Obstetricians and Gynaecologists have received wide support. These guidelines, encompassing the earlier suggestions of Grimes (1982), state that uterine investigation is justifiable for young women under 40 years who have failed to respond to medical treatment or who describe intermenstrual bleeding. Women over 40 who report significant menstrual disturbance warrant further evaluation. Hysteroscopy complemented with endometrial biopsy is the investigation of choice.

Acknowledgements

Thanks are due to Mr Tom McFetters for assistance with the photomicrographs and also to Mrs Vicky Watters for secretarial support.

References

Andolf, E. and Jorgensen, C. (1988). A prospective comparison of clinical ultrasound and operative examination of the female pelvis. *Journal of Ultrasound in Medicine*, **7**, 617–20.

Bridgman, S.A. (1994). Increasing operative rates for dysfunctional uterine bleeding. *Lancet*, **344**, 893.

Cameron, I.T. (1989). Dysfunctional uterine bleeding. *Baillière's Clinical Obstetrics and Gynaecology*, **3**, 315–27.

Cameron, I.T., Irvine, G., and Norman, J.E. (1996). Menstruation. In *Scientific essentials of reproductive medicine*. (ed. S.G. Hillier, H. Kitchener, and J.P. Neilson), pp. 208–18. W.B. Saunders London.

Chimbira, T.H., Anderson, A.B.M., and Turnbull, A.C. (1980). Relation between measured menstrual bood loss and the patient's subjective assessment of loss, duration of bleeding, number of sanitary towels used, uterine weight and endometrial surface area. *British Journal of Obstetrics and Gynaecology*, **87**, 603–9.

Cole, S.K., Billiwicz, W.Z., and Thomson, A.M. (1971). Sources of variation in menstrual blood loss. *British Journal of Obstetrics and Gynaecology*, **78**, 933–9.

Coulter, A. (1994). Trends in gynaecological surgery. *Lancet*, **344**, 1367.

Coulter, A., Klassen, A., Mackenzie, I.Z., and McPherson, K. (1993). Diagnostic dilatation and curettage: is it used appropriately. *British Medical Journal*, **306**, 236–9.

Dorum, A., Kristensen, G.B., Langebrekke, A., Sornes, T., and Skaar, O. (1993). Evaluation of endometrial thickness measured by endovaginal ultrasound in women with post menopausal bleeding. *Acta Obstetrica et Gynecologica Scandinavica*, **72**, 116–19.

Effective Health Care Bulletin (1995). *The management of menorrhagia*, No. 9. The University of Leeds.

Fraser, I.S., McCarron, G., and Markham, R. (1984). A preliminary study of factors influencing perception of menstrual blood loss volume. *American Journal of Obstetrics and Gynecology*, **149**, 788–93.

Fraser, I.S., McCarron, G., Markham, R., and Resta, T. (1985). Blood and fluid content of menstrual discharge. *Obstetrics and Gynecology*, **65**, 194–8.

Gillespie, A. and Nichols A. (1994). The value of hysteroscopy. *Australian and New Zealand Journal of Obstetrics and Gynaecology*, **34**, 85–7.

Gimpelson, R.J. and Rappold, H.O. (1988). A comparative study between panoramic hysteroscopy with directed biopsies and dilatation and curettage. *American Journal of Obstetrics and Gynecology*, **158**, 489–92.

Goldstein, S.R., Nachtigall, M., Snyder, J.R., and Nachtigall, L. (1990). Endometrial assessment by vaginal ultrasonography before endometrial sampling in patients with post menopausal bleeding. *American Journal of Obstetrics and Gynecology*, **163**, 119–23.

Grimes, D.A. (1982). Diagnostic dilatation and curettage: a reappraisal. *American Journal of Obstetrics and Gynecology*, **142**, 1–6.

Hallberg, L. and Nilsson, L. (1964). Determination of menstrual blood loss. *Scandinavian Journal of Clinical and Laboratory Investigation*, **16**, 244–8.

Hallberg, L., Högdahl, A.M., Nilsson, L., and Rybo G. (1966). Menstrual blood loss – a population study. *Acta Obstetrica et Gynecologica Scandinavica*, **45**, 320–51.

Haynes, P.J., Anderson, A.B.M., and Turnbull, A.C. (1979). Patterns of menstrual blood loss in menorrhagia. *Research and Clinical Forums*, **1**, 73–8.

Higham, J.M., O'Brien, P.M.S., and Shaw, R.W. (1990). Assessment of menstrual loss using a pictorial chart. *British Journal of Obstetrics and Gynaecology*, **97**, 734–9.

Jacobs, A. and Butler, E.B. (1965). Menstrual blood loss in iron deficiency anaemia. *Lancet*, **ii**, 407–9.

Janssen, C.A.H., Scholten, P.C., and Heintz A.P.M. (1995). A simple visual assessment technique to discriminate between menorrhagia and normal menstrual blood loss. *Obstetrics and Gynecology*, **85**, 977–82.

Kasonde, J.M. and Bonnar, J. (1975). Effect of ethamsylate and aminocaproic acid on menstrual blood loss in women using intrauterine devices. *British Medical Journal*, **4**, 21–2.

Kaunitz, A.M., Maciello, A., Ostrowski, M., Rovira, E.Z., and Stat, M. (1988). Comparison of endometrial biopsy with the endometrial pipelle and the Vabra aspirator. *Journal of Reproductive Medicine*, **33**, 427–31.

Lewis, B.V. (1990). Hysteroscopy for the investigation of abnormal uterine bleeding. *British Journal of Obstetrics and Gynaecology*, **97**, 283–4.

Lewis, B.V. (1993). Diagnostic dilatation and curettage in young women. *British Medical Journal*, **306**, 225–6.

Loffer, F.D. (1989). Hysteroscopy with selective endometrial sampling compared with D&C for abnormal uterine bleeding: the value of a negative hysteroscopic view. *Obstetrics and Gynecology*, **73**, 16–20.

Mackenzie, I.Z. and Bibby, J.G. (1978). Critical assessment of dilatation and curettage in 1029 women. *Lancet*, **i**, 566–8.

Mencaglia, L., Perino, A., and Hamou, J. (1987). Hysteroscopy in perimenopausal women with abnormal uterine bleeding. *Journal of Reproductive Medicine*, **32**, 577–82.

Nasri, M.N. and Coast, G.J. (1989). Correlation of ultrasound findings and endometrial histopathology in post menopausal women. *British Journal of Obstetrics and Gynaecology*, **96**, 1333–8.

Novak, E. (1935). A suction curette apparatus for endometrial biopsy. *Journal of the American Medical Association*, **104**, 1497–8.

Rees, M.C.P. and Turnbull, A.C. (1989). Menstrual disorders – an overview. *Baillière's Clinical Obstetrics and Gynaecology*, **3**, 217–26.

Rodriguez, G.C., Yaqub, N., and King, M.E. (1993). A comparison of the pipelle device and the Vabra aspirator as measured by endometrial denudation in hysterectomy specimens. *American Journal of Obstetrics and Gynecology*, **168**, 55–9.

Royal College of Obstetricians and Gynaecologists (1994). In-patient treatment – D&C in women age 40 or less. *Royal College of Obstetricians and Gynaecologists, Guidelines*, **3**, 1–4.

Rybo, G. (1966). Clinical and experimental studies on menstrual blood loss. *Acta Obstetrica et Gynecologica Scandinavica*, **45** (Suppl.), 1–23.

Schild, R. and Kutta, T. (1992). Ranking of cervical cytology and uterine curettage in diagnosis of endometrial carcinoma. *Geburtshilfe und Frauenheilkunde*, **52**, 467–70.

Short, R.V. (1984). Oestrus and menstrual cycles. In *Hormonal control of reproduction* (ed. C.R. Austin and R.V. Short), pp. 115–52. Cambridge University Press.

Smith, S.K. and Haining, R.E.B. (1994). The investigation and management of excessive menstrual bleeding. In *Proceedings of a Seminar on Dysfunctional Uterine Bleeding*, pp. 109–27. Royal Society Medical Press Ltd, London.

Stock, R.J. and Kanbour, A. (1975). Pre hysterectomy curettage. *Obstetrics and Gynecology*, **45**, 537–41.

Taylor, P.J. and Hamou, J. (1983). Hysteroscopy. *Journal of Reproductive Medicine*, **28**, 359–89.

Teo, P.Y.K. (1991). Hysterectomy in Scotland. *Health Bulletin*, **49**, 226–43.

van Eijkeren, M.A., Christiaens, G.C.M.L., Sixma, J.J., and Haspels, A.A. (1989). Menorrhagia: a review. *Obstetrics and Gynecology Survey*, **44**, 421–9.

Vessey, M., Clarke, J., and MacKenzie, I. (1979). Dilatation and curettage in young women. *Health Bulletin*, **39**, 59–62.

Vessey, M.P., Villard-Mackintosh, L., McPherson, K., Coulter, A., and Yeates, D. (1992). The epidemiology of hysterectomy: findings in a large cohort study. *British Journal of Obstetrics and Gynaecology*, **99**, 402–7.

Warner, P. (1994). Preferences regarding treatment for period problems: relationship to menstrual and demographic factors. *Journal of Psychosomatic Obstetrics and Gynaecology*, **15**, 93–110.

Warner, P. (1995). Characteristics of women referred for menstrual problems. In *Psychosomatic obstetrics and gynaecology* (ed. J. Bitzer and M. Stauber), pp. 335–42. Proceedings of 11th International Congress of Psychosomatic Obstetrics and Gynaecology, Basel, 1995. Mondnzzi Editore, Bologna, Italy.

11 Office hysteroscopy and suction curettage in the evaluation of abnormal uterine bleeding

Milton Goldrath

Introduction

The dilatation and curettage (D&C) has long been considered the method of choice for investigating abnormal uterine bleeding and obtaining samples of endometrium for histologic examination. In 1975, approximately 977, 000 patients underwent diagnostic D&C in short stay, non-federal hospitals (Grimes 1982). This number had dropped by 65 per cent by 1991 according to data from the National Health Survey. This probably still makes D&C one of the most commonly performed operations in the United States today. Because of the current emphasis on cost containment for health care there has been increasing motivation to find less expensive procedures to substitute for the routine hospital diagnostic curettage. In addition, a hospital procedure is inconvenient and time-consuming. Initially we moved to outpatient procedures instead of the usual two-day admission. This has reduced costs. However, the increasing costs of hospital operation necessitated raising the charges even for out patient surgery to very high levels.

Aspiration curettage without cervical dilatation, in an office setting, has been shown to be a reliable and acceptable method of endometrial sampling (Hofmeister 1974; Smith *et al.* 1974; Creasman and Weed 1976; Hale *et al.* 1976; Lutz *et al.* 1977; MacKenzie and Bibby 1978; Grimes 1982). As the menopause approaches, the incidence of atypical adenomatous hyperplasia and endometrial carcinoma increases. It is, of course, the gynaecologist's prime responsibility to rule out endometrial carcinoma and precursor lesions in patients who have abnormal bleeding. The various studies mentioned above show that aspiration curettage equals and, perhaps, surpasses conventional dilatation and curettage in its ability to diagnose endometrial carcinoma. Smith *et al.* (1974), in their study of endometrial carcinoma, thought that the Gravlee jet washer was superior to both curettage and endometrial biopsy as a diagnostic procedure. It is noted in these various studies that on rare occasions, endometrial carcinoma may be missed by all the methods described previously.

It is recognized by gynaecologists that the incidence of carcinoma, especially in younger women, is very low. The primary reason for diagnostic curettage in these patients is to find causes for menstrual abnormalities that can be remedied, i.e. endometrial polyps and submucous leiomyomata. A large number of symptomatic endometrial polyps and submucous leiomyomata may be missed by endometrial biopsy and aspiration curettage. It has long been the gynaecologist's view that the conventional D&C was more likely to result in the discovery of submucous leiomyomata because one can 'feel' with the curette while one cannot feel with the usual suction cannula. In addition, at conventional dilatation and curettage, exploration with a polyp forceps will often result in the removal of endometrial polyps which were missed with the curette.

In reality, experience has shown that many submucous leiomyomata were missed by repeated curettages, that many leiomyomata 'found' at curettage were not present at the time of hysterectomy, and that many endometrial polyps not discovered at dilatation and curettage were present in hysterectomy specimens when hysterectomy was eventually performed to relieve patients' symptoms. MacKenzie and Bibby (1978), in a retrospective study of over 1000 diagnostic curettages, found that unsuspected pelvic or endometrial lesions were present in 34 of 160 patients who underwent hysterectomy after the initial curettage.

Although most gynaecologists maintain that D&C is by far the most reliable technique for diagnosing endometrial abnormalities, the sensitivity and specificity of a D&C are difficult to assess because unless the uterus is removed the true incidence of lesions in the uterus is unknown. Stock and Kanbour (1975) evaluated the completeness of curettage performed immediately before hysterectomy. They found that in 60 per cent of the patients, less than half of the uterine cavity was curetted and in 16 per cent of the specimens less than one-quarter of the cavity had been curetted. It is therefore not unusual to miss endometrial polyps, submucous myomata, or small endometrial carcinomas at routine curettage. Word *et al.* (1958) demonstrated that 49 of 512 patients who had a hysterectomy following a curettage had residual endometrial polyps. Clearly the curette left many polyps undetected.

Hysteroscopy is indicated in any situation in which intrauterine visualization will enhance diagnostic accuracy and define therapy (Valle 1978). The most common indication for hysteroscopy is abnormal uterine bleeding.

Surgical technique

Hysteroscopy is performed with a 4 mm hysteroscope in a 5 mm sheath using CO_2 as a distending medium. Rarely, a low viscosity medium (saline) is used in patients who are bleeding. A small flexible hysteroscope is used by some authors. Paracervical block with 5 ml of 1 per cent mepivacaine injected into the base of each cardinal ligament decreases the patient's discomfort. *One should wait at least two minutes after injection before beginning the hysteroscopy.* There have been no untoward effects from the paracervical block.

The patient is placed in the usual position on a regular examination table. Bimanual examination is done to determine the position of the uterus. A Graves speculum, a double Sims speculum, or other open-sided speculum is used to visualize the cervix. The cervix is grasped with a single tooth tenaculum and the vagina and cervix are wiped with an antiseptic solution.

It is helpful and much more comfortable for the operator if the patient's buttocks are elevated. Most gynaecological examination tables allow this. Carbon dioxide is delivered through the hysteroscope sheath, using one of various types of purpose-designed hysteroscopic delivery systems. It is important that laparoscopic insufflating machines *not* be used, for these may deliver large amounts of carbon dioxide under pressure and may prove disastrous. A 150 watt light source delivers light through the fibre optic cable. This is not adequate for photographic purposes. With a flow rate of 30–35 ml CO_2 per minute, and a maximum pressure of 50–100 mm Hg, the hysteroscope is advanced through the endocervical canal. The canal is seen ahead of the 'scope and under direct vision the endometrial cavity is entered. The entire cavity is inspected including the cornual regions, the fundus, and the anterior and posterior walls, down to the isthmus. With moderate experience, this procedure may only take 30–40 seconds. Usually the 'scope is then removed and a 6 mm flexible suction cannula on a 50 ml syringe is inserted. The uterine cavity is aspirated thoroughly by suction while slowly scraping and rotating the cannula over the entire surface of the uterus. It was found that small polyps could often be removed with this size cannula. All patients with abnormal uterine bleeding have endometrial sampling by suction curettage immediately following the hysteroscopy.

If a small discrete lesion is to be biopsied, the hysteroscope can be used with an operating sheath through which a small biopsy forceps may be introduced. This is rarely used in clinical practice.

Patients experience minimal discomfort and this is further decreased by the paracervical block. Rarely, patients have severe discomfort. In general, patients have more discomfort from the suction curettage than from hysteroscopy. Patients are discharged immediately following the procedure. A few patients have shoulder pain due to carbon dioxide passing through the Fallopian tubes and rising to the diaphragm. Although gynaecologists are aware of this phenomenon, the patient should be warned, as it is often frightening.

Goldrath and Sherman (1985) reported on 423 procedures. Some patients had the procedure twice and one patient three times. Their ages ranged from 24 to 94 years. This age distribution was similar to that of patients having hospital dilatation and curettage. The indications for the hysteroscopy and suction curettage are the same as the standard indications for dilatation and curettage which have been used by gynaecologists for many years. It should be noted that 149 (37 per cent) of the patients were seen for menorrhagia. This reflected the large number of patients referred for laser ablation of the endometrium (Goldrath *et al.* 1981). Eighty four of the patients had post-menopausal bleeding or spotting. Ten of these post-menopausal patients had an endometrial carcinoma. One had an adenocarcinoma high in the endocervix. Two additional patients with intermenstrual spotting also had adenocarcinoma of the endometrium.

Corson and Brooks (1983) reported significant findings in 64 per cent of their patients with abnormal and/or menopausal bleeding whom they examined hysteroscopically. Goldrath and Sherman's (1985) hysteroscopic and/or pathologic diagnoses as related to the presenting symptoms are seen in Table 11.1. In addition to the miscellaneous findings unrelated to the patient's symptoms, i.e. synechiae, diethylstilboestrol (DES) uterus, septate uterus, and hemiuterus, significant hysteroscopic diagnoses were made in 181 of the 406 procedures (45 per cent). This is an extremely high diagnostic yield compared to other published reports for diagnostic dilatation and curettage (MacKenzie and Bibby 1978) and even more significant when considering the definitions used for normal hysteroscopic and/or pathologic diagnoses. Normal hysteroscopy was defined as the absence of submucous leiomyomata, polyps, or hysteroscopically abnormal endometrium. A large uterine cavity associated with intramural leiomyomata was not considered an abnormal hysteroscopic finding in this study. Atrophic endometrium was considered normal. Minute polyps which are often seen hysteroscopically were also considered a normal variant and not significant. Similarly, secretory appearing endometrium, which is often polypoid, was not considered abnormal. The pathological diagnosis of 'dyshormonal' patterns of the endometrium was also considered normal. This includes the occasional reports of decidual reactions, irregular shedding, and mixed endometrium. Endometritis was not found in this series.

The abnormal findings merit further discussion. The most common abnormality seen hysteroscopically in this series was submucous leiomyomata (n = 87). It should be noted that in 28 of these cases there were no palpable myomata on bimanual examination. In 59 cases palpable myomata were associated with the submucous leiomyomata. In 16 of these, the uterus was larger than a 10 week size pregnancy. In 43 cases the uterus was smaller than this. Four of these were thought to have adenomyosis.

Table 11.1 Indication for hysteroscopy

Hysteroscopic and/or pathologic diagnosis	**Intermenstrual bleeding** (n = 56)	**Dysfunctional bleeding** (n = 54)	**Post-menopausal bleeding** (n = 84)	**Menorrhagia** (n = 149)	**Menometrorrhagia** (n = 23)	**Other** (n = 40)
Normal (n = 219)	35	34	48	67	12	23
Submucous (n = 87)	5	5	7	59	8	3
Carcinoma (n = 12)	2	0	10	0	0	0
Hyperplasia (n = 14)	3	5	4	1	1	0
Endometrial polyp (n = 38)	10	5	10	11	0	2
Adenomyosis (n = 3)	0	0	0	3	0	0
Miscellaneous* (n = 27)	1	4	1	8	2	11
Failure to complete hysteroscopy (n = 6)	0	1	4	0	0	1
Total	56	54	84	149	23	40

* Synechiae, 14; adenocarcinoma of the cervix, 1; T-shaped uterus in patients exposed to diethylstilboestrol, 4; septate uteri, 4; hemipterous, 1; imbedded intrauterine device, 2; vascular anomaly, 1

Failure to complete hysteroscopy occurred infrequently. Cervical stenosis was responsible for four cases. Another was in a patient with a myoma greater than 10 weeks gestational size whose cervical canal was so distorted that the hysteroscope could not be inserted. The sixth was a patient with marked vaginal distortion due to scarring from a vaginal plastic procedure. In four cases, the hysteroscopic examination was considered unsatisfactory because of large amounts of secretory endometrium present. Towards the end of a normal menstrual cycle the profuse amount of succulent secretory endometrium prevents proper examination. These four patients returned after their menstrual period and in all four a satisfactory examination was accomplished. Hysteroscopic examinations in the proliferative phase of the cycle are strongly advised. The procedure is much more satisfactory in the presence of flattened endometrium and, when performed in the follicular phase of the cycle, will not interfere with a luteal phase pregnancy.

Of interest was the fact that in five patients, hysteroscopic examination failed to show the submucous myomata previously diagnosed by D&C. MacKenzie and Bibby (1978) similarly reported seven *disappearing leiomyomata* in their large series of diagnostic curettages.

The incidence of adenocarcinomas of the endometrium (3 per cent) was consistent with the incidence of endometrial carcinoma found by D&C in other series. A similar incidence of endometrial hyperplasia was found. It should be noted that in each of these carcinoma cases the isthmus and cervix were examined. One showed involvement by carcinoma; this was confirmed histologically at hysterectomy. Usually patients with post-menopausal bleeding have their endocervix curetted separately prior to the D&C. However, with the presently described technique, fractional curettage can probably be carried out after the hysteroscopic portion of the procedure without risking contamination from endometrial fragments. This should confirm the hysteroscopic impression of presence or absence of cervical involvement which is considered important in staging endometrial carcinoma.

To answer the question, 'Can we eliminate the hospital diagnostic D&C?', we must address the following points: safety; adequacy of specimen and diagnostic accuracy; convenience; discomfort; benefits of examination under anaesthesia; and the evaluation of therapeutic effects. These parameters were thoroughly discussed by Grimes (1982) in his excellent reappraisal of the diagnostic dilatation and curettage. In comparing the safety and adequacy of specimens, the Vabra aspiration compared very favourably with the D&C.

It is only logical to expect that combining CO_2 hysteroscopy with suction curettage will improve results. Lindemann (1979) reported no infections in 1500 consecutive CO_2 hysteroscopies. Taylor and Hamou (1983) reported no infections in their last 3000 CO_2 hysteroscopies. Perforations of the uterus are very rare in all series. It seems that the risk of perforation is greater when *operative* procedures are being performed through the hysteroscope. The technique of passing the hysteroscope through the cervix into the endometrial cavity under direct vision seems greatly to reduce the risk of perforation. Perforation at the time of hysteroscopy seems to be less than at the time of dilatation and curettage.

Grimes (1982) in comparing the diagnostic accuracy of Vabra aspiration versus D&C states that Vabra aspiration appears to be sensitive in diagnosing adenocarcinoma but less sensitive in detecting polyps. This decreased sensitivity of aspiration curettage to detect polyps can certainly be remedied by the use of carbon dioxide hysteroscopy prior to suction aspiration. In addition, utilizing a 6 mm suction curette often results in the removal of polyps and negates the necessity of doing a therapeutic curettage. In many cases the cervix can be dilated and a forceps inserted for removal of visualized endometrial polyps. There is no doubt that hysteroscopy reveals many more submucous leiomyomata than suction curettage or D&C. In addition, hysteroscopy should avoid the mistaken 'finding' of submucous leiomyomata that are not actually present.

Hale *et al.* (1976) compared the adequacy of specimens obtained for histopathologic examination by routine dilatation and curettage with those collected using a flexible suction cannula. They found the suction cannula far superior for adequacy of sampling as well as adequacy of specimen obtained. They also stated that the technique minimizes damage to the basal endometrium, and perhaps decreases synechiae.

Though general anaesthesia for dilatation and curettage is a very safe procedure, there are certainly complications associated with it. No complications were associated with the use of paracervical block in Goldrath and Sherman's (1985) series.

When the cost of office hysteroscopy combined with suction curettage is compared with an outpatient diagnostic curettage there is no contest. As previously stated, the hospital charge for this procedure, including pre-operative care, operating room, and post-anaesthetic recovery room, is very high. To this is added the anaesthetist's professional fee and the gynaecologist's professional fees. The pathologist's fee must also be added. Suction D&C with hysteroscopy in an office setting only incurs a surgical fee, and a fee for pathologic examination of tissue removed. Compared to hospital procedures, the savings would be enormous.

In discussing convenience, of course, there is no comparing an office visit with a trip to the hospital, even for out patient surgery. The procedure is done on a routine office visit and it adds about 5–10 minutes to the total time of the visit. A trip to the hospital entails at least one day out of a person's usual routine. If a general anaesthetic is used, the patient is often groggy the following day. In addition, she needs someone to accompany her to the hospital and to take her home from the hospital. Patients, after office hysteroscopy and suction curettage, leave and drive themselves home or to work with no after-effects from the procedure.

Although examination under anaesthesia will occasionally yield findings that are beneficial to the patient, I do not believe they are germane to this discussion. Usually the findings have nothing to do with the reason for the dilatation and curettage. In present day gynaecological practice, there are certainly ample methods for the diagnosis of hidden pathology other than examination under anaesthesia, i.e. ultrasound, CT scans, etc.

In discussing the therapeutic effects of diagnostic D&Cs, any direct effect is inconceivable unless some pathology is discovered and removed. Grimes (1982) is of the same opinion. It is more likely that the improvement of menstrual disturbances which occasionally occurs following diagnostic curettage is more coincidental than causal. Haynes *et al.* (1977) measured blood loss in women who had a dilatation and curettage for menorrhagia and found that after the first month there was no improvement in the amount of blood loss. This has also been our impression. The combined use of CO_2 hysteroscopy and suction curettage will yield many more cases of endometrial polyps and submucous myomas amenable to proper treatment by therapeutic curettage, myomectomy, or by other appropriate means.

Although hysteroscopy is a new procedure to most gynaecologists, its use is proliferating. It is a procedure which is readily learned in a short period of time. It should be taught to residents during their training. Graduate courses in hysteroscopy are available and it is highly recommended that one be taken by gynaecologists who plan to use this procedure. The clarity of view with CO_2 hysteroscopy is quite astounding. Most gynaecologists are familiar with the appearance of the uterine cavity and its possible contents and, therefore, rapidly become secure with hysteroscopic observations. As with most new diagnostic procedures, errors may be made at first, but ample safeguards are provided by following up with suction curettage in all of these cases.

In conclusion, carbon dioxide hysteroscopy in combination with suction curettage using a flexible cannula of 6 mm is a superior alternative to routine dilatation and curettage. It provides, at a greatly diminished cost, greater accuracy, convenience, safety, and degree of comfort. Currently it is used as the primary diagnostic procedure in all patients where a diagnostic dilatation and curettage had previously been indicated. In those few instances where hysteroscopy and suction curettage cannot be completed as an office procedure, the same operation should be performed in a hospital operating room.

References

Corson, S.L., and Brooks, P.G. (1983). Experience with the Hamou colpomicrohysteroscope. *Journal of Reproductive Medicine*, **28**, 654–8.

Creasman, W.T. and Weed, J.C. (1976). Screening techniques in endometrial cancer. *Cancer*, **38**, 436–40.

Goldrath, M.H., Fuller, T.A., and Segal, S. (1981). Laser photovaporization of endometrium for the treatment of menorrhagia. *American Journal of Obstetrics and Gynecology*, **140**, 14–19.

Goldrath, M.H. and Sherman, A.I. (1985). Office hysteroscopy and suction curettage: can we eliminate the hospital diagnostic dilation and curettage? *American Journal of Obstetrics and Gynecology*, **155**, 202–29.

Grimes, D.A. (1982). Diagnostic dilatation and curettage: a reappraisal. *American Journal of Obstetrics and Gynecology*, **142**, 1–6.

Hale, R.W., Reich, L.A., Joiner, J.M., Pion, R.J., and Kobara, T. (1976). Histophathologic evaluation of uteri curetted by flexible suction cannula. *American Journal of Obstetrics and Gynecology*, **125**, 805–8.

Haynes, P.J., Hodgson, H., Anderson, A.B., and Turnbull, A.C. (1977). Measurement of menstrual blood loss in patients complaining of menorrhagia. *British Journal of Obstetrics and Gynaecology*, **84**, 763–8.

Hofmeister, F.J. (1974). Endometrial biopsy: another look. *American Journal of Obstetrics and Gynecology*, **118**, 773–7.

Lindemann, H.J. (1979). CO_2 hysteroscopies today. *Endoscopy*, **11**, 94–100.

Lutz, M.H., Underwood, P.B. Jr, Kreutner, A., and Mitchell, K.S. (1977). Vacuum aspiration: An efficient out-patient screening technique for endometrial disease. *Southern Medical Journal*, **70**, 393–5.

MacKenzie, I.Z., and Bibby, J.G. (1978). Critical assessment of dilatation and curettage in 1029 women. *Lancet*, **ii**, 566–8.

Smith, J.P., Ehrlich, C.E., and Lukeman, J.M. (1974). Detection of endometrial adenocarcinoma using a jet washer. *Obstetrics and Gynecology*, **43**, 522–6.

Stock, R.J., and Kanbour, A. (1975). Pre-hysterectomy curettage. *Obstetrics and Gynecology*, **45**, 537–41.

Taylor, P.J., and Hamou, J.E. (1983). Hysteroscopy. *Journal of Reproductive Medicine for the Obstetrician and Gynaecologist*, **28**, 359–89.

Valle, R.F. (1978). Hysteroscopy. In *Obstetrics and gynecology annual* (ed. R.M. Wynn), Vol. 7, pp. 245–83. Appleton-Century-Crofts, New York.

Word, B., Gravlee, L.C., and Wideman, G.L. (1958). The fallacy of simple uterine curettage. *Obstetrics and Gynecology*, **12**, 642–8.

12 The medical management of menorrhagia

Margaret C.P. Rees

Introduction

Menorrhagia is one of the most common reasons for women to consult their general practitioners and be referred to gynaecologists. This is not surprising since on average Western women will experience about 400 menstruations between the menarche and the menopause. In a national community survey where 1069 women were interviewed in their own homes, 31 per cent reported heavy periods and 38 per cent painful periods (Corrado 1990). Of these, one third had consulted a doctor within the past four months. It has been estimated that 5 per cent of women aged 30–49 consult their general practitioners for complaints of excessive menstrual bleeding in one year in the UK (Coulter *et al.* 1995*a*).

The treatment options are medical or surgical, but counselling is an important adjunct. Hysterectomy is the most common surgical treatment but the number of endometrial resections or laser ablations is increasing. While hysterectomy provides a definitive solution to menorrhagia it has a significant morbidity and a small mortality rate. A recent study has estimated the mortality rate in women under 50 undergoing surgery for benign conditions to be 4.2 per 10 000. It is also of concern that hysterectomy, even with ovarian conservation, advances the age of the menopause with potential adverse effects on the cardiovascular and skeletal systems. Not all women will be rendered amenorrhoeic by endometrial ablative techniques and re-treatment rates of 16 per cent have been reported at one year (reviewed by Coulter *et al.* 1995*a*): furthermore, little is known about the long term effects of these procedures. Thus it is not surprising that some women will wish to avoid surgery.

The first line of treatment should be medical, especially in primary care. A wide variety of options is now available. Each year about £7 million is spent on primary care prescribing for menorrhagia in the UK; 822 000 prescriptions were issued to 345 225 women for this condition in 1993 (Coulter *et al.* 1995*a*). Medical therapy is indicated when there is no obvious pelvic abnormality and the woman wishes to retain her fertility. Since menstrual loss, in the absence of pathology, does not change markedly, treatment is long term. Thus the drug regimen chosen must be effective, have few or mild side-effects and must be acceptable to the patient.

The aims of therapy are to reduce blood loss, reduce the risk of anaemia and improve quality of life. Menorrhagia is the commonest cause of iron deficiency anaemia in Western women and thus iron therapy should be used as well as the options discussed below. It could be argued that blood loss should be reduced to be within the normal range (i.e. less than 80 ml per period). However, women who are keen to avoid surgery may accept a higher loss if they can cope with the flow and any anaemia is controlled with iron.

Assessment of efficacy of medical treatments

It is essential that drug therapies are assessed in terms of reduction of measured menstrual blood loss. Patients' estimations have been repeatedly shown to be inaccurate indicators of menstrual blood loss in several studies where subjective and objective assessments have been compared (Chimbira *et al.* 1980; Preston *et al.* 1995). In general it has been estimated that only 40 per cent of women complaining of menorrhagia have a blood loss greater than 80 ml per period. The most commonly used method of measuring blood loss is the non-invasive alkaline haematin method. Various visual scoring techniques have been devised, but they do not provide an objective measure.

Well designed, randomized controlled trials provide the best evidence of the efficacy of any intervention, as any differences between groups can be more confidently attributed to differences in treatment. Thirty-one randomized controlled trials of medical treatments for menorrhagia with objective measurement of menstrual blood loss have recently been identified (Coulter *et al.* 1995*a*, *b*).

The trials have a variety of designs which makes comparisons difficult. For example, the designs used include cross-over, double blind, placebo controlled, and double-dummy. Many have not used placebo; however, there is good evidence that placebo does not appear to have a significant effect (Nilsson and Rybo 1967; Chimbira *et al.* 1980; Varygas *et al.* 1987; Turnbull and Rees 1990). Different levels of blood loss have been used as entry criteria with some studies using 60 ml or 75 ml rather than 80 ml. Indeed some studies have also included women with normal blood loss (Fraser *et al.* 1981). Some trials compared the effects of different dosages; in others the doses varied from study to study. The duration of each phase of a study (pre-treatment baseline, placebo active treatment), needs to cover at least two cycles to allow for the natural variation in menstrual loss. Side-effects have not been consistently reported and there is a paucity of data on quality of life. Follow-up in general has been short, usually being confined to two months, thus limiting the amount of long-term data. Finally, although menstrual blood loss has a skewed distribution where medians and ranges would provide a more appropriate measure, many studies report only mean loss.

In routine clinical practice menstrual blood loss measurements are not available, and thus over half the women complaining of menorrhagia have a blood loss within normal limits. Here it is the woman's perception and the effect of her menstrual flow on her quality of life which are the reasons for seeking medical help. These factors must be taken into account when discussing treatment options. A trial in Oxford is currently examining the reasons for consultation by women with objectively normal blood loss.

Treatment options

Medical treatments for menorrhagia can be divided into two main classes: non-hormonal and hormonal. The former includes prostaglandin synthetase inhibitors and antifibrinolytic agents; the latter includes progestogens, combined oral contraceptives, hormone replacement therapy, danazol, gestrinone, and GnRH analogues. Non-hormonal treatment is taken during menstruation itself which avoids any possible teratogenic effects, and is therefore suitable for women who wish to conceive. Treatment for ovulatory dysfunctional uterine bleeding (or essential menorrhagia), anovulatory dysfunctional uterine bleeding, and IUCD-induced menorrhagia will be discussed where appropriate. Most women with regular excessive menstrual bleeding have normal ovulatory cycles (Haynes *et al.* 1980). Non-hormonal treatments for menorrhagia are summarized below:

- Prostaglandin synthetase inhibitors:
  mefenamic acid
  meclofenamic acid
  naproxen
  ibuprofen
  flurbiprofen
  diclofenac
- Antifibrinolytics:
  tranexamic acid
  epsilon-amino caproic acid
- Ethamsylate

Non-hormonal treatments

Prostaglandin synthetase inhibitors

Inhibitors of prostaglandin synthesis can be classified chemically into four main groups: salicylates (aspirin), indolacetic acid analogues (indomethacin), aryl proprionic acid derivatives (naproxen, ibuprofen), and fenamates (mefenamic acid, flufenamic acid, meclofenamic acid). Of the four groups, the fenamates have been the most extensively studied for the treatment of menorrhagia.

The use of prostaglandin synthetase inhibitors is based on the observations showing that prostaglandin (PG) biosynthesis is altered in menorrhagia. The levels of PGs in menstrual fluid suggest increased uterine $PGF_{2\alpha}$ and PGE_2 production during menstruation itself (Rees *et al.* 1984*a*). However, studies of endometrial and myometrial PGs have principally examined other phases of the menstrual cycle using hysterectomy specimens. In general, PG production by uterine tissues collected throughout the menstrual cycle from menorrhagic women is not increased and does not correlate with menstrual blood loss (MBL) (Rees *et al.* 1984*b*). However, in samples collected during the first two days of menstruation, when the largest volume of menstrual flow occurs, the data are suggestive of a relationship between the volume of blood loss and PGE_2, PGF_2, and 6-keto-$PGF_{1\alpha}$ release by endometrium and myometrium (Rees *et al.* 1984*b*). A shift in endometrial synthesizing capacity towards PGE_2 in menorrhagic women was originally suggested by Smith *et al.* in 1981, but was not subsequently confirmed (Rees *et al.* 1984*b*; Cameron *et al.* 1987). As well as inhibiting prostaglandin synthesis the fenamates bind to prostaglandin receptors. PG receptors have been detected principally in myometrium rather than endometrium and are occupied by PGs of the E series in preference to $PGF_{2\alpha}$ (Adelantado *et al.* 1988). Furthermore, PGE receptor concentrations are significantly higher in women with menorrhagia (Adelantado *et al.* 1988). Fenamates inhibit the binding of radiolabelled PGE_2 to its receptor in membrane preparations of human myometrium (Rees *et al.* 1988). Sodium meclofenamate was the most potent compound tested, followed by mefenamic acid. Other PG synthesis inhibitors had no effect. Sodium meclofenamate affects PGE receptor activation in that it inhibits

PGE-stimulated cAMP generation in myometrium. Thus the fenamates are the only inhibitors of PG synthesis which also bind to PGE receptors.

The fenamates have also been found to affect haemostasis in endometrium during menstruation (van Eijkeren *et al.* 1992). In women with menorrhagia endometrium contains two forms of haemostatic plugs which are not found in normally menstruating women (van Eijkeren *et al.* 1992): large fragile plugs protruding into the extravascular space reflecting decreased platelet aggregation and degranulation, and plugs with extensive re-canalization, possibly due to increased fibrinolysis. In women treated with mefenamic acid before hysterectomy performed during the first 24 hours of menstruation, there were fewer large haemostatic plugs, the plugs were further transformed, and there were fewer vessels without a plug compared to a group given placebo. The authors concluded that mefenamic acid may act through an improvement of platelet aggregation and degranulation and through increased vasoconstriction (van Eijkeren *et al.* 1992).

Fenamates

The ability of mefenamic acid to reduce excessive menstrual bleeding was first described by Anderson *et al.* (1976). In this preliminary report, five women were treated with mefenamic acid, 500 mg three times daily, on the first three days of menstruation when heavy blood loss was anticipated by the patient. Measured menstrual loss was reduced from a pre-treatment mean of 119 ml to 60 ml. Subsequently, a larger open study was reported by Haynes *et al.* (1980) in which 22 women with true menorrhagia were treated with mefenamic acid, 500 mg four times daily, during the first three days of menstruation. This again confirmed the findings of the earlier study, median menstrual loss being reduced from 137 ml before treatment to 76 ml on treatment.

The effect of fenamates was then examined using randomized placebo-controlled trials. Fraser *et al.* (1981) examined women complaining of menorrhagia but not all of whom had objective menorrhagia; in 30 MBL exceeded 80 ml, in 39 it was less than 80 ml, and of these, 14 had losses less than 35 ml. Overall, mefenamic acid treatment reduced menstrual loss by 28 per cent; 30 per cent for those with MBL $>$ 80 ml and 19 per cent for those whose MBL was $<$ 80 ml. The women with MBL $<$ 35 ml did not show any significant change in blood loss, indeed a small increase was recorded. Muggeridge and Elder (1983) found a 30 per cent reduction with mefenamic acid versus a 12 per cent reduction for placebo, which is within normal cycle to cycle variation. With regards to long-term efficacy, follow-up 12–15 months after commencing treatment showed that mefenamic acid continued to be effective (Fraser *et al.* 1983).

The effects of mefenamic acid have been compared to other treatments: naproxen, the combined contraceptive pill, norethisterone, danazol, tranexamic acid, and ethamsylate (Hall *et al.* 1987; Dockeray *et al.* 1989; Cameron *et al.* 1990; Chamberlain *et al.* 1991; Fraser and McCarron 1991; Bonnar 1994). Mefenamic acid and naproxen produced virtually identical reduction in loss, being 46 per cent and 47 per cent respectively (Hall *et al.* 1987). Comparison of several agents in one study showed overall MBL reductions of 31 per cent on mefenamic acid, 12 per cent on naproxen, 43 per cent on oral contraceptives, and 50 per cent on danazol (Fraser and McCarron 1991). Mefenamic acid and norethisterone reduced MBL in women with ovulatory dysfunctional bleeding by 24 per cent and 20 per cent respectively (Cameron *et al.* 1990). The percentage reduction in menstrual loss after mefenamic acid and danazol was 22 per cent and 56 per cent, but the authors concluded that mefenamic acid was a better initial treatment because of fewer side-effects (Dockeray *et al.* 1989).

One study has examined the effect of sodium meclofenamate using a double blind, placebo-controlled cross-over design (Varygas *et al.* 1987). Here meclofenamate reduced blood loss by 49 per cent compared with only 4 per cent for placebo, which is well within the normal cycle-to-cycle variation in MBL.

Other prostaglandin synthetase inhibitors

Reductions in menstrual loss have also been documented for other PG synthetase inhibitors such as naproxen, ibuprofen, sodium diclofenac, and flurbiprofen (reviewed by Coulter *et al.* 1995*a*). The percentage reduction in blood loss varied from 25 to 47 per cent depending on the agent and dose used. It was also commented that naproxen and ibuprofen were ineffective in women with leiomyomas.

Prostaglandin synthetase inhibitors and intrauterine contraceptive devices

In women with intrauterine contraceptive devices mefenamic acid, naproxen, and ibuprofen have demonstrated reductions in blood loss varying from 22 to 34 per cent, again depending on the agent and dose used. Furthermore, greater reductions were found in women with heavier loss; mefenamic acid reduced MBL by 34 per cent in women with objective menorrhagia and by 23 per cent in those with MBL < 80 ml (Guillebaud *et al.* 1978).

Side-effects

Various, generally mild, side-effects have been reported, mostly related to the gastrointestinal tract, such as nausea, dyspepsia, and diarrhoea. Others have included headaches and dizziness.

Thus PG synthetase inhibitors should be considered as a first line treatment in ovulatory dysfunctional uterine bleeding or essential menorrhagia since they are well tolerated and suitable for long term treatment. An added factor is that these drugs will also deal with menstrual pain.

Antifibrinolytic agents

The use of antifibrinolytic agents is based on the observation of increased levels of fibrinolytic activity in endometrium in women with menorrhagia. The effect of tranexamic acid was first reported in 1967 by Nilsson and Rybo. They compared two doses of tranexamic acid, 250 mg four-hourly and 500 mg four-hourly, which reduced MBL by 38 and 51 per cent respectively, compared to 8 per cent by placebo. Further studies have confirmed similar reductions in MBL (Callender *et al.* 1970; Milsom *et al.* 1991; Bonnar and Sheppard 1996; Preston *et al.* 1995). Tranexamic acid has been compared to PG synthetase inhibitors such as mefenamic acid (Bonnar 1994) and progestogens such as norethisterone (Preston *et al.* 1995). Tranexamic acid (1 g, four times daily) produced a greater reduction in MBL than mefenamic acid (500 mg, three times daily), the reduction in loss being 58 and 25 per cent, respectively. In a comparison with luteal phase administration of norethisterone, the same dose of tranexamic acid reduced MBL by 45 per cent and the progestogen increased MBL by 20 per cent. Thus antifibrinolytic agents should be considered as a first line treatment for menorrhagia, but unlike PG synthetase hihibitors they do not deal with any attendant dysmenorrhoea.

The incidence of side-effects is related to dose and about one third of women receiving 3–6 g daily experience gastrointestinal symptoms. Nevertheless, a recent study has shown no patient withdrawals as a result of side-effects (Preston *et al.* 1995). Serious side-effects have also been suggested, including cerebral sinus thrombosis and central venous stasis retinopathy. However, over a 19-year time span and 238 000 woman-years of treatment with tranexamic acid from the late 1960s, no increase of thrombotic events over and above that of the general population of the same age was observed in Scandinavia (Rybo 1991).

Ethamsylate

Ethamsylate is thought to act by reducing capillary fragility, though the precise mechanisms are uncertain. It is not widely used to treat menorrhagia. While one comparative study has shown a 20 per cent reduction in blood loss, another has shown none (Chamberlain *et al.* 1991; Bonnar and Sheppard 1996).

Hormonal treatments

Hormonal treatments for menorrhagia are summarized below:

- progestogens
  - norethisterone
  - medroxyprogesterone acetate
  - dydrogesterone
- intrauterine progestogens
  - levonorgestrel IUCD
  - progestasert IUCD
- combined oestrogen/progestogens
  - oral contraceptives
  - hormone replacement therapy
- other
  - danazol
  - gestrinone
  - GnRH analogues

Progestogens

These will only be discussed briefly here (see Chapter 13). The use of progestogens is based on the concept that women with menorrhagia principally have anovulatory cycles and that a progestogen supplement is required. However, many studies have shown that most women with regular excessive menstrual bleeding have normal ovulatory cycles (Haynes *et al.* 1980). Progestogens are the commonest prescription for women in the United Kingdom complaining of menorrhagia. The first report of their use was in 1960 in a study where menstrual blood loss was not measured, and the conclusions were based on a subjective response (Bishop and de Almeida 1960). However, studies where MBL has been objectively measured following luteal phase administration for seven days with 5 mg twice daily demonstrate either a 20 per cent decrease or even an increase in blood loss (Cameron *et al.* 1990; Preston *et al.* 1995). Thus, with current evidence, the short term use of norethisterone for ovulatory menorrhagia cannot be justified. There is some evidence that if given for a longer time, say 14 or 21 days, or in higher dose, progestogens may be effective. In a study of 10 women with ovulatory menorrhagia, three experienced dramatic reductions in MBL, four experienced moderate reductions, and three showed no improvement over two months following treatment with norethisterone 15 mg daily or medroxyprogesterone acetate 30 mg daily from day 5 of the cycle for 21 days (Fraser 1990). In the same study, in six women with anovulatory menorrhagia, reductions in MBL from 131 ± 40 ml to 64 ± 14 ml were found after using the same gestagens at the same doses, for 14 days from day 12 of the cycle.

Intrauterine progesterone or, more especially, levonorgestrel are much more successful. With progesterone, released at 125 μg daily (Progestasert), MBL was significantly reduced after one month but the duration of bleeding was somewhat prolonged. Twelve months after insertion, MBL was 35 per cent of the blood loss before insertion (Berqvist and Rybo 1983). The results were more impressive with the levonorgestrel-releasing IUCD (20 μg daily) where a reduction of MBL of 88 and 96 per cent was found after six months and 12 months respectively. This compares with 21 per cent for flurbiprofen and 44 per cent for tranexamic acid (Milsom *et al.* 1991). The levonorgestrel IUCD also provides very effective contraception. It could now be considered to be a serious candidate as an alternative to surgical management for menorrhagia.

Oestrogen/progestogen

The combined oral contraceptive pill is often used clinically to reduce MBL. In general the reduction in loss is about 50 per cent (Nilsson and Rybo 1971; Fraser and McCarron 1991). The mechanism of action is probably related to the induced endometrial atrophy resulting in decreased PG synthesis and decreased fibrinolysis. Hormone replacement therapy is also used to treat menorrhagia in perimenopausal women. While no studies have examined the effect on blood loss, it is known that with at least with one preparation containing oestradiol valerate 2 mg daily continuously and levonorgestrel 75 g for 12 days each 28 day cycle, median blood loss after 12 months' treatment was 16 ml (Rees and Barlow 1991).

Danazol

Danazol is an isoxazol derivative of 17-ethinyl-testosterone which acts on the hypothalamic–pituitary–ovarian axis as well as on the endometrium to produce histological atrophy. Studies have shown MBL reductions ranging from 50 to 85 per cent (Chimbira *et al.* 1980; Dockeray *et al.* 1989; Fraser and McCarron 1991). However, the clinical use of danazol is limited by its androgenic side-effects which include weight gain and skin rashes, as well as its long-term metabolic side-effects. The use of danazol is probably best restricted to women awaiting surgery.

Gestrinone

Gestrinone is a 19-nortestosterone derivative which has antiprogestogenic, antioestrogenic, and androgenic activity. In a placebo-controlled study of gestrinone 2.5 mg twice weekly for 12 weeks for 19 women with proven menorrhagia (Turnbull and Rees 1990), ten women became amenorrhoeic and a marked reduction in MBL was seen in five. Placebo had no effect. In three of the non-responders submucous fibroids were found at subsequent hysterectomy. The therapy was well tolerated since all women completed the trial. However, gestrinone's androgenic side-effects preclude long term therapy.

GnRH analogues

These agents can be used to reduce MBL by pituitary downregulation and subsequent inhibition of ovarian activity resulting in amenorrhoea. However, the induced hypo-oestrogenic state with its adverse effects on bone metabolism limits the use of these agents beyond six months. When cyclical oestrogen/progestogen hormone replacement therapy has been used in conjunction with GnRH analogues, median MBL after three months' treatment in the women with objective menorrhagia was 74 ml (Thomas *et al.* 1991). This treatment combination is expensive and should not be used as a first line.

Other treatments

Acute bleeds have been stopped with intravenous infusions of conjugated equine oestrogens, but this therapy is not a suitable long term strategy (DeVore *et al.* 1982). Some women may be keen to avoid drug therapy altogether. Diet and exercise have been proposed to influence blood loss, but no controlled trials have been undertaken.

What happens in current practice

Current management in primary care has been examined recently in Oxford and in a national survey (Coulter *et al.* 1995*a*, *b*). In the Oxford study of six general practices with 4977 registered female patients in the 30–49 year age group, 6.5 per cent consulted during 1991 for menorrhagia. Only 15 per cent had a pelvic examination and 13 per cent a blood test. Sixty-three per cent were given drug therapy and 30 per cent were referred to a specialist. In those given drug therapy, 41 per cent were prescribed norethisterone, 35 per cent mefenamic acid, and 1 per cent tranexamic acid. A similar pattern was found in the national survey of 518 general practitioners. It is of concern that the most frequently prescribed drug is norethisterone when scientific evidence shows that it is the least effective therapy for ovulatory menorrhagia.

The role of patients' preferences and the decision to treat by general practitioners is another important issue. Women are more likely to continue long-term medical treatment if their preferences and the options have been explored. In a recent survey in primary care only 36 per cent of patients indicated that they had a strong treatment preference (Coulter *et al.* 1994). The best predictors of having a treatment preference were higher education and previous consultation for gynaecological problems. Women with higher education were more likely to choose medical treatment; and female general practitioners were more inclined than their male counterparts to instigate drug treatment rather than refer for surgery. A history of prior surgery and a male general practitioner increased the likelihood of referral to a gynaecologist. This survey shows there is a significant scope for improvement in providing information on treatment options especially since one of the goals of treatment is to produce better long-term quality of life.

Treatment failures

Several options have to be considered when the patient says that the treatment has failed. First, her loss may be so excessive that, unless the treatment produces amenorrhoea, it has been insufficiently controlled. For example, with tranexamic acid where pre-treatment blood loss is less than 200 ml per menstruation, 92 per cent of women will have their blood loss reduced to less than 80 ml on therapy. However, if blood loss exceeds 250 ml, tranexamic acid is very unlikely to achieve a loss within normal limits (Preston *et al.* 1995). A similar pattern would be expected with PG synthetase inhibitors. Second, she may have a pre-treatment blood loss of less than 80 ml and the perceived reduction in loss on therapy is not sufficient for her. It is significant that in a study which included women with subjective menorrhagia but with normal objective MBL, therapy with mefenamic acid did not reduce loss and actually increased it (Fraser *et al.* 1981). Lastly, the patient may have unsuspected uterine pathology such as a submucous fibroid or endometrial polyp which makes medical treatment ineffective (Turnbull and Rees 1990). It is unfortunate that many studies do not follow up their treatment failures with hysteroscopy to check for such pathology.

Counselling

It is of concern that only 40 per cent of women complaining of menorrhagia actually have objective menorrhagia (Haynes *et al.* 1980; Chimbira *et al.* 1980; Fraser *et al.* 1984; Preston *et al.* 1995). Thus the majority of women could be considered to have inappropriate treatment, and that counselling might be a better option. A study of 17 women referred for hospital treatment for menorrhagia, in whom blood loss was less than 80 ml, shows that counselling is effective (Rees 1991). A three-year follow-up of these women showed that only one woman had opted for hysterectomy, two had taken drug therapy, and the remainder had accepted the advice. The effectiveness of reassurance and counselling is not known; it is currently being examined in a randomized controlled trial in Oxford.

Conclusion

The ideal management of complaints of menorrhagia should be based on objective menstrual blood loss measurements. Thus, treatment could be tailored to the loss. In women with a normal pelvic examination and normal blood loss, reassurance and counselling would be the most appropriate option. This would reduce the need for unnecessary treatment. If blood loss is less than 200 ml, effective drug therapy such as tranexamic acid or mefenamic acid should be employed. Norethisterone, in short courses, should not be used as it is ineffective. A good candidate for blood losses greater than 200 ml would be the levonorgestrel-releasing IUCD. Women in whom treatment does not reduce blood loss, should be investigated for previously unsuspected uterine pathology. It must be remembered that any medical treatment is usually long term and must not have unacceptable side-effects. Information packages need to be improved, and patient preferences need to be examined. Options must be discussed with the woman so that she can make an informed decision as to the best treatment for her as an individual.

References

Adelantado, J.M., Rees, M.C.P., Lopez-Bernal, A., and Turnbull, A.C. (1988). Increased uterine prostaglandin E receptors in menorrhagic women. *British Journal of Obstetrics and Gynaecology*, **95**, 162–5.

Anderson, A.B.M., Haynes, P.J., and Turnbull, A.C. (1976). Reduction in menstrual blood loss by prostaglandin synthetase inhibitors. *Lancet*, **i**, 774–6.

Berqvist, A. and Rybo, G. (1983). Treatment of menorrhagia with intrauterine release of progesterone. *British Journal of Obstetrics and Gynaecology*, **90**, 255–8.

Bishop, P.M.F. and de Almeida, J.C.C. (1960). Treatment of menstrual disorders with norethisterone. *British Medical Journal*, **1**, 1103–5.

Bonnar, J. and Sheppard, B.L. (1996). Treatment of menorrhagia during menstruation: randomised controlled trial of ethamsylate, mefenamic acid and tranexamic acid. *British Medical Journal*, **313**, 579–82.

Callender, S.T., Warner, G.T., and Cope, E. (1970). Treatment of menorrhagia with tranexamic acid. A double-blind trial. *British Medical Journal*, **4**, 214–16.

Cameron, I.T., Leask, R., Kelly, R., and Baird, D.T. (1987). Endometrial prostaglandins in women with abnormal menstrual bleeding. *Prostaglandins, Leukotrienes and Medicine*, **29**, 249–57.

Cameron, I.T., Haining, R., Lumsden, M.-A., Thomas, V.R., and Smith, S.K. (1990). The effects of mefenamic acid and norethisterone on measured menstrual blood loss. *Obstetrics and Gynecology*, **76**, 85–8.

Chamberlain, G., Freeman, R., Price, F., Kennedy, A., Green, D., and Eve, L. (1991). A comparative study of ethamsylate and mefenamic acid in dysfunctional uterine bleeding. *British Journal of Obstetrics and Gynaecology*, **98**, 707–11.

Chimbira, T.H., Anderson, A.B.M., Naish, C., Cope, E., and Turnbull, A.C. (1980). Reduction of menstrual blood loss by danazol in unexplained menorrhagia: lack of effect of placebo. *British Journal of Obstetrics and Gynaecology*, **87**, 1152–8.

Corrado, M. (1990). *Women's health in 1990*. Research study conducted on behalf of Parke-Davies Research Laboratories. MORI (Market Opinion and Research International).

Coulter, A., Peto, V., and Doll, H. (1994). Patients' preferences and general pracitioners' decisions in the treatment of menstrual disorders. *Family Practice*, **11**, 67–74.

Coulter, A., Kelland, J., Long, A., Melville, A., O'Meara, S., Sculpher, M. *et al.* (1995*a*) The managment of menorrhagia. *Effective health care bulletin*, No 9. Stott Bros, Halifax.

Coulter, A., Kelland, J., Peto, V., and Rees, M. (1995*b*). Treating menorrhagia in primary care: an overview of drug trials and a survey of prescribing practice. *International Journal of Health Technology Assessment in Health Care*, **11**, 456–71.

DeVore, G.R., Owens, O., and Kase, N. (1982). Use of intravenous Premarin in the treatment of dysfunctional uterine bleeding – a double-blind randomised controlled study. *Obstetrics and Gynecology*, **59**, 285–91.

Dockeray, C.J., Sheppard, B.L., and Bonnar, J. (1989). Comparison between mefenamic acid and danazol in the treatment of established menorrhagia. *British Journal of Obstetrics and Gynaecology*, **96**, 840–4.

Fraser, I.S. (1990). Treatment of ovulatory and anovulatory dysfunctional uterine bleeding with oral progestogens. *Australia and New Zealand Journal of Obstetric and Gynaecology*, **30**, 353–6.

Fraser, I.S. and McCarron, G. (1991). Randomised trial of two hormonal and two prostaglandin-inhibiting agents in women with a complaint of menorrhagia. *Australia and New Zealand Journal of Obstetrics and Gynaecology*, **31**, 66–70.

Fraser, I.S., Pearse, C., Shearman, R.P., Elliott, P.M., Mcllveen, J., and Markham, R. (1981). Effect of mefenamic acid in patients with a complaint of menorrhagia. *Obstetrics and Gynecology*, **58**, 543–51.

Fraser, I.S., McCarron, G., and Markham, R., Robinson, M., and Smyth, E. (1983). Long-term treatment of menorrhagia with mefenamic acid. *Obstetrics and Gynecology*, **61**, 109–12.

Fraser, I.S., McCarron, G., and Markham, R. (1984). A preliminary study of factors influencing the perception of menstrual blood volume. *American Journal of Obstetrics and Gynecology*, **149**, 788–93.

Guillebaud, J., Anderson, A.B.M., and Turnbull, A.C. (1978). Reduction by mefenamic acid of increased menstrual blood loss associated with intrauterine contraception. *British Journal of Obstetrics and Gynaecology*, **85**, 53–62.

Hall, P., Maclachlan, N., Thorn, N., Nudd, M.W.E., Taylor, C.G., and Garrioch, D.B. (1987). Control of menorrhagia by the cyclooxygenase inhibitors naproxen sodium and mefenamic acid. *British Journal of Obstetrics and Gynaecology*, **94**, 554–8.

Haynes, P.J., Flint, A.P.F., Hodgson, H., Anderson, A.B.M., Dray, F., and Turnbull, A.C. (1980). Studies in menorrhagia: a) mefenamic acid, b) endometrial prostagladin concentrations. *International Journal of Obstetrics and Gynecology*, **17**, 567–72.

Milsom, I., Andersson, K., Andersch, B., and Rybo, G. (1991). A comparison of flubiprofen, tranexamic acid, and a levonorgestrel-releasing intrauterine contraceptive device in the treatment of idiopathic menorrhagia. *American Journal of Obstetrics and Gynecology*, **164**, 879–83.

Muggeridge, J. and Elder, M.G. (1983). Mefenamic acid in the treatment of menorrhagia. *Research and Clinical Forums*, **5**, 83–8.

Nilsson, L. and Rybo, G. (1967). Treatment of menorrhagia with an antifibrinolytic agent, tranexamic acid (AMCA). *Acta Obstetrica et Gynecologica Scandinavica*, **90**, 78–83.

Nilsson, L. and Rybo, G. (1971). Treatment of menorrhagia. *American Journal of Obstetrics and Gynecology*, **110**, 713–20.

Preston, T.J., Cameron, I.T., Adams, E.J., and Smith, S.K. (1995). Comparative study of tranexamic acid and norethisterone in the treatment of ovulatory menorrhagia. *British Journal of Obstetrics and Gynaecology*, **102**, 401–6.

Rees, M. (1991). Role of menstrual blood loss measurement in management of complaints of excessive menstrual bleeding. *British Journal of Obstetrics and Gynaecology*, **98**, 327–8

Rees, M.C.P. and Barlow, D.H. (1991). Quantitation of hormone replacement induced withdrawal bleeds. *British Journal of Obstetrics and Gynaecology*, **98**, 106–7.

Rees, M.C.P., Anderson, A.B.M., Demers, L.M., and Turnbull, A.C. (1984*a*). Prostaglandins in menstrual fluid in menorrhagia and dysmenorrhoea. *British Journal of Obstetrics and Gynaecology*, **91**, 673–80.

Rees, M.C.P., Anderson, A.B.M., Demers, L.M., and Turnbull, A.C. (1984*b*). Endometrial and myometrial prostaglandin release during the menstrual cycle in relation to menstrual blood loss. *Journal of Clinical Endocrinology and Metabolism*, **58**, 813–18.

Rees, M.C.P., Canete-Soler, R., Lopez-Bernal, A., and Turnbull, A.C. (1988). Effect of fenamates on prostaglandin E receptor binding. *Lancet*, **ii**, 541–2.

Rybo, G. (1991). Tranexamic acid therapy: effective treatment in heavy menstrual bleeding. Clinical update on safety. *Therapeutic Advances*, **4**, 1–8.

Smith, S.K., Abel, M.H., Kelly, R.W., and Baird, D.T. (1981). Prostaglandin synthesis in the endometrium of women with ovular dysfunctional uterine bleeding. *British Journal of Obstetrics and Gynaecology*, **88**, 434–42.

Thomas, E.J., Okuda, K.J., and Thomas, N.M. (1991). The combination of depot gonadotrophin releasing hormone agonist and cyclical hormonal replacement therapy for dysfunctional uterine bleeding. *British Journal of Obstetrics and Gynaecology* **98**, 1155–9.

Turnbull, A.C. and Rees, M.C.P. (1990). Gestrinone in the treatment of menorrhagia. *British Journal of Obstetrics and Gynaecology*, **97**, 713–15.

van Eijkeren, M.A., Christiaens, G.C.M.L., Gueze, J.J., Haspels, A.A., and Sixma, J.J. (1992). Effects of mefenamic acid on menstrual haemostasis in essential menorrhagia. *American Journal of Obstetrics and Gynecology*, **166**, 1419–28.

Varygas, J.M., Campeau, J.D., and Mishell, D.R. (1987). Treatment of menorrhagia with meclofenamate sodium. *American Journal of Obstetrics and Gynecology*, **157**, 944–50.

13 The role of synthetic progestogens in the medical management of menorrhagia

Kerstin Andersson and Göran Rybo

Synthetic progestogens have been widely used in the treatment of heavy menstrual bleeding. The physiological background for this is the change of the endometrium which occurs after administration of progestogens indicative of endometrial suppression: small depleted glands lined with a thin epithelium and a more or less pronounced decidual transformation of the stroma.

Various administration regimens of progestogens are used:

- cyclic administration of progestogens alone
- continuous administration of progestogens alone
- intrauterine administration from a progestogen-releasing device.

The use of progestogens in combination with oestrogens to treat menorrhagia is considered in Chapter 12.

Cyclic administration

Usually, cyclic administration is given during the luteal phase. In one study (Cameron *et al.* 1990) 5 mg of norethisterone was given twice daily on days 19–26 of the cycle to menorrhagic women with ovulatory cycles whose menstrual blood loss (MBL) was objectively measured. Using this regimen a 20 per cent reduction in blood loss was achieved. However, in another study (Preston *et al.* 1995) using the same progestogen and the same dosage and administration regimen no significant change in blood loss was seen. In a third study (Higham and Shaw 1993) the effect of 5 mg of norethisterone given three times daily on days 19 through 26 was evaluated in menorrhagic women using objective blood loss measurement. Again no significant reductions in blood loss were seen. Bonduelle *et al.* (1991), using a questionnaire for bleeding intensity score, did not find any significant reduction of the blood loss using the same progestogen, dosage, and administration regimen. Finally, Cameron *et al.* (1987) studied the effects of 5 mg of norethisterone given twice daily from days 15 to 25 of the cycle. No significant reduction of menstrual blood loss was seen in menorrhagic women.

However, when norethisterone was given for more days during the cycle (from days 5 to 26) to menorrhagic women in a non-randomized open study, blood loss reductions of 30 per cent were achieved (Fraser 1990). It can be concluded that oral cyclic progestogens given for short periods in the luteal phase of the cycle are not effective in reducing the degree of menstrual blood loss in women with menorrhagia. It is possible that if progestogen is given for a longer time (21 days of a 28 day cycle) some blood loss reductions might be achieved.

Continuous administration

Progestagens can be administered continuously as oral tablets, long-acting intramuscular injections, or as subdermal implants which can last for many years. In the literature, however, no studies are published which present results of treatment of menorrhagia with continuous administration of progestogens. When women with normal menstrual blood loss used subdermal 70 μg/24 hours levonorgestrel-releasing implants (Norplant®) for contraception, Nilsson and Holma (1981) did not find any reduction of objectively measured MBL.

Continuous administration of progestogen has been used extensively for contraception and for the treatment of other gynaecological disorders such as endometriosis. From clinical experience it is well known that irregular bleeding and oligomenorrhoea (and in many cases amenorrhoea) are common consequences of this form of treatment. In addition, women taking contraceptive pills containing low dose progestogen only may also report diminished menstrual blood loss. As continuous administration of progestogen causes endometrial suppression it is reasonable to assume that this administration route may be an effective means to reduce menstrual blood loss in menorrhagic women.

Danazol is a derivative of the synthetic steroid 17-ethinyltestosterone. It is a weak androgen with little oestrogenic and progestotional activity which inhibits gonadotrophin release and steroidogenesis, resulting in endometrial suppression. Several studies have demonstrated the beneficial effect of continuous administration of 200 mg danazol in menorrhagic women whose menstrual blood loss was reduced by 40–80 per cent (Chimbira *et al.* 1980; Higham and Shaw 1993; Shaw 1994). Given in the luteal phase or during menstruation, danazol had no effect on blood loss (Chimbira *et al.* 1980). However, many women experience side-effects with danazol such as weight gain, acne, headache, and depression. In many women, these side-effects prevent long-term use and result in poor compliance.

Intrauterine administration of progestogen

Progestogens can be released directly into the uterine cavity from an intrauterine device (IUCD) and a pronounced endometrial suppression can be obtained even though the dose of hormone is so low that ovarian function is hardly affected.

Initially, intrauterine release of progestogen from an IUCD was thought to reduce uterine contractility and thus prevent expulsion of the device (Doyle and Clewe 1968). However, in clinical trials it was found that the steroid did not affect expulsion rates (Scommegna *et al.* 1970) but that contraceptive efficacy was increased (Pharriss *et al.* 1974). Moreover, the problem of increased menstrual blood loss, common when inert and copper IUCDs were used, was diminished. A device which released 65 μg of progesterone daily into the uterine cavity (Progestasert®) was found to reduce menstrual blood loss by 65 per cent after 12 months of use, and increase serum iron concentrations (Bergqvist and Rybo 1983). A disadvantage of this device was its short lifetime; it had to be replaced at approximately 12 months intervals.

Animal experiments showed that of the synthetic progestogens, levonorgestrel had the slowest release rate from an IUCD (Doyle 1975; Doyle *et al.* 1975). Different release rates of levonorgestrel were subsequently studied. One pregnancy occurred with release of 10–12 μg per day in a pilot study, and a release of 65–100 μg daily, which could only be maintained for less than a year, suppressed ovulation (Nilsson *et al.* 1980). A device releasing 30 μg levonorgestrel daily

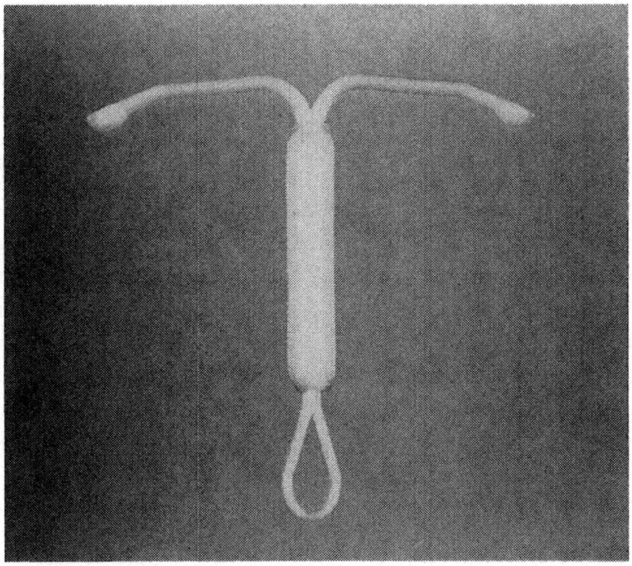

Fig. 13.1 The 20 μg/24 hours levonorgestrel-releasing intrauterine device has a Nova-T polyethylene frame and the steroid is dispersed in a polydimethyl-siloxane reservoir covered by a rate-limiting membrane on the vertical arm.

had no advantages in terms of contraceptive efficacy compared with a 20 μg releasing device (Luukkainen *et al.* 1986). Thus a release rate of 20 μg daily was selected for further development.

The levonorgestrel-releasing IUCD (LNG-IUCD) consists of a plain Nova-T device and a silastic rod, impregnated with 50 per cent levonorgestrel by weight attached to the vertical arm of the device and covered by a rate-limiting Silastic membrane (Fig. 13.1). The theoretical backgound for controlling the release of steroid from an insoluble polymeric membrane matrix is described by Fick's law of diffusion, which states that the amount of material transported across a polymeric membrane is proportional to the surface area of the membrane and inversely proportional to its thickness.

The life-span of the LNG-IUCD is at least five years (Luukkainen *et al.* 1986).

Mode of action

The effect of the LNG-IUCD is mainly local. There is only an occasional and weak effect on ovarian function. Intrauterine release of levonorgestrel causes endometrial glandular atrophy, stromal decidualization, and epithelial cell inactivation. These histological changes are seen within a month of insertion and the endometrial changes are independent of ovarian activity (Nilsson *et al.* 1978; Silverberg *et al.* 1986).

Stromal infiltration of leukocytes and some lymphocytes, a 'foreign body reaction', has been found to the same extent as with inert IUCDs (Nilsson *et al.* 1978). Compared with progesterone-releasing IUCDs, the endometrial effects seen during LNG-IUCD use are more uniform and profound because levonorgestrel is not metabolized by the endometrium as rapidly as progesterone (Nilsson *et al.* 1978). When the IUCD is removed, the endometrium recovers quickly and Silverberg *et al.* (1986) showed that biopsies obtained 1–3 months after IUCD removal were normal with no signs of progestagen administration or IUCD use, even when the device had been in place for more than five years.

Concentrations of levonorgestrel in endometrium, myometrium, Fallopian tubes, and fatty tissue from the abdominal wall have been compared following a 30 μg per 24 hour LNG-IUCD or after the oral administration of 250 μg of levonorgestrel (Nilsson *et al.* 1982). In the endometrium, levonorgestrel concentrations were 100-fold higher in the LNG-IUCD group, but in the myometrium and the Fallopian tube the levonorgestrel concentration was similar irrespective of the mode of administration. However, in the fatty tissue there was a significantly different and higher concentration in women given levonorgestrel orally compared with LNG-IUCD users. This reflects the high plasma concentrations of levonorgestrel in the orally treated group which were 2.5 times greater than the IUCD group.

Nilsson *et al.* (1984) studied ovarian function in 20 women who had used the LNG-IUCD for four years. Eight women were amenorrhoeic and 12 had regular but scanty bleeding. Seventy-five per cent of the women ovulated, whether menstruating or amenorrhoeic. There were no differences in oestradiol concentrations between the two groups.

Therapeutic use

The marked suppression of the endometrium and the development of oligo-/amenorrhoea, leads to a significant decrease in menstrual blood loss (MBL) (Nilsson 1977; Scholten 1989). In a population with a high incidence of anaemia (Dominian Republic) it has been shown that the use of the LNG-IUCD reduced the risk of iron deficiency anaemia and depletion of body iron stores compared with non-IUCD users (Faundes *et al.* 1988). These observations were the reason for evaluating the use of LNG-IUCD in the treatment of menorrhagia.

So far, three studies have been published in which the effect of the LNG-IUCD has been assessed objectively in women with menorrhagia. Menorrhagia was defined as regular menstrual bleeding with menstrual blood loss $>$ 80 ml. Menstrual blood loss was measured objectively as described by Hallberg and Nilsson (1964) and modified by Newton *et al.* (1977). Scholten (1989) studied 11 women 7–12 months after insertion of the LNG-IUCD. Blood loss decreased more that 75 per cent in all women and haemoglobin and serum ferritin concentrations had increased significantly. Similar results were presented in a Chinese trial (Tang and Lo 1995). In a study from our clinic, 20 women with menorrhagia were treated with the LNG-IUCD. After 12 months, menstrual blood loss had decreased by 97 per cent and haemoglobin and serum ferritin had increased significantly (Figs 13.2 and 13.3). One woman with a mean MBL of 501 ml prior to IUCD insertion experienced an expulsion of the IUCD a couple of weeks after insertion and was excluded from the study. She later had a hysterectomy, at which time submucous fibroids were noted. Another three women withdrew from the study because of intermenstrual bleeding and/or progestogenic side-effects (Andersson and Rybo 1990).

All women will notice a change of bleeding pattern after insertion of LNG-IUCD and intermenstrual bleeding and spotting are frequent during the initial months. The number of bleeding/spotting days will gradually decrease and an increasing number of women will become amenorrhoeic. Some women will notice progestogenic side-effects such as breast tenderness, headache, or acne initially but these side-effects mostly disappear after 3–6 months. However, counselling is extremely important if good compliance is to be achieved.

So far the LNG-IUCD is one of the most effective reversible long-term treatments for menorrhagia (Milsom *et al.* 1991). In the studies mentioned above only women with a normal sized or

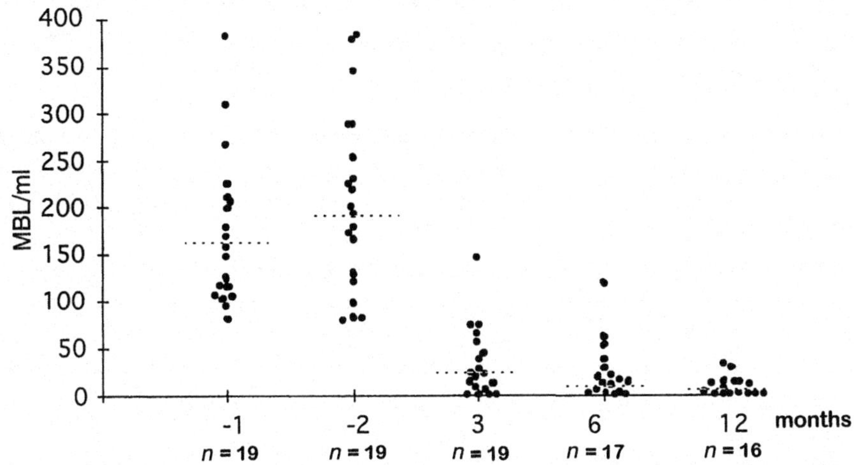

Fig. 13.2 Menstrual blood loss (MBL) in menorrhagic women during two control periods before LNG-IUCD insertion and after 3, 6, and 12 months of use. All individual values are indicated, and the median values are marked. (Modified from Andersson and Rybo 1990.)

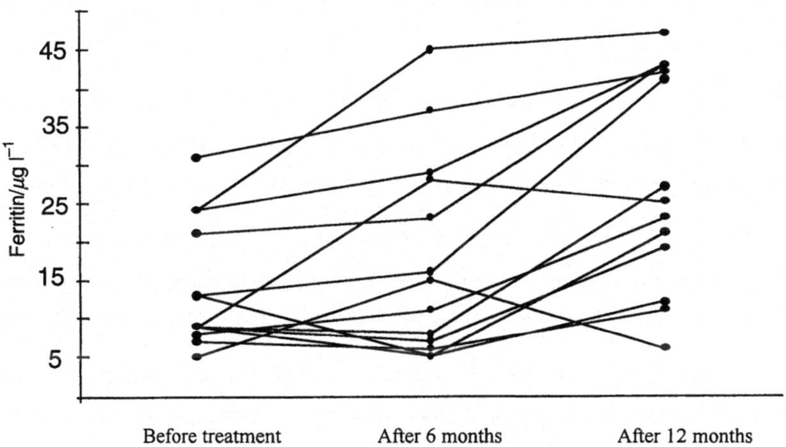

Fig. 13.3 Changes in serum ferritin concentrations in 13 menorrhagic women before LNG-IUCD insertion and after 6 and 12 months. Only women whose serum ferritin was determined all three occasions are included in the figure. (Modified from Andersson and Rybo 1990.)

minimally enlarged uterus were treated. It is not known whether MBL is affected by the presence of fibroids. However, in a recent publication Sivin and Stern (1994) indicated that the development of fibroids was decreased in LNG-IUCD users compared to copper IUCD users.

Besides reducing MBL, the LNG-IUCD is a highly effective method of contraception, comparable to female sterilization, with a cumulative gross pregnancy rate of 0.5 per cent after five years (Andersson *et al.* 1994). The contraceptive effect is rapidly reversible and after removal of a LNG-IUCD women conceive within the same period as after removal of a copper IUCD (Nilsson 1982; Anderson *et al.* 1992 *a*). The reason for the rapid return to fertility is that LNG-IUCD has a strong suppressive effect on the endometrium but hardly affects ovarian function. Compared to copper IUCDs there is a significantly reduced risk of pelvic inflamatory disease during LNG-IUCD use (Toivonen *et al.* 1991). Heavy MBL is more common in women aged

40–50 years than in younger women (Hallberg *et al.* 1966), and as the LNG-IUCD effectively decreases MBL this may be advantageous in perimenopausal women. Furthermore, in the perimenopausal period contraception might be a problem which could be resolved by the LNG-IUCD.

In addition it is likely that the development of endometrial hyperplasia might be prevented by use of a LNG-IUCD. Two reports have shown that even in combination with atypia, endometrial hyperplasia can be treated with the intrauterine insertion of levonorgestrel (Perino *et al.* 1987; Scarselli *et al.* 1988).

Levonorgestrel can now be used to provide endometrial protection for perimenopausal women receiving continuous oestradiol for climacteric symptoms. The mean number of bleeding and/or spotting days gradually decreased and the bleeding pattern was well tolerated (Andersson *et al.* 1992 *a*, *b*). No case of endometrial proliferation was seen after 12 months. Other investigators have shown that the LNG-IUCD is well accepted for this indication (Suhonen *et al.* 1995; Raudaskoski *et al.* 1995).

It can be concluded that the LNG-IUCD can be used successfully throughout the reproductive period for effective contraception and the treatment of menorrhagia. Moreover, use of the device can be continued after the climacteric to provide progestagenic protection to the endometrium in women receiving exogenous oestrogens.

References

Andersson, K. and Rybo, G. (1990). Levonorgestrel-releasing intrauterine device in the treatment of menorrhagia. *British Journal of Obstetrics and Gynaecology*, **97**, 690–4.

Andersson, K., Batar, I., and Rybo, G. (1992*a*). Return to fertility after removal of a levonorgestrel-releasing intrauterine device and Nova-T. *Contraception*, **46**, 575–84.

Andersson, K., Mattsson, L.-Å., Rybo, G., and Stadberg, E. (1992*b*). Intrauterine release of levonorgestrel – a new way of adding progestogen in hormone replacement therapy. *Obstetrics and Gynecology*, **79**, 963–7.

Andersson, K., Odlind, V., and Rybo, G. (1994). Levonorgestrel-releasing and copper-releasing (Nova T) IUCDs during five years of use: a randomized comparative trial. *Contraception*, **49**, 56–72.

Bergqvist, A. and Rybo, G. (1983). Treatment of menorrhagia with intrauterine release of progesterone. *British Journal of Obstetrics and Gynaecology*, **90**, 255–8.

Bonduelle, M., Walker, J.J., and Calder, A.A. (1991). A comparative study of danazol and norethisterone in dysfunctional bleeding presenting as menorrhagia. *Postgraduate Medical Journal*, **67**, 833–6.

Cameron, I.T., Leask, R., Kelly, R.W., and Baird, D.T. (1987). The effects of danazol, mefenamic acid, norethisterone and a progesterone-impregnated coil on endometrial prostaglandin concentrations in women with menorrhagia. *Prostaglandins*, **34**, 99–110.

Cameron, I.T., Haining, R., Lumsden, M.A., Thomas, V.R., and Smith, S.K. (1990). The effects of mefenemic acid and norethisterone on measured menstrual blood loss. *Obstetrics and Gynecology*, **76**, 85–8.

Chimbira, T.H., Anderson, A.B., Naish, C., Cope, E., and Turnbull, A.C. (1980). Reduction of menstrual blood loss by danazol in unexplained menorrhagia: lack of effect of placebo. *British Journal of Obstetrics and Gynaecology*, **87**, 1152–8.

Doyle, L.L. (1975). Hormone-releasing silicon-rubber intrauterine contraceptive devices. *American Journal of Obstetrics and Gynecology*, **121**, 405–11.

Doyle, L.L. and Clewe, T.H. (1968). Preliminary studies on the effect of hormone-releasing intrauterine devices. *American Journal of Obstetrics and Gynecology*, **101**, 564–8.

Doyle, L.L., Stryker, J.C., Clewe, T.H., and Harrison, R.A. (1975). Selection of steroids for incorporation into silastic intrauterine devices. *Journal of Steroid Biochemistry*, **6**, 885–8.

Faundes, A., Alvarez, F., Brache, V., and Tejada, A.S. (1988). The role of the levonorgestrel intrauterine device in the prevention and treatment of iron deficiency anemia during fertility regulation. *International Journal of Gynecology and Obstetrics*, **26**, 429–33.

Fraser, I.S. (1990). Treatment of ovulatory and anovulatory dysfunctional uterine bleeding with oral progestogens. *Australia and New Zealand Journal of Obstetrics and Gynaecology*, **30**, 353–6.

Hallberg, L. and Nilsson, L. (1964). Determination of menstrual blood loss. *Scandinavian Journal of Clinical and Laboratory Investigation*, **16**, 244–8.

Hallberg, L., Högdal, A.-M., Nilsson, L., and Rybo, G. (1966). Menstrual blood loss – a population study. *Acta Obstetrica et Gynecologica Scandinavica*, **43** (Suppl. 7), 320–52.

Higham, J.M. and Shaw, R.W. (1993). A comparative study of danazol and norethindrone in the treatment of objectively proven unexplained menorrhagia. *American Journal of Obstetrics and Gynecology*, **169**, 1134–9.

Luukkainen, T., Allonen, H., Haukkamaa, M., Lähteenmäki, P., Nilsson, C.G., and Toivonen, J. (1986). Five years experience with levonorgestrel-releasing IUCDs. *Contraception*, **33**, 139–48.

Milsom, I., Andersson, K., Andersch, B., and Rybo, G. (1991). A comparison of flurbiprofen, tranexamic acid and a levonorgestrel-releasing intrauterine contraceptive device in the treatment of idiopathic menorrhagia. *American Journal of Obstetrics and Gynecology*, **164**, 879–83.

Newton, J., Barnard, G., and Collins, W. (1977). A rapid method for measuring menstrual blood loss using automatic extraction. *Contraception*, **16**, 269–82.

Nilsson, C.G. (1977). Comparative quantitation of menstrual blood loss with a D-norgestrel-releasing IUCD and a Nova-T copper device. *Contraception*, **15**, 379–87.

Nilsson, C.G. (1982). Fertility after discontinuation of levonorgestrel-releasing intrauterine devices. *Contraception*, **25**, 273–8.

Nilsson, C.G. and Holma, P. (1981). Menstrual blood loss with contraceptive subdermal levonorgestrel implants. *Fertility and Sterility*, **35**, 304–6.

Nilsson, C.G., Luukkainen, T., and Arko, H. (1978). Endometrial morphology of women using a D-norgestrel-releasing intrauterine device. *Fertility and Sterility*, **29**, 397–401.

Nilsson, C.G., Lähteenmäki, P., Robertson, D.N., and Luukkainen, T. (1980). Plasma concentration of levonorgestrel as a function of the release rate of levonorgestrel from medicated intrauterine devices. *Acta Endocrinologica*, **93**, 380–4.

Nilsson, C.G., Haukkamaa, M., Vierola, H., and Luukkainen, T. (1982). Tissue concentrations of levonorgestrel in women using a levonorgestrel-releasing IUCD. *Clinical Endocrinology*, **17**, 529–36.

Nilsson, C.G., Lähteenmäki, P., and Luukkainen, T. (1984). Ovarian function in amenorrheic and menstruating users of a levonorgestrel-releasing intrauterine device. *Fertility and Sterility*, **41**, 52–5.

Perino, A., Quartararo, P., Catinella, E., Genova, G., and Cittadini, E. (1987). Treatment of endometrial hyperplasia with levonorgestrel releasing intrauterine devices. *Acta Europea Fertilitatis*, **18**, 137–40.

Pharriss, B.B., Erickson, R., Bashaw, J., Hoff, S., Place, V.A., and Zaffaroni, A. (1974). Progestasert: a uterine therapeutic system for long-term contraception. Philosophy and clinical efficacy. *Fertility and Sterility*, **25**, 915–21.

Preston, J.T., Cameron, I.T., Adams, E.J., and Smith, S.K. (1995). Comparative study of tranexamic acid and norethisterone in the treatment of ovulatory menorrhagia. *British Journal of Obstetrics and Gynaecology*, **102**, 401–6.

Raudaskoski, T., Lahti, E., Kauppila, A., Apaja-Sarkkinen, M., and Laatikainen, T. (1995). Transdermal estrogen with a levonorgestrel-releasing intrauterine device for climacteric complaints: clinical and endometrial responses. *American Journal of Obstetrics and Gynecology*, **172**, 114–19.

Scarselli, G., Tantini, C., Colafranceschi, M., Taddei, G.L., Bargelli, G., Venturini, N., and Branconi, F. (1988). Levonorgestrel-Nova T and precancerous lesions of the endometrium. *European Journal of Gynaecological Oncology*, **9**, 284–6.

Scholten, P.C. (1989). The levonorgestrel IUCD, clinical performance and impact on menstruation. Dissertation, University of Utrecht, Holland.

Scommegna, A., Pandya, G.N., Christ, M., Lee, A.W., and Cohen, M.R. (1970). Intrauterine administration of progesterone by a slow releasing device. *Fertility and Sterility*, **21**, 201–10.

Shaw, R.W. (1994). Assessment of medical treatments for menorrhagia. *Journal of Obstetrics and Gynecology*, **101** (Suppl. 11), 15–18.

Silverberg, S.G., Haukkamaa, M., Arko, H., Nilsson, C.G., and Luukkainen, T. (1986). Endometrial morphology during long-term use of levonorgestrel-releasing intrauterine devices. *International Journal of Gynecological Pathology*, **5**, 235–41.

Sivin, I. and Stern, J. (1994). Health during prolonged use of levonorgestrel 20 μg/d and the Copper TCu 380 Ag intrauterine contraceptive devices: a multicenter study. *Fertility and Sterility*, **61**, 70–7.

Suhonen, S., Holmström, T., Allonen, H., and Lähteenmäki, P. (1995). Intrauterine and subdermal progestin administration in postmenopausal hormone replacement therapy. *Fertility and Sterility*, **63**, 336–42.

Tang, G.W.K. and Lo, S.S.T. (1995). Levonorgestrel releasing intrauterine device in the treatment of menorrhagia in Chinese women: efficacy versus acceptability. *Contraception*, **51**, 231–5.

Toivonen, J., Luukkainen, T., and Allonen, H. (1991). Protective effect of intrauterine release of levonorgestrel on pelvic infection: three years experience of levonorgestrel- and copper-releasing intrauterine devices. *Obstetrics and Gynecology*, **77**, 261–4.

14 Hysteroscopic endometrial ablation

Milton Goldrath

Menorrhagia represents a widespread clinical problem, and is the leading cause of elective hysterectomy in women with a normal uterus (D'Esopo 1962; Cole and Berlin 1977; Dyck *et al.* 1977). Various methods are used to treat this condition, including dilatation and curettage (D&C), hormone therapy, ergot derivatives, anti-fibrinolytic agents, and non-steroidal anti-inflammatory drugs (Nilsson and Rybo 1971). While oral contraceptives appear to be the most effective approach to medical treatment, their usefulness is limited by side-effects and contraindications to therapy. Until recently, women who did not respond to pharmacologic intervention were limited to one of two options: hysterectomy or continued cycles of heavy menstrual bleeding.

The primary objective of endometrial ablation is to limit uterine bleeding and produce amenorrhoea – in essence, replicating Asherman's syndrome. First described by Fritch in 1894, Asherman (1948) identified this syndrome as a condition involving intrauterine synechiae, which usually results from post-abortal or post-partum uterine curettage. The syndrome is associated with amenorrhoea and infertility.

It soon became apparent that any technique capable of reproducing Asherman's syndrome might be used to correct excessive uterine bleeding. In subsequent years, a variety of chemical and physical methods were used for this purpose, the majority of which proved unsuccessful. While radium and cryocoagulation were both associated with some limited success, radium is no longer used in the absence of malignancy, and the cryocoagulation procedure described by Droegemueller *et al.* (1971*a,b*) was abandoned because of the potential for producing painful haematometra.

With the advent of hysteroscopic laser surgery in 1979 (Goldrath *et al.* 1981), women with menorrhagia refractory to other methods of therapy were offered an alternative to hysterectomy. For the first time, it was possible to predictably destroy the endometrium: producing amenorrhoea or hypomenorrhoea. Thus, the number of patients for whom this procedure is potentially beneficial is quite sizable.

Subsequent to the introduction of hysteroscopic laser ablation of the endometrium, DeCherney and Polan (1983) successfully destroyed the endometrium and produced amenorrhoea through the hysteroscopic use of high-frequency coagulating current. Vancaillie (1989, 1993) and also Townsend *et al.* (1990) described the use of the 'rollerball' electrode to facilitate electrosurgical endometrial ablation. In 1978, Neuwirth (1983) had used the urologic resectoscope to resect submucous myomas in women with abnormal bleeding. This led to his description of transcervical resection of the endometrium utilizing the cutting loop of the resectoscope in 1983. Hamou (1993) introduced endometrial resection in France utilizing a low viscosity fluid (1.5 per cent glycine) for irrigation. These hysteroscopic electrosurgical methods will be described in greater detail later in this chapter.

Other endometrial ablative techniques include radio-frequency induced thermal ablation (Phipps *et al.* 1990) and more recently, Neuwirth *et al.* (1994) and Singer *et al.* (1994) reported the use of a water heated intrauterine balloon to destroy the endometrium. These two techniques do not utilize the hysteroscope and, therefore, will not be further described in this chapter – but, they are indicative of a continuing quest for effective and simpler means of endometrial ablation.

Laser ablation of the endometrium

With the development of optical fibers capable of transmitting laser energy, lasers have steadily gained acceptance over the past two decades for use in performing endoscopic and hysteroscopic surgical procedures. One such laser, the neodymium:yttrium–aluminum–garnet (Nd:YAG), is particularly well suited to photocoagulation of the endometrium as a result of its high power and transmission through fibre optics. Its deep tissue penetration (up to 4 mm beneath the surface) and extensive coagulation distinguish it from the carbon dioxide and argon lasers.

Only a small percentage of the power of the Nd:YAG laser is absorbed by the tissue, the majority being diffused backwards (30–40 per cent) and forwards (25–30 per cent) as the laser energy scatters. Because of the danger posed to the surgeon from backscatter after tissue impact, use of special safety lenses or a protective filter over the eyepiece of the hysteroscope is essential, unless the procedure is done under video visualization.

The human uterus is characterized by a relatively thick myometrium (usually > 15 mm) and thin endometrium (usually < 1 mm), thus providing an ideal environment for laser surgery. The fact that only about 5 per cent of the uterine thickness must be ablated in order to destroy the endometrium provides a substantial safety factor.

Physiologic saline is currently used to distend the uterus and has proven an excellent visualizing medium. The use of an electrolyte solution has great advantage. With the large amounts that may occasionally be absorbed, there is no danger of dilutional hyponatremia. Previous experience with 32 per cent dextran (Hyskon) demonstrated that its high viscosity was associated with large bubbles that obscured viewing. In addition, it often discolours with the heat of the laser. Gaseous distending media may be useful for diagnostic purposes, but should not be used as a medium for therapeutic hysteroscopic surgery because of the risk of fatal gas emboli. It should be stated that Gallinat (1992) has devised an ingenious continuous flow system to use CO_2 as a distending medium for Nd:YAG ablation. In his hands it has proved safe and effective but it is not commercially available. *The reader should be warned not to use conventional CO_2* hysteroscopic distending systems as they can be extremely hazardous and could yield fatal results.

The procedure is performed with the patient under general or spinal anaesthesia. Alternatively, local anaesthesia with sedation may be used. A continuous-flow hysteroscope is used. The saline flows in by gravity only and is removed by low suction to provide a constant flow of fluid at low pressure. This is important not only for the removal of blood and gas bubbles from the operative field, but also for the prevention of earlier problems with excess fluid absorption.

Endometrial photovaporization and photocoagulation are performed under direct visualization using a power output of 50 watts, continuous wave. The entire endometrial lining is treated, commencing in the cornual areas and extending across the fundus and down the anterior and posterior walls to the isthmus, terminating 4 cm from the external cervical os (Fig. 14.1). To avoid treating

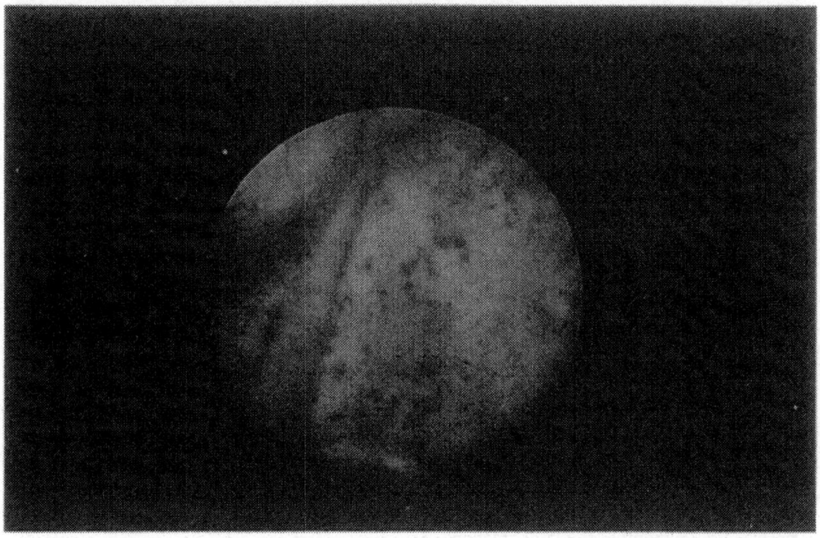

Fig. 14.1 Danazol-prepared endometrium prior to treating with laser. Note the atrophy and telangiectasia. Quartz fibre in view.

the endocervix, the level of the internal os (4 cm) is marked on the sheath of the hysteroscope. Care is also taken to avoid perforation near the tubal ostia, the thinnest portion of the uterus. This procedure takes 30 minutes in a normal size uterus, longer in a larger uterus.

Endometrial ablation results in pitting and charring of the treated areas (Fig. 14.2). After a long healing period, synechiae develop that are similar to those described by Asherman (1948) (Fig. 14.3). In many instances complete obliteration of the endometrial cavity eventually ensues (Fig. 14.4).

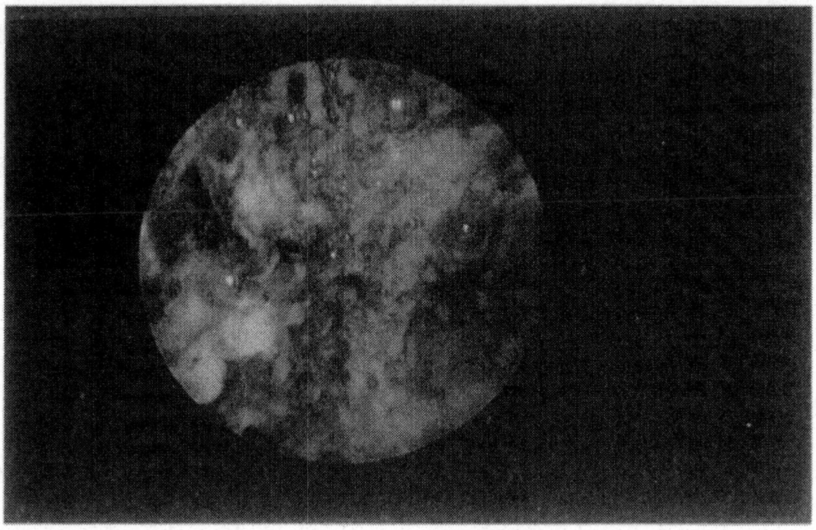

Fig. 14.2 A view of completely ablated endometrium. Note the pitted appearance and marked carbonization. Gas bubbles are visible.

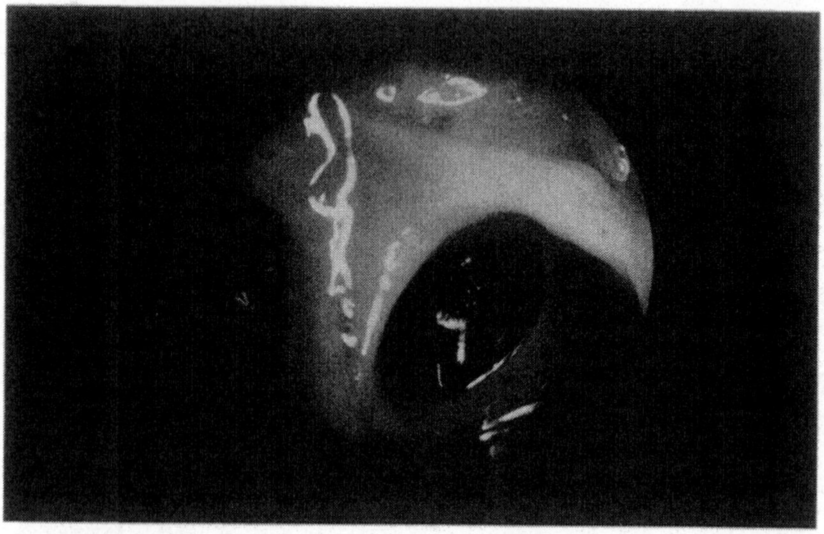

Fig. 14.3 Synechiae twelve months after laser ablation.

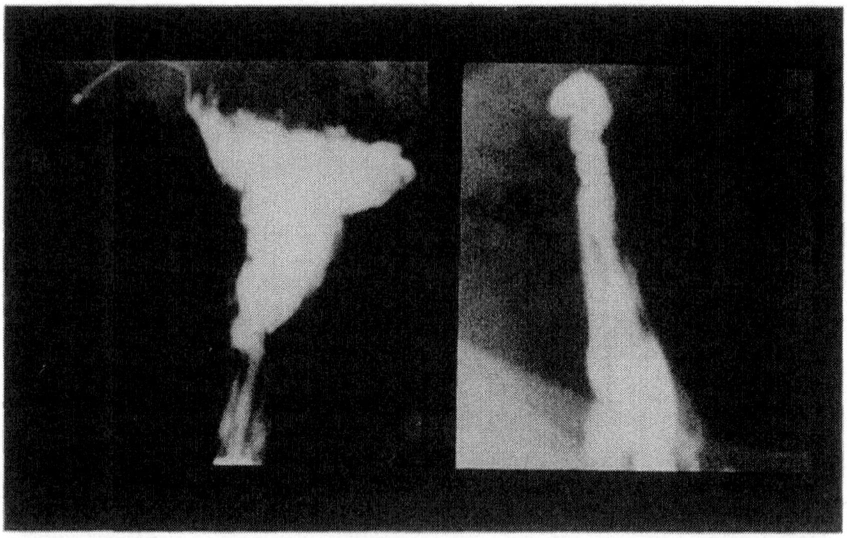

Fig. 14.4 Hysterosalpingograms performed three months and one year after laser ablation. Note the complete obliteration of the cavity.

Pre-operative preparation of the endometrium

Danazol was initially used in an attempt to duplicate the hormonal state of a patient who develops Asherman's syndrome (Goldrath *et al.* 1981). Since post-abortal or post-partum endocrine activity is negligible, it was believed that by treating a patient with danazol for three weeks prior to surgery and for two weeks following surgery, healing might occur before the endometrium had an opportunity to regenerate. Danazol is an effective inhibitor of normal follicular maturation and thus inhibits endogenous oestrogen production. It has been widely used for the treatment of endometriosis and has been shown to suppress menstrual bleeding (Greenblatt *et al.* 1971; Chimbira *et al.* 1979, 1980; Luciano 1982; Fraser 1985).

It has subsequently been discovered that healing takes up to six months following the procedure. Thus, danazol is no longer used post-operatively. However, the preoperative use of danazol greatly facilitates ablation of the endometrium, since the steroid decreases the thickness of the endometrial lining. GnRH analogues also produce endometrial atrophy and have been utilized for preoperative preparation (Brooks *et al.* 1991). Postoperative hormonal manipulation will be discussed later in this chapter.

Clinical experience

To date, over 600 women have been operated upon in the author's series. The following 407 women aged 12 to 53 years have undergone 427 hysteroscopic laser ablation procedures for the treatment of menorrhagia in the 11 years ending January 1990. Twenty patients had the procedure performed twice. They were initially classified as failures (to be described later). More than 60 per cent of the patients ($n = 274$) had fibroids, most of which were submucous fibroids or possibly adenomyosis. The criteria for patient selection include:

(1) excessive and disabling bleeding;

(2) inability or unwillingness to use other therapies;

(3) candidacy for hysterectomy;

(4) future childbearing not desired; and

(5) D&C within six months of the surgical procedure to rule out adenocarcinoma of the endometrium or cancer precursors. For the last eight years of the 11 year period, all patients had preoperative office hysteroscopic evaluation coupled with thorough suction curettage (Goldrath and Sherman 1985).

Most patients have fared extremely well post-operatively. The procedure is usually performed on an ambulatory basis, with the patients discharged two to three hours later. Although severe cramping typically occurs for the first two hours following surgery, it has recently been noted that the use of bupivacaine hydrochloride (Marcaine) 0.25 per cent paracervical block with epinephrine 1:400 000 at the beginning of the procedure greatly reduces the postoperative pain and seems to decrease intraoperative bleeding. A number of patients have had the procedure performed with only this anaesthetic in addition to intravenous sedation.

Overall, the postoperative symptoms resemble those associated with a D&C. All patients have experienced varying degrees of serosanguinous discharge that lasts for up to four weeks. None of the patients has become febrile.

Results

The results have been excellent in 379 (89 per cent) of the 427 procedures, 70 per cent of which produced amenorrhoea, with the remainder of these patients experiencing only a few days of spotting per cycle (Table 14.1). In ten patients (2.3 per cent) the procedure produced *only* 'good

Table 14.1 Results of 427 laser ablations in 407 women (over six months after laser ablation)

Outcome		Number of patients
Excellent		379 (89%)
Good		10 (2.3%)
Poor		35 (8.2%)
Early failure	17%	
Late failure (1.5 to 8 years)	18%	

results', meaning the patients were satisfied with treatment and experienced what they considered to be normal menstrual bleeding. Of the 35 procedures which had poor results (8.2 per cent), retreatment in 19 of 22 patients resulted in amenorrhoea (86 per cent) and three failed, necessitating hysterectomy. Of the remaining 13 failed patients, 12 underwent hysterectomy, without retreatment. One patient elected to put up with her symptoms. The designation as '*good*' or '*poor*' results requires some explanation. You will note that only 10 patients had what we consider '*good*' results. By our definition, this means that the patient has 'normal menses' and is satisfied with the degree of relief of her symptoms. The physician should not object to this. It is not difficult to quantify the blood loss from a patient who says she is amenorrhoeic or has a few days of spotting with a menstrual cycle. These are considered excellent. 'Poor' results are more difficult. I have decided to use the patient's perception of her results, as I did with 'good' results, rather than attempt to quantify her blood loss. If she was unhappy she was offered retreatment.

Fifty-five of the patients had clotting disorders, all of whom did well following surgery (Table 14.2). The procedure can be performed without correction of the clotting disorder, making these patients ideal candidates for endometrial ablation. However, *intracervical* injection of local anaesthetic agents should be substituted for *paracervical* block because of the hazard of haematoma formation. Spinal and epidural anaesthesia are contraindicated in these patients. Twenty-two of the patients were receiving warfarin therapy; 14 had von Willebrand's disease; five were renal transplant patients; five had immunologic thrombocytopenic purpura; three were dialysis patients; an additional three had storage-pool disease, a platelet disorder; and one had

Table 14.2 Clotting disorders in patients having laser ablation

Warfarin treatment	22
von Willebrand's disease	14
Idiopathic thrombocytopenic purpura (ITP)	5
Storage-pool disease	3
Bernard–Soulier syndrome	1
Polycythaemia/thrombocytosis	1
Antithrombin III deficiency	1
Renal transplant	5
Dialysis	3
Total	55

Table 14.3 Reasons for hysterectomies after successful laser ablation

Large myomas (4–5 months)	4
Ovarian cyst	3
Endometriosis	3
Marshall–Marchetti–Kranz (MMK)	2
Adenomyosis (pain)	1
Mittleschmerz (haemophiliac)	1
Haematometra (pain)	1
Bilateral hydrosalpinx	1
Retroperitoneal sarcoma	1
Cyclic spotting (HRT)	1
Total	18

Bernard–Soulier syndrome, another platelet disorder. One was a symptomatic haemophilia carrier, and one had antithrombin III deficiency.

Out of a total of 31 hysterectomies, 18 were laser successes (i.e. no excessive bleeding) and 13 laser failures (excessive bleeding). The indications for the hysterectomy in the patients who did not have excessive bleeding are shown in Table 14.3.

It must be realized that patients who have a uterus and adnexa are still subject to diseases of these and associated organs even though the endometrium has been successfully ablated. The procedure does not prevent fibroids from becoming very large. It may not prevent the development or progression of endometriosis. The patient who had the retropubic urethrovesical suspension (Marshall–Marchetti–Kranz procedure) had a hysterectomy at the time because her surgeon thought it was so indicated. The patient with haematometra and cyclic pain could probably have been easily treated by dilation of the cervix as will be described later in this chapter under complications. The patient with bilateral hydrosalpinges which were diagnosed as bilateral ovarian cysts approximately two years after the endometrial ablation presents an interesting thought. Presumably she had a distal tubal occlusion and the endometrial ablation occluded the uterotubal junctions bilaterally which then led to the hydrosalpinges. The patient who had cyclic spotting when placed on hormonal replacement therapy subsequently had hysterectomy recommended and performed by her personal physician because he did not believe that patients who had endometrial ablation should have any bleeding. This is not my opinion.

Of the early failures, 13 had hysterectomies for bleeding. One had large submucous myomas. Five had adenomyosis. Among the seven patients who had hysterectomy for late failures, two involved significantly enlarged fibroids, two had submucous myomas, and three had adenomyosis. Thus, eight of the 13 hysterectomies that failed (i.e. for bleeding) had adenomyosis.

Post-operative hormonal manipulation

Because of the possibility that adenomyosis was associated with a greater risk of endometrial regeneration, it was decided to administer a single dose of medroxyprogesterone acetate (Depo-Provera), 150 mg, to patients with suspected adenomyosis or submucous fibroids on the day of surgery in order to delay ovarian cycling until scarring could occur. Sixty-nine per cent of the

Table 14.4 Effects of single-dose medroxyprogesterone acetate: numbers of patients, with number of patients (%) percentages in parentheses

Administration of medroxyprogesterone acetate	No* bleeding	Scant flow	Normal flow	Heavy** flow	Total no. of patients
No	79 (37.3)	115 (54.2)	5 (2.4)	13 (6.1)	212
Yes	70 (69.3)	28 (27.7)	2 (2.0)	1 (1.0)	101
Total	149	143	7	14	213

*$p < 0.0001$ ($\chi^2 = 29.4$; DF = 1).
**$p < 0.0396$ ($\chi^2 = 4.23$; DF = 1).

patients treated with medroxyprogesterone acetate became amenorrhoeic and remained so, as compared with only 37 per cent of those who did not receive treatment (Table 14.4). This difference is highly significant ($p < 0.00001$). It should also be noted that the difference in failures (heavy flow) is also significant ($p < 0.0396$) (Goldrath 1990). Quite probably, the use of danazol or GnRH analogue for 4–5 months following surgery might also inhibit endometrial regeneration, but this requires additional study, and, of course, would result in considerably greater expense than would medroxyprogesterone acetate.

Complications

The complications encountered with laser ablation are summarized in Table 14.5. The major complication observed with this procedure has been fluid overload, which led to frank pulmonary oedema in two cases. However, it should be noted that this problem occurred early when a 'push' infusion method was used to distend the uterus. We now use a continuous irrigation technique that involves gravity feed of fluid into the uterus and active suction out of the uterus, with the rate of outflow adjusted by increasing or decreasing the suction to distend the uterus and control any bleeding. Very accurate measurement of the amount of fluid absorbed is essential to prevent this potentially disastrous complication. If excess fluid is absorbed a diuretic should be used. The use of physiologic saline solution as a distending medium obviates the risk of dilutional hyponatraemia, but massive fluid overload itself can be hazardous.

Table 14.5 Complications from laser ablation

Excess fluid (two with pulmonary oedema)	6
Profuse bleeding (tamponade)	15
Urinary tract infection	3
Drug reaction	3
Uterine perforation	1
Cervical bleeding (hysterectomy)	1
(Endo)myometritis	1
Haematometra	20

Following surgery, profuse bleeding developed in 15 patients after withdrawal of irrigating pressure. The bleeding was controlled by balloon tamponade using a Foley catheter inserted into the uterus (Goldrath 1983).

Three patients had post-operative urinary tract infections related presumably to intraoperative catheter drainage. In one patient, endomyometritis developed one week post-operatively, manifested by a profuse purulent cervical discharge. Although afebrile and otherwise asymptomatic, she was hospitalized for two days and treated with intravenous antibiotics. The purulent discharge stopped immediately.

One and three months post-procedure, all patients underwent a suction curettage; if haematometra was found, suction curettage was performed weekly until the condition resolved. Routine suction curettage revealed 11 cases of post-operative haematometra. This was not surprising in view of data reported by Droegemueller *et al.* (1971*a*,*b*). Early experience suggested that if haematometra had not developed within three months following laser ablation, it would not develop subsequently. However, we have since discovered nine cases of delayed haematometra. One was diagnosed nine years following laser therapy coincident with starting hormonal replacement therapy (HRT). Four patients with recurrent haematometra were treated by insertion of an IUCD, the tail of which keeps the cervix open. One had hysterectomy performed at the time of an operation for stress urinary incontinence. If a patient develops cyclic pain or other symptoms of hematometra, ultrasonic examination should be diagnostic. Indeed, we are now routinely performing transvaginal ultrasound examination at one and three months post-operatively rather than suction curettage to gain assurance that haematometra are not present.

Three patients had allergic reactions to danazol. The reaction was mild in two cases, and therapy was continued. Only one patient had to discontinue treatment because of a severe allergic reaction.

Laser ablation was not completed in one patient due to an instrument-related uterine perforation. The patient returned to the hospital two months later, at which time the laser procedure was completed.

One patient had an emergency hysterectomy for cervical bleeding. This complication deserves special comment. At the time, it was our practice to continue administering danazol for two weeks after the procedure. The patient was taking warfarin. Ten days following surgery, excessive, uncontrollable bleeding occurred, necessitating hysterectomy. It has since been published that the dose of warfarin must be reduced in patients receiving danazol therapy (Goulbourne and Macleod 1981). This underscores an important precaution in the prescribing of danazol: co-administering with warfarin may now be relatively contraindicated. Danazol potentiates the action of warfarin, greatly increasing the prothrombin time. Prior to the introduction of GnRH analogues, if the two drugs had to be administered concomitantly, the warfarin dosage was reduced by half. It was also advisable to monitor prothrombin times every three days through the course of combination therapy. The use of GnRH analogues for preparation of the endometrium in patients receiving warfarin has obviated this incompatibility.

Conclusion

The data accumulated over 16 years indicate that hysteroscopic laser ablation offers a highly viable alternative to hysterectomy in patients with menorrhagia who are not good candidates for simpler forms of treatment. Our current experience indicates that this procedure can be remarkably safe and effective and involves minimal post-operative morbidity and discomfort. The preoperative use of danazol or GnRH analogue to enhance endometrial atrophy has greatly facilitated the success of this endoscopic intervention.

I have discussed, briefly, the history of endometrial ablation and given a detailed description of laser ablation of the endometrium. This was done in great detail because it is where my expertise lies and is the description of the longest running personal series of endometrial ablations.

Electrosurgical endometrial ablation methods

Although the hysteroscopic use of electrosurgery for endometrial ablation is relatively recent, attempts to destroy the endometrium using electrocoagulation date back to the 1930s and 1940s (Baumann 1948). These were crude techniques that were done blindly by inserting a large ball electrode into the uterus. According to Vancaillie (1993) the results were reasonable and the complications fairly low. Vancaillie believes that these procedures were abandoned for social and economic reasons coupled with the increased safety of major operative procedures and anaesthesia. It is my belief that the procedures were abandoned because of a basic distrust of blind procedures and I would surmise that such procedures would probably give temporary rather than permanent relief.

The impetus to diagnostic hysteroscopy provided by Lindemann (1972) eventually allowed us to avoid blind procedures for therapeutic as well as diagnostic intervention. This is what led to the performance of endometrial ablation first by laser and subsequently by electrosurgical instrumentation. Electrosurgical instrumentation has been used by urologists for decades and it was a natural progression to adapt these instruments for operative hysteroscopy. It must be kept in mind that the early hysteroscope was only an adaptation of the urologic cystoscope.

Both the Nd:YAG laser and electrosurgery utilize heat for the operative destruction or coagulation of tissue. Both produce enough heat to coagulate the endometrium and superficial myometrium. Coincidentally, intraoperative bleeding is controlled by both modalities. This is very important as a small amount of bleeding within the confined space of the uterus would impair vision and make surgical procedures extremely difficult. In theory, both modalities are capable of producing complete endometrial destruction and, therefore, amenorrhoea. In practice amenorrhoea is demonstrated in all series of endometrial ablation. However, it is not uniformly attained. There is great variation in the percentage of procedures resulting in amenorrhoea in various series utilizing the laser and various series utilizing the electrosurgical techniques that will presently be described. Presumably this is due to different levels of operative skill and the amount of time and the technique used in these somewhat difficult operations. It should be pointed out that trying to destroy all visible endometrium meticulously will yield a higher amenorrhoea rate. The same meticulous attention to detail will help reduce the complications of excessive fluid intravasation as well as uterine perforation with possible disastrous consequences.

The two methods of hysteroscopic electrosurgical ablation of the endometrium in use at the present time are trans-cervical resection of the endometrium (TCRE) and 'rollerball' electrocoagulation (RBE). As mentioned previously, Amin and Neuwirth (1983) deserve the credit for the initial use of the urologic resectoscope for hysteroscopic surgery. In 1979, they described the resection of submucous fibroids in women with abnormal bleeding. In 1983, they suggested the use of the cutting loop resectoscope to cause the destruction of the entire endometrium (Neuwirth 1983). DeCherney and Polan (1983) also performed coagulation of the endometrium using a modified cutting loop of the resectoscope. Hallez *et al.* (1987) used the urologic resectoscope as it was designed (as a cutting instrument for resecting the prostate) to resect the endometrium. Although both methods are similar uses of electrosurgical techniques, there are essential differences and, therefore, they will be discussed separately.

Hamou, at the same time, suggested partial endometrial resection because of the desire of French women to continue normal menses (J. Hamou; personal communication 1985). Hamou also suggested the use of low viscosity fluids such as are used in transurethral resection of the prostate.

The 'rollerball' was also a urologic instrument used on resectoscopes. This proved a natural adaptation for hysteroscopic endometrial ablation in that it could be used as a coagulator without the cutting associated with resection of the endometrium. This has proved an advantage in that it is a more easily used instrument and would not be as likely to penetrate the uterine wall.

Trans-cervical resection of the endometrium (TCRE)

This procedure is analogous to transurethral resection of the prostate. It involves the use of a standard, continuous flow resectoscope. The use of continuous flow instruments is essential in preventing absorption of a large amount of distending fluid, which in distinction to the electrolyte solution used in laser procedures, must be non-conductive (electrolyte free). This is essential because an electrolyte solution will disperse the high frequency current and there will be little or no thermal effect. The hazard of absorption of electrolyte-free solutions with resulting hyponatraemia will be discussed later. Intrauterine pressure can be maintained by gravity alone and it is the author's preference. The flow of fluid through the outflow channel of the continuous flow resectoscope is maintained by low suction which can be varied to raise or lower the intrauterine pressure to remove gas bubbles, control bleeding, and provide adequate distension. Other authors have described various pumps which will regulate the intrauterine pressure to provide sufficient distension for visualization and yet keep the pressure low enough to prevent excessive intravasation of fluid (Hamou 1993).

As with laser ablation of the endometrium, preparation of the endometrium utilizing danazol (Goldrath *et al.* 1981) or GnRH analogue (Brooks *et al.* 1991; Serden and Brooks 1992) greatly facilitates the procedure. If the endometrium is thinner, much less has to be resected and an adequate depth of resection will be much easier to attain. It is thought that the endometrium should be resected to a depth of 3 mm which roughly corresponds to the 4 mm coagulation that is obtained with laser ablation of the endometrium considering that if the area resected is 3 mm, there will be approximately a 1 mm zone of coagulation beyond that. If submucous myomas are present in the cavity, these can be resected, as indicated, in order to give good exposure to the entire endometrial cavity.

It is essential that the resection be done in a systematic manner otherwise large areas may be left untreated. The resection should extend to the isthmus. The 'chips' which accumulate in the uterus present an annoying problem. They must be removed at some point during the procedure, in most cases, in order to get good exposure. This could be done with a small polyp forceps. We have had great difficulty removing the chips by washing them out as has been done in transurethral resection of the prostate.

This removal of chips points out a great advantage of TCRE – that is, the ability to get histological sections of the excised tissue. In general, this is not necessary in most ablative procedures, as the endometrium should have been well sampled prior to the operation by hysteroscopy and endometrial biopsy in order to rule out endometrial cancer and its precursors. However, there is an ability to examine the superficial myometrium which perhaps could give an indication of whether adenomyosis is present. The dilemma is whether 3 mm is sufficient depth to diagnose adenomyosis. Most authors think that it is. The ability to diagnose adenomyosis definitively would be of interest. There is some evidence that patients with adenomyosis are more likely to have failure of endometrial ablation. As noted in our data from laser ablation failures, this does not seem to be the case. However, we do not know for sure the denominator (i.e. how many patients actually had adenomyosis and were successfully treated). The collective data from five European series (two unpublished) representing over 1000 patients presented by Broadbent and Magos (1993) showed an improvement rate in over 90 per cent of patients with adenomyosis and a small failure rate. The amenorrhoea rates were considerably lower than those reported in series of laser ablation of the endometrium except for the two unpublished series which showed amenorrhoea rates of 59 and 42 per cent. In these two series, medroxyprogesterone acetate was used postoperatively.

Rollerball electroablation (RBE)

Other than the actual operative technique and the instrument used on the resectoscope (i.e. the rollerball or rollerbar for RBE and the cutting loop for TCRE), the procedures are quite similar. It is difficult to quantify the actual results as many of the procedures have not been done for a long time but I presume that they would also be quite similar.

Complications of electrosurgical ablation methods

The complications observed with each procedure are of a similar nature and because of their importance will be described in some detail. The complication rate is much higher with TCRE than RBE. The most important complication of electrosurgical endometrial ablation (TCRE or RBE) is excessive intravasation of the distending medium. Some intravasation must occur in all cases. Because the myometrium is invaded with TCRE, more fluid will be absorbed than with RBE. When it occurs in great volume, it leads to a complication that may be disastrous. It is far more important with electrosurgical ablation than with laser ablation because of the necessity to use solutions that are electrolyte free. As stated previously, electrolyte-containing solutions will not interfere with laser use, but with electrosurgical techniques, the fluid must be non-conductive. The absorption of large amounts of this fluid can lead to dilutional hyponatraemia. There have been numerous reports of deaths due to this very serious complication. The work of Arief is particularly frightening. He studied extensively the hazards of hyponatraemia in menstruating (reproductive age) females (Arieff 1986, 1993; Arieff *et al.* 1993; Ayus *et al.* 1992; Fraser *et al.* 1989).

Arief's observation that hyponatraemia is far more serious in menstruating females than in males or postmenopausal females is a startling one. Indeed, patients who had symptomatic hyponatraemia (manifested by headache, nausea, vomiting, or weakness, and progressing to cerebral impairment and/or coma and eventual respiratory arrest) induced by intravenous administration of hypotonic solutions, had a 25-fold increased risk of mortality if they were females of reproductive age when compared to males. A study by Fraser *et al.* (1989) demonstrated that the marked impairment of the ability of the female rat brain to defend against hyponatraemia progressing into cerebral oedema is often associated with elevated plasma vasopressin levels. There is a distinct difference between the response in male and female rats. They suggested that the circulating levels of vasopressin may contribute to the genesis of cerebral oedema by disrupting normal phosphorous metabolism in the female brain. They were primarily describing endogenous arginine vasopressin, but the current practice of many gynaecologists doing resectoscopic hysteroscopic surgery is to use injections of vasopressin for haemostasis. If this were coupled with dilutional hyponatraemia the results could perhaps be worsened. It is this author's belief that all gynaecologists doing resectoscopic surgery should be familiar with Arief's observations. For the above reasons, it is my practice *not* to use vasopressin with this type of surgery. In addition there is concern with the direct cardiovascular effects of vasopressin, which are purported to decrease coronary artery perfusion as well to raise blood pressure and cause bradycardia (Martin and Shenk 1994). Many women undergoing hysteroscopic surgery are perimenopausal and may be more likely to have coronary artery disease.

It is crucial, in light of the above information, that meticulous detail be observed in accurately determining *and* limiting the amount of fluid absorption occurring during hysteroscopic surgery. If the amount of absorption is excessive, one should abandon the procedure and have the patient return for a second attempt at ablation, rather than risk the disastrous complications mentioned above. This presupposes a degree of experience and judgement that will allow a surgeon to take such a step. Many authors believe that it is wise to determine sodium levels following the procedure when electrolyte-free solutions are used. This could be done in the recovery room.

It is possible that if a large amount of electrolyte-free distending medium were to be absorbed from the peritoneal cavity, such as would occur following an unrecognized perforation, rather than by intravasation or passage along patent Fallopian tubes, as is the usual route, hyponatraemia could occur several hours after the procedure, by which time the patient may have been discharged. The amount of fluid absorbed to create such a situation would, by necessity, be quite large and should have easily been discovered during computation of the inflow and outflow differential. Indeed, our studies of the amount of the fluid 'lost' or absorbed during laser ablation of the endometrium showed no significant difference in patients who had prior tubal ligation when compared to those whose tubes were presumably patent (Table 14.6).

Uterine perforation has been documented in all types of hysteroscopic surgery. It was documented in laser ablation of the endometrium as well as series of resectoscopic TCRE procedures.

Table 14.6 Fluid absorbed during laser ablation: numbers of patients, percentages in parentheses (K = 1000 ml)

Volume absorbed	Tubal ligation	No tubal ligation
None	13 (13.5)	31 (25.6)
0–1 K	45 (46.9)	54 (44.6)
1–2 K	21 (21.9)	24 (19.9)
2–3 K	9 (9.4)	8 (6.6)
> 3 K	8 (8.3)	4 (3.3)
Total	96 (100)	121 (100)

$\chi^2 = 6.9$; DF = 4; $p > 0.1366$.

In our institution we have had two perforations with RBE. Perforation most commonly occurs early in the experience of the operator, as noted by several authors (Magos *et al.* 1991; Macdonald and Phipps 1992; Broadbent and Magos 1993). What is important is what is happening when the perforation occurs. If the perforation occurs instrumentally when power is not being applied – and this pertains to both electrosurgical and laser power – it is of much less importance as there is little possibility of damaging abdominal organs (i.e. as when dilating the cervix, inserting the hysteroscope initially, removing chips with a polyp forceps). These types of perforations can be treated much like a perforation at the time of a D&C. The patient can either be observed for evidence of bleeding or, if the surgeon feels insecure, laparoscopy would suffice to see if there was any bleeding or gross trauma to abdominal viscera. However, if perforation occurs by direct action of the resectoscope perforating the uterine wall while power is being applied, or if perforation of the uterine wall with a laser fibre occurs when power is being applied, laparotomy is probably necessary with very careful inspection of the bowel wall in the area to be sure there is no damage. If damage occurs it must be treated appropriately and if small bowel is involved resection may be necessary. Resectoscopic injury to the urinary tract as well as major vascular structures has also been reported.

As important as recognizing a perforation is its prevention. The surgeon *must* at all times apply electrical power only when the tip of the resectoscope, rollerball, or laser fibre is in full view. Doing this procedure blindly is extremely hazardous. In addition, resectoscopic power should only be applied with the loop being pulled towards the operator, never when moving away. The same applies to the laser fibre and the rollerball.

Infection is very unusual following hysteroscopic endometrial ablation, though authors (Broadbent and Magos 1993; Townsend *et al.* 1990) have suggested the use of prophylactic antibiotics. It has *not* been our policy to use prophylactic antibiotics with these procedures, except when otherwise indicated. In over 600 patients with laser ablation of the endometrium, we have had only one intrauterine infection.

Pregnancy following endometrial ablation has been reported on several occasions. This is not very common, but when it does occur it is most distressing. The complications of pregnancy in patients with clinical Asherman's syndrome are well reported and include prematurity, early abortion, and mid-trimester abortion. Pregnancies reported after laser ablation of the endometrium have largely been normal if they were not terminated, or spontaneously aborted. Tubal ectopic pregnancies have been reported. I think a common sense approach to this problem would be to advise patients that we cannot guarantee sterility following endometrial ablation, although the incidence of pregnancy is very low. If tubal ligation has not been previously or concomitantly performed, use of contraception may be advisable. This is especially important if the patient continues to menstruate following the endometrial ablation.

Summary

The addition of endometrial ablation to the gynaecological surgeon's armamentarium seems to be changing gynaecological practice rapidly. The attraction to patients of an outpatient procedure that has very limited disability is quite evident. Although the very long term data regarding these procedures are not yet available, this laser ablation series dates back to 1979 and to date there have been no adverse late complications.

References

Amin, H.K. and Neuwirth, R.S. (1983). Operative hysteroscopy utilizing dextran as distending medium. *Clinical Obstetrics and Gynecology*, **26**, 277–84.

Arieff, A.I. (1986). Hyponatremia, convulsion, respiratory arrest, and permanent brain damage after elective surgery in healthy women. *New England Journal of Medicine*, **314**, 1529–33.

Arieff, A.I. (1993). Management of hyponatremia. *British Medical Journal*, **307**, 305–8.

Arieff, A.I., Kozniewska, E., Roberts, T.P., (ed.), Vexler, Z.S., Kanda, F., and Kucharczyk, J. (1993). Role of vasopressin in brain damage from hyponatremic encephalopathy. In *Vasopressin* (eds. P. Gross, D. Richter, and G.L. Robertson), pp. 243–57. John Libbey Eurotext, Montrouge, France.

Asherman, J.G. (1948). Amenorrhoea traumatica (atretica). *Journal of Obstetrics and Gynecology of the British Empire*, **55**, 23–30.

Ayus, J.S., Wheeler, J.M., and Arieff, A.I. (1992). Postoperative hyponatremia encephalopathy in menstrual women. *American Journal of Internal Medicine*, **117**, 891–7.

Baumann, A. (1948). Über die Electrokoagulation des Endometriums sowie der Zevikalscheimhaut. *Geburtshilfe und Frauenheilkunde*, **8**, 221–6.

Broadbent, J.A. and Magos, A.L. (1993). Transcervical resection of the endometrium (TCRE). In *Endoscopic surgery for gynaecologists*, (ed. C. Sutton and M. Diamond), pp. 294–306. W.B. Saunders, London.

Brooks, P.G., Serden, S.P., and Davos, I. (1991). Hormonal inhibition of the endometrium for resectoscopic endometrial ablation. *Americal Journal of Obstetrics and Gynecology*, **164**, 1601–8.

Chimbira, T.H., Cope, E., Anderson, A.B.M., and Bolton, F.G. (1979). The effect of danazol on menorrhagia, coagulation mechanisms, haematological indices and body weight. *British Journal of Obstetrics and Gynaecolgy*, **86**, 46–50.

Chimbira, T.H., Anderson, A.B.M., Naish, C., Cope, E., and Turnbull, A.C. (1980). Reduction of menstrual blood loss by danazol in unexplained menorrhagia: lack of effect of placebo. *British Journal of Obstetrics and Gynaecology*, **87**, 1152–8.

Cole, P. and Berlin, I. (1977). Elective hysterectomy. *American Journal of Obstetrics and Gynecology*, **129**, 117–23.

D'Esopo, D.A. (1962). Hysterectomy when the uterus is grossly normal. *American Journal of Obstetrics and Gynecology*, **83**, 113–22.

DeCherney, A. and Polan, M.L. (1983). Hysteroscopic management of intrauterine lesions and intractable uterine bleeding. *Obstetrics and Gynecology*, **61**, 392–7.

Droegemueller, W., Greer, B., and Makowski, E. (1971*a*). Cryosurgery in patients with dysfunctional uterine bleeding. *Obstetrics and Gynecology*, **38**, 256–8.

Droegemueller, W., Makowski, E., and Macsalka, R. (1971*b*). Destruction of the endometrium by cryosurgery. *American Journal of Obstetrics and Gynecology*, **110**, 467–9.

Dyck, F.J., Murphy, F.A., Murphy, J.K., Road, D.A., Boyd, M.S., Osborne, E. *et al.* (1977). Effect of surveillance in the number of hysterectomies in the Province of Saskatchewan. *New England Journal of Medicine*, **296**, 1326–8.

Fraser, I.S. (1985). Treatment of dysfunctional uterine bleeding with danazol. *Australian and New Zealand Journal of Obstetrics and Gynaecology*, **25**, 224–6.

Fraser, C.L., Kucharczyk, J., Arieff, A.I., Rollin, C., Sarnacki, P., and Norman, D. (1989). Sex differences result in increased morbidity from hyponatremia in female rats. *American Journal of Physiology*, **256**, R880–5.

Gallinat, A. (1992). Endometrial ablation using the Nd:YAG laser in CO_2 hysteroscopy. In *Endoscopic surgery in gynecology*, (ed. R.P. Lueken and A. Gallinat), pp. 109–16. Demeter, Grafelfing.

Goldrath, M.H. (1983). Uterine tamponade for the control of acute uterine bleeding. *American Journal of Obstetrics and Gynecology*, **147**, 869–72.

Goldrath, M.H. (1990). Use of danazol in hysteroscopic surgery for menorrhagia. *Journal of Reproductive Medicine for the Obstetrician and Gynaecologist*, **35**, 91–6.

Goldrath, M.H. and Sherman, A.I. (1985). Office hysteroscopy and suction curettage: can we eliminate the hospital diagnostic dilatation and curettage? *American Journal of Obstetrics and Gynecology*, **155**, 220–9.

Goldrath, M.H., Fuller, T.A., and Segal, S. (1981). Laser photovaporization of endometrium for the treatment of menorrhagia. *American Journal of Obstetrics and Gynecology*, **140**, 14–19.

Goulbourne, I.A. and Macleod, D.A.D. (1981). Interaction between danazol and warfarin. Case report. *British Journal of Obstetrics and Gynaecology*, **88**, 950–1.

Greenblatt, R.B., Dmowski, W.P., Mahesh, V.B., and Scholer, H.F. (1971). Clinical studies with an antigonadotropin, danazol. *Fertility and Sterility*, **22**, 102–12.

Hallez, J.P., Netter, A., and Cartier, R. (1987). Methodical intrauterine resection. *American Journal of Obstetrics and Gynecology*, **156**, 1080–4.

Hamou, J. (1993). Electroresection of fibroids. In C. Sutton and M. Diamond, *Endoscopic surgery for gynaecologists*, pp. 327–30. W.B. Saunders, London.

Lindeman, H.J. (1972). The use of CO_2 in the uterine cavity for the hysteroscopy. *International Journal of Fertility*, **17**, 221–4.

Luciano, A.A. (1982). A guide to managing endometriosis. *Contemporary Obstetrics and Gynecology*, **19**, 211–34.

Macdonald, R. and Phipps, J. (1992). Endometrial ablation: a safe procedure. *Gynaecological Endoscopy*, **1**, 7–9.

Magos, A.L., Baumann, R., Lockwood, G.M., and Turnbull, A.C. (1991). Experience with the first 250 endometrial resections for menorrhagia. *Lancet*, **337**, 1074–8.

Martin, J.D. and Shenk, L.G. (1994). Intraoperative myocardial infarction after paracervical vasopressin infiltration. *Anesthesia and Analgesia*, **79**, 1201–2.

Neuwirth, R.S. (1983). Hysteroscopic management of symptomatic submucous fibroids. *Obstetrics and Gynecology*, **62**, 509–11.

Neuwirth, R.S., Duran, A.A., Singer, A., MacDonald, R., and Bolduc, L. (1994). The endometrial ablator: a new instrument. *Obstetrics and Gynecology*, **83**, 792–6.

Nilsson, L. and Rybo, G. (1971). Treatment of menorrhagia. *American Journal of Obstetrics and Gynecology*, **110**, 713–20.

Phipps, J.H., Lewis, B.V., Prior, M.V., and Roberts, T. (1990). Experimental and clinical studies with radio frequency-induced thermal endometrial ablation for functional menorrhagia. *Obstetrics and Gynecology*, **76**, 876–81.

Serden, S.P. and Brooks, P.G. (1992). Preoperative therapy in preparation of endometrial ablation. *Journal of Reproductive Medicine for the Obstetrician and Gynaecologist*, **37**, 679–81.

Singer, A., Almanza, R., Gutierrez, A., Haber, G., Bolduc, L.R., and Neuwirth, R. (1994). Preliminary clinical experience with a thermal balloon endometrial ablation method to treat menorrhagia. *Obstetrics and Gynecology*, **83**, 732–4.

Townsend, D.E., Richart, R.M., Paskowitz, R.A., and Woolfork, R.E. (1990). 'Rollerball' coagulation of the endometrium. *Obstetrics and Gynecology*, **76**, 310–13.

Vancaillie, T. (1989). Electrocoagulation of the endometrium with the ball-end resectoscope. *Obstetrics and Gynecology*, **74**, 425–7.

Vancaillie, T. (1993). Endometrial electroablation. In *Endoscopic surgery for gynaecologists*, (ed. C. Sutton and M. Diamond), pp. 307–16. W.B. Saunders, London.

15 The role of hysterectomy for menorrhagia

Oswald M. Petrucco

Introduction

Disorders of menstruation resulting in excessive menstrual loss, or menorrhagia, affect up to 20 per cent of otherwise healthy women. At a rate of 20–30 per 1000 these women will seek the help of primary care physicians and when referred to gynaecologists they will represent up to 12 per cent of all gynaecological consultations (Bradlow *et al.* 1992). The health care costs of abnormal menstruation and associated anaemia, when related to loss of productivity in the work force and home and utilization of medical services, are considerable even before expenditure is considered for investigating and treating this disorder. Medication prescribed for women suffering from menorrhagia for 1993 in England and Wales resulted in 821 700 prescriptions at a cost of £7 176 596. In the same year 128 000 diagnostic procedures and 73 000 hysterectomies were performed for the management of menorrhagia (Nuffield Institute for Health 1995).

Despite the reviews, articles, and editorials over the past 20 years which have examined the indications, appropriateness, complications, and cost effectiveness of hysterectomy, there is still a need for assessing how this procedure will affect the quality of women's health care as we approach the next century. A second primary goal of health care provision is the need to contain health care costs, particularly in relation to surgical procedures. More recently, laparoscopic associated hysterectomy has led to further debate on the current utilization and cost effectiveness of this high-technology related procedure.

Incidence

In Western societies hysterectomy is usually the second most common major operation performed after Caesarean section. The prevalence of hysterectomy varies widely in different parts of the world and also within regions with as much as a six-fold variance for different countries. The highest rates have been recorded in the United States of America, Canada, and Australia and the lowest in Scandinavian countries (Table 15.1).

The incidence of hysterectomy has fallen from a peak in 1975 in the USA and since 1985 in Canada (Lalonde 1994). In Australia as well there has been a decline in hysterectomies performed for privately insured patients in the decade between 1976 and 1986 (Wood *et al.* 1992). Despite these trends the lifetime risk of having a hysterectomy is 22 per cent in Europe and almost 50 per cent in the United States of America (Bunker 1976). Australian studies have indi-

Table 15.1 Incidence of hysterectomy in different regions (Adapted from Hirsch 1993 and Van Keep *et al.* 1983)

Country	Rate (per thousand women)
United States	5.56
Canada	4.70
Australia	3.97
New Zealand	2.50
United Kingdom	1.45
Sweden	1.32
Netherlands	0.38

cated that 16.9 per cent of all women and 34.2 per cent of women in the over 50 age group had undergone this procedure (Schofield *et al.* 1991).

Factors influencing prevalence of hysterectomy

Factors unrelated to primary indications for hysterectomy which have been found to influence hysterectomy rates are summarized in Fig. 15.1.

Sterilization

The relationship between sterilization and subsequent menstrual abnormality and the need to perform hysterectomy has been a much discussed, but, until the last decade or so, poorly studied subject. Disruption to ovarian blood supply and thus ovarian function has not been substantiated by luteal phase and endometrial maturation studies (Donnez *et al.* 1981).

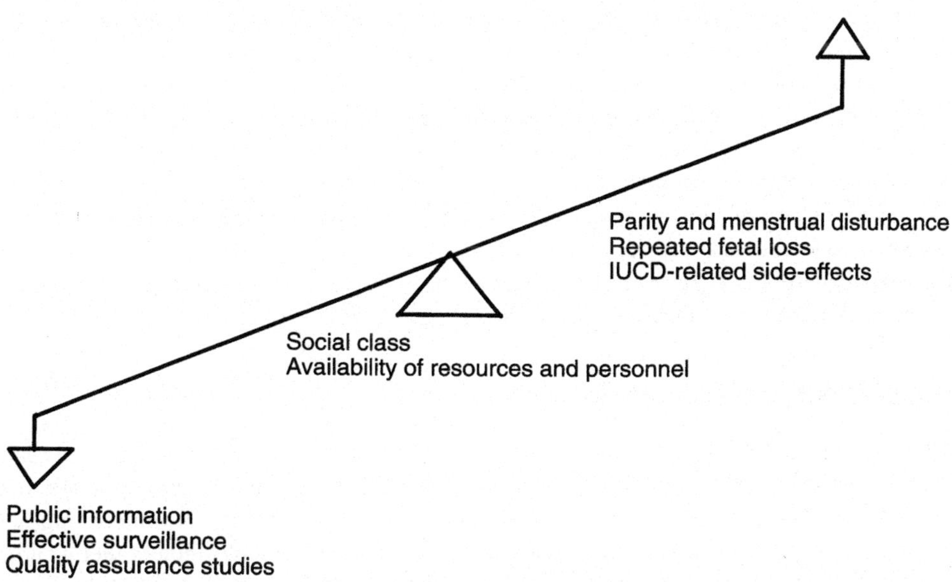

Fig. 15.1 Factors influencing hysterectomy rates.

A multicentre study involving 2500 women having electrocautery and Fallope® ring sterilization revealed in a two year follow-up no increase in the prevalence of abnormal menstrual function except for dysmenorrhoea associated with the electrocautery group (DeStefano *et al.* 1983). Fifty per cent of women who had experienced menstrual problems pre-operatively reported an improvement following sterilization. Santow and Bracher (1992) found that the incidence of hysterectomy was less in women who had been sterilized than in those who had experienced repeated fetal loss or side-effects related to intrauterine device usage.

Publicity and public awareness campaigns

Public awareness campaigns, quality assurance studies, and the effect of surveillance of hysterectomy rate in a community are known to influence the incidence of hysterectomy. Dyck *et al.* (1977) in a Saskatchewan study found that public awareness of indications for hysterectomy reduced the 'unjustified rate' from 23.7 per cent to 7.8 per cent. Gambone *et al.* (1990) similarly found that standardization of indications for hysterectomy in quality assurance programmes was associated with a reduction in incidence of both abdominal and vaginal hysterectomy. Vessey *et al.* (1992) found, in a large cohort study, that social class has only a slight influence on having a hysterectomy whereas menstrual disturbances have a strong positive influence. An Australian community survey has indicated that the availability of hospital beds and trained personnel did not significantly influence hysterectomy rates (Schofield *et al.* 1991).

Indications for hysterectomy

The principal reason gynaecologists advise hysterectomy for the management of menorrhagia is the effectiveness of the operation in coping with a symptom which has not responded to medical therapy. Some women choose surgery rather than medical management because of perceived or experienced side-effects of medication or because of the unwillingness to consider prolonged medical treatment. Coexistent disease with associated pelvic pain, pelvic mass, symptoms of prolapse, or urinary incontinence often influence doctor and patient to favour hysterectomy. An important prerequisite to decision-making therefore must be an adequate assessment by history, examination, and investigations which evaluate the presence of organic pathology.

In reviewing non-malignant indications for hysterectomy Carlson *et al.* (1993) have found that uterine leiomyomas account for 30 per cent of hysterectomies, dysfunctional uterine bleeding 20 per cent, endometriosis and adenomyosis 20 per cent, chronic pelvic pain 10 per cent, and endometrial hyperplasia 6 per cent. Other studies have indicated a hysterectomy incidence of 30–50 per cent for dysfunctional uterine bleeding (Fraser 1989).

Alternative surgical approaches

Alternative approaches to the management of leiomyomas with gonadotrophin-releasing hormone agonists, hysteroscopic resection of submucosal myomas, and myomectomy are more commonly considered for younger women wanting to preserve fertility. An interesting new approach to defunctioning uterine fibroids has been the radiologic embolization of uterine arteries, thus achieving a decrease in uterine and fibroid blood flow (Ravina *et al.* 1995). More conservative surgery has also been advocated for the treatment of adenomyosis. Doppler flow vaginal ultrasound diagnosis and laparoscopic electrocautery of adenomyotic foci has been advocated by Wood *et al.* (1993).

Endometrial destructive procedures

The majority of women investigated for menorrhagia, however, have no demonstrable organic pathology with currently available investigative procedures and are classified as having dysfunctional uterine bleeding. This group in particular are thought to be the most eligible for transcervical endometrial ablation or resection. These procedures are associated with a shorter hospitalization, and convalescence, but the need to carry out further surgery, either repeat ablation or resection or hysterectomy, has been reported in up to 23 per cent of patients, particularly in the longest follow-up studies (Dwyer *et al.* 1993; Pinion *et al.* 1994). An Australian study on the outcome of 1853 privately insured patients having endometrial ablation in 1991 reported that in a 20–26 month follow-up period, 10 per cent had hysterectomy, 6 per cent repeat endometrial ablation, and 5 per cent other gynaecological procedures (Molloy and Taylor 1994). The incidence of endometrial ablation procedures on privately insured patients in Australia reached a peak in 1992–1993, with an overall decline in incidence of 46 per cent over the next two years (Molloy and Crosdale 1996). Data from the same group of patients indicated an almost three-fold increase in the number of laparoscopic-assisted vaginal hysterectomies from 1993 to 1995.

Surgical methods and complications

Once a decision to opt for hysterectomy has been made, the type of procedure chosen will greatly depend on the attitude and operative skill of the surgeon in performing vaginal hysterectomy. There is reasonable agreement by gynaecologists trained in British, European, and United States hospitals that the vaginal route provides a safe and cost-effective way of removing the uterus with least morbidity and mortality. Except for the very accomplished and motivated vaginal surgeon, however, the presence of a large uterine mass (greater than 12 weeks' gestational size), associated endometriosis, pelvic adhesions, the need to carry out bilateral oophorectomy, vaginal scarring, and nulliparity are usually considered contraindications to vaginal surgery and the abdominal route is chosen.

The fact remains, however, that the majority of hysterectomies are performed abdominally. In the UK in 1993/94 only 19.2 per cent of hysterectomies were performed vaginally (Nuffield Institute for Health 1995). Australian Health Insurance Commission data (Hirsch 1993) indicate that Medicare benefit payments in 1991/92 accounted for 68.7 per cent abdominal and 28.5 per cent vaginal hysterectomies. The same source (Hirsch 1993) revealed a slight increase in vaginal and decrease in abdominal hysterectomies between 1989 and 1992.

The impact of laparoscopic-associated hysterectomy

Since being introduced in 1989 laparoscopic-associated hysterectomy procedures have been performed by surgeons skilled in endoscopic surgery. Although carried out in increasing numbers it is still early to assess whether this procedure will reduce the number of abdominal hysterectomies performed in the same centre. The impact of laparoscopic surgery on vaginal hysterectomy was assessed by Querleu *et al.* (1993). Over a one year period, by excluding malignant disease and vaginal prolapse requiring colporrhaphy and sacrospinous fixation, 149 patients had hysterectomy performed by surgeons experienced in both vaginal and laparoscopic surgery. Vaginal hysterectomy was achieved in 114 cases (77 per cent), laparoscopic-assisted vaginal hysterectomy (LAVH) in 26 (17 per cent), and abdominal hysterectomy was necessary in only 9 cases (6 per cent). Following retrospective comparison of the first 115 laparoscopic-assisted vaginal hysterectomies with vaginal and abdominal hysterectomies at one medical centre, Casey *et al.* (1994) concluded that LAVH was performed for cases that would have been otherwise selected for abdominal rather than vaginal hysterectomy and that LAVH was expected to replace many abdominal hysterectomies in the future. Findings from a retrospective study involving 2563 hysterectomies performed in a large metropolitan nil-for-profit hospital involving 37 gynaecologists over a three year period (1991–93) also indicated a reduction in abdominal hysterectomy from 65 to 36 per cent (Johns *et al.* 1995). Unlike the French study, however, LAVH increased from 12 to 45 per cent and vaginal hysterectomy varied from 19 to 23 per cent.

The conclusion reached by Richardson *et al.* (1995) from a prospective, randomized controlled study to assess whether most women offered abdominal hysterectomy could have the procedure performed vaginally, was that up to 75 per cent of their patients could be treated by vaginal surgery. They suggested that previous pelvic surgery, mild endometriosis, history of pelvic sepsis, or uterine fibroids need not be contraindications to vaginal surgery. These authors also indicated that to reduce operating time, when laparoscopy is initially used to diagnose or treat suspected pelvic pathology, the subsequent LAVH should be converted to a vaginal procedure at the earliest opportunity. The series presented by Browne and Frazer (1991) (349 cases) and Kovac (1995) (617 cases) attest to the fact that dedicated vaginal surgeons can perform hysterectomy in 79–89 per cent of patients.

Hospital stay and costs

Early reports of increased cost and longer operating time for laparoscopic procedures were compensated by reduced hospital stay and quicker recuperation and return to work. Utilization of reusable endoscopy equipment and traditional surgical electrocautery rather than disposable stapling methods has considerably reduced the cost of laparoscopic hysterectomy.

The randomized prospective study of laparoscopic vaginal hysterectomy versus abdominal hysterectomy of Raju and Auld (1994), hopefully to be followed by similar randomized studies from other centres, has helped to clarify the issue of cost and acceptance of this new procedure. The laparoscopic procedures took longer (100 vs 57 min), but patients had 3.5 versus 6 days in hospital and recovered in 3 versus 6 weeks. There were minimal and insignificant differences in complications in both groups. Because disposable instruments were used, the cost of LAVH was greater; however, the total cost of treatment was less because of a shortened post-operative stay in hospital. By using reusable laparoscopic instruments and electrosurgery and suturing for haemostasis, Johns *et al.* (1995) found an identical hospital cost when performing abdominal hysterectomy (68 h hospital stay) and LAVH (44 h hospital stay), with a lower cost for vaginal hysterectomy (43 h hospital stay). The argument of shorter hospital stay will probably not be so significant in the future because of the trend, on the basis of costs, for earlier discharge from hospital for all categories of surgical patients.

Nevertheless, proponents of vaginal hysterectomy have demonstrated that early discharge is also appropriate following this procedure. Stovall *et al.* 1992, Summit *et al.* (1992), and Ng and

Hogston (1994) have reported an 8–12 h stay in hospital and Youssif and Ledward (1993) a 48–72 h discharge interval. Patients discharged within 12 h were contacted by telephone by surgeons and qualified nurse practitioners for the first three postoperative days and appropriate investigations were performed at home when required. In an unselected group of patients Rankin (1992) found that the mean length of hospital stay for vaginal hysterectomy patients was 2.4 days and for abdominal hysterectomy 2.8 days. In a series of 50 patients having abdominal hysterectomy for benign bleeding disorders, Bennett (1994) noted a mean operating time of 49 minutes and postoperative in-patient stay of 3.7 days (range 2.75–6.1 days).

Using the criteria of apyrexia, urination, ambulation, and lack of need for strong analgesic, Jackson *et al.* (1995) found that the median post-operative stay for abdominal hysterectomy was reduced to three days (range 1–7 days). The case – control comparative study of Carter *et al.* (1994) reported that women having abdominal hysterectomy had reported significantly more pain after discharge from hospital than women having had LAVH.

Morbidity and mortality of hysterectomy procedures

Hysterectomy procedures are associated with mortality and significant morbidity. Review of various studies has indicated mortality rates for hysterectomy to vary between 0.4 and 2 per 1000 women with lower mortality rates having been reported for vaginal (1 per 1000) than abdominal hysterectomy (2 per 1000) (Nuffield Institute for Health 1995). Deaths are commonly associated with cardiac or pulmonary arrest and pulmonary emboli (Martin and Benson 1987; Osborne *et al.* 1991).

Vaginal and abdominal hysterectomy

Short and long term complication rates of up to 45 per cent for abdominal hysterectomy compared to 24 per cent for vaginal hysterectomy were reported by Dicker *et al.* (1982). Morbidity is associated with bowel injury (1–2 per cent of complications), ureteric injury (0.1–1 per cent of cases), haemorrhage (0.2–2 per cent of all cases), and infections (10–20 per cent of cases), the latter usually related to urinary tract, chest, wound, and pelvic cavity. Paralytic ileus, deep venous thrombosis, and need for transfusion are less common with vaginal hysterectomy, but voiding difficulties and urinary tract injuries occur more frequently following this procedure. A review of 10 000 vaginal hysterectomies over a 30 year period indicated a major complication rate of only 0.5 per cent up to two weeks postoperatively (Gitsch *et al.* 1991).

Laparoscopic-associated hysterectomy

Morbidity associated with laparoscopic hysterectomy procedures was recently reviewed by meta-analysis of 29 studies (Garry and Phillips 1995) in which 3184 cases were contributed by what the authors considered 'most skilled gynaecological laparoscopists'. Febrile morbidity (4.3 per cent) and need to convert to laparotomy (3.45 per cent) were the most common complications. Trochar injuries (2.57 per cent), bowel injury (0.47 per cent), and urinary tract damage occurred in 1.38 per cent of cases. Comparison with the Dicker *et al.* (1982) study of complications of vaginal and abdominal hysterectomy indicated a lower febrile morbidity and need for transfusion and comparable rates for unintended major surgery, bowel and urinary tract trauma, and incidence of pulmonary embolus. The overall complication rate per 1000 women for laparoscopic-associated hysterectomy was 15.6 compared to 24.5 for vaginal and 42.8 for abdominal hysterectomy.

To assess the complication rate of laparoscopic-assisted vaginal hysterectomy during the learning phase, the incidence of major and minor complications experienced by gynaecologists in South Australia was analysed from medical records of all private and public hospitals in South Australia where the procedures had been performed (O'Shea and Petrucco 1995). The initial audit of 482 cases from 1991 to 1993 revealed a mean operating time of 137 min (range 25–300 min) and mean hospital stay of four days (range 2–16 days). An overall major complication rate of 110 per thousand included haemorrhage (35/1000), febrile morbidity (41.5/1000), bowel injury (6.2/1000) and a requirement for unintended transfusions in eight cases. Bladder damage occurred in 2.3 per cent of cases and ureteric injury in 2 per cent, which represents 4–10 times the injury rate expected for abdominal and vaginal hysterectomy.

The results of this audit support the contention that occlusion of the uterine artery, particularly in the learning phase, is associated with greater morbidity due to damage to the ureter and bladder or by causing excessive haemorrhage than would be expected for abdominal hysterectomy. Attempts to simplify the laparoscopic procedure include the modifications of laparoscopic Doederlein (LD) laparovaginal and laparoscopic supracervical hysterectomy (LSH). The LD procedure involves division of the upper pedicles and parametrium laparoscopically to the level of the uterine arteries. The uterine fundus is then extracted vaginally by traction via an anterior colpotomy incision. The uterine and cardinal/uterosacral ligament pedicles are then secured vaginally. This modification combines an easier approach to the upper pedicles with vaginal suturing of the lower pedicles, utilizing techniques which are safe and well known to all gynaecologists (Garry 1994*a*).

In an effort to reduce prolonged raised intraperitoneal pressure and to compensate for loss of pneumoperitoneum when the vagina is opened, Maher *et al.* (1994) have utilized an abdominal wall elevator and a combined laparoscopic and vaginal application of a stapling gun to secure all pedicles.

Subtotal hysterectomy

A recent editorial (Garry 1994*b*) and commentary (Drife 1994) have refocused attention on conservation of the cervix at hysterectomy. The issue of cervical conservation at hysterectomy for benign bleeding disorders is particularly relevant as the cervix is usually found to be normal. For women with a documented history of negative cervical cytology, the incidence of subsequent cervical cancer has been documented to be less than 0.3 per cent (Drife 1994). Cervical cancer can be further prevented by electrocoagulation or resection of the transformation zone to cervical canal in the remaining cervical stump. Other reasons for removing the cervix include the occurrence of cervical stump prolapse, vaginal discharge, bleeding, and dyspareunia. Potential advantages for cervical conservation (Sutton 1995) are listed below:

- less injury to ureters and bladder
- reduced wound and pelvic infection
- reduced haematoma formation
- avoidance of vault granulation

- preservation of pelvic floor support
- reduced bladder dysfunction
- improved sexual response.

The laparoscopic approach to subtotal hysterectomy was first described by Semm (1993) and subsequently by Donnez and Nisolle (1993), Lyons (1993), Hasson (1993), and Ewen and Sutton (1994). The reason given for using the laparoscopic subtotal approach is related to the perception that the operation is made easier, safer, and quicker to perform. The above authors have noted operating times varying between 60 and 188 minutes which seem comparable to mean operating times reported for laparoscopic-assisted vaginal hysterectomy (64 min) (Phipps *et al.* 1993) and Doederleins hysterectomy (59 min) (Saye *et al.* 1993).

Removal of the uterus by morcellation or via a posterior colpotomy has in the past prolonged the subtotal operation. The ability to morcellate large quantities of tissue laparoscopically has been significantly improved with the introduction of electric morcellators.

Sutton (1995), reporting an initial experience of 58 patients having laparoscopic subtotal hysterectomy with removal of the transformation zone, found that the mean hospital stay was 2.8 days with return to full activity by 20 days. The mean operating time of 75 minutes compares favourably with abdominal hysterectomy. Apart from two cases of secondary haemorrhage, there were no major complications in this series. When compared to 50 patients having abdominal hysterectomy, included in a case-controlled study by the same author, two ureteric and one bladder injury occurred in the latter group which had a much higher morbidity rate overall and a six-week interval for return to full activity. The issue of length of convalescence and ability to return to work are significantly influenced, however, by the attitude of the surgeon concerned and the patient's expectations of a prolonged convalescence which, historically, has been associated with laparotomy procedures.

Long-term sequelae of hysterectomy

Ovarian function

Hysterectomy has been shown to have an acute effect on ovarian blood flow possibly due to ligation of the adnexal branches of the uterine vessels (Janson and Jansson 1977). A transient post-operative drop in circulating ovarian steroids lasting approximately 48 h may be related to the above findings (Stone *et al.* 1975). Ovarian function and ovulation usually return to normal after hysterectomy (Doyle *et al.* 1971). Premature ovarian failure following this procedure may occur, however, in a subgroup of women (Siddle *et al.* 1987).

Bowel and urinary tract function

Dysfunction of both bladder and bowel have been reported following hysterectomy. A prospective study including subjective and urodynamic findings pre- and post-operatively led Parys *et al.* (1989) to conclude that urinary symptoms increased significantly because of vesicourethral functional changes and pelvic neuropathy. Subtotal hysterectomy, which is unlikely to alter autonomic nerve supply to the bladder, has been reported to be associated with reduced urinary symptoms in the year following surgery (Kilkku 1985).

Psychological sequelae

Unlike earlier, less well designed studies, three recent prospective studies found no evidence of adverse psychological sequelae following hysterectomy for benign conditions (Martin *et al.* 1980; Gath *et al.* 1982*a*, *b*; Ryan *et al.* 1989). These studies involved the use of standardized psychiatric interviews and psychological rating scales administered pre- and post-operatively with allowance for adequate recovery from the operation. Between 55 and 58 percent of women studied had evidence of psychological morbidity before surgery. The studies by Gath *et al.* (1982*a*) and Ryan *et al.* (1989) demonstrated considerable reduction in the incidence of psychiatric disorder post-operatively from 55 to 32 per cent of patients studied. The overall conclusion was that hysterectomy was not associated with an increased incidence of psychological sequelae.

Psychological distress, however, may be precipitated by gynaecological symptoms as demonstrated in the longitudinal study of Slade and Anderton (1992). The prospective, randomized controlled trial of Alexander *et al.* (1996) which compared psychiatric and psychosocial aspects of hysterectomy with endometrial ablation also found that 'both treatments reduced the anxiety and depression present before the operation and there were no differences in mental health between the groups at 12 months. Hysterectomy did not lead to post-operative psychiatric illness'. Patients suffering from depression, however, may develop menstrual changes secondary to altered hypothalamic–pituitary control of ovarian function.

The psychologically disadvantaged patients may also not be able to tolerate menstrual disorders as readily or be as objective in utilizing hysterectomy as a treatment option. Adequate assessment and treatment of psychological distress must be contemplated before offering surgical remedies for benign bleeding disorders.

Sexuality issues and hysterectomy

Studies of the effect of hysterectomy on sexuality have also been plagued by methodological difficulties. The use of informal postal questionnaires and use of ambiguous terms such as 'sexual response' and 'libido' have contributed to the difficulties encountered in assessing reports. Studies which have included women in the climacteric age group at which sexuality may be influenced by menopausal changes are similarly more difficult to interpret. For similar reasons, pre-menopausal women having bilateral oophorectomy performed may develop adverse sexuality responses if there has been failure to provide adequate hormone replacement therapy. A retrospective study by Jorgen and Alhorst-Boos (1992) confirmed a significant adverse effect on sexuality in women having had oophorectomy performed compared to women retaining their ovaries who, overall, found an improvement in their sexual life.

Studies carried out in the 70s in general tended to indicate that hysterectomy was unlikely to cause a deterioration in sexual outcome while more recent prospective studies (Coppen *et al.* 1981; Gath *et al.* 1992*b*) suggest either improvement or similar sexual status for the majority of patients with an adverse outcome in about 20 per cent of women studied. The study of Alexander *et al.* (1996) found that neither hysterectomy nor endometrial ablation affected sexual interest with equal numbers reporting loss of sexual interest (25 per cent) and increased sexual interest (27 per cent).

Cervix preservation and subsequent sexuality response

The prospective study by Kilkku (1983) and Kilkku *et al.* (1983) comparing women having total and supracervical hysterectomy showed no differences in coital frequency and libido. Almost 50 per cent of the total hysterectomy group and just over 30 per cent of the supracervical group noted a reduction in the frequency of orgasm one year after their operation. This was a non-randomized study and therefore prone to recruitment bias and overall the response of the two groups was not statistically different.

The supposition that total hysterectomy causes damage to the autonomic innervation of the proximal vagina and thus influences orgasmic response has not been proven by physiological or clinical studies. The corollary that cervical preservation (which is often associated with destruction of the cervical canal) improves orgasmic response is similarly flawed. The prospective study of Helstrom *et al.* (1993) of women's sexuality after subtotal hysterectomy indicated results similar to other conventional hysterectomy studies. Half of the women in this study reported improvement, 21 per cent deterioration, and 20 per cent reported no change. These authors concluded that preoperative sexual activity was an important predictor of post-operative sexuality outcome. Wierrani *et al.* (1995) also found no significant differences in quality of libido and genital sexual sensitivity following subtotal hysterectomy when compared to vaginal, abdominal, and LAVH surgical techniques.

Hysterectomy towards 2000

The holistic approach

Primary care physicians and gynaecologists will play a significant role in determining health care costs related to benign bleeding disorders. The decision to investigate and then treat menorrhagia by either medical or surgical means will influence the incidence of hysterectomy in their region.

Easier methods to assess quantitatively menstrual blood loss, as suggested by Higham *et al.* (1990), have simplified the diagnosis of abnormal menstruation. The majority of women complaining of menorrhagia, however, are found not to have excessive menstruation and yet feel that their quality of life is affected by their altered menstruation. Each patient should be provided with understandable information on the range of treatments available. The role the patient plays in decision making has justifiably become even more relevant in view of the improved understanding of menstrual physiology by women in general.

Adequate discussion of psychological, sexuality-related, and physical change following hysterectomy must be part of the counselling required to enable individuals to give informed consent. The involvement of a partner will often obviate difficulties encountered during convalescence particularly in relation to the resumption of a sexual relationship. By observing these requirements, patient expectations, quality assessment, and improved quality of care will all be fulfilled.

Cost-effective care and hysterectomy

The provision of cost-effective care related to hysterectomy must depend on adequate studies by health care providers to assess overall cost and net health effects to arrive at a calculation of effectiveness to cost ratio (Keeler 1994).

The type of hysterectomy chosen

The procedure performed by an individual gynaecologist will be dependent as much on the adequacy of their training to perform vaginal and endoscopic surgery as the pathology encountered. More emphasis should be placed in training programmes to learn vaginal surgery. The higher morbidity rate currently documented for LAVH during the learning phase of experience must be counteracted by training and accreditation procedures currently recommended by parent bodies in the UK, Canada, USA, and Australia. Prospective, randomized, and preferably multicentre studies are still required to answer the question 'which type of hysterectomy is best suited for this patient?'.

Studies should encompass quality-of-life issues including sexuality, as well as recovery time to full activity. Assessment of patients' ability to cope with early discharge programmes will influence the need to provide domiciliary care and the overall cost effectiveness of a particular procedure.

The results of these studies will play a significant role in the future and determine the conjoint choice by patient and gynaecologist of the type of hysterectomy performed.

I was reminded of the relevance and acceptance of hysterectomy by an artist who painted two flowers, one before and one after surgery (see plates 3 and 4). In the letter accompanying the pictures she wrote 'When I was feeling wretchedly anaemic I painted a vase of flowers which resembled a witch's cauldron and, to me, symbolic of my dreaded menstruation. The black vase represented a womb and the mass of disorganised flowers my blurred, weakened state. A few weeks after hysterectomy I painted a single, beautiful flower, symbolising my new found strength and good general health'.

References

Alexander, D.A., Naji, A.A., Pinion, S.B., Mollison, J., Kitchener, H.C., and Parkin, D.E. (1996). Randomised trial comparing hysterectomy with endometrial ablation for dysfunctional uterine bleeding: psychiatric and psychosocial aspects. *British Medical Journal*, **312**, 280–4.

Bennett, M.J. (1994). Laparoscopic hysterectomy. *The Medical Journal of Australia*, **161**, 282.

Bradlow, J., Coulter, A., and Brooks, P. (1992). *Patterns of referral: a studv of referrals to outpatient clinics from general practices in the Oxford region.* Health Services Research Unit, Department of Public Health and Primary Care, University of Oxford.

Browne, D.S. and Frazer, M.I. (1991). Hysterectomy revisited. *Australian and New Zealand Journal of Obstetrics and Gynaecology*, **31**, 148–52.

Bunker, J. (1976). Elective hysterectomy: pro and con. Public health rounds at the Harvard School of Public Health. *New England Journal of Medicine*, **295**, 264–8.

Carlson, K.J., Nichols, D.H., and Schiff, I. (1993). Indications for hysterectomy. *The New England Journal of Medicine*, **328**, 856–60.

Carter, J.E., Ryoo, J., and Katz, A. (1994). Laparoscopic-assisted vaginal hysterectomy: a case control comparative study with total abdominal hysterectomy. *The Journal of the American Association of Gynecologic Laparoscopists*, **1**, 116–21.

Casey, M.J., Garcia-Padial, J., Johnson, C., Osborne, N.G., Sotolongo, J., and Watson, P. (1994). A critical analysis of laparoscopic assisted vaginal hysterectomies compared with vaginal hysterectomies unassisted by laparoscopy and transabdominal hysterectomies. *Journal of Gynecologic Surgery*, **10**, 7–14.

Coppen, A., Bishop, M., Beard, R., Barnard, G., and Collins, W. (1981). Hysterectomy, hormones and behaviour. *Lancet*, **i**, 126–8.

DeStefano, F., Huezo, C.M., Peterson, H.B., Layde, P.M., Ong, H.W., and Rubin, G.L. (1983). Menstrual changes after tubal ligation. *Obstetrics and Gynecology*, **62**, 673–81.

Dicker, R.C., Greenspan, J.R., Strauss L.T., Cowatt, M.R., Scally, M.J., Peterson, H.B. *et al.* (1982). Complications of abdominal and vaginal hysterectomy among women of reproductive age in the United States. *American Journal of Obstetrics and Gynecology*, **144**, 841–8.

Donnez, J. and Nisolle, M. (1993). Laparoscopic subtotal hysterectomy (LASH). *Gynaecological Endoscopy*, **2**, 77–8.

Donnez, J., Wauter, S.M., and Thomas, K. (1981). Luteal function after tubal sterilization. *Obstetrics and Gynecology*, **57**, 65–8.

Doyle, L.L., Barclay, D.L., Duncan, G.W., and Kirton, K.T. (1971). Human luteal function following hysterectomy as assessed by plasma progestin. *American Journal of Obstetrics and Gynecology*, **101**, 92–7.

Drife, J. (1994). Conserving the cervix at hysterectomy. *British Journal of Obstetrics and Gynaecology*, **101**, 563–4.

Dwyer, N., Hutton, J., and Stirrat, G.M. (1993). Randomised controlled trial comparing endometrial resection with abdominal hysterectomy for the surgical treatment of menorrhagia. *British Journal of Obstetrics and Gynaecology*, **100**, 237–43.

Dyck, F.J., Murphy, F.A., Murphy, K.J., Road, D.A., Boyd, M.S., Osborne, E., *et al.* (1977). Effect of surveillance on the number of hysterectomies in the province of Saskatchewan. *New England Journal of Medicine*, **296**, 1326–8.

Ewen, S.P. and Sutton, C.J.G. (1994). Initial experience with supracervical laparoscopic hysterectomy and removal of the cervical transformation zone. *British Journal of Obstetrics and Gynaecology*, **101**, 225–8.

Fraser, I.S. (1989). Treatment of menorrhagia. *Baillière's Clinical Obstetrics and Gynecology*, **3**, 391–401.

Gambone, J.C., Reiter, R.C., Lench, J.B., and Moore, J.G. (1990). The impact of a quality assurance process on the frequency and histologic verification rate of hysterectomy. *American Journal of Obstetrics and Gynecology*, **163**, 545–9.

Garry, R. (1994*a*). The evolution of a technique for laparoscopic hysterectomy: laparoscopic-assisted Doederlein's hysterectomy. *Gynaecological Endoscopy*, **3**, 123–8.

Garry, R. (1994*b*). What to do with the cervix. *Gynaecological Endoscopy*, **3**, 139–41.

Garry, R. and Phillips, G. (1995). How safe is the laparoscopic approach to hysterectomy? *Gynaecological Endoscopy*, **4**, 77–9.

Gath, D., Cooper, P., and Day, A. (1982*a*). Hysterectomy and psychiatric disorders: I. Levels of psychiatric morbidity before and after hysterectomy. *British Journal of Psychiatry*, **140**, 335–42.

Gath, D., Cooper, P., and Bond, A. (1982*b*). Hysterectomy and psychiatric disorder: II. Demographic psychiatric and physical factors in relation to psychiatric outcome. *British Journal of Psychiatry*, **140**, 342–50.

Gitsch, G., Berger, E., and Tatra, G. (1991). Trends in 30 years of vaginal hysterectomy. *Surgical Gynecology and Obstetrics*, **172**, 207–10.

Hasson, H. (1993). Experience with laparoscopic hysterectomy. *Journal of American Association of Gynecologic Laparoscopists*, **1**, 1–11.

Helstrom, L., Lundberg, P.O., Sorbom, D., and Backstrom, T. (1993). Sexuality after hysterectomy: a factor analysis of women's sexual lives before and after subtotal hysterectomy. *Obstetrics and Gynecology*, **81**, 357–62.

Higham, J.M., O'Brien, P.M.S., and Shaw, R.W. (1990). Assessment of menstrual blood loss using a pictorial chart. *British Journal of Obstetrics and Gynaecology*, **97**, 734–9.

Hirsch, N.A. (1993). Technologies for the treatment of menorrhagia and uterine myomas. *Australian Institute of Health and Welfare: health care technology series*, Vol. 10. Australian Government Printing Service Canberra.

Jackson, S., Draycott, T., and Read, M. (1995). Laparoscopic vaginal hysterectomy versus abdominal hysterectomy. *British Joumal of Obstetrics and Gynaecology*, **102**, 511–12.

Janson, O. and Jansson, I. (1977). The acute effect of hysterectomy on ovarian blood flow. *American Journal of Obstetrics and Gynecology*, **127**, 349–52.

Johns, D.A., Carrera, B., Jones, J., DeLeon, F., Vincent, R., and Safely, C. (1995). The medical and economic impact of laparoscopically assisted vaginal hysterectomy in a large, metropolitan, not-for-profit hospital. *American Journal of Obstetrics and Gynecology*, **172**, 1709–19.

Jorgen, N. and Alhorst-Boos, S. (1992). Psychological reactions and sexual life after hysterectomy with and without oophorectomy. *Gynecologic and Obstetric Investigation*, **34**, 97–101.

Keeler, E.B. (1994). Decision analysis and cost-effectiveness analysis in women's health care. *Clinical Obstetrics and Gynecology*, **37**, 207–15.

Kilkku, P. (1983). Supravaginal uterine amputation vs. hysterectomy: effects on coital frequency and dyspareunia. *Acta Obstetrica et Gynecologica Scandinavica*, **62**, 141–5.

Kilkku, P. (1985). Supravaginal uterine amputation vs. hysterectomy with reference to subjective bladder symptoms and incontinence. *Acta Obstetrica et Gynecologica Scandinavica*, **64**, 375–9.

Kilkku, P., Gronross, M., Hirvonen, T., and Rauramo, L. (1983). Supravaginal uterine amputation vs. hysterectomy: effects on libido and orgasm. *Acta Obstetrica et Gynecologica Scandinavica*, **62**, 147–52.

Kovac, S.R. (1995). Guidelines to determine the route of hysterectomy. *Obstetrics and Gynecology*, **85**, 18–23.

Lalonde, A. (1994). Evaluation of surgical options in menorrhagia. *British Journal of Obstetrics and Gynaecology*, **10**, 8–14.

Lyons, T.L. (1993). Laparoscopic supracervical hysterectomy using the contact Nd: YAG laser. *Gynaecological Endoscopy*, **2**, 79–81.

Maher, P., Hill, D., and Wood, C. (1994). Laparovaginal hysterectomy – a new approach. *Gynaecological Endoscopy*, **3**, 129–32.

Martin, L. and Benson, R.C. (1987). Preoperative and postoperative care. In *current obstetrics and gynaecologic diagnosis and treatment* (6th edn), (ed. M.L. Pernoll and R.C. Benson), pp. 798–816. Appleton and Lange, New York.

Martin, R.L., Roberts, W.V., and Cayton, P.J. (1980). Psychiatric status after hysterectomy: a one year follow up. *Journal of the American Medical Association*, **244**, 350–3.

Molloy, D. and Crosdale, S. (1996). National trends in gynaecological endoscopic surgery. *Australian and New Zealand Journal of Obstetrics and Gynaecology*, **36**, 27–31.

Molloy, D. and Taylor, P.T. (1994). Gynaecological surgery after endometrial ablation. *The Medical Journal of Australia*, **161**, 604–6.

Ng, P.H. and Hogston, P. (1994). Early discharge following major gynaecological surgery. *Australian and New Zealand Journal of Obstetrics and Gynaecology*, **34**, 474–6.

Nuffield Institute for Health, NHS Centre for Reviews and Dissemination, Royal College of Physicians (1995). *Effective health care*. Churchill Livingstone, London.

Osborne, G.A., Rudkin, G.E., and Moran, P. (1991). Fluid uptake in laser endometrial ablation. *Anaesthesia Intensive Care*, **19**, 217–19.

O'Shea, R.T. and Petrucco, O.M. (1995). Laparoscopically-assisted vaginal hysterectomy, Adelaide complication audit 1991–94. Abstract 23. In *Programme and Abstract book*, 5th Annual Scientific Meeting of the Australian Gynaecological Endoscopy Society, Melbourne.

Parys, B.T., Haylen, B.T., Hutton, J.L., and Parsons, K.F. (1989). The effects of simple hysterectomy on vesicourethral function. *British Journal of Urology*, **64**, 594–9.

Phipps, J.H., Hassanaien, J.M., and Saeed, M. (1993). Laparoscopic and laparoscopic assisted vaginal hysterectomy: a series of 114 cases. *Gynaecological Endoscopy*, **3**, 7–12.

Pinion, S.B., Parkin, D.E., Abramovich, D.R., Naji, A., Alexander, D.A., Russell, I.T., *et al.* (1994). Randomised trial of hysterectomy, endometrial laser ablation, and transcervical endometrial resection for dysfunctional uterine bleeding. *British Medical Journal*, **309**, 979–83.

Querleu, D., Cosson, M., Parmentier, D., and Debodinance, P. (1993). The impact of laparoscopic surgery on vaginal hysterectomy. *Gynaecological Endoscopy*, **2**, 89–91.

Raju, K.S. and Auld, B.J. (1994). A randomised prospective study of laparoscopic vaginal hysterectomy versus abdominal hysterectomy each with bilateral salpingo-oophorectomy. *British Journal of Obstetrics and Gynaecology*, **101**, 1068–71.

Rankin, G.L.S. (1992). Laparoscopically assisted vaginal hysterectomy. *Lancet*, **339**, 501.

Ravina, J.H., Bouret, J.M., Fried, D., Benifla, J.L., Darai, E., Pennehouat, G., *et al.* (1995). Value of pre-operative embolization of uterine fibroma: report of a multicenter series of 31 cases. *Contraception Fertilite et Sexualite*, **23**, 45–9.

Richardson, R.E., Bournas, N., and Magos, A.L. (1995). Is laparoscopic hysterectomy a waste of time? *Lancet*, **345**, 36–41.

Ryan, M.M., Dennerstein, L., and Pepperell, R. (1989). Psychological aspects of hysterectomy. A prospective study. *British Journal of Psvchiatry*, **154**, 516–22.

Santow, G. and Bracher, M. (1992). Correlates of hysterectomy in Australia. *Social Science in Medicine*, **34**, 929–42.

Saye, W.B., Espy G.B., Bishop, M.R., and Miller, W. (1993). Laparoscopic Doederlein hysterectomy: a rational alternative to traditional abdominal hysterectomy. *Surgical Laparoscopy and Endoscopy*, **2**, 88–94.

Schofield, M.J., Hennrikus, D.J., Redman, S., and Sanson-Fisher, R.W. (1991). Prevalence and characteristics of women who have had a hysterectomy in a community survey. *Australian and New Zealand Journal of Obstetrics and Gynaecology*, **31**, 153–8.

Semm, K. (1993). Hysterectomy by pelviscopy: an alternative approach without colpotomy (CASH). In *Laparoscopic hysterectomy* (ed. R. Garry and H. Reich), pp. 118–32. Blackwell Scientific, Oxford.

Siddle, N., Sarrel, P., and Whitehead, M. (1987). The effect of hysterectomy on the age at ovarian failure: identification of a subgroup of women with premature loss of ovarian function and literature review. *Fertility and Sterility*, **47**, 94–100.

Slade, P. and Anderton, K.J. (1992). Gynaecological symptoms and psychological distress: a longitudinal study of their relationship. *Journal of Psychosomatic Obstetrics and Gynaecology*, **13**, 51–63.

Stone, S.C., Dickey, R.P., and Mickal, A. (1975). The acute effect of hysterectomy on ovarian function. *American Journal of Obstetrics and Gynecology*, **121**, 193–7.

Stovall, T.G., Summitt, R.L., and Ling, F.W. (1992). Outpatient vaginal hysterectomy: a pilot study. *Obstetrics and Gynecology*, **80**, 145–9.

Summitt, R.L., Stovall, T.G., Lipscombe, G.H., and Ling, F.W. (1992). Randomized comparison of laparoscopy-assisted vaginal hysterectomy with standard vaginal hysterectomy in an outpatient setting. *Obstetrics and Gynecology*, **80**, 895–901.

Sutton, C. (1995). Laparoscopic hysterectomy. *Current Obstetrics and Gvnaecology*, **5**, 142–6.

Van Keep, P.A., Wildemeersch, D., and Lehert, P. (1983). Hysterectomy in six European countries. *Maturitas*, **5**, 69–75.

Vessey, M.P., Villard-Mackintosh, L., McPherson, K., Coulter, A., and Yeates, D. (1992). The epidemiology of hysterectomy: findings in a large cohort study. *British Journal of Obstetrics and Gynaecology*, **99**, 402–7.

Wierrani, F., Huber, M., Grin, W., Henry, M., and Grunberger, W. (1995). Postoperative libido and genital sexual sensitivity following various forms of hysterectomy. *Journal of Gynecologic Surgery*, **11**, 127–32.

Wood, C., Maher, P., Hill, D., and Sellwood, T. (1992). Hysterectomy: a time of change. *The Medical Journal of Australia*, **157**, 651–3.

Wood, C., Maher, P., and Hill, D. (1993). Biopsy diagnosis and conservative surgery in the treatment of adenomyosis. *Australian and New Zealand Journal of Obstetrics and Gynaecology*, **3**, 319–21.

Youssif, S.N.M. and Ledward, R.S. (1993). Vaginal hysterectomy. Study of early discharge and implications. *Journal of Obstetrics and Gynaecology*, **13**, 355–7.

16 Pathophysiology and medical treatment of uterine fibroids

Beverley J. Vollenhoven and David L. Healy

Introduction

Uterine leiomyomas are the commonest solid tumours in women. They are tumours of the smooth muscle of the uterus, but they also contain varying amounts of fibrous tissue. They are said to occur in 20–25 per cent of females over the age of 30 years. However, the figure is probably an underestimate and they are more likely to occur in about 50 per cent of women (Thompson and Rock 1992).

The clinical features of uterine fibroids are variable. If symptoms are present, their type and severity usually depend on the size, site, and the number of fibroids present. The most common symptom reported by women with fibroids is menorrhagia (Buttram and Reiter 1981). Other symptoms include dysmenorrhoea and pressure symptoms such as frequency of micturition due to bladder pressure from an anteriorly placed fibroid. Fibroids may also be a contributing factor in infertility as well as recurrent miscarriage, although this remains controversial. Fibroids are a well recognized risk factor in an ongoing pregnancy. They are associated with preterm labour, abnormal presentation, outlet obstruction, post-partum haemorrhage, and puerperal sepsis (Buttram and Reiter 1981).

Aetiology

There have been recent advances regarding the aetiology of fibroids. These tumours are only known to occur during the reproductive years and to regress after the menopause – whether this is a natural event, induced by surgery, or mimicked by repetitive administration of luteinizing hormone-releasing hormone agonists (LHRHa). This circumstantial evidence suggests that oestrogen (E) plays a part in fibroid growth and this is further strengthened by the risk factors for the growth of these tumours as well as results from steroid binding studies.

Risk factors for fibroid growth

Nulliparity

There is a definite association between nulliparity and the incidence of fibroids. The relative risk of fibroids has been shown to decrease with each additional term pregnancy, the risk being reduced to one fifth with five term pregnancies, compared with the nulliparous woman (Ross *et al.* 1986). Therefore, continuous oestradiol (E_2) secretion, uninterrupted by pregnancy and lactation, is a risk factor for fibroid growth. It is an increased number of cycles rather than increase in serum E_2 per cycle that is the risk factor, as it has been shown that women with fibroids have similar circulating E_2 levels to women who do not have fibroids (Spellacy *et al.* 1972).

Obesity

Obesity increases the risk of fibroid development by 21 per cent with each 10 kg weight gain (Ross *et al.* 1986). There may be two reasons for this. Firstly, there is peripheral conversion of circulating androgens to E by fat aromatase. Secondly, in the obese, there is a decrease in the hepatic production of sex-hormone-binding globulin (SHBG) – a carrier for E_2. Therefore, obesity confers a relative hyper-oestrogenic state which may predispose to fibroid growth.

Race

From clinical and epidemiological surveys, in the USA, it is known that fibroids are 3–9 times more common in blacks than in whites (Ross *et al.* 1986). This may be due to genetic factors as, anecdotally, there is often a positive family history in women who develop fibroids. Recent molecular endocrinology has shown that uterine fibroids have frequent chromosomal abnormalities involving chromosome 12, in particular 12q13–15. Sequencing of clones from a 40 kb portion of the abnormal region has led to the identification of a candidate gene related to the genesis of fibroids (Bullerdiek *et al.* 1995).

Protective factors against fibroid growth

Cigarette smoking

Women who smoke 10 cigarettes per day have an 18 per cent lowered risk of fibroid development compared with non-smokers (Ross *et al.* 1986). Smoking is regarded as anti-oestrogenic and smokers undergo menopause, on average, three years earlier than non-smokers.

Combined oral contraceptive pills

The combined oral contraceptive pill reduces the risk of fibroids by approximately 17 per cent with each five years of usage. It is thought that this is due to the progestogenic component (Ross *et al.* 1986).

Steroid factors

Oestrogen has been implicated in the growth of fibroids, because

(1) fibroids only grow in the reproductive years and regress after the menopause;

(2) E and progesterone (P) receptor (ER, PR) concentrations (both cytosolic and nuclear) have been shown to be greater in fibroids than in surrounding myometrium, although others have contradicted these findings; and

(3) immunohistochemistry has shown a greater staining intensity and a greater ER:PR ratio in fibroids than myometrium (reviewed by Vollenhoven *et al.* 1994*a*).

A recent study shows that there may be two forms of the PR. Receptor A is 94 kDa and receptor B is 120 kDa. They both result from the same gene by transcription from different promoters which are regulated independently *in vitro*. In the presence of P the two forms activate transcription but are functionally different. In the presence of a P antagonist, the B form activates transcription inappropriately so that the antagonist behaves as a partial agonist. Oestrogen responsiveness is conferred on the part of the gene from which the A form is produced and therefore there most likely will be consequences for the regulation of PR by E (Viville *et al.* 1995).

In women treated with LHRHa, steroid receptor binding studies are conflicting. This conflict may have arisen due to the presence of two different forms of the PR (Viville *et al.* 1995). With this background Pasqualini and associates (1990) showed a significant decrease in PR content in both tissues after treatment with these agents. However, Rein and colleagues (1990*a*) showed that the PR content was unchanged and that the fibroid ER content was six times greater than in the fibroids from untreated women. There was no statistically significantly different myometrial ER and PR content between pre-treated and untreated women. They explained the increased ER content in pre-treated fibroids as possibly being due to an altered receptor metabolism causing an increased sensitivity of fibroids to low levels of E. This, acting in conjunction with the low P levels, in LHRHa pre-treated women, may then result in overexpression of the ER. Lumsden and co-workers (1989) confirmed increased ER levels in women pre-treated with LHRHa, but showed that the PR content was decreased. Vollenhoven and associates (1994*a*) showed that there was no difference in ER or PR binding between treated and untreated fibroids and that there was also no difference in the mRNA expression of either of the receptors in these tissues. We postulated that fibroids shrink on application of these agents because of a decrease in the ligand concentration (E_2 and P) available to react with their respective receptors.

Peptide growth factors

Peptide growth factors may also have a role in the growth of fibroids.

Insulin-like growth factors (IGFs)

Serum IGF-1 levels in women with fibroids have been found to be similar to the levels in fibroid-free women (Dawood and Khan-Dawood 1991). As with serum E_2 levels, if these factors contribute to fibroid growth, it would seem that they do so at a local paracrine or autocrine level rather than at an endocrine level.

The mRNA expression of IGF-1 and IGF-2 in fibroids and myometrium have been investigated by Hoppener and associates (1988), Boehm and colleagues (1990) and Vollenhoven and co-workers (1993*a*). The first two studies found that IGF-1 and IGF-2 mRNA expression was greater in fibroids than in myometrium. However, neither addressed the very important issue of the expression of the IGFBPs, which are known to modulate IGF action, at least *in vitro*. We investigated the mRNA expression of IGF-1, IGF-2, and IGFBP-1–3 in fibroids and corresponding myometrium. In fibroids compared with myometrium from 20 untreated women, there was a 12-fold increase in IGF-2 mRNA abundance and there was a two-fold decrease in IGFBP-3 mRNA abundance, although protein levels appeared to be similar. IGF-1 and IGFBP-2 mRNA expression was also present in these tissues with no difference in the mRNA expression between fibroids and myometrium. We postulated that the differential expression of IGF-2 and IGFBP-3 mRNA between fibroids and myometrium led to an increase in the bioavailability of IGF-2 in these tissues thereby promoting fibroid growth. In nine women pre-treated with LHRHa, there was no difference in the relative abundance of each of the factors between treated and untreated fibroids. We concluded that LHRHa have no effect on the IGFs and that their action on fibroid shrinkage is via the induction of a hypo-oestrogenic state (Vollenhoven *et al.* 1994*b*). Other findings show that growth hormone (GH) is probably not the regulatory factor of IGF-1 and IGFBP-3 in these tissues, as the mRNA for its receptor was not present when examined by Northern blot analysis.

Receptor studies for both IGF-1 and IGF-2 have also been reported. IGF-1 receptor (type 1) numbers, but not IGF-2 receptors (type 2), have been found to be greater in fibroids compared with myometrium (Tommola *et al.* 1989). Recent evidence suggests that most of the actions of IGF-1 and IGF-2 are mediated by the type 1 receptor while the type 2 receptor may be involved in the uptake and degradation of IGF-2 (Jones and Clemmons 1995). IGF-2, therefore, remains an important factor in fibroid growth.

Explant cultures of fibroid and myometrium have been shown to secrete IGF-1 and IGF-2. Cultures from both tissues from LHRHa pre-treated women have been shown to secrete significantly less IGF-1 and IGF-2 compared with untreated fibroids and myometrium. The secretion of IGF-1 from all fibroid samples was no different to that from all myometrial specimens but the mean secretion of IGF-2 from all fibroids was greater than that from myometrium (Rein *et al.* 1990*b*).

Platelet derived growth factor (PDGF)

PDGF binding sites have been found in greater numbers in fibroids than in normal myometrium but the receptor affinity was found to be greater in myometrium than fibroids (Fayed *et al.* 1989). However, mRNA expression of PDGF has been found to be the same in fibroid and myometrium (Boehm *et al.* 1990). We have also concluded that PDGF is probably not important in fibroid growth as the mRNA in these tissues is only present at extremely low levels.

Epidermal growth factor (EGF) and transforming growth factor α (TGFα)

Hofmann and others (1984) and Lumsden and associates (1988) showed the presence of high affinity binding sites for EGF but no significant variation in EGF binding between myometrium and fibroid. Conversely, Tommola and colleagues (1989) and Fayed and others (1989) showed a decreased binding of EGF, due to decreased receptor concentration, in fibroid membranes compared with normal myometrial membranes. In women pre-treated with LHRHa, binding of EGF to fibroid cell membranes has been shown to be lower compared with fibroids from untreated patients. However, EGF binding to the myometrium was found to be unchanged (Lumsden *et al.* 1988).

Using immunohistochemistry, Leone and others (1991) showed EGF receptor localization to be mainly in endothelial cell membranes in both fibroids and myometrium. They also showed, in women pre-treated with LHRHa, that there was a decrease in fibroid EGF binding. They concluded, therefore, that the reduction in fibroid size in LHRHa pre-treated women may be related to a decrease in the blood supply in these tumours and that this may be EGF-mediated. In fact, Matta and others (1988) demonstrated, by Doppler ultrasound, that hypo-oestrogenism leads to a decrease in uterine arterial blood flow. EGF may play a role in fibroid growth by an angiogenic mechanism.

The mRNA expression of EGF, the EGF receptor, and TGFα were examined by Yeh and co-workers (1991), in pure monolayer cultures of fibroid and myometrium. Using the technique of reverse transcriptase polymerase chain reaction (RT-PCR) they showed that mRNA expression of EGF and the EGF receptor, but not TGFα, was present in fibroids and myometrium. We have shown that the mRNA expression of EGF as well as TGFβ was present in fibroids and myometrium from untreated women as well as in fibroids from LHRHa pre-treated women (Vollenhoven *et al.* 1995). There was no difference in expression of either of these factors between the three tissues studied. However, given the decrease in EGF binding in fibroids compared with myometrium there may be less bioactive EGF in fibroids compared with myometrium. TGFβ and EGF together cause a growth inhibition in transformed fibroblasts (Sporn and Roberts 1988). If this were extended to include fibroids it may mean that there is less growth inhibition in fibroids compared with myometrium. By quantitative RT-PCR it has been shown that EGF mRNA expression in fibroids was greater than that in myometrium but only in the secretory phase of the cycle and myometrium from uteri without fibroids had similar levels of EGF mRNA in the proliferative and secretory phases. Untreated fibroids, only in the secretory phase, had greater levels of EGF mRNA than LHRHa pre-treated fibroids. This further raises the possibility that P may also be an important mediator in fibroid growth (Harrison-Woolrych *et al.* 1994).

Uncharacterized fibroid mitogens

Koutsilieris and others (1990) have shown that mitogens are present in fibroid extracts. These mitogens were shown to stimulate cells with the fibroblast, myoblast, and osteoblast phenotype. The addition of FGF, EGF, and insulin caused a dose-dependent cell stimulation. These mitogens, as yet uncharacterized, may be acting in conjunction with both steroid and peptide growth factors and may therefore be partly responsible for fibroid growth.

Medical management

The treatment of fibroids has traditionally been surgical. Where once a woman had no choice other than hysterectomy, particularly if the fibroids were symptomatic, recent medical advances using LHRHa pre-treatment followed by surgical advances of hysteroscopic laser resection and/or abdominal myolysis, are becoming increasingly the management of these patients. These advances have been paralleled by advances in women's rights and the increasing demands of women for alternatives to hysterectomy.

Luteinizing hormone-releasing hormone agonists

LHRHa are a group of drugs which are derivatives of hypothalamic LHRH. Peptide substitutions in the amino acid structure make them 40–200 times more potent than native LHRH. The peptide modifications cause both an increase in binding affinity to pituitary LHRH receptors and an increase in resistance to proteolytic degradation. On initial exposure to the drugs there is elevation of serum gonadotrophin levels and subsequently plasma sex steroid levels, which may last several hours. However, with continuous administration there is suppression of the pituitary–ovarian axis with the induction of a state of menopause which is readily reversible on cessation of the medication. The mechanism of this suppression is thought to be due to down-regulation of the pituitary LHRH binding sites.

The agonists cannot be administered orally because of inactivation by gastric peptidases. They may be given by nasal spray, subcutaneous injection, and in slow release preparations such as depot injections or implants. The use of implants and injections is the most convenient for the patient as they are given at monthly intervals and do not require self-administration and, therefore, compliance by the patient. Intranasal preparations are as effective as subcutaneous preparations in causing fibroid shrinkage (Vollenhoven *et al.* 1990).

The timing of administration of LHRHa in relation to the menstrual cycle is an important consideration. When the drug is begun in the first half of the cycle, ideally days 2–4, there will be an E withdrawal bleed 10–14 days later as well as the normal period at the expected time. This time of commencement rules out the possibility of accidental administration during pregnancy. When begun in the second phase of the menstrual cycle, day 21 if possible, the elevation of gonadotropins and sex steroids is restricted to this phase and normal menstruation occurs at the expected time without a subsequent withdrawal bleed in the following cycle. This is advantageous in a woman who suffers from heavy menstrual loss as a result of fibroids.

Side-effects

The side-effects of prolonged LHRHa administration are well tolerated and mainly due to the menopausal state. All patients suffer from hot flushes. Mood changes, vaginal dryness, arthralgias, and decreased libido are reported by 32.5 per cent, 27.5 per cent, 22.5 per cent and 12.5 per cent of patients respectively (Vollenhoven *et al.* 1990).

The more worrying sequel to hypo-oestrogenism is the potential development of osteoporosis. Reported studies have shown a significant bone loss (6 per cent) in trabecular bone of the lumbar vertebrae, when measured by computerized tomography, after six months of treatment. This loss, however, has been shown to be reversible six months after the cessation of treatment (Matta *et al.* 1987). The studies differ in their site of bone density measurement and in their method of measuring the bone density. If assessed in the distal radius, composed of cortical bone, bone loss is generally not seen, but if measured in trabecular bone (more rapid turnover than cortical bone), loss is more likely to be reported. Biochemical markers of bone metabolism, such as alkaline phosphatase and hydroxyproline, have also been shown to be significantly increased during therapy and decreased with therapy cessation (Eckstein *et al.* 1992). The side-effect of osteoporosis is the limiting factor in the long term usage of LHRHa.

Rationale for use

The rationale behind the usage of LHRHa in fibroids is that the smaller the fibroid the less likely it is to cause symptoms and the less the blood loss at myomectomy or hysterectomy. Since the first case report was published showing successful treatment of fibroids with LHRHa (Filicori *et al.* 1983), there have been multiple studies, including randomized, double-blind placebo-controlled trials that have attested to the potential use of LHRHa, not only as an initial option, but also now as an adjunct to surgical management. There has been regression of fibroids typically to 50 per cent of their initial volume, complete regression only occurring with smaller tumours.

Women with the greatest initial fibroid volume are most likely to experience the greatest shrinkage of their tumours, this usually occurring in the first 12 weeks of therapy, further significant reduction being unlikely with continuing treatment (Vollenhoven *et al.* 1990). The reduction in total fibroid/uterine volume seems to be dependent on the level of E suppression. Moreover, Friedman and others (1992*a*) have shown a statistically significant negative correlation between the precentage reduction in uterine volume and the serum E_2 concentration at week 12. They also showed a significant negative correlation between the percentage reduction in uterine volume and the pre-treatment weight of the patient.

One of the major advantages of the menopausal state induced by LHRHa is that menstrual bleeding may cease completely or become scant. This is a great advantage for the anaemic woman. It allows her to restore her haemoglobin concentration to normal thereby preventing blood transfusion prior to surgery and it gives her symptomatic relief from monthly heavy blood loss (Candiani *et al.* 1990; Vollenhoven *et al.* 1990). Once normal concentrations are restored, blood is able to be stored if the need for autologous transfusion arises at surgery.

Invariably, however, after therapy is stopped there is regrowth of the fibroids. Long-term follow-up studies have shown regrowth in all cases with symptom recurrence in a smaller percentage of women (Matta *et al.* 1989). The regrowth usually occurs within the first year after treatment.

Add-back therapy

Since fibroid recurrence after LHRHa treatment is inevitable and as long-term therapy (two years or more) with these drugs is not possible because of the risk of osteoporosis, several studies have added P and/or E at the same time as LHRHa treatment or after three months of therapy and once fibroid shrinkage has occurred. The latter regimen is now called steroid 'add-back' therapy.

Studies using a progestogen beginning at the same time as LHRHa treatment have shown that fibroid shrinkage does not occur (West *et al.* 1992). However, if the progestogen is begun three months after the agonist treatment alone has started and once fibroid shrinkage has occurred, there are fewer hypo-oestrogenic side-effects and this sequential therapy also seems to be successful in preventing fibroid regrowth for longer (West *et al.* 1992). It is thought that this therapy combination is successful because, once E_2 levels are suppressed after three months agonist treatment alone, the introduction of a progestogen results in decreased P binding to its receptor. Oestrogen is known to cause production of the PR. If a hypo-oestrogenic state exists, then the PR numbers will also be low. Whereas, when a progestogen is introduced at the same time as the LHRHa, the initial E surge causes production of PR and with the introduction of a progestogen, the P/PR binding probably prevents fibroid shrinkage (West *et al.* 1992). However, a study using progestogen alone as add-back therapy showed that it was not as effective when compared with combined hormone replacement therapy (HRT) add-back treatment in maintaining fibroid shrinkage. The former regimen may also cause a detrimental effect on lipid profiles (Friedman *et al.* 1993).

Combined E and P treatment or HRT, begun after fibroid shrinkage has occurred and continuing with the LHRHa, seems successful in maintaining shrinkage, relieving hypo-oestrogenic side-effects, and, importantly, maintaining bone density (Friedman 1989). Protocols of initial LHRHa therapy with the addition of HRT or progestogen treatment alone, once fibroid shrinkage has occurred, may be the answer to long-term agonist use.

Pre-surgical therapy

Because of the regrowth of these tumours after therapy cessation, the major therapeutic situation for the use of LHRHa is prior to hysterectomy, hysteroscopic or abdominal myomectomy, or before laparoscopic myolysis. Studies have concluded that pre-treatment prior to hysterectomy results in reduced blood loss and easier operations, more often performed through transverse abdominal incisions, or more often performed vaginally (especially if pre-treatment uterine size was 14–18 weeks' gestational size) than abdominally (Golan *et al.* 1993; Lumsden *et al.* 1994). This final consequence is an advantage for the patient as vaginal hysterectomy is associated with a lower morbidity compared with abdominal hysterectomy – 24.5 per cent versus 42.8 per cent (Dicker *et al.* 1982). The pre-operative haemoglobin concentration is also usually higher in the LHRHa treated women so that if considerable blood loss occurs, it is better tolerated and less likely to result in transfusion.

Pre-treatment with LHRHa before abdominal or hysteroscopic myomectomy confers benefits to the patient and the surgeon, in terms of ease of operation, reduced blood loss (especially with large fibroid uteri > 10 weeks' gestational size at abdominal myomectomy or approximately 5 cm diameter at hysteroscopic myomectomy), and consequently less post-operative pelvic adhesion formation (Golan *et al.* 1993). It has been shown that the size of the fibroid prior to myomectomy is an important prognostic factor for subsequent fertility (Buttram and Reiter 1981). Therefore, if the fibroid is shrunk prior to surgery, theoretically, there should be an improved postoperative pregnancy rate. We reported a 50 per cent post-myomectomy pregnancy rate in infertile women, whose sole cause for infertility was fibroids (Vollenhoven *et al.* 1993*b*). These women had been pre-treated with LHRHa and then underwent abdominal myomectomy. This figure for post-myomectomy pregnancy rate is consistent with other reported series in which women have no pre-treatment (reviewed by Vollenhoven *et al.* 1993*b*). The only method of investigating whether LHRHa have any effect on the post-myomectomy pregnancy rate is to perform a randomized trial (treatment versus no treatment) in women whose only cause for infertility is the presence of fibroids. This has never been reported.

Disadvantages of pre-treatment with LHRHa have also been addressed. Fedele and others (1990) reported that six months after operation, significantly more women who had been pre-treated, compared with untreated women, had small fibroids, < 1.5 cm, when examined by trans-vaginal ultrasonography. This may occur because the smaller fibroids shrink to such an extent prior to surgery that they are missed at operation. As the effect of the LHRHa reverses, these small fibroids re-grow. It may be that women with small fibroids should be treated for a shorter time-period if the ultimate aim is to remove all fibroids at surgery. However, this finding has been disputed by another study which showed that LHRHa pre-treatment made no difference to the post-operative recurrence rate of fibroids (Friedman *et al.* 1992*b*). Some surgeons report that pre-operative LHRHa treatment creates a hard, fibrotic nodule of leiomyoma that makes surgery difficult. We have not found such difficulty and believe the advantage of a 'bloodless' field at hysteroscopy or laparoscopy/laparotomy is a great advantage.

Other medical management

Mifepristone (RU 486)

RU486 is a PR antagonist. It has recently been used with success to shrink fibroids, with few side-effects (Murphy *et al.*, 1993). Its mode of action in shrinking fibroids is thought to occur via a decrease in blood flow to the uterus. It has been shown that this reduction is about 40 per cent and is greater than the reduction that occurs on LHRHa (21 per cent) (Reinsch *et al.*, 1994).

Progestogens

In an older study, Goldzieher and others (1966) treated 46 women with 25 mg medrogestone and reported fibroid shrinkage after just 14 days of treatment. They showed that marked degenerative changes, similar to 'red degeneration' of pregnancy, were induced in the fibroids. It was thought that progestogens had the potential to decrease the size of uterine fibroids but this has not been further substantiated.

Gestrinone

Gestrinone is a synthetic trienic 19 norsteroid which has mild androgenic side-effects. It too has been successful in shrinking fibroids (Coutinho and Goncalves 1989).

Anti-progestogen/Anti-oestrogen combinations

Medicines, such as tamoxifen, are now widely used by women at mid-life for prevention or treatment of breast cancer. Endocrine actions of tamoxifen are complex. Anti-oestrogenic activities of tamoxifen suggest it may be useful in shrinking fibroids. Long-term administration of tamoxifen is known to be well tolerated.

Combinations of anti-steroid hormones merit testing for the treatment of fibroids. Mifepristone–tamoxifen would be one possible combination. Such medical treatment might be equally effective as LHRHa at a cheaper cost.

References

Boehm, K.D., Daimon, M., Gorodeski, I.G., Sheean, I.A., Utian, W.H., and Ilan, J. (1990). Expression of insulin – like and platelet derived growth factor genes in human uterine tissues. *Molecular Reproduction and Development*, **27**, 93–101.

Bullerdiek, J., Hennig, Y., Deichert, U., Heilmann, I., Thode, B., Schoenmakers, E., *et al.* (1995). A common molecular basis of leiomyomas and endometrial polyps. *Abstracts of the 11th annual meeting of the European Society of Human Reproduction and Embryology*, Abstract 077. Hamburg, Germany.

Buttram, V.C. and Reiter, R.C. (1981). Uterine leiomyomata: etiology, symptomatology and management. *Fertility and Sterility*, **36**, 433–45.

Candiani, G.B., Vercellini, P., Fedele, L., Arcaini, L., Bianchi, S., and Candiani M. (1990). Use of Goserelin depot, a gonadotropin-releasing hormone agonist, for the treatment of menorrhagia and severe anaemia in women with leiomyomata uteri. *Acta Obstetrica et Gynecological Scandinavica*, **69**, 413–15.

Coutinho, E.M. and Goncalves, M.T. (1989). Long-term treatment of leiomyomas with gestrinone. *Fertility and Sterility*, **51**, 939–46.

Dawood, M.Y. and Khan-Dawood, F.S. (1991). Plasma insulin like growth factor-I (IGF I), CA 125, estrogen and progesterone in women with leiomyomas. In *Abstracts of the 47th annual meeting of the American Fertility Society*. Abstract P-205. The American Fertility Society, Orlando, Florida.

Dicker, R.C., Greenspan, J.R., Strauss, L.T., Cowart, M.R., Scaly, M.J., Peterson, H.B., *et al.* (1982). Complications of abdominal and vaginal hysterectomy among women of reproductive age in the United States. *American Journal of Obstetrics and Gynecology*, **144**, 841–8.

Eckstein, N., Foldes, J., Feinstein, Y., Vagman, I., Eshel, A., Steinberg, R., *et al.* (1992). Calcium homeostasis, bone metabolism and safety aspects during long-term treatment with a GnRH agonist. *Maturitas*, **15**, 25–32.

Fayed, Y.M., Tsibris, J.C.M., Langenberg, P.W., and Robertson, A.L. Jr (1989). Human leiomyoma cells: binding and growth responses to epidermal growth factor, platelet derived growth factor and insulin. *Laboratory Investigation*, **60**, 30–7.

Fedele, L., Bianchi, S., Baglioni, A., Arcaini, I., Marchini, M., and Bocciolone, I. (1990). Intranasal buserelin versus surgery in the treatment of uterine leiomymata: long term follow-up. *European Journal of Obstetrics, Gynecology and Reproductive Biology*, **38**, 53–7.

Filicori, M., Hall, D.A., Loughlin, J.S., Rivier, J., Vale, W., and Crowley, W.F. Jr (1983). A conservative approach to the management of uterine leiomyoma: pituitary desensitization by a luteinizing hormone-releasing hormone analog. *American Journal of Obstetrics and Gynecology*, **147**, 726–7.

Friedman, A.J. (1989). Treatment of leiomyomata uteri with short-term leuprolide followed by estrogen-progestin hormone replacement therapy for two years: a pilot study. *Fertility and Sterility*, **51**, 526–8.

Friedman, A.J., Daly, M., Juneau-Norcross, M., and Rein, M.S. (1992*a*). Predictors of uterine volume reduction in women with myomas treated with a gonadotropin-releasing hormone agonist. *Fertility and Sterility*, **58**, 413–15.

Friedman, A.J., Daly, M., Juneau-Norcross, M., Fine, C., and Rein, M.S. (1992*b*). Recurrence of myomas after myomectomy in women pre-treated with leuprolide acetate depot or placebo. *Fertility and Sterility*, **58**, 205–8.

Friedman, A.J., Daly, M., Juneau-Norcross, M., Rein, M.S., Fince, C., Gleason, R, *et al.* (1993). A prospective, randomized trial of gonadotropin-releasing hormone agonist plus estrogen-progestin or progestin 'add-back' regimens for women with leiomyomata uteri. *Journal of Clinical Endocrinology and Metabolism*, **76**, 1439–45.

Golan, A., Bukovsky, I., Pansky, M., Schneider, D., Weinraub, Z., and Caspi, E. (1993). Preoperative gonadotrophin-releasing hormone agonist treatment in surgery for uterine leiomyomata. *Human Reproduction*, **8**, 450–2.

Goldzieher, J.W., Maqueo, M., Ricaud, L., Aguilar, J.A., and Canales, E. (1996). Induction of degenerative changes in uterine myomas by high dose progestin therapy. *American Journal of Obstetrics and Gynecology*, **96**, 1078–87.

Harrison-Woolrych, M.L., Charnock-Jones, D.S., and Smith, S.K. (1994). Quantification of messenger ribonucleic acid for epidermal growth factor in human myometrium and leiomyomata using reverse transcriptase polymerase chain reaction. *Journal of Clinical Endocrinology and Metabolism*, **78**, 1179–84.

Hofmann, G.E., Rao, V., Barrows, G.H., Schultz, G.S., and Sanfilippo, J.F. (1984). Binding sites for epidermal growth factors in human uterine tissues and leiomyomas. *Journal of Clinical Endocrinology and Metabolism*, **58**, 880–3.

Hoppener, J.W.M., Mosselman, S., Roholl, P.J.M., Lambrechts, C., Slebos, R.J.C., de Pagter-Holthuizen P., *et al.* (1988). Expression of insulin-like growth factors-I and -II genes in human smooth muscle tumours. *EMBO Journal*, **7**, 1379–85.

Jones, J.I. and Clemmons, D.R. (1995). Insulin like growth factors and their binding proteins: biological actions. *Endocrine Reviews*, **16**, 3–34.

Koutsilieris, M., Michaud, J., and Nikolis, A. (1990). Preferential mitogenic activity for myoblast-like cells can be extracted from uterine leiomyoma tissues. *American Journal of Obstetrics and Gynecology*, **163**, 1665–70.

Leone, M., Cuccuccio, S., Venturini, P.L., Valenzano-Menada, M., Messeni, I.M., and De-Cesso, I. (1991). Immunohistochemical localization of epidermal growth factor receptor in leiomyomas from women treated with Goserelin depot. *Hormone and Metabolism Research*, **23**, 442–5.

Lumsden, M.A., West, C.P., Bramley, J., Rumgay, L., and Baird, D.T. (1988). The binding of epidermal growth factor to the human uterus and leiomyomata in women rendered hypo-oestrogenic by continuous administration of an LHRH-agonist. *British Journal of Obstetrics and Gynaecology*, **95**, 1299–304.

Lumsden, M.A., West, C.P., Hawkins, R.A., Branley, T.A., Rumgay, L., and Baird, D.T. (1989). The binding of steroids to myometrium and leiomyomata (fibroids) in women treated with the gonadotrophin releasing hormone agonist Zoladex (ICI 118630). *Journal of Endocrinology*, **121**, 389–96.

Lumsden, M.A., West, C.P., Thomas, E., Coutts, J., Hillier, H., Thomas, N. *et al.* (1994). Treatment with the gonadotrophin releasing hormone agonist goserelin before hysterectomy for uterine fibroids. *British Journal of Obstetrics and Gynaecology*, **101**, 438–42.

Matta, W.H., Shaw, R.W., Hesp, R., and Katz, D. (1987). Hypogonadism induced by luteinizing hormone releasing hormone analogues: effects on bone density in premenopausal women. *British Medical Journal*, **294**, 1523–4.

Matta, W.H.M., Stabile, I., Shaw, R.W., and Campbell, S. (1988). Doppler assessment of uterine blood flow changes in patients with fibroids receiving the gonadotrophin releasing hormone agonist buserelin. *Fertility and Sterility*, **49**, 1083–5.

Matta, W.H.M., Shaw, R.W., and Nye, M. (1989). Long-term follow-up of patients with uterine fibroids after treatment with the LHRH agonist buserelin. *British Journal of Obstetrics and Gynaecology*, **96**, 200–6.

Murphy, A.A., Kettel, L.M., Morales, A.J., Roberts, V.J., and Yenn, S.S.C. (1993). Regression of uterine leiomyomata in response to the antiprogesterone RU486. *Journal of Clinical Endocrinology and Metabolism*, **76**, 513–17.

Pasqualini, J.R., Vella, C., Cornier, E., Grenier, J., Vella, C., Schatz, B., *et al.* (1990). Effect of Decapeptyl, an agonist analog of gonadotropin-releasing hormone on estrogens, estrogen sulfates, and progesterone receptors in leiomyoma and myometrium. *Fertility and Sterility*, **53**, 1012–17.

Rein, M.S., Friedman, A.J., Stuart, J., and MacLaughlin, D.T. (1990*a*). Fibroid and myometrial steroid receptors in women treated with a gonadotrophin-releasing hormone agonist leuprolide acetate. *Fertility and Sterility*, **53**, 1018–23.

Rein, M.S., Friedman, A.J., Pandian, M.R., and Heffner, I.J. (1990*b*). The secretion of insulin-like growth factors I and II by explant cultures of fibroids and myometrium from women treated with a gonadotropin-releasing hormone agonist. *Obstetrics and Gynaecology*, **76**, 388–94.

Reinsch, R.C., Murphy, A.A., Morales, A.J., and Yen, S.S.C. (1994). The effects of RU486 and leuprolide acetate on uterine artery blood flow in the fibroid uterus: a prospective randomized study. *American Journal of Obstetrics and Gynaecology*, **170**, 1623–8.

Ross, R.K., Pike, M.C., Vessey, M.P., Bull, D., Yeates, D., and Casagrande, J.T. (1986). Risk factors for uterine fibroids: reduced risk associated with oral contraceptives. *British Medical Journal*, **293**, 359–63.

Spellacy, W.N., Le Maire, W.J., Buhi, W.C., Birk, S.A., and Bradley, B.A. (1972). Plasma growth hormone and estradiol levels in women with uterine myomas. *Obstetrics and Gynaecology*, **40**, 829–34.

Sporn, M.B. and Roberts, A.B. (1988). Peptide growth factors are multifunctional. *Nature*, **332**, 217–19.

Thompson, J.D. and Rock, J.A. (eds) (1992). *Te Linde's operative gynecology*, (7th edn). JB Lippincott, London.

Tommola, P., Pekonen, F., and Rutanen, E. (1989). Binding of epidermal growth factor, insulin-like growth factor I in human myometrium and leiomyomata. *Obstetrics and Gynaecology*, **74**, 658–62.

Viville, B., Charnock-Jones, D.S., Sharkey, A.M., and Smith, S.K. (1995). Progesterone A and B receptors in fibroids and normal myometrium. *Abstracts of the 11th annual meeting of the European Society of Human Reproduction and Embryology*. Abstract 349. Hamburg, Germany.

Vollenhoven, B.J., Shekleton, P., McDonald, J., and Healy, D.L. (1990). Clinical predictors of buserelin acetate treatment of uterine fibroids: a prospective study of 40 women. *Fertility and Sterility*, **54**, 1032–8.

Vollenhoven, B.J., Herington, A.C., and Healy, D.L. (1993*a*). Messenger ribonucleic acid expression of the insulin-like growth factors and their binding proteins in uterine fibroids and myometrium. *Journal of Clinical Endocrinology and Metabolism*, **76**, 1106–10.

Vollenhoven, B.J., McCloud, P., Shekleton, P., McDonald, J., and Healy, D.L. (1993*b*). An open study of luteinizing hormone-releasing agonists (LHRHa) in infertile women with uterine fibroids. *Gynaecological Endocrinology*, **7**, 57–61.

Vollenhoven, B.J., Pearce, P., Herington, A.C., and Healy, D.L. (1994*a*). Steroid receptor binding and messenger RNA expression in fibroids from untreated and luteinizing hormone-releasing hormone agonist pre-treated women. *Clinical Endocrinology*, **40**, 537–44.

Vollenhoven, B.J., Herington, A.C. and Healy, D.L. (1994*b*). Messenger RNA encoding the insulin-like growth factors and their binding proteins, in women with fibroids, pre-treated with luteinizing hormone-releasing hormone agonist. *Human Reproduction*, **9**, 214–19.

Vollenhoven, B.J., Herington, A.C., and Healy, D.L. (1995). Epidermal growth factor and transforming growth factor β in uterine fibroids and myometrium. *Gynaecologic and Obstetric Investigation*, **40**, 120–4.

West, C.P., Lumsden, M.A., Hillier, H., Sweeting, V., and Baird, D.T. (1992). Potential role for medroxyprogesterone acetate as a adjunct to goserelin (Zoladex) in the medical management of uterine fibroids. *Human Reproduction*, **7**, 328–32.

Yeh, J., Rein, M., and Nowak, R. (1991). Presence of messenger ribonucleic acid for epidermal growth factor (EGF) and EGF receptor demonstrable in monolayer cell cultures of myometrium and leiomyomata. *Fertility and Sterility*, **56**, 997–1000.

17 Surgical treatment of submucous fibroids

Jacques Donnez, Michelle Nisolle, Stephane Gillerot, Salim Bassil, Roland Polet, and Mireille Smets

Introduction

Dysfunctional uterine bleeding and fibroids are the major reasons for hysterectomy in women over 40 years of age. Since 1985, gonadotrophin releasing hormone (GnRH) agonists have been recognized as a possible medical management for these conditions (Maheux *et al.* 1985). Nevertheless, because of the bone loss induced by the hypoestrogenic state, this therapy must be considered as either a temporary medical approach before endoscopic surgery, or as a long-term therapy combined with 'add-back' therapy (Friedman *et al.* 1988; Maheux *et al.* 1991).

Hysteroscopic surgical techniques have proved to be successful in the control of menorrhagia (Goldrath 1985; Loffer 1988). The hysteroscope allows destruction of the endometrium to be carried out under direct vision. Both the electrical current of the resectoscope (Neuwirth 1983; De Cherney and Polan 1983; Hallez *et al.* 1987; Van Caillie 1989; Hamou 1993) and the energy of the neodymium:yttrium–aluminium–garnet (Nd:YAG) laser (Goldrath 1985; Donnez and Nisolle 1989, 1992; Dequesne 1989; Nisolle *et al.* 1991) have been effective tools for the destruction of endometrial tissue to a sufficient depth to avoid regeneration. The aim of this procedure is to decrease menstrual flow sufficiently to allow patients to avoid hysterectomy. Indeed, amenorrhoea and hypomenorrhoea are recognized sequelae of intrauterine adhesions (see Chapter 14). Other methods that have been used in an attempt to create endometrial destruction and scarring include cryotherapy, superheated steam, intracavitary radium, rigorous curettage, quinocrine methyl cyanoacrylate, oxalic acid, paraformaldehyde, and silicone rubber. However, only the Nd:YAG laser and the resectoscope have provided acceptable results (Goldrath 1985; Loffer 1988; Van Caillie 1989; Donnez *et al.* 1990*a*, 1994*a*, *b*; Garry *et al.* 1991; Hamou 1993). Laser energy has the advantage of precision of tissue destruction when compared with the electrical energy used in the resectoscope. Unlike electricity, laser energy does not travel through tissue. Its tissue effects depend on the amount of power used, and its effects are quite reproducible.

Classification of myomas

The classification of submucous fibroids according to hysterosalpingography and echography is listed below (Donnez *et al.* 1989*a*; Donnez 1993).

(1) submucous fibroids, the greatest diameters of which are inside the uterine cavity (Fig.17.1(a));

(2) submucous fibroids, the largest portions of which are located in the myometrium (Fig.17.1(b));

(3) multiple (> 2) submucous fibroids (myofibromatous uterus with submucous fibroids and intramural fibroids – Fig.17.1(c)).

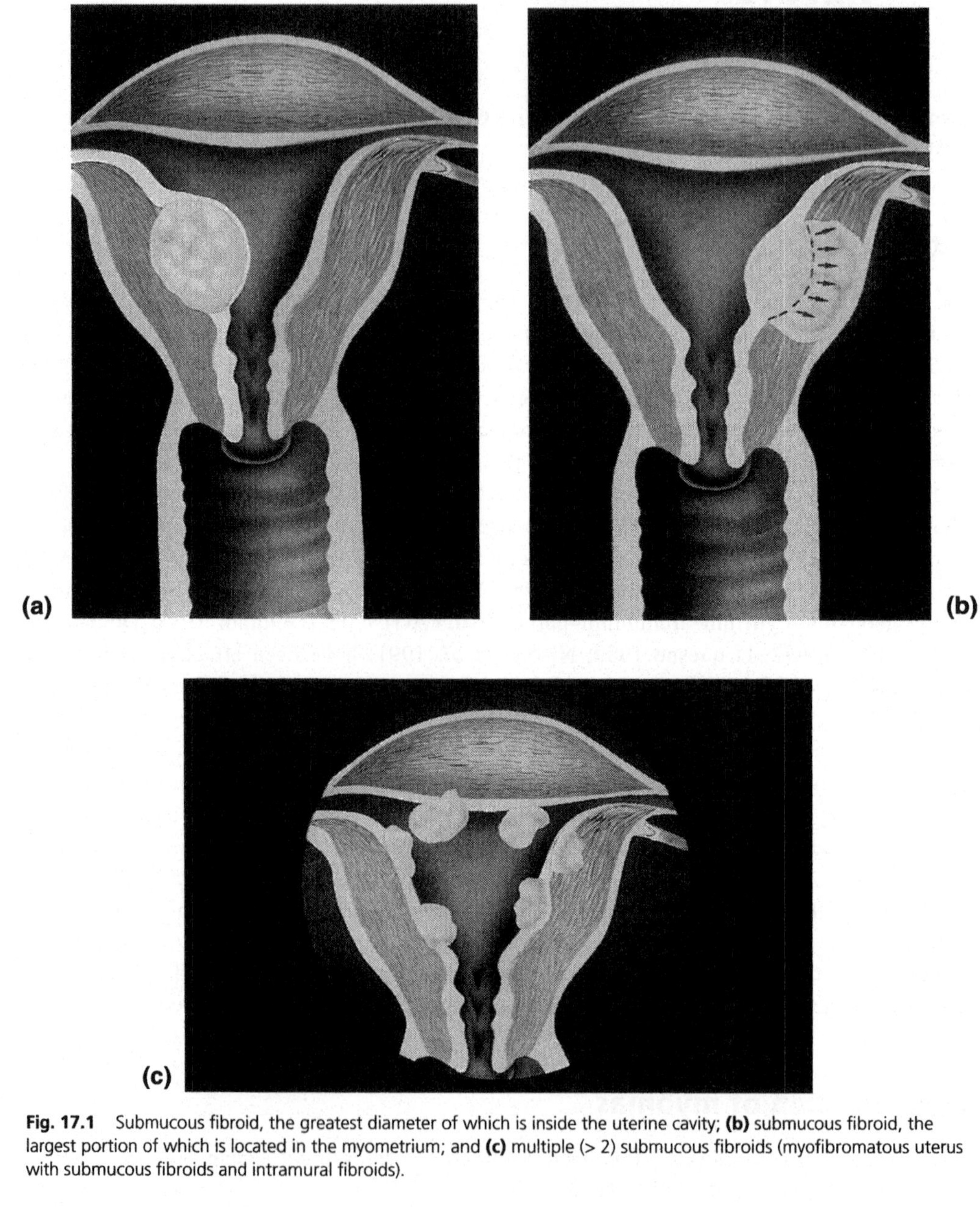

Fig. 17.1 Submucous fibroid, the greatest diameter of which is inside the uterine cavity; **(b)** submucous fibroid, the largest portion of which is located in the myometrium; and **(c)** multiple (> 2) submucous fibroids (myofibromatous uterus with submucous fibroids and intramural fibroids).

Hysteroscopic myomectomy: techniques

In our department, 366 women aged between 23 and 43 years (mean age 33 years) with symptomatic submucous uterine fibroids were treated with a biodegradable GnRH agonist (Zoladex, Zeneca, Macclesfield, UK). One implant was inserted at weeks 0, 4, and 8. Hysteroscopic myomectomy was carried out at 8 weeks.

Patients with submucous fibroids with their greatest diameter inside the uterine cavity underwent myomectomy using hysteroscopy and Nd:YAG laser. The myometrium overlying the myoma was less vascular following pretreatment with GnRH agonist, and 'shrinkage' of the uterine cavity may have accounted for the relative ease of separating the myomas from the surrounding myometrium.

For women with very large submucous fibroids, the largest portion of which was not inside the uterine cavity but inside the uterine wall, two-step operative hysteroscopy has been proposed (Donnez *et al.* 1990*a*). After eight weeks of pre-operative GnRH agonist therapy, partial myomectomy was carried out by resecting the protruding portion of the myoma. Thereafter, the laser fibre was directed as perpendicularly as possible at the remaining (intramural) fibroid portion, and was introduced into the fibroid to a depth of 5–10 mm. During the application of laser energy, the fibre was slowly removed so that the deeper areas were coagulated. The aim of this procedure was to decrease the size of the remaining myoma by decreasing the vascularity. This technique induces a myoma necrobiosis and can be called 'transhysteroscopic myolysis' (Donnez *et al.* 1990*a*).

Gonadotrophin-releasing hormone agonist therapy was given for another eight weeks and a second-look hysteroscopy was then performed. In all cases, myomas were found to protrude inside the uterine cavity. They appeared very white and without any apparent vessels on their surface. Shrinkage of the uterine cavity allowed these residual myoma portions to be separated easily from the surrounding myometrium and dissected off. Myomectomy was then carried out. In all cases (except when no decrease in the myoma size was observed), the detached myoma was left in the uterine cavity. There were no complications, and the necrotic myoma was probably eventually ejected with the menstrual blood.

In cases of multiple submucous fibroids, each myoma was either separated from the surrounding myometrium or totally photocoagulated. The myomas were then systematically destroyed, following which, endometrial ablation was carried out with the Nd:YAG laser.

Hysteroscopic myomectomy: treatment outcome

Using the method previously described, the reduction of very large submucous fibroid areas was calculated (Donnez *et al.* 1989*a*, *b*, 1990*a*, *b*). When more than one fibroid was present, only the largest was evaluated (Table 17.1). In all but four cases, fibroid area decreased by an average of 38 per cent. However, the response was variable, ranging from 4 to 95 per cent. Fibroid area was found to decrease significantly from the baseline area of $7.2 \pm 4.7\ cm^2$ to $4.4 \pm 3.5\ cm^2$ ($p < 0.01$) after eight weeks of GnRH agonist therapy. However, about 10 per cent of myomas did not respond well to GnRH agonist.

Table 17.2 shows long-term results according to myoma classification. In cases with large submucous fibroids, the greatest diameter of which was inside the uterine cavity ($n = 233$), surgery

Table 17.1 Submucous fibroid areas as assessed by hysterosalpingography before and after an eight week course of GnRH agonist

Size	Area (cm²)		Percentage reduction
	Pre-agonist	Post-agonist	
> 10 cm² (*n* = 34)	14.5 ± 6.5	9.7 ± 5.6	34.4
5–10 cm² (*n* = 36)	6.9 ± 1.3	4.5 ± 1.9	34.9
< 5 cm² (*n* = 80)	2.5 ± 1.2	1.7 ± 0.9	34.4
Total (*n* = 150)	6.3 ± 5.8	4.7 ± 3.8	34.5

Table 17.2 Surgical procedures and long-term results according to the site of myomas.

	Greatest diameter inside the uterine cavity	Largest portion located in the uterine wall	Multiple submucous myomas (myomectomy and endometrial ablation)
Surgical procedures			
Total number	233	78	55
Successful	230	74	51
Failed	3*	4**	4†
Recurrence of menorrhagia	5 (2%)	4 (5%)	15 (27%)

* Stromal tumour.
** A third-look hysteroscopy allowed the myoma to be removed.
† Myomectomy was not totally successful (in two cases, second-look laser hysteroscopy was successfully performed – in the other two cases, vaginal hysterectomy was proposed and successfully performed).

was carried out successfully in 230 cases. In three cases, an endometrial stromal tumour was diagnosed after histologic examination of the removed 'myomas', which had appeared benign during hysteroscopy. Thus, the incidence of 'stromal tumours' in apparently benign myomas was 1.2 per cent (3/233). It is important to note that there had been a poor response to treatment with GnRH agonist (less than 10 per cent decrease in size) in all three cases.

When successfully performed, myomectomy results in the restoration of normal menstrual flow. Long-term evaluation of the clinical outcome following hysteroscopic myomectomy has shown that menorrhagia recurred most often (27 per cent) in women who had had multiple submucous myomas (Donnez 1993). Hysterosalpingography and hysteroscopy revealed that the recurrence of menorrhagia was associated with the growth of new myomas at new sites.

Because most leiomyomata return to pretreatment size within four months of cessation of GnRH agonist therapy, these agents cannot be used as definitive medical therapy (Healy *et al.* 1984; Maheux *et al.* 1985; Andreyko *et al.* 1988; Friedman *et al.* 1988). Several reports have demonstrated reductions in uterine and fibroid volumes of 52 to 77 per cent after six months of GnRH agonist therapy, as assessed by ultrasound imaging. In our studies using hysterographic imaging, an average decrease in size of 35 per cent was found (Donnez *et al.* 1989*a*, *b*). Another study demonstrated reductions in fibroid area of 38 per cent after eight weeks of GnRH agonist therapy. However, the response was variable, ranging from 4 to 95 per cent (Donnez *et al.* 1990*a*). Reduction in size was not related to the pretreatment fibroid area.

Perioperative blood loss during hysteroscopic myomectomy is minimal, possibly because of the decreased vascularity of the myometrium, which has been demonstrated by a significant reduction in uterine arterial blood flow (Doppler) after treatment with GnRH agonists (Matta *et al.* 1988).

Conclusion

Gonadotrophin-releasing hormone agonists offer an effective adjunct for preoperative reduction of fibroid size, so that subsequent surgical treatment by hysteroscopy is possible. Even when the largest diameter of the fibroids was in the myometrium itself, the two-step hysteroscopic therapy combined with GnRH agonist represented an ideal management of large submucous myomas, reducing the need for myomectomy by laparotomy, and in turn reducing the associated problems of increased operative blood loss and post-operative adhesion formation (Donnez *et al.* 1990*a*, *b*; Donnez and Nisolle 1992). Because of the cessation of uterine bleeding, pre-operative therapy resulted in the restoration of a normal haemoglobin concentration, which also allows for the possibility of later autologous transfusion, if required.

The amount of fluid absorbed during the hysteroscopic procedure was lower if the endometrium was atrophic. By reducing the amount of fluid absorbed, preoperative GnRH agonist therapy reduced the risk of fluid overload and this represents another major advantage of this combined medical and surgical approach to therapy (Van Boven *et al.* 1989).

A stromal tumour was found in our series in 1.2 per cent of cases. In all three women, the 'myoma' did not respond to GnRH agonist. Finally, recurrence of fibroids was more likely in women with numerous submucous and intramural myomas, when compared with patients with only one submucous myoma. Because of this high rate of recurrence, we now prefer to perform a laparoscopic supracervical hysterectomy (LASH), rather than a hysteroscopic multiple myomectomy (Donnez and Nisolle 1993).

References

Andreyko, J.L., Blumenfeld, Z., Marschall, L.A., Monroe, S.E., Hricak, H., and Jaffe, R.B. (1988). Use of an agonistic analog of gonadotropin-releasing hormone (nafarelin) to treat leiomyomas: assessment by magnetic resonance imaging. *American Journal of Obstetrics and Gynecology*, **158**, 903–10.

De Cherney, A. and Polan, M.L. (1983). Hysteroscopic management of intrauterine lesions and intractable uterine bleeding. *Obstetrics and Gynecology*, **61**, 392–6.

Dequesne, J. (1989). Focal treatment of uterine bleeding and infertility with Nd:YAG laser and flexible hysteroscope. *Journal of Gynecology Surgery*, **5**, 177–82.

Donnez, J. and Nisolle, M. (1989). Laser hysteroscopy in uterine bleeding: endometrial ablation and polypectomy. In Donnez J Ed : *Laser operative laparoscopy and hysteroscopy* (ed. J. Donnez), pp. 277–88. Nauwelaerts, Louvain.

Donnez, J., Schrurs, B., Gillerot, S., Sandow, J., and Clerckx, F. (1989*a*). Treatment of uterine fibroids with implants of gonadotropin-releasing hormone agonist: assessment by hysterography. *Fertility and Sterility*, **51**, 947–50.

Donnez, J., Schrurs, B., Clerckx, F., and Nisolle, M. (1989*b*). Les agonistes de la LH-RH une alternative dans le traitement de la myomatose uterine. *Contraception Fertility Sex*, **17**, 47–9.

Donnez, J., Gillerot, S., Bourgonjon, D., Clerckx, F., and Nisolle, M. (1990*a*). Neodynium: YAG laser hysteroscopy in large submucous fibroids. *Fertility and Sterility*, **54**, 999–1003.

Donnez, J., Malvaux, V., Nisolle, M., and Casanas-Roux, F. (1990*b*). Hysteroscopic sterilization with the Nd:YAG laser. *Journal of Gynecological Surgery*, **6**, 149–53.

Donnez, J. and Nisolle, M. (1992). Hysteroscopic surgery. *Current Opinion in Obstetrics and Gynecology*, **4**, 439–46.

Donnez, J. and Nisolle, M. (1993). LASH: laparoscopic supracervical hysterectomy. *Journal of Gynecological Surgery*, **9**, 91–4.

Donnez, J. (1993). Nd:YAG laser hysteroscopic myomectomy. In *Endoscopic surgery for gynaecologists* (ed C. Sutton and M. Diamond), pp. 331–7. W.B. Saunders,

Donnez, J., Nisolle, M., Clerckx, F., Casanas-Roux, F., Saussoy, P., and Gillerot, S. (1994*a*). Advanced endoscopic techniques used in dysfunctional bleeding, fibroids and endometriosis and the role of gonadotrophin-releasing hormone agonist treatment. *British Journal of Obstetrics and Gynaecology*, **101**(Suppl. 10), 2–9.

Donnez, J., Nisolle, M., Clerckx, F., Gillerot, S., and Saussoy, P. (1994*b*). Hysteroscopic myomectomy. In *Atlas of laser operative laparoscopy and hysteroscopy* (ed. J. Donnez and M. Nisolle), pp. 323–35. Parthenon, New York.

Friedman, A.J., Barbieri, R.L., Doubilet, P.M., Fine, C., and Schiff, I. (1988). A randomized, double-blind trial of gonadotropin releasing hormone agonist (leuprolide) with or without medroxyprogesterone acetate in the treatment of leiomyomata uteri. *Fertility and Sterility*, **49**, 404–409.

Garry, R., Erian, J., and Grochmal, S. (1991). A multicentre collaborative study into the treatment of menorrhagia by Nd–YAG laser ablation of the endometrium. *British Journal of Obstetric and Gynaecology*, **98**, 357–62.

Goldrath, M.H. (1985). Hysteroscopic laser surgery. In *Basic and advanced laser surgery in gynecology* (ed. M.S. Baggish), p. 357. Appleton-Century-Crofts, Norwalk, CT.

Hallez, J.P., Cetteer, A., and Cartier, R. (1987). Methodical intrauterine resection. *American Journal of Obstetric and Gynecology*, **156**, 1080–4.

Hamou, J. (1993). Electroresection of fibroids. In *Endoscopic surgery for gynecologists* (ed. C. Sutton and M. Diamond), pp. 327–30. W.B. Saunders, Philadelphia.

Healy, D.L., Fraser, H.M., and Lawson, S.L. (1984). Shrinkage of a uterine fibroid after subcutaneous infusion of a LH-RH agonist. *British Medical Journal*, **289**, 1267–8.

Loffer, F.D. (1988). Laser ablation of the endometrium. *Obstetric and Gynecology Clinics of North America*, **15**, 77–89.

Maheux, R., Guilloteau, C., Lemay, A., Bastide, A., and Fazekas, A.T.A. (1985). Luteinizing hormone-releasing hormone agonist and uterine leiomyoma: pilot study. *American Journal of Obstetric and Gynecology*, **152**, 1034–8.

Maheux, R., Lemay, A., Blanchet, P., Friede, J., and Pratt, X. (1991). Maintained reduction of uterine leiomyoma following addition of hormonal replacement therapy to a monthy luteinizing hormone-releasing hormone agonist implant: a pilot study. *Human Reproduction*, **6**, 500–5.

Matta, W.H.M., Stabile, I., Shaw, R.S., and Campbell, S. (1988). Doppler assessment of uterine blood flow changes in patients with fibroids receiving the gonadotropin-releasing hormone agonist buserelin. *Fertility and Sterilinity*, **49**, 1083–5.

Neuwirth, R.S. (1983). Hysteroscopic management of symptomatic submucous fibroids. *Obstetric and Gynecology*, **62**, 509–11.

Nisolle, M., Grandjean, P., Gillerot, S., and Donnez, J. (1991). Endometrial ablation with the Nd:YAG laser in dysfunctional bleeding. *Min. and Investigation Therapy*, **1**, 35–9.

Van Boven, M., Singelyn, F., Donnez, J., and Gribomont, B. (1989). Dilution hyponatremia associated with intrauterine endoscopic laser surgery. *Anesthesiology*, **71**, 449–50.

Van Caillie, T. (1989). Electrocoagulation of the endometrium with the ball-end resectoscope. *Obstetrics and Gynecol*, **74**, 425–7.

III

Amenorrhoea, oligomenorrhoea, and irregular bleeding

18 Amenorrhoea

Tony G. Zreik and David L. Olive

Amenorrhoea, defined as the absence or cessation of menstrual flow, is the end result of a number of different pathological states, some congenital, others benign, and occasionally one of several that are life-threatening. For this reason, correct diagnosis is of critical importance. Amenorrhoea is a relatively common disorder, with an estimated prevalence of 1.8–3 per cent in the general female population during the reproductive years (Petterson *et al.* 1973), and as high as 8.5 per cent in an unselected adolescent population (Johnson and Whitaker 1992). Although a number of classification schemes for amenorrhoea are available, it is conventional to subdivide the patients initially into those with primary versus those with secondary amenorrhoea.

Primary amenorrhoea

The incidence of primary amenorrhoea is estimated to be less than 1 : 1000, and is defined as no spontaneous menses by the age of 16; however, a diagnostic work-up should be initiated by age 14 in the girl who has delayed puberty (absent menstruation and failure of development of secondary sexual characteristics). Similarly, evaluation should be performed in the girl who has failed to menstruate within four years following the onset of thelarche and adrenarche. Patients with primary amenorrhoea and normal external genitalia can be placed in one of four diagnostic categories depending on the presence or absence of breast development, and whether or not a uterus is present. Patients with ambiguous genitalia or cryptomenorrhoea will not be considered here. A scheme for elucidating primary amenorrhoea is illustrated in Fig. 18.1.

No breast development, uterus present

In this category, the abnormality may be due to a hypothalamic failure to release gonadotrophin-releasing hormone (GnRH), or to a failure of pituitary or gonadal function. Hypothalamic amenorrhoea implies a normally responsive pituitary–ovarian axis to GnRH. GnRH pulsatile release is an intrinsic property of the GnRH neurones (Weiner and Martinez de la Escalera 1993), with numerous neuropeptides and transmitters modulating its release. A decreased or acyclic release of GnRH from the hypothalamus may be mediated by catecholamines such as noradrenaline, dopamine, or β-endorphin. In addition, enkephalins, endorphins, and opiate receptors have been found in the arcuate nucleus and median eminence as well as on dopamine-secreting neurones (Pollard *et al.* 1977; Wilkes *et al.* 1980), thus raising the possibility that the expression of receptors on GnRH neurones may be mediated by direct neuronal inputs or by paracrine interactions with glial elements.

Hypogonadotrophic eunuchoidism or Kallmann's syndrome, also called De Morsier–Gauthier syndrome, is an inherited autosomal dominant or X-linked autosomal recessive anomaly with gonadotrophin deficiency resulting from the incapacity to activate the frequency of pulsatile

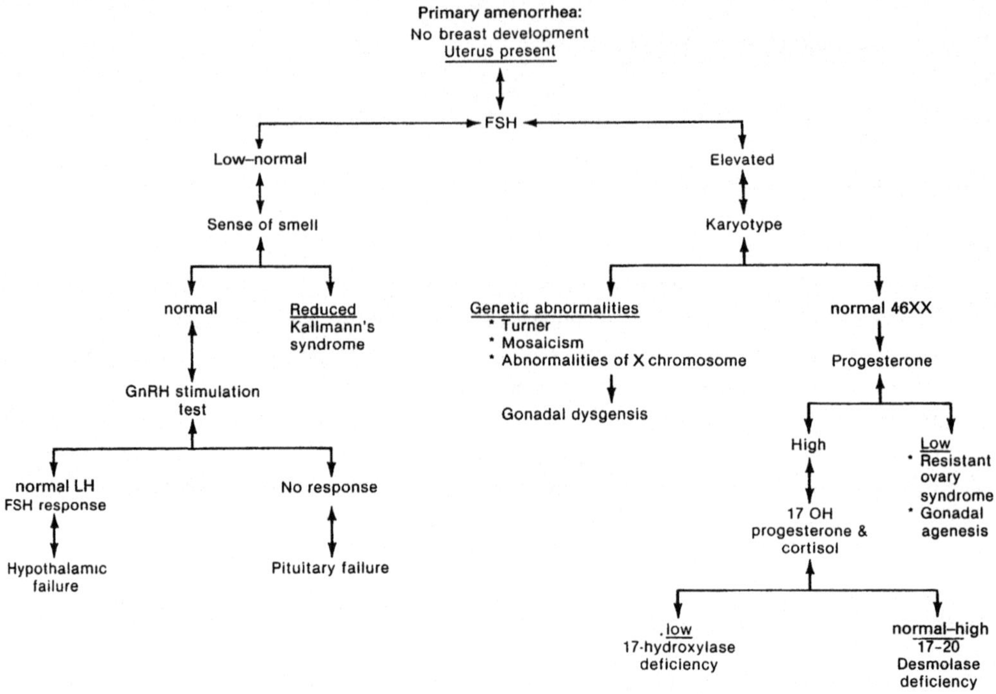

Fig. 18.1 Investigation of primary amenorrhoea.

GnRH secretion (Santen and Paulsen 1973; Leiblish *et al.* 1982). The most characteristic feature of this syndrome is anosmia, related to agenesis of the olfactory lobe in the central nervous system. Other associated anomalies include cryptorchidism, congenital deafness, colour blindness, midline defects such as cleft lip or palate, renal agenesis, and mental retardation in some patients. Hypogonadotrophic hypogonadism may also occur in women who do not have anosmia.

Pituitary failure, on the other hand, may occur sporadically or as an inherited disorder in patients exhibiting a normal sense of smell and none of the dysmorphic features that characterize Kallmann's syndrome. In patients with multiple pituitary hormone deficiencies, either idiopathic or secondary to organic aetiologies, gonadotrophin deficiency is noted along with a lack of growth hormone, thyroid-stimulating hormone, and adrenocorticotrophic hormone. In addition, pituitary adenomas, mumps, encephalitis, or prepubertal hypothyroidism may lead to failure of pituitary secretion of gonadotrophins.

Individuals with gonadal failure cannot synthesize ovarian steroids; thus these patients have elevated gonadotrophins as they lack the negative feedback of sex steroids on the hypothalamic–pituitary axis (hypergonadotrophic hypogonadism). Gonadal failure is generally due to chromosomal abnormalities or to enzyme deficiency states. The former group is the most common cause of primary amenorrhoea, and consists of Turner's syndrome patients, women with Turner's mosaicism, or structural abnormalities of the X chromosome (Turner 1938; Ford *et al.* 1959; Simpson 1975). These patients have streak gonads that lack primary follicles, with a resulting lack of ovarian steroid synthesis; thus, the negative feedback on the hypothalamic–pituitary axis is missing, leading to elevated gonadotrophins (Conte *et al.* 1975). Enzyme deficiency states such as 17-hydroxylase deficiency and 17–20 desmolase deficiency will also produce gonadal failure. Such patients present with a 46XX karyotype, primary amenorrhoea, no breast development, a prepubertal uterus, and slightly eunuchoid habitus. 17-hydroxylase deficiency results in a relative reduction in cortisol production, per unit of adrenocorticotrophic hormone (ACTH) secretion which in turn causes an increase in ACTH release to maintain appropriate cortisol levels. This may lead to excessive production of mineralocorticoids (deoxycorticosterone (DOC), corticosterone), which in turn can result in sodium retention, hypertension, and hypokalaemia. The diagnosis of 17-hydroxylase deficiency should be suspected when a high serum progesterone level, a low 17α hydroxyprogesterone level, and an elevated serum DOC level are obtained. The diagnosis can then be confirmed by performing an ACTH stimulation test, which induces markedly elevated progesterone levels with little change in the serum 17α hydroxyprogesterone levels.

Arrest of ovarian maturation at puberty may also result from a lack of ovarian response to gonadotrophin stimulation. This condition has been labelled ovarian dysgenesis despite the normal XX karyotype (Simpson *et al.* 1971), and has recently been linked to a mutation in exon 7 of the follicle-stimulating hormone (FSH) receptor gene, adjacent to a glycosylation site of the receptor that is essential for FSH binding (Aittomäki *et al.* 1995). The resulting low FSH binding capacity causes failure of ovarian follicle development in the face of elevated circulating levels of FSH and luteinizing hormone (LH). Clinically, in conjunction with poorly developed streak ovaries, this condition is characterized by normal prepubertal development with variably developed secondary sex characteristics and primary amenorrhoea.

The work-up of these patients with primary amenorrhoea, no breast development, and uterus present, begins with a serum FSH. This value distinguishes central (hypothalamic and pituitary) abnormalities from primary gonadal failure; an elevated FSH points to an ovarian aetiology, whereas a low or normal FSH indicates a hypothalamic or pituitary disorder. When primary gonadal failure is suspected following an elevated FSH serum level, a karyotype evaluation is necessary to rule out genetic abnormalities.

The central nervous system (CNS) abnormalities can be sorted into hypothalamic versus pituitary in origin by performing a GnRH stimulation test (100 μg s.c.) following a week of priming with oestrogen (ethinyl estradiol in a dose of 5–10 μg given orally each day). An elevation of FSH and LH in response to GnRH stimulation indicates hypothalamic failure. These patients should be evaluated via imaging studies for a central nervous system neoplasm (such as craniopharyngioma) and a qualitative test for olfaction should be performed to rule out Kallmann's syndrome. Treatment consists of hormonal replacement therapy (HRT) or ovulation induction with gonadotrophins or pulsatile GnRH if the patient is trying to conceive.

In rare instances, GnRH elicits no response, even after proper pre-treatment with oestradiol, indicating a pituitary failure. Evaluation of these patients consists of a computerized tomography (CT) scan or magnetic resonance imaging (MRI) to rule out pituitary tumours. Treatment consists of cyclic oestrogen and progestogen therapy to develop the breast and other secondary sexual characteristics as well as to prevent osteoporosis. If pregnancy is desired, the treatment of choice is exogenous gonadotrophin therapy.

Breast development, uterus absent

Two disorders lead to this clinical scenario: androgen insensitivity (testicular feminization), and congenital absence of the uterus (Mayer–Rokitansky–Kuster–Hauser syndrome, or Müllerian agenesis).

The former is an X-linked inherited disorder: patients have a 46XY karyotype, testes, and female phenotype, with such clinical features as sparse axillary and pubic hair, abnormal but well developed breasts, and a blind vaginal pouch. The prevalence of this condition is estimated to be 1 in 20 000 to 1 in 64 000 male births (Jagiello and Atwell 1962). A variety of defects have been noted ranging from the complete absence of androgen receptors to abnormal binding of androgens to the receptors, as well as post-receptor-binding abnormalities (Keenan *et al.* 1974). Characteristically, elevation of serum levels of oestradiol and gonadotrophins are noted. In addition, elevation in serum testosterone is used in conjunction with the physical examination to differentiate these individuals from patients with other abnormalities of Müllerian development (Table 18.1).

Management consists of removing the gonads postpubertally and placing the patient on hormone replacement therapy once full development is attained. This is the only exception to the rule that gonads, in the presence of a Y chromosome, should be removed prior to puberty. The reasoning behind this is that pubertal development is better achieved with endogenous hormones, while gonadal tumours in these patients have not been encountered prior to puberty (Manuel *et al.* 1976).

Congenital absence of the uterus is due to a failure of development of the Müllerian system and is one of the most common causes of primary amenorrhoea. This disorder is characterized by a 46XX karyotype, the presence of ovaries and normal secondary sex characteristics along with an absent uterus, and an absent or hypoplastic vagina. The clinical diagnosis can be confirmed by ultrasonography or magnetic resonance imaging of the pelvis. These patients with Müllerian agenesis should also be evaluated with an intravenous urogram to rule out associated extragenital anomalies. Up to 40 per cent of patients will have associated renal anomalies with absence of a kidney or the presence of a pelvic kidney being the most common defects (Fore *et al.* 1975). Moreover, 12 per cent of patients will have skeletal abnormalities, mostly involving the spine: examples include spina bifida, scoliosis, and congenital fusion of the cervical spine (the Klippel–Feil anomaly). Additional extragenital anomalies include rib and limb abnormalities, congenital heart disease, and inguinal hernias (Griffin *et al.* 1976).

Treatment of the genital anomalies of patients with Müllerian agenesis consists of development of an artificial or pseudo-vaginal pouch. This is occasionally performed via surgical reconstruction. Surgery, however, should be reserved for those cases in which the use of vaginal dilators has failed.

Table 18.1 Differentiating congenital absence of the uterus from androgen-insensitivity syndrome

	Müllerian agenesis	**Testicular feminization**
Hereditary pattern	Sporadic	X linked
Karyotype	46XX	46XY
Gonads	Ovaries	Testes
Sexual hair	Normal female	Absent to sparse
Associated anomalies	Present	Absent
Testosterone	Low	Normal male

Differences between Müllerian agenesis and testicular feminization include a 46XX karyotype and normal female sexual hair in the former, as opposed to a 46XY karyotype and absent to sparse sexual hair seen with testicular feminization. The simplest, least expensive test used to differentiate the two conditions is a serum testosterone level. A normal male testosterone concentration is consistent with androgen insensitivity; however, a testosterone level in the normal female range indicates congenital absence of the uterus. For more definitive evaluation, a karyotype evaluation may be used to distinguish the two conditions.

No breast development, no uterus

The combination of no breast development and absence of a uterus in a phenotypic female is extremely rare: all reported cases have a male karyotype, elevated gonadotrophins, and female levels of serum testosterone. Two enzyme defects in the male have been reported to cause this condition: 17α-hydroxylase deficiency and 17–20 desmolase deficiency, both leading to failure of androgen and oestrogen synthesis. These 46XY patients have abdominal testes that require removal followed by oestrogen replacement therapy (ERT).

In addition to these enzyme defects in the male, a case of agonadism presenting with primary amenorrhoea, no breast development, and uterine agenesis has been reported. The absence of the uterus in this patient was thought to be secondary to vanishing testicular tissue possibly present early in embryonic life; thus this syndrome of agonadism is also referred to as the vanishing testes syndrome. When a 46XX karyotype is obtained in women presenting with absence of a uterus and lack of female secondary characteristics, Müllerian agenesis along with another disorder such as primary ovarian failure or hypothalamic amenorrhoea should be suspected.

Breast development, uterus present

This diagnostic category comprises one-third of patients with primary amenorrhoea. Approximately 20 per cent of patients in this group have elevated prolactin levels and should be evaluated for hyperprolactinaemia. The remaining 80 per cent have the same disorders seen with secondary amenorrhoea, and should be evaluated accordingly.

Secondary amenorrhoea

Secondary amenorrhoea is defined as the absence of menses for six months in a woman previously having regular menses, or 12 months if previously oligomenorrhoeic. The prevalence of secondary amenorrhoea is reported to be about 5 per cent (Petterson *et al.* 1973; Münster *et al.* 1992).

Initial investigation should rule out pregnancy and thyroid disease. Amenorrhoea secondary to excess cortisol or androgen excess states will not be discussed in this section. Included here will be conditions involving abnormalities of the hypothalamic–pituitary–ovarian axis as well as intrauterine synechiae. A scheme for elucidating secondary amenorrhoea is shown in Fig. 18.2.

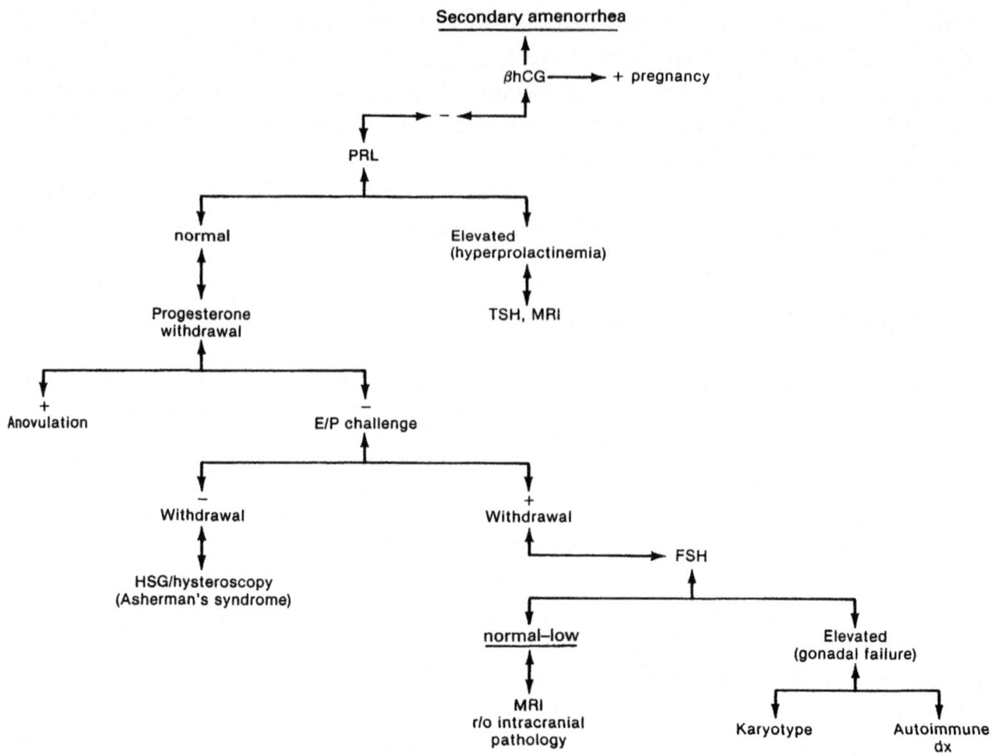

Fig. 18.2 Investigation of secondary amenorrhoea.

Hypothalamic dysfunction

The patient with secondary amenorrhoea for whom no organic cause can be detected is often considered to fall into the category of hypothalamic amenorrhoea. In most instances, serum gonadotrophin levels may be normal; however, there are abnormalities of GnRH pulsatile release as determined by abnormalities in LH pulses. In addition, many of these patients have a pattern of decreased gonadotrophin secretion which appears to be related to either a CNS neurotransmitter alteration or a hypothalamic derangement, most commonly idiopathic in nature, leading to a hypothalamic hypogonadal amenorrhoea. Other causes include medications (phenothiazines and other psychotropic drugs), stress, exercise, weight loss, and anorexia nervosa, along with hypothalamic lesions such as craniopharyngiomas, tuberculous granulomas, sarcoidosis, and meningoencephalitis.

Pituitary dysfunction

Amenorrhoea resulting from pituitary abnormalities may either be due to destruction of the LH- and FSH-secreting cells, or to the production of a hormone (e.g. prolactin, PRL) that affects reproductive function. As such, amenorrhoea may be the first symptom of a pituitary tumour, most commonly a prolactin secreting adenoma. These tumors may be microadenomas (less than 1 cm) or macroadenomas (greater than 1 cm), and are often treated medically with a dopamine agonist such as bromocriptine. In addition, 'non-secreting' pituitary tumours or chromophobe adenomas (which may secrete substances with no detectable physiological effect such as α-subunits or endorphins), along with non-neoplastic lesions of the pituitary, such as Sheehan's syndrome (post-partum pituitary necrosis) have also been shown to cause secondary amenorrhoea, mainly by compressing or destroying the LH and FSH-producing cells or by compressing the pituitary stalk, leading to elevated prolactin levels.

Ovarian dysfunction

Ovarian failure can occur before the onset of menses or any time after the menstrual cycle has been initiated. It is characterized by low oestrogen levels and elevated FSH levels. The aetiology of premature ovarian failure, which is defined as menopause prior to the age of 40, is unknown in many cases but may be due to specific sex chromosome anomalies (45X, 47XXY, and mosaicism), or to autoimmune antibodies directed against steroid producing cells of the ovary. Other rare genetic associations include galactosaemia and blepharophimosis.

The association between premature ovarian failure and autoimmune disease entities is well established; these entities include Hashimoto's thyroiditis, Grave's disease, hypoparathyroidism, hypoadrenalism, juvenile onset diabetes mellitus, myasthenia gravis, pernicious anaemia, and idiopathic thrombocytopenic purpura. The diagnosis of autoimmune oophoritis requires the demonstration of circulating tissue-specific antiovarian antibodies.

Loss of ovarian function may also be secondary to castration, haemorrhage, infection (including mumps), or destruction of follicles by physical insult such as irradiation (with as little as 0.5 Gy (50 rads) to the ovaries in older women) or chemotherapy (especially alkylating agents such as cyclophosphamide).

Multicomponent dysfunction of the hypothalamic–pituitary–ovarian axis

Patients with this abnormality are commonly referred to as having polycystic ovarian disease (PCO) because of the presence of multiple small (2–10 mm) subcortical follicular structures in both ovaries. Such patients have normal or elevated serum oestrogen levels, but are usually chronically anovulatory. All components of the hypothalamic–pituitary–ovarian axis may be functional but dyssynchronous; thus the polycystic ovary is the result of a functional derangement rather than a specific deficiency state.

Most patients present with obesity, hirsutism, and oligomenorrhoea but some may have secondary or even primary amenorrhoea. Serum oestradiol levels are generally greater than 120 pmol/l; thus bleeding will occur in response to progestogen withdrawal. In addition, an increased LH-to-FSH ratio is usually noted along with elevated dihydroepiandrosterone (DHEA), DHEAS, testosterone, and androstenedione levels. The ovarian follicular structures can be well demonstrated by vaginal ultrasound scanning. It is important to differentiate this condition from hypo- or hyperthyroidism, and from benign or neoplastic conditions of adrenal or ovarian origin (such as late onset congenital adrenal hyperplasia or androgen secreting tumours).

Treatment of polycystic ovarian disease should be tailored to the appropriate concern and presenting symptoms. Oral contraceptives may be used to regulate menstrual disturbances when fertility is not a current goal. Clomiphene citrate is usually given to women who desire fertility. Ovulation follows in approximately 75 per cent of cases (Garcia *et al.* 1977) although pregnancy rates may be lower. Patients who are found to have increased levels of DHEAS often respond to the addition of dexamethasone (Lobo *et al.* 1982). When ovulation is not achieved with high dose clomiphene or clomiphene citrate combined with dexamethasone and/or bromocriptine, a combination of a GnRH agonist and human menopausal gonadotrophins, or gonadotrophins alone may be used (Lanzone *et al.* 1987). Ovarian wedge resection has been reported to cause spontaneous ovulation (Judd *et al.* 1976), but it is infrequently used today because of the significant incidence of post-operative adhesions (Buttram and Vaquero 1975). In recent years, several studies have reported the use of electrocautery or laser drilling of ovarian cysts to treat anovulatory women with PCO but these may also cause some ovarian adhesions. Interestingly, unilateral diathermy can result in bilateral ovarian activity, probably by correcting the abnormalities in ovarian–pituitary feedback that are observed in such patients (Balen and Jacobs 1994). *In vitro* fertilization is reserved for the difficult patients or those who do not readily ovulate with the previously mentioned therapies.

Uterine dysfunction

The formation of intrauterine adhesions or synechiae, Asherman's syndrome, is often due to dilatation and curettage performed either to terminate pregnancy or in the immediate post-partum or post-abortal period in the presence of retained products. It may also be due rarely to severe endometritis following uterine surgery such as Caesarean section, myomectomy, or metroplasty. Such patients will ovulate normally but menses will not occur. The diagnosis can be suspected by hysterosalpingography, ultrasonography, or sonohysterography, and can be confirmed by hysteroscopy. Although treatment consists of hysteroscopic resection of the intrauterine adhesions, a preoperative vaginal sonographic measurement of the endometrial pattern may be beneficial in predicting the outcome of the surgical repair, and thus may be helpful in selecting the appropriate candidates for the procedure (Schlaff and Hurst 1995).

Diagnosing the cause of secondary amenorrhoea

After adequate history and physical examination are obtained, including nutritional and exercise habits, a serum pregnancy test should be obtained.

Once pregnancy is excluded, a serum prolactin level is obtained. If elevated, the patient should be evaluated for causes of hyperprolactinaemia including hypothyroidism, drugs, and renal failure. A CT scan or MRI may also be necessary to rule out pituitary adenomas.

In North America, if a normal serum prolactin is obtained, menses are attempted to be induced at this point by administration of a progestotional agent. If a positive withdrawal bleed is noted, anovulation with some spontaneous oestrogen secretion should be suspected and evaluated accordingly. If no withdrawal bleeding is achieved with a progestotional agent, an oestrogen/progestogen challenge is initiated (conjugated oestrogen 0.625 mg orally per day for 25 days, with 10 mg orally of medroxyprogesterone acetate daily for the final 5–10 days). If menses again fail to occur, end organ dysfunction (Asherman's syndrome) is suspected and can be diagnosed by hysterosalpingography or hysteroscopy.

However, if withdrawal bleeding occurs following an oestrogen/progestogen challenge, a serum FSH should be obtained. A low to normal FSH indicates a central (hypothalamic or pituitary) origin of the amenorrhoea, and necessitates a CT scan or an MRI to rule out intracranial pathology. When elevated levels of FSH are obtained in a patient less than 40 years of age, the diagnosis is premature ovarian failure. This warrants further evaluation: a karyotype test to rule out sex chromosome anomalies, and thyroid function tests with thyroid antibodies, cortisol, rheumatoid factor, and antinuclear antibodies to rule out a possible autoimmune origin of the ovarian failure.

In many other countries serum levels of FSH, LH, oestradiol, and TSH will be measured at the same time as serum prolactin. High levels of prolactin will usually be associated with low-to-normal levels of FSH, LH, and oestradiol signifying hypogonadism secondary to hyperprolactinaemia; normal prolactin with low-to-normal FSH, LH and oestradiol signifies hypothalamic amenorrhoea; high LH with low-to-normal FSH, LH, and variable oestradiol and prolactin is compatible with PCO; high FSH and LH will usually be associated with low oestradiol and prolactin indicating premature ovarian failure (usually premature menopause, but occasionally resistant ovary syndrome). Serum TSH is a sensitive screening test for hypothyroidism and elevated levels of free circulating thyroid hormones will indicate hyperthyroidism. Further investigations may sometimes be necessary to elucidate individual cases.

References

Aittomäki, K., Diegnez Lucena, J.L., Pakarinen, P., Sistonen, P., Tapanainen, J., Gromoll, J., *et al.* (1995). Mutation in the follicle-stimulating hormone receptor gene causes hereditary hypergonadotropic ovarian failure. *Cell*, **82**, 959–68.

Balen, A.H. and Jacobs, H.S. (1994). A prospective study comparing unilateral and bilateral ovarian diathermy in women with PCO syndrome. *Fertility and Sterility*, **62**, 921–5.

Buttram, V.C. Jr and Vaquero, C. (1975). Post-ovarian wedge resection adhesive disease. *Fertility and Sterility*, **26**, 874–6.

Conte, F.A., Grumbach, M.M., and Kaplan, S.L. (1975). A diphasic pattern of gonadotrophin secretion in patients with the syndrome of gonadal dysgenesis. *Journal of Clinical Endocrinology and Metabolism*, **40**, 670–4.

Ford, C.E., Jones, K.W., Polani, P.E., DeAlmeida, J.C., and Briggs, J.H. (1959). A sex chromosome anomaly in a case of gonadal dysgenesis. *Lancet*, **i**, 711–13.

Fore, S.R., Hammond, C.B., Parker, R.T., and Anderson, E.E. (1975). Urologic and genital anomalies in patients with congenital absence of the vagina. *Obstetrics and Gynecology*, **46**, 410–16.

Garcia, J., Jones, G.S., and Wentz, A.C. (1977). The use of clomiphene citrate. *Fertility and Sterility*, **28**, 707–17.

Griffin, J.E., Edwards, C., Madden, J.D., Harrod, M.J., and Wilson, J.D. (1976). Congenital absence of the vagina. The Mayer–Rokitansky–Kuster–Hauser syndrome (review). *Annals of Internal Medicine*, **85**, 224–36.

Jagiello, G. and Atwell, J.D. (1962). Prevalence of testicular feminisation. *Lancet*, **i**, 329.

Johnson, J. and Whitaker, A.H. (1992). Adolescent smoking, weight changes, and binge–purge behavior: association with secondary amenorrhea. *American Journal of Public Health*, **82**, 47–54.

Judd, H.L., Rigg, L.A., Anderson, D.C., and Yen, S.S. (1976). The effects of ovarian wedge resection on circulating gonadotropin and ovarian steroid levels in patients with PCO. *Journal of Clinical Endocrinology and Metabolism*, **43**, 347–55, 1976.

Keenan, B.S., Meyer, W.J., Hadjian, A.J., Jones, H.W., and Migeon, C.J. (1974). Syndrome of androgen insensitivity in man: absence of 5α-dihydrotestosterone binding protein in skin fibroblasts. *Journal of Clinical Endocrinology and Metabolism*, **38**, 1143–6.

Lanzone, A., Fulghesu, A.M., Spina, M.A., Apa, R., Menini, E., Caruso, A., and Mancuso, S. (1987). Successful induction of ovulation and conception with combined GnRH agonist plus highly purified FSH in patients with PCO disease. *Journal of Clinical Endocrinology and Metabolism*, **65**, 1253–8.

Leiblish, J.M., Rogol, A.D., White, B.J., and Rosen, S.W. (1982). Syndrome of anosmia with hypogonadotropic hypogonadism (Kallman syndrome). *American Journal of Medicine*, **73**, 506–20.

Lobo, R.A., Paul, W., March, C.M., Granger, L., and Kletzky, O.A. (1982). Clomiphene and dexamethasone in women unresponsive to clomiphene alone. *Obstetrics and Gynecology*, **60**, 497.

Manuel, M., Katayama, K.P., and Jones, H.W. (1976). The age of occurrence of gonadal tumours in intersex patients with a Y chromosome. *American Journal of Obstetrics and Gynecology*, **124**, 293.

Münster, K., Helm, P., and Schmidt, L. (1992). Secondary amenorrhea: Prevalence and medical contact – a cross sectional study from a Danish county. *British Journal of Obstetrics and Gynaecology*, **99**, 430–3.

Petterson, F., Fries, H., and Nillius, S.J. (1973). Epidemiology of secondary amenorrhea. I. Incidence and prevalence rates. *American Journal of Obstetrics and Gynecology*, **117**, 80–6.

Pollard, H., Lioreus-Cortes, C., and Schwartz, J.C. (1977). Enkephalin receptors on dopamine neurones in rat striatum. *Nature*, **268**, 745–7.

Santen, R.J. and Paulsen, C.A. (1973). Hypogonadotropic eunuchoidism. I: clinical study of the mode of inheritance. *Journal of Clinical Endocrinology and Metabolism*, **36**, 47–54.

Schlaff, W.D. and Hurst, B.S. (1995). Preoperative sonographic measurement of endomentrial pattern predicts outcome of surgical repair in patients with severe Asherman's syndrome. *Fertility and Sterility*, **63**, 410–13.

Simpson, J. (1975). Gonadal dysgenesis and abnormalities of the human sex chromosomes: current status of the phenotypic–karyotypic correlations. *Birth Defects*, **11**, 23–9.

Simpson, J.L., Christakes, A.C., Horwith, M., and Silverman, F.S. (1971). Gonadal dysgenesis in individuals with apparently normal chromosomal complements: tabulation of cases and compilation of genetic data. *Birth Defects*, **7**, 215–28.

Turner, H.H. (1938). A syndrome of infantilism, congenital webbed-neck, and cubitus valgus. *Endocrinology*, **23**, 566–8.

Weiner, R.I. and Martinez de la Escalera G. (1993). Pulsatile release of GnRH is an intrinsic property of GT1 neuronal cell lines. *Human Reproduction*, **8** (suppl. 2), 13–17.

Wilkes, M.M., Watkins, W.B., Stewart, R.D., and Yen, S.S.C. (1980). Localization and quantitation of β-endorphin in human brain and pituitary. *Neuroendocrinology*, **30**, 113–21.

19 Oligomenorrhoea and polycystic ovary syndrome

Stephen Franks

Oligomenorrhoea

Oligomenorrhoea is conventionally defined as an intermenstrual interval of greater than 42 days and is usually indicative of anovulation. Although the focus of this chapter is on oligomenorrhoea, it should be noted that its causes and management are very similar to those of secondary amenorrhoea or irregular menses which are also manifestations of anovulation. Anovulatory menses carries the implication that the ovary is producing oestrogen concentrations which are in the mid-follicular phase range but that progesterone secretion will be deficient. A series of anovulatory menses may, however, be interspersed by the occasional ovulatory cycle, a phenomenon which is relevant when considering the management of patients with oligomenorrhoea, as will be discussed later.

Causes of anovulation and oligomenorrhoea

The causes of anovulation can be classified, functionally, into three major groups: primary ovarian failure, deficiency or disordered regulation of gonadotrophins, and polycystic ovary syndrome (Table 19.1).

In a series of 75 consecutive patients presenting to a gynaecological endocrine clinic with oligomenorrhoea (Table 19.2), two ('perimenopausal') had evidence of primary ovarian failure (raised serum FSH) and two had disorders of gonadotrophin regulation (one hyperprolactinaemic, one partially recovered weight loss). In a further six subjects the cause was unknown, although it was associated with obesity in three of these women. However, the largest group by far (87 per cent of subjects) was that of polycystic ovary syndrome (Adams *et al.* 1986).

Investigation of oligomenorrhoea

The procedure for investigation of patients with oligomenorrhoea is essentially very simple. A single blood sample is taken for the measurement of follicle-stimulating hormone (FSH), luteinizing hormone (LH), and prolactin and a detailed pelvic ultrasound scan is performed to assess ovarian and endometrial morphology. If patients are also complaining of symptoms of hyperandrogenism (acne, hirsutism, alopecia), serum testosterone should be measured (see below under 'investigation of polycystic ovary syndrome'). It is debatable whether thyroid function tests (i.e. a baseline serum measurement of TSH) should be performed routinely in women with

Table 19.1 Causes of anovulation

Classification	Causes
Primary ovarian failure	Genetic (e.g. Turner's syndrome)
	Autoimmune
	Irradiation or chemotherapy
Second ovarian dysfunction	Disorders of gonadotrophin regulation
	Specific:
	Hyperprolactinaemia
	Kallmann's syndrome
	Functional:
	Weight loss
	Exercise
	Idiopathic
	Gonadotrophin deficiency
	Pituitary tumour
	Pituitary surgery or irradiation
Polycystic ovary syndrome	

Table 19.2 Causes of oligomenorrhoea in 75 consecutive subjects (from Adams *et al.* 1986)

Diagnosis	Number (%)
Polycystic ovaries	65 (87)
Obese (no polycystic ovaries)	3 (4)
Hyperprolactinaemia	1 (1)
Perimenopausal	2 (3)
Recovered weight loss	1 (1)
Unknown	3 (4)

oligomenorrhoea. Many centres will include this test in the programme of investigation but the rationale is uncertain. In a recent analysis of the results from our own centre, we found that abnormal thyroid function tests were no more common in women with oligomenorrhoea than in an age-matched, female population with regular, ovulatory menses (M. Foster, D. White, and S. Franks, unpublished observations).

Management of oligomenorrhoea

The management of patients with oligomenorrhoea can be categorized under three headings: treatment of infertility, treatment of hormone (progesterone) deficiency, and treatment of possible hormone excess (e.g. hyperandrogenism and hyperprolactinaemia) (Table 19.3). These factors are discussed below in the context of treatment of polycystic ovary syndrome.

Table 19.3 Management of oligomenorrhoea

Category	Treatment
Infertility	Induction of ovulation
Hormone deficiency	Progesterone replacement
	Cyclic progestogens
	Combined oral contraceptive pill
Hormone excess	
Hyperandrogenism	Anti-androgens
Hyperprolactinaemia	Dopamine agonists

Polycystic ovary syndrome

Polycystic ovary syndrome is one of the most common endocrine disorders but its aetiology remains uncertain (Franks 1995). The apparent heterogeneity of the clinical presentation has inevitably raised the question as to whether polycystic ovary syndrome is one disorder or whether its origins are as variable as its manner of presentation. It is now recognized that not only is polycystic ovary syndrome the most frequent cause of anovulatory infertility and of hirsutism (Adams *et al.* 1986; Hull 1987; Franks 1989, 1995) but it is also associated with characteristic metabolic abnormalities which may carry an increased risk, in the long term, for the development of non-insulin dependent diabetes and cardiovascular disease (Dahlgren *et al.* 1992*a*, *b*; Franks 1995).

Definition and diagnosis of polycystic ovary syndrome

There has always been vigorous debate about the definition of polycystic ovary syndrome and it seems likely to remain so until the specific aetiology (ies) of the syndrome can be elucidated. The classic definition includes the clinical manifestations of anovulation and hyperandrogenism in women with bilateral polycystic ovaries; obesity is a common but not universal accompaniment (Givens 1976; Yen 1980). Typically, but not exclusively, these features are associated with hypersecretion of luteinizing hormone (LH) and androgens but with normal, or slightly low, serum concentrations of follicle-stimulating hormone (FSH) (Gambrell *et al.* 1973; Rebar *et al.* 1976; Holte *et al.* 1994*a*). In recent years, the ability to identify polycystic ovaries by pelvic ultrasonography has provided new insight into the spectrum of clinical and biochemical presentation of women with a polycystic morphology of the ovaries (Swanson *et al.* 1981; Parisi *et al.* 1984; Adams *et al.* 1985, 1986). It is now evident that this spectrum includes both anovulatory women without hirsutism (but who are usually hyperandrogenaemic) and, conversely, those who are hirsute and have regular, ovulatory cycles (but may also have elevated serum LH concentrations) (Adams *et al.* 1986; Franks 1989). Thus, irrespective of clinical presentation, there is a typical pattern of biochemical abnormalities which seems to unite these subgroups of women with ultrasound evidence of polycystic ovaries.

In our own department the diagnosis of polycystic ovary syndrome is based primarily on the ultrasound definition of polycystic ovaries in patients with anovulation and/or hyperandrogenism. We have excluded patients who have polycystic ovaries on ultrasound but in whom the primary diagnosis is of pituitary or adrenal diseases such as hyperprolactinaemia, acromegaly, and classical or non-classical congenital adrenal hyperplasia (Zawadzki and Dunaif 1992). Neither have we included subjects with clinical and endocrine features suggesting polycystic ovary syndrome but who have normal ovarian morphology – less than ten per cent of such patients, in our experience. Many groups have relied mainly on clinical and biochemical criteria to make the diagnosis of polycystic ovary syndrome. The term 'ovarian hyperandrogenism' (Lobo 1991; Ehrmann *et al.* 1992) has been suggested to encompass, in addition to those with polycystic ovaries, women with biochemical evidence of ovarian androgen excess but who have apparently normal ovarian morphology. Despite some inconsistencies in results between groups which can be attributed to different methods of diagnosis, comparative studies have demonstrated that there is a high degree of concordance of ultrasound with histological features of polycystic ovaries and with clinical and endocrine evidence of the syndrome (Adams *et al.* 1986; Fox *et al.* 1991; Takahashi *et al.* 1992).

In summary, the classic (and perhaps most widely accepted) definition of polycystic ovary syndrome is the association of hyperandrogenism with chronic anovulation in patients without specific diseases of the adrenal or pituitary glands (Zawadzki and Dunaif 1992). We, and others, would argue that the definitions should be modified in the light of the ultrasonographic studies cited above. Thus the term 'polycystic ovaries' refers to the ovarian morphology which may occur regardless of symptoms and 'polycystic ovary syndrome' can be defined as the typical ovarian morphology plus at least one presenting symptom of hyperandrogenism (hirsutism, acne, alopecia), anovulation (oligomenorrhoea or non-oestrogen deficient), or amenorrhoea (Franks 1989; Conway *et al.* 1989). This definition would therefore include women with polycystic ovaries and regular menses who present with hirsutism or acne.

Prevalence and presentation of polycystic ovary syndrome

It has been recognized for more than fifty years that polycystic ovary syndrome is an important cause of anovulation and of hirsutism but the prevalence of polycystic ovaries in women with these problems has rarely been studied. In our centre, 221 patients presenting consecutively to the gynaecological–endocrine clinic were evaluated by ultrasonographic, clinical, and endocrine criteria (Adams *et al.* 1986). Thirty of 100 women with secondary amenorrhoea and, as indicated above, 65 of 75 (87 per cent) with oligomenorrhoea were found to have polycystic ovaries. Of the women with oligomenorrhoea and polycystic ovaries, 54 per cent had hirsutism or acne (Table 19.4).

Surprisingly, 40 out of 46 (87 per cent) of women with hirsutism and regular menses had polycystic ovaries on ultrasound. Although there was a spectrum of gonadotrophin and androgen concentrations in women with polycystic ovaries, each clinical subgroup was characterized by a significant increase in serum concentrations of LH and the androgens, testosterone and androstenedione, compared with control subjects. In the women with oligomenorrhoea, 61 per cent had an elevated serum LH concentration, 84 per cent had an LH:FSH ratio in excess of 3, and 64 per cent had a raised serum testosterone concentration (Table 19.4). Overall, more than 90 per cent of women with oligomenorrhoea and polycystic ovary syndrome, as diagnosed by ultrasonography, had at least one abnormal biochemical test which would be considered characteristic of the classic definition of the syndrome. In addition, amongst anovulatory women with polycystic ovaries, concentrations of LH and androgens were equally elevated in those with hirsutism and those without. In other words, polycystic ovaries was a better marker of hyperandro-

Table 19.4 Clinical and endocrine presentation of 65 women with oligomenorrhoea who had ultrasound evidence of polycystic ovaries (from Adams *et al.* 1985)

Presentation	Percentage
Hirsutism and/or acne	54%
Elevated serum LH concentration	61%
LH:FSH ratio > 3	84%
At least one biochemical abnormality	90%*

* Of the five women with oligomenorrhoea with polycystic ovaries and normal hormones, four had hirsutism.

genaemia than the presence of hirsutism in this group. Polycystic ovaries have also been noted to be common in hyperandrogenic women presenting with acne or androgen-dependent alopecia (Conway *et al.* 1989; Franks 1989; Bunker *et al.* 1991).

Obesity occurs in 35–40 per cent of women with polycystic ovary syndrome (Goldzieher and Green 1962; Conway *et al.* 1989; Kiddy *et al.* 1990). Its presence influences the clinical presentation, with hirsutism and menstrual disturbances being significantly more common in obese compared with lean subjects (Conway *et al.* 1989; Kiddy *et al.* 1990).

The finding of an unexpectedly high prevalence of polycystic ovaries in women with anovulation is supported by studies from a regional infertility centre in south-west England. Using clinical and biochemical criteria, rather than ultrasonography, to make the diagnosis, Hull (1987) reported that 37 per cent of women with amenorrhea and 90 per cent of women with oligomenorrhoea had polycystic ovary syndrome. These figures are remarkably similar to those reported above. Overall 73 per cent of cases of anovulatory infertility were estimated to have polycystic ovary syndrome. In a subsequent study, the Bristol group has shown concordance between these clinical and biochemical markers of polycystic ovary syndrome and ultrasonographic results (Fox *et al.* 1991).

The characteristic endocrinopathy of raised mean levels of serum androgens and LH has been reported in all published series of women with polycystic ovary syndrome (Yen 1980; Franks 1989) but the variation in LH levels between individuals (which depends not only on the criteria for diagnosis but also the method of measurement) means that the diagnostic value of a single hormone measurement is limited (Franks 1995).

Similarly, although serum concentrations of testosterone and androstenedione are elevated in women with polycystic ovary syndrome there is a good deal of variation from patient to patient (Givens 1976; Conway *et al.* 1989; Franks 1989). This is illustrated by the observation that anovulatory but non-hirsute women with polycystic ovaries may have hyperandrogenaemia whilst hirsute women with polycystic ovaries may have normal serum androgen levels (Conway *et al.* 1989; Franks 1989; Lobo 1991). This phenomenon may be explained by the fact that both production and clearance of androgens are increased in women with hirsutism (Bardin and Lipsett 1967; Kirschner *et al.* 1983). Low serum concentrations of sex-hormone-binding globulin (SHBG) – the principal transport protein for testosterone in the blood – may contribute to increased clearance of testosterone (Anderson 1974).

Blood levels of SHBG are inversely correlated with body mass index (BMI; calculated from the quotient of weight [kg] and height squared [m^2]) which may help to explain why obese subjects with polycystic ovary syndrome are more likely to be hirsute than their lean counterparts, despite similar serum levels of testosterone (Kiddy *et al.* 1990). The effects of obesity on SHBG are likely to be mediated by insulin (Plymate *et al.* 1988; Kiddy *et al.* 1989, 1992; Nestler and Strauss 1991; Pugeat *et al.* 1991). The role of hyperinsulinaemia and insulin resistance in the aetiology and presentation of polycystic ovary syndrome has been the subject of intensive research over the last few years and will be discussed in detail below.

Other hormonal abnormalities including hyperprolactinaemia and impaired secretion of growth hormone have been described in women with polycystic ovary syndrome (Franks 1989, 1995). Moderate hyperprolactinaemia occurs in 5–10 per cent of women with typical clinical and biochemical features of polycystic ovary syndrome. The significance of hyperprolactinaemia in polycystic ovary syndrome remains unclear. Impaired growth hormone secretion in women with polycystic ovaries may simply be a function of accompanying obesity rather than a specific feature of the syndrome (Slowinska-Srzednicka *et al.* 1992).

Hyperinsulinaemia, insulin resistance, and polycystic ovary syndrome

Women with polycystic ovary syndrome are both hyperinsulinaemic (Burghen *et al.* 1980; Chang *et al.* 1983; Dunaif *et al.* 1987) and insulin resistant (Dunaif *et al.* 1989; Robinson *et al.* 1992; Holte *et al.* 1994*b*) compared to weight-matched control groups. Both lean and obese women with polycystic ovary syndrome show evidence of decreased insulin sensitivity but there is an interaction between obesity and polycystic ovary syndrome so that this metabolic disorder is excacerbated in obese subjects with the syndrome (Dunaif *et al.* 1989; Robinson *et al.* 1992; Holte *et al.* 1994*b*). There is a close correlation between body fat topography and both hyperinsulinaemia and insulin resistance, so that if polycystic ovary and non-polycystic ovary groups are matched for waist–hip ratio rather than body mass index, the difference in insulin concentrations and sensitivity between women with polycystic ovary syndrome and controls is no longer significant (Robinson *et al.* 1992; Holte *et al.* 1994*b*). The complex interrelationship of hyperandrogenism, central adiposity, and insulin resistance remains to be unravelled. Supression of ovarian androgen production does not change the pattern of insulin secretion (Dunaif *et al.* 1990; Dale *et al.* 1992) and although a longer term effect of androgens on adipocyte biology and glucose homeostasis cannot be ruled out, the evidence points to insulin being the cause rather than the consequence of disturbances of androgen metabolism (Dunaif 1993). Insulin stimulates androgen production by human ovarian theca-interstitial tissue *in vitro* (Barbieri *et al.* 1984; Bergh *et al.* 1993). There is also evidence, from clinical studies, of a positive correlation between serum androgens and the level of insulin in the circulation (Conway *et al.* 1990; Nestler and Strauss 1991) although not all groups have observed this (Sharp *et al.* 1991; Toscano *et al.* 1992). It can be argued that the effect of insulin on androgen clearance is perhaps of more clinical significance. There is an inverse correlation of SHBG with fasting and glucose-stimulated insulin which appears to account, predominantly, for the effect of body weight on SHBG concentrations in hyperandrogenaemic women (Sharp *et al.* 1991; Pugeat *et al.* 1991). Further evidence that insulin is an important regulator of SHBG secretion comes from studies which report a direct suppressive effect of insulin on the synthesis and secretion of this binding protein (Plymate *et al.* 1988).

Insulin resistance in women with polycystic ovary syndrome is characterized by peripheral but not hepatic resistance. The underlying cellular mechanism(s) remain unclear but there is evidence for a post-insulin receptor defect which implicates impaired insulin-mediated glucose uptake by adipose and muscle cells (Dunaif 1993).

Relationship of insulin resistance to menstrual pattern in hyperandrogenaemic women

Hyperinsulinaemia and insulin resistance are not universal features of women with hyperandrogenism. Hyperandrogenaemic women with polycystic ovaries who have regular menstrual cycles have fasting and glucose-stimulated serum insulin concentrations which are indistinguishable from those in weight-matched normal subjects (Dunaif *et al.* 1987; Conway *et al.* 1990; Robinson *et al.* 1993). Likewise, reduced insulin sensitivity is characteristic of women with polycystic ovaries who have oligo- or amenorrhoea but equally hyperandrogenaemic, weight- and age-matched polycystic ovaries patients with regular cycles have normal insulin-mediated glucose disposal (Robinson *et al.* 1993). What is the significance of the association of insulin resistance with menstrual pattern in hyperandrogenaemic women? There is little to suggest that anovulation, itself, can affect insulin sensitivity but, conversely, hyperinsulinaemia/insulin resistance may affect menstrual function. For example, changes in insulin concentrations during calorie restriction precede resumption of ovulatory cycles in obese women with polycystic ovary syndrome (Kiddy *et al.* 1992).

The distinction in insulin dynamics between anovulatory and ovulatory women with equal degrees of hyperandrogenaemia is of some importance, both in assessing the role of insulin resistance in the aetiology of polycystic ovary syndrome and in determining which hyperandrogenic women may be at long-term risk of the metabolic and cardiovascular sequelae of insulin resistance. Thus it seems unlikely that insulin resistance has an *obligatory* role in development of ovarian hyperandrogenism although its presence may determine whether a woman with this condition becomes anovulatory (Robinson *et al.* 1993; Franks 1995). From another viewpoint, the pattern of menstruation in a patient with hyperandrogenism and polycystic ovaries may allow one to identify, clinically, the likely presence of insulin resistance and its metabolic and clinical consequences.

Metabolic abnormalities and their clinical consequences in women with polycystic ovaries

What, therefore, are the metabolic abnormalities in women with polycystic ovary syndrome, how are they related to insulin resistance, and what are the implications for long-term health? As might be predicted, women with polycystic ovary syndrome appear to be at increased risk of non-insulin dependent diabetes mellitus (NIDDM) in later life. Dunaif and colleagues (1987) reported that 20 per cent of obese young women with polycystic ovary syndrome had either impaired glucose tolerance (IGT) or frank diabetes. These figures are consistent with recent data from an important, follow-up study of a cohort of women who, 20–30 years earlier, had undergone ovarian wedge resection for symptoms of polycystic ovary syndrome. Dahlgren and co-workers (1992*a*) found that 13 per cent of the polycystic ovary group had previously diagnosed diabetes mellitus, compared with 2.3 per cent in a carefully matched, large reference population.

Abnormalities of lipid and lipoprotein metabolism have been reported in a number of studies of women with polycystic ovary syndrome (Mattsson *et al.* 1984; Wild and Bartholomew 1988; Conway *et al.* 1992; Robinson *et al.* 1996). Although not all such studies have been able to discern an adverse effect of polycystic ovary syndrome on lipid profiles which was independent of the effects of obesity (Graf *et al.* 1990), recent data suggest that the presence of polycystic ovaries, particularly if associated with insulin resistance, has a deleterious impact on lipid metabolism. Higher serum concentrations of triglycerides and lower levels of HDL-cholesterol (and the HDL2-C subfraction) have been noted in women with polycystic ovary syndrome compared with weight-matched controls (Wild and Bartholomew 1988; Conway *et al.* 1990).

Does this dyslipidaemia in young women with polycystic ovary syndrome imply an increased risk of cardiovascular disease in middle age? An early indication that women with polycystic ovary syndrome might be at risk of premature cardiovascular disease came from a retrospective analysis of patients undergoing cardiac catheterization (Wild *et al.* 1990). The prevalence of hirsutism was much higher in those with evidence of coronary artery disease than in those without. More recently, Dahlgren's long-term follow-up study of women with a proven diagnosis of polycystic ovary syndrome indicates that although few patients had reached the age at which overt cardiovascular disease is prevalent, the computed risk of coronary artery disease was seven times higher than that of the reference population (Dahlgren *et al.* 1992*b*). The implications of these findings are enormously important. If they can be supported by other prospective studies, they suggest that we may be able to identify, in young women presenting with hirsutism and menstrual disturbances, those who would be at long-term risk of coronary artery disease, and intervene accordingly.

The aetiology of polycystic ovaries and polycystic ovary syndrome

At first sight the heterogeneity of clinical presentation of women with polycystic ovaries would appear to support the notion that polycystic ovaries, as defined by sonography, can result from a variety of separate causes. However, if one excludes discrete disorders – Cushing's disease for example – which may masquerade as polycystic ovary syndrome ('polycystic ovary-like syndromes'), the common biochemical feature which links the spectrum of symptoms and signs is elevated serum concentrations of testosterone (Franks 1991).

Characterization of ovarian hyperandrogenism

The ovary, rather than the adrenal, appears to be the major source of excess androgen secretion (Couzinet *et al.* 1986; Steingold *et al.* 1987; Barnes *et al.* 1989). Rosenfield and colleagues have postulated that ovarian hyperandrogenism in polycystic ovary syndrome is caused by dysregulation of cytochrome P450$c_{17\alpha}$, which catalyses both 17α-hydroxylase and 17–20 lyase activities (Barnes *et al.* 1989; Rosenfield *et al.* 1990). This is based on their findings in women with polycystic ovary syndrome who, following suppression of adrenal steroidogenesis by dexamethasone, have received a single (and therefore stimulatory) dose of GnRHa. The serum concentrations of androstenedione and 17α-hydroxyprogesterone were higher than in control subjects both before and after GnRHa. These observations have been confirmed in subsequent studies from our own department in which we, in addition, found evidence of a similar pattern of ovarian hyperandrogenism in *ovulatory*, hyperandrogenic women with polycystic ovaries (White *et al.* 1995).

Data from *in vitro* studies comparing ovarian androgen production by theca cells from normal ovaries with polycystic ovaries provide supportive evidence that dysregulation of P450$c_{17\alpha}$ may be an important (but probably not the only) factor in the aetiology of abnormal androgen biosynthesis in polycystic ovary syndrome (Gilling-Smith *et al.* 1994). A striking feature of these results was that both basal and LH-stimulated androstenedione production, per theca cell, was some 20-fold higher in polycystic ovaries than normal ovaries, irrespective of whether the polycystic ovary theca was obtained from anovulatory or ovulatory hyperandrogenaemic women and regardless of the degree of elevation of serum LH.

An explanation of hypersecretion of LH in polycystic ovary syndrome

The interrelation of hyperandrogenism and excessive secretion of LH in all groups of women with polycystic ovaries is so intimate that it becomes almost impossible to determine cause and effect. It can be argued that analyses of data from both *in vivo* and *in vitro* studies favour the abnormality of androgen biosynthesis as the primary factor in this equation. In particular, some 20 per cent of women with all the other clinical and biochemical feaures of polycystic ovary syndrome have a normal LH secretory pattern (Yen 1980; Franks 1989). LH concentrations are much higher in anovulatory than ovulatory women with polycystic ovaries but are significantly reduced during spontaneous or induced ovulatory cycles (Franks 1989). The lack of cyclical progesterone secretion may therefore be an important factor in hypersecretion of LH but the moderate and more subtle elevation of LH in ovulatory women with polycystic ovaries remains unexplained (Franks 1989). A primary abnormality of the hypothalamic regulation of LH seems unlikely (Stanhope *et al.* 1987) and it has been suggested that the secretion of LH in women with polycystic ovaries may represent conditioning or 'masculinization' of the pituitary by exposure to excessive androgen levels during development (Rosenfield *et al.* 1990). The recent observation that patients with a history of neonatal exposure to hyperandrogenaemia due to classic 21-hydroxylase deficiency have a similarly enhanced LH response to GnRHa lends further weight to the hypothesis (Barnes *et al.* 1993).

The high prevalence of symptomatically affected siblings in the families of women with polycystic ovary syndrome (Hague *et al.* 1988) suggests a genetically determined disorder and although the mode of inheritance remains controversial (Simpson 1992), the results of recently published studies (Carey *et al.* 1993, 1994) suggest that at least one gene affecting androgen production is involved in the aetiology of the syndrome.

Management of polycystic ovary sydrome

In this section the focus will be on the management of women with polycystic ovary syndrome who present with oligomenorrhoea. As summarized in Table 19.3, treatment is essentially symptomatic and includes treatment of infertility, menstrual regulation in women not desiring pregnancy, and treatment of associated symptoms of hyperandrogenism. In addition, some thought should be given to the prevention of the possible long-term consequences of the metabolic disturbance characteristic of anovulatory women with polycystic ovary syndrome.

Induction of ovulation

The treatment of choice for induction of ovulation in polycystic ovary syndrome is anti-oestrogen therapy. Clomiphene citrate is the most commonly used anti-oestrogen, producing rates of ovulation of 75–80 per cent (Franks *et al.* 1985). The cumulative conception rate has been calculated to be around 75 per cent after 12 cycles of treatment (Hull 1992). There is, therefore, a significant minority of women with polycystic ovary syndrome who remain infertile after anti-oestrogen treatment and management of this group may be difficult (Franks 1992).

Ovulation can be induced by administration of gonadotrophins (usually urinary-derived preparations) but the particular hazard of such treatment is the development of multiple follicles and patients with polycystic ovary syndrome seem more likely to respond in this way to FSH than do patients with gonadotrophin deficiency. Consequently, the rates of multiple pregnancy (30 per cent) and hyperstimulation syndrome (2 per cent with severe symptoms) are worryingly high following conventional dosage regimens for gonadotrophins (Lunenfeld and Insler 1978; Wang and Gemzell 1980).

In the light of these observations, a number of centres have used regimens which involve giving lower than usual doses of gonadotrophins to clomiphene-resistant women with polycystic ovary syndrome (Kamrava *et al.* 1982; Polson *et al.* 1987; Hamilton-Fairley *et al.* 1991). At our centre, we start with a low dose (50–75 International Units (iv)/day) and make small incremental increases reaching towards a notional 'threshold' level of FSH (Brown 1978) which facilitates the maturation of a single pre-ovulatory follicle but above which multiple follicle development is more likely to occur. This treatment has proved successful in achieving pregnancy rates of around 45 per cent with a relatively low multiple pregnancy rate of 5 per cent (Hamilton-Fairley *et al.* 1991).

Unfortunately low-dose gonadotrophin treatment does not appear to affect the high prevalence (25–30 per cent) of miscarriage (usually early pregnancy loss) common to all forms of treatment of anovulatory women with polycystic ovary syndrome. The main factors which influence the rate of miscarriage are the age of the patient, persistent elevation of LH during ovulatory cycles, and obesity (Hamilton-Fairley *et al.* 1991, 1992). It has been suggested that concurrent administration of GnRH analogues, by suppressing endogenous LH levels, improves the chance of successful pregnancy following gonadotrophin treatment (whether given in low doses or conventional doses). However, there has been, as yet, no publication of the outcome of an appropriately designed, randomized, controlled study of sufficient power to demonstrate differences in miscarriage rates between treatment groups.

Strikingly, women with moderate obesity (BMI 25–28 kg/m^2) suffered twice the rate of pregnancy loss as lean women with polycystic ovary syndrome (Hamilton-Fairley *et al.* 1992). The mechanism of this effect is not yet clear and it remains to be determined whether weight reduction will improve outcome.

Surgical treatment of polycystic ovary syndrome can be considered either as an alternative to gonadotrophin therapy or as an additional option for treatment if gonadotrophins have not been effective. Although the traditional operation of ovarian wedge resection is now rarely performed, modern laparasopic techniques have been popular in recent years (Gjonnaess 1990; Armar *et al.* 1990; Abdel Gadir *et al.* 1990). The results of laparascopic diathermy or laser 'drilling' of the ovaries have been encouraging although only one controlled trial comparing surgical with gonadotrophin treatment has been published (Abdel Gadir *et al.* 1990). This showed no statistically significant difference in pregnancy and miscarriage rates between patients receiving surgery and those treated with conventional doses of gonadotrophins. Surgery has the advantage of a single treatment which may lead to a succession of ovulatory cycles but many patients appear to require adjuvant medical treatment for induction of ovulation and there is a significant risk of pelvic adhesions (Gurgan *et al.* 1991).

Menstrual regulation

Oligomenorrhoeic patients with polycystic ovary syndrome who do not wish to conceive may still require treatment (Franks *et al.* 1985; Franks 1995). Many patients have episodes of prolonged and/or heavy vaginal bleeding and although, by definition, these may occur infrequently, they are nevertheless distressing. Even in subjects without menstrual symptoms, treatment may be advisable because of the long term risks of unopposed oestrogen predisposing to endometrial hyperplasia and cancer. A low-dose (20–35 μg ethinyl oestradiol) combined oral contraceptive may be the most convenient form of treatment although the choice of a suitable progestogen has become a little more difficult, given the recent disquiet regarding the use of gestodene or desogestrel (which have proved particularly useful in the management of women with symptoms of hyperandrogenism). Our policy is to advise such patients about the increased (but still small) risk of thromboembolism which is associated with the use of these progestagens but to support their continued use if there are no other risk factors for thromboembolic disease. Oral contraceptives containing L-norgestrel or norethisterone can excacerbate hirsutism or acne but may be satisfactory in oligomenorrhoeic women without these symptoms.

Cyclical progestagens are a useful alternative to the combined oral contraceptive, particularly in women who do not need the 'pill' for contraceptive purposes (it must be emphasized that although oligomenorrhoeic women with polycystic ovaries obviously have reduced fertility, they may ovulate spontaneously and conceive). A suitable (non-androgenic) progestagen (e.g. medroxyprogesterone acetate) is given for 12 days per month.

In patients who are reluctant to have monthly cycles or do not want medical treatment, we advise that a pelvic ultrasound scan be performed at regular (perhaps three monthly) intervals to monitor endometrial thickness.

Hirsutism and acne

It is beyond the scope of this chapter to review, in detail, the management of symptoms of hyperandrogenism. Treatment of hirsutism usually involves a combination of cosmetic treatment to remove unwanted hair and, in more severe cases, anti-androgen therapy. In Europe, the most commonly used anti-androgen is cyproterone acetate. This also has progestagenic activity and can be combined with ethinyl oestradiol to provide cycle control as well as management of hyperandrogenic symptoms. This treatment is equally effective in treatment of acne but other options include antibiotics and retinoic acid derivatives.

Conclusion

In summary, polycystic ovary syndrome is the most common cause of oligomenorrhoea. The diagnosis is often obvious clinically because of associated symptoms of hyperandrogenism and can be confirmed by a small number of simple investigations, including a pelvic ultrasound scan. Management is essentially empirically based and may be directed towards induction of ovulation, regulation of menses, and control of associated symptoms such as hirsutism and acne. As far as the metabolic implications of polycystic ovary syndrome are concerned, there are, as yet, insufficient data to allow informed management but it would seem sensible to ensure that obese subjects with polycystic ovary syndrome are given suitable dietary advice.

References

Abdel Gadir, A., Mowafi, R.S., Alnaser, H.M., Alrashid, A.H., Alonezi, O.M., and Shaw, R.W. (1990). Ovarian electrocautery versus human menopausal gonadotrophins and pure follicle stimulating hormone therapy in the treatment of patients with polycystic ovarian disease. *Clinical Endocrinology*, **33**, 585–92.

Adams, J., Franks, S., Polson, D.W., Mason, H.D., Abdulwahid, N.A., Tucker, M., *et al.* (1985). Multifollicular ovaries: clinical and endocrine features and response to pulsatile gonadotropin releasing hormone. *Lancet*, **ii**, 1375–9.

Adams, J., Polson D.W., and Franks, S. (1986). Prevalence of polycystic ovaries in women with anovulation and idiopathic hirsutism. *British Medicine Journal*, **293**, 355–9.

Anderson, D.C. (1974). Sex hormone-binding globulin. *Clinical Endocrinology*, **3**, 69–96.

Armar, N.A., McGarrigle, H.H., Honour, J., Holownia, P., Jacobs, H.S., and Lachelin, G.C. (1990). Laparoscopic ovarian diathermy in the management of anovulatory infertility in women with polycystic ovaries: endocrine changes and clinical outcome. *Fertility and Sterility*, **53**, 45–9.

Barbieri, R.L., Makris, A., and Ryan, K.J. (1984). Insulin stimulates androgen accumulation in incubations of human ovarian stroma and theca. *Obstetrics and Gynecology*, **64**, 73S–80S.

Bardin, C.W. and Lipsett, M.B. (1967). Testosterone and androstenedione blood production rates in normal women and women with idiopathic hirsutism or polycystic ovaries. *Journal of Clinical Investigation*, **46**, 891–902.

Barnes, R.B., Rosenfield, R.L., Burstein, S., and Ehrmann, D.A. (1989). Pituitary–ovarian responses to nafarelin testing in the polycystic ovary syndrome. *New England Journal of Medicine*, **320**, 559–65.

Barnes, R.B., Ehrmann, D.A., and Rosenfield, R.L. (1993). Ovarian hyperandrogenism in 'late-onset' congenital adrenal hyperplasia. *Proceedings of the Endocrine Society 75th Annual Meeting 1993*, Abstract 128.

Bergh, C., Carlsson, B., Olsson, J.-H., Selleskog, U., and Hillensjo, T. (1993). Regulation of androgen production in cultured human theca cells by insulin-like growth factor-1 and insulin. *Fertility and Sterility*, **59**, 323–31.

Brown, J.B. (1978). Pituitary control of ovarian function – concepts derived from gonadotrophin therapy. *Australian and New Zealand Journal of Obstetrics and Gynaecology*, **18**: 47–54.

Bunker, C.B., Newton, J.A., Conway, G.S., Jacobs, H.S., Greaves M.W., and Dowd, P.M. (1991). The hormonal profile of women with acne and polycystic ovaries. *Clinical and Experimental Dermatology*, **16**, 420–3.

Burghen, G.A., Givens, J.R., and Kitabachi, A.E. (1980). Correlations of hyperandrogenism with insulin resistance in polycystic ovarian disease. *Journal of Clinical Endocrinology and Metabolism*, **50**, 113–16.

Carey, A.H., Chan, K.L., Short, F., White, D.M., Williamson, R., and Franks, S. (1993). Evidence for a single gene effect in polycystic ovaries and male pattern baldness. *Clinical Endocrinology*, **38**, 653–8.

Carey, A.C., Waterworth, D., Patel, K., White, D., Little, J., Novelli, P., *et al.* (1994). Polycystic ovaries and premature male pattern baldness are associated with one allele of the steroid metabolism gene CYP17. *Human Molecular Genetics*, **10**, 1873–6.

Chang, R.J., Nakamura, R.M., Judd, H.L., and Kaplan, S.A. (1983). Insulin resistance in non-obese patients with polycystic ovarian disease. *Journal of Clinical Endocrinology and Metabolism*, **57**, 356–9.

Conway, G.S., Honour, J.W., and Jacobs, H.S. (1989). Heterogeneity of the polycystic ovary syndrome: clinical, endocrine and ultrasound features in 556 patients. *Clinical Endocrinology*, **30**, 459–70.

Conway, G.S., Jacobs, H.S., Holly, J.M.P., and Wass, J.A.H. (1990). Effects of luteinizing hormone, insulin-like growth factor-1 and insulin-like growth factor binding protein 1 in the polycystic ovary syndrome. *Clinical Endocrinology*, **33**, 593–603.

Conway, G.S., Agrawal, R., Betteridge, D.J., and Jacobs, H.S. (1992). Risk factors for coronary artery disease in lean and obese women with the polycystic ovary syndrome. *Clinical Endocrinology*, **37**, 119–25.

Couzinet, B., Le Strat, N., Brailly, S., and Schaison, G. (1986). Comparative effects of cyproterone acetate or a long-acting gonadotropin-releasing hormone agonist in polycystic ovarian disease. *Journal of Clinical Endocrinology and Metabolism*, **63**, 1031–5.

Dahlgren, E., Johansson S., Lindstedt G., Knotsson, F., Oden, A., Janson, P.O., *et al.* (1992*a*). Women with polycystic ovary syndrome wedge resected in 1956 to 1965: a long-term follow-up focusing on natural history and circulating hormones. *Fertility and Sterility*, **57**, 505–13.

Dahlgren, E., Janson P.O., Johansson, S., Lapidus, L., Oden, A., Janson P.O., *et al.* (1992*b*). Polycystic ovary syndrome and risk for myocardial infarction – evaluated from a risk factor model based on a prospective study of women. *Acta Obstetrica et Gynecologica Scandinavica*, **71**, 599–604.

Dale, P.O., Tanbo, T., Djoseland, O., Jervell, J., and Abyholm, T. (1992). Persistence of hyperinsulinemia in polycystic ovary syndrome after ovarian suppression by gonadotropin-releasing hormone agonist. *Acta Endocrinologica, Copenhagen*, **126**, 132–6.

Dunaif, A. (1993). Insulin resistance and ovarian dysfunction. In *Insulin resistance*, (ed. D. Moller pp. 301–25. John Wiley, New York.

Dunaif, A., Graf, M., Mandeli, J., Laumas, V., and Dobrjansky, A. (1987). Characterization of groups of hyperandrogenic women with acanthosis nigricans, impaired glucose tolerance, and/or hyperinsulinemia. *Journal of Clinical Endocrinology and Metabolism*, **65**, 499–507.

Dunaif, A., Segal, K.R., Futterweit, W., and Dobrjansky, A. (1989). Profound peripheral insulin resistance, independent of obesity, in polycystic ovary syndrome. *Diabetes*, **38**, 1165–74.

Dunaif, A., Green, G., Futterweit, W., and Dobrjansky, A. (1990). Suppression of hyperandrogenism does not improve peripheral or hepatic insulin resistance in the polycystic ovary syndrome. *Journal of Clinical Endocrinology and Metabolism*, **70**, 699–704.

Ehrmann, D.A., Rosenfield, R.L., Barnes, R.B., Brigell, D.F., and Sheikh, Z. (1992). Detection of functional ovarian hyperandrogenism in women with androgen excess. *New England Journal of Medicine*, **327**, 157–62.

Fox, R., Corrigan, E., Thomas, P.A., and Hull, M.G. (1991). The diagnosis of polycystic ovaries in women with oligo-amenorrhoea: predictive power of endocrine tests. *Clinical Endocrinology (Oxford)*, **34**, 127–31.

Franks, S. (1989). Polycystic ovary syndrome: a changing perspective. *Clinical Endocrinology Oxford*, **31**, 87–120.

Franks, S. (1991). The ubiquitous polycystic ovary. *Journal of Endocrinology*, **129**, 317–19.

Franks, S. (1992). Induction of ovulation. In: Templeton A.A., Drife, J.O., eds. *Infertility*, (ed. A.A. Templeton and J.O. Drife), pp. 237–50. Springer, London.

Franks, S. (1995). Medical progress article: polycystic ovary syndrome. *New England Journal of Medicine*, **333**, 853–61.

Franks, S., Adams, J., Mason, H., and Polson, D. (1985). Ovulatory disorders in women with polycystic ovary syndorme. *Clinical Obstetrics and Gynaecology*, **12**, 605–32.

Gambrell, R.D., Jr, Greenblatt, R.B., and Mahesh, V.B. (1973). Inappropriate secretion of luteinizing hormone in the Stein Leventhal syndrome. *Obstetrics and Gynecology*, **42**, 429–40.

Gilling-Smith, C., Willis, D.S., Beard, R.W., and Franks, S. (1994). Hypersecretion of androstenedione by isolated theca cells from polycystic ovaries. *Journal of Clinical Endocrinology and Metabolism*, **79**, 1158–65.

Givens, J.R. (1976). Hirsutism and hyperandrogenism. *Advances in Internal Medicine*, **21**, 221–47.

Gjonnaess, H. (1990). A simple treatment for polycystic ovarian syndrome. *World Health Forum*, **11**, 214–17.

Goldzieher, J.W. and Green, J.A. (1962). The polycystic ovary. 1 clinical and histological features. *Journal of Clinical Endocrinology and Metabolism*, **22**, 325–38.

Graf, M.J., Richards, C.J., Brown, V., Meissner, L., and Dunaif, A. (1990). The independent effects of hyperandrogenaemia, hyperinsulinaemia and obesity in lipid and lipoprotein profiles in women. *Clinical Endocrinology*, **33**, 119–31.

Gurgan, T., Kisnisci, H., Yarali, H., Develioglu, O., Zeyneloglu H., and Aksu, T (1991). Evaluation of adhesion formation after laparoscopic treatment of polycystic ovarian disease. *Fertility and Sterility*, **56**, 1176–8.

Hague, W.M., Adams, J., Reeders, S.T., Peto T.E., and Jacobs, H.S. (1988). Familial polycystic ovaries: a genetic disease? *Clinical Endocrinology Oxford*, **29**, 593–605.

Hamilton-Fairley, D., Kiddy, D., Watson, H., Sagle, M., and Franks, S. (1991). Low-dose gonadotrophin therapy for induction of ovulation in 100 women with polycystic ovary syndrome. *Human Reproduction*, **6**, 1095–9.

Hamilton-Fairley, D., Kiddy, D., Watson, H., Paterson, C., and Franks, S. (1992). Association of moderate obesity with a poor pregnancy outcome in women with polycystic ovary syndrome treated with low dose gonadotrophin. *British Journal of Obstetrics and Gynaecology*, **99**, 128–31.

Holte, J., Bergh, T., Gennarelli, G., and Wide, L. (1994*a*). The independent effects of polycystic ovary syndrome and obesity on serum concentrations of gonadotrophins and sex steroids in premenopausal women. *Clinical Endocrinology*, **41**, 473–82.

Holte, J., Bergh, T., Berne, C., Berglund, L., and Lithell, H. (1994*b*). Enhanced early insulin response to glucose in relation to insulin resistance in women with polycystic ovary syndrome and normal glucose tolerance. *Journal of Clinical Endocrinology and Metabolism*, **78**, 1052–8.

Hull, M.G. (1987). Epidemiology of infertility and polycystic ovarian disease: endocrinological and demographic studies. *Gynecological Endocrinology*, **1**, 235–45.

Hull, M.G.R. (1992). The causes of infertility and relative effectiveness of treatment. In *Infertility* (ed. A.A. Templeton and J.O. Drife, pp. 33–62. Springer, London.

Kamrava, M.M., Seibel, M.M., Berger, M.J., Thompson, I., and Taymor, M.L. (1982). Reversal of persistent anovulation in polycystic ovarian disease by administration of chronic low-dose follicle-stimulating hormone. *Fertility and Sterility*, **37**, 520–3.

Kiddy, D.S., Hamilton-Fairley, D., Seppala, M., Koistinen, R., James V.H.T., Reed, M.J., and Franks, S. (1989). Diet-induced changes in in sex hormone-binding globulin and free testosterone in women with normal and polycystic ovaries: correlation with serum insulin and insulin-like growth factor I. *Clinical Endocrinology*, **31**, 757–63.

Kiddy, D.S., Sharp, P.S., White, D.M., Scanlon, M.F., Mason, H.D., Bray, C.S., *et al.* (1990). Differences in clinical and endocrine features between obese and non-obese subjects with polycystic ovary syndrome: an analysis of 263 consecutive cases. *Clinical Endocrinology*, **32**, 213–20.

Kiddy, D.S., Hamilton-Fairley, D., Bush, A., Short, F., Anyaoku, Reed, M.J., and Franks, S. (1992). Improvement in endocrine and ovarian function during dietary treatment of obese women with polycystic ovary syndrome. *Clinical Endocrinology*, **36**, 105–11.

Kirschner, M.A., Samojlik, E., and Silber, D. (1983). A comparison of androgen production and clearance in obese and hirsute women. *Journal of Steroid Biochemistry*, **19**, 607–14.

Lobo, R.A. (1991). Hirsutism in polycystic ovary syndrome: current concepts. *Clinical Obstetrics and Gynecology*, **34**, 817–26.

Lunenfeld, B. and Insler, V. (1978). *Diagnosis and trèatment of functional infertility*. Gross, Berlin.

Mattsson, L.A., Cullberg, G., Hamberger, L., Samsioe, G., and Silfverstople, G. (1984). Lipid metabolism in women with polycystic ovary syndrome: possible implications for increased risk of coronary heart disease. *Fertility and Sterility*, **42**, 579–84.

Nestler, J.E. and Strauss, J. (1991). Insulin as an effector of human ovarian and adrenal steroid metabolism. *Endocrinology and Metabolism Clinics of North America*, **20**, 807–23.

Parisi, L., Tramonti, M., Derchi, L.E., Casciano, S., Zurli, A., and Rocchi, P. (1984). Polycystic ovarian disease: ultrasonic evaluation and correlations with clinical and hormonal data. *Journal of Clinical Ultrasound*, **12**, 21–6.

Plymate, S.R., Matej, L.A., Jones, R.E., and Friedl, K.E. (1988). Inhibition of sex hormone-binding globulin production in human hepatoma (Hep G2) cell line by insulin and prolactin. *Journal of Clinical Endocrinology and Metabolism*, **67**, 460–4.

Polson, D.W., Mason, H.D., Saldahna, M.B., and Franks, S. (1987). Ovulation of a single dominant follicle during treatment with low-dose pulsatile follicle stimulating hormone in women with polycystic ovary syndrome. *Clinical Endocrinology*, **26**, 205–12.

Pugeat, M., Crave, J.C., Elmidani, M., Crave, J.C., Elmidami, M., Nicolas, M.H., *et al.* (1991). Pathophysiology of sex hormone binding globulin (SHBG): relation to insulin. *Journal of Steroid Biochemistry and Molecular Biology*, **40**, 841–9.

Rebar, R., Judd, H.L., Yen, S.S.C., Rakoff, J., Vandenberg, G., and Naftolin, F. (1976). Characterization of inappropriate gonadotropin secretion in polycystic ovary syndrome. *Journal of Clinical Investigation*, **57**, 1320–9.

Robinson, S., Chan, S.-P., Spacey, S., Anyaoku, V., Johnson, D.G., and Franks, S. (1992). Post prandial thermogenesis is reduced in polycystic ovary syndrome and is associated with increased insulin resistance. *Clinical Endocrinology*, **36**, 537–43.

Robinson, S., Kiddy, D., Gelding, S.V., Willis, D., Niththyananathan, R., Bush, A., Johnston, D.G., and Franks, S. (1993). The relationship of insulin sensitivity to menstrual pattern in women with hyperandrogenism and polycystic ovaries. *Clinical Endocrinology*, **39**, 351–5.

Robinson, S., Henderson, A.D., Gelding, S.V., Kiddy, D.S., Niththyananathan, R., Bush, A., *et al.* (1996). Dyslipidaemia is associated with insulin resistance in women with polycystic ovary syndrome. *Clinical Endocrinology*, **44**, 259–68.

Rosenfield, R.L., Barnes, R.B., Cara, J.F., and Lucky, A.W. (1990). Dysregulation of cytochrome P450c 17 alpha as the cause of polycystic ovarian syndrome. *Fertility and Sterility*, **53**, 785–91.

Sharp, P.S., Kiddy, D.S., Reed, M.J., Anyaoku, V., Johnston, D.G., and Franks, S. (1991). Correlation of plasma insulin and insulin-like growth factor-I with indices of androgen transport and metabolism in women with polycystic ovary syndrome. *Clinical Endocrinology Oxford*, **35**, 253–7.

Simpson, J.L. (1992). Elucidating the genetics of polycystic ovary syndrome. In *Polycystic ovary syndrome* (ed. A. Dunaif, J.R. Givens, F.P. Haseltine, and G.R. Merriam, pp. 59–77. Blackwell Scientific, Oxford.

Slowinska-Srzednicka, J., Zgliczynski, W., Makowska, A., Jeske, W., Brzezinska, A., Soszynski, P., and Zgliczynski, S. (1992). An abnormality of the growth hormone/insulin-like growth factor-I axis in women with polycystic ovary syndrome due to coexistent obesity. *Journal of Clinical Endocrinology and Metabolism*, **74**, 1432–5.

Stanhope, R., Adams, J., Pringle, J.P., Jacobs, H.S., and Brook, C.G. (1987). The evolution of polycystic ovaries in a girl with hypogonadotropic hypogonadism before puberty and during puberty induced with pulsatile gonadotropin-releasing hormone. *Fertility and Sterility*, **47**, 872–5.

Steingold, K., De Ziegler, D., Cedars, M., Meldrum, D.R., Lu, J.K.H., Vale, W., *et al.* (1987). Clinical and hormonal effects of chronic gonadotropin-releasing hormone agonist treatment in polycystic ovarian disease. *Journal of Clinical Endocrinology and Metabolism*, **65**, 773–8.

Swanson, M., Sauerbrei, E.E., and Cooperberg, P.L. (1981). Medical implications of ultrasonically detected polycystic ovaries. *Journal of Clinical Ultrasound*, **9**, 219–22.

Takahashi, K., Yoshino, K., Nishigaki, A., Eda, Y., and Kitao, M. (1992). On the relationship between endocrine and ovulatory abnormalities, and polycystic ovaries as diagnosed by ultrasonography. *International Journal of Fertility*, **37**, 222–6.

Toscano, V., Bianchi, P., Balducci, R., Guglielmi, R., Mangiantini, A., Lubrano, C., and Sciarra, F. (1992). Lack of linear relationship between hyperinsulinaemia and hyperandrogenism. *Clinical Endocrinology (Oxford)*, **36**, 197–202.

Wang, C.F. and Gemzell, C. (1980). The use of human gonadotropins for induction of ovulation in women with polycystic ovarian disease. *Fertility and Sterility*, **33**, 479–86.

White, D.W., Leigh, A., Wilson, C., Donaldson, A., and Franks, S. (1995). Gonadotrophin and gonadal steroid response to a single dose of a long-acting agonist of gonadotrophin-releasing hormone in ovulatory and anovulatory women with polycystic ovary syndrome. *Clinical Endocrinology*, **42**, 475–81.

Wild, R.A. and Bartholomew, M.J. (1988). The influence of body weight on lipoprotein lipids in patients with polycystic ovary syndrome. *American Journal of Obstetrics and Gynecology*, **159**, 423–7.

Wild, R.A., Van Nort, J.J., Grubb, B., Bachman, W., Hartz, A., and Bartholomew, M. (1990). Clinical signs of androgen excess as risk factors for coronary artery disease. *Fertility and Sterility*, **54**, 255–9.

Yen, S.S.C. (1980) The polycystic ovary syndrome. *Clinical Endocrinology*, **12**, 177–207.

Zawadzki, J.K. and Dunaif, A. (1992). Diagnostic criteria for polycystic ovary syndrome: towards a rational approach. In *Polycystic ovary syndrome* (ed.) A. Dunaif, J.R. Givens, F.P. Haseltine and G.R. Merriam pp. 337–840. Blackwell Scientific, Oxford.

20 Intermenstrual and post-coital bleeding

Britt-Marie Landgren and Bo von Schoultz

Disruption of the cyclical pattern of menstrual bleeding may occur at any age and for a variety of reasons. An understanding of the physiological life cycle variations is essential to determine whether a pattern of bleeding episodes should be regarded as normal or abnormal. Normal menstruation occurs in response to the decline in progesterone following the regression of the corpus luteum. Any alteration in the cyclical exposure of the endometrium first, to unopposed oestrogen during the follicular phase and, after ovulation, to oestrogen and progesterone, is likely to result in disturbances in the menstrual pattern. Intermenstrual bleeding may last only a few hours or persist for several days. Bleeding perceived as abnormal or unusual evokes fear and anxiety and is a common reason for gynaecological consultation.

Inter-menstrual bleeding, defined as bleeding episodes occurring between otherwise normal regular bleeding periods, can occur alone or overlap with pre- and post-menstrual spotting. Post-coital bleeding occurs only after coitus, but may accompany intermenstrual bleeding. Post-coital bleeding begins at the time of coitus, and the woman is usually aware of it immediately or as soon as she gets up from bed.

Causes of intermenstrual and post-coital bleeding

Abnormal bleeding of these types can be caused by completely benign or by serious malignant conditions (Table 20.1). Bleeding mimicking intermenstrual bleeding can occur during early pregnancy and can be caused by spontaneous abortion or ectopic pregnancy. Other aetiologies include uterine and cervical polyps, anovulatory conditions such as functional ovarian cysts or polycystic ovarian disease, and corpus luteum insufficiency. Genital infections, especially cervicitis, can induce intermenstrual bleeding and spotting. Breakthrough bleeding can occur in women using exogenous hormonal preparations for contraception. Intermenstrual bleeding and spotting are important early symptoms of gynaecological malignancies such as endometrial and cervical cancer (Fraser and Petrucco 1996). Pre-menstrual spotting can be caused by endometriosis or use of an intrauterine device.

Endometrial response in the normal menstrual cycle

In order to understand the mechanism of bleeding irregularities associated with hormonal abnormalities, one has to consider the endometrial response to hormonal stimulation during the normal cycle (Fig. 20.1). The morphological criteria of a normal menstrual cycle are still based on the idealized

Table 20.1 Causes of inter-menstrual and post-coital bleeding

Complications of pregnancy	Ectopic pregnancy Abortion: threatened, inevitable, complete, incomplete
Coagulopathies	
Ovarian dysfunction	Anovulation Luteal phase deficiency
Breakthrough bleeding during use of hormonal contraceptives	Combined oestrogen-progestogen pill Progestogen-only methods
Breakthrough bleeding with intrauterine contraceptive devices	
Benign surface abnormalities of the genital tract	Cervical ectropion Cervical polyp Endometrial polyp
Inflammatory conditions	Cervicitis Endometritis Atrophic vaginitis and cervicitis Endometriosis
Malignant neoplasm	Vulvar and vaginal Cervical Endometrial

cycle of 28 days as introduced by Noyes *et al.* in 1950 in which ovulation occurs on day 14 and divides the cycle into proliferative and secretory phases of equal length. Specific day to day changes could allow dating of the endometrium in relation to the cycle days selected for biopsy. During the follicular phase of the cycle oestrogen increases the thickness of the endometrial tissue. After ovulation, progesterone stimulates secretory activity of the endometrium. At menstruation, sloughing of the functional layer of the endometrium occurs (Ferenczy *et al.* 1979; Genz *et al.* 1980; Daly *et al.* 1982; Flowers and Wilborn 1982).

Menstrual cycle length

Menstrual cycle length is determined by the rate and quality of follicle growth and development, and it is normal for the cycle to vary in individual women. Our best information on cycle length comes from two longitudinal studies. Vollman (1977) reported on mid-cycle bleeding in confirmed normal cycles in only 35 women, making a total of about 100 out of 30 000 cycles (a frequency of approximately 0.3 per cent). The study by Treloar *et al.* (1967) covered more than 25 000 woman-years of menstrual experience in over 2700 women. These studies clearly established that there are systematic age-related changes in menstrual cycle length. About 20 per cent of patients presenting with dysfunctional irregular bleeding are adolescent and about half are over the age of 40 (Zimmermann 1988). The years immediately after menarche are characterized by a high incidence of irregular cycles which is followed by a pattern of much more regular cycles during the age interval of 20–40 years. The number of irregular cycles again increases

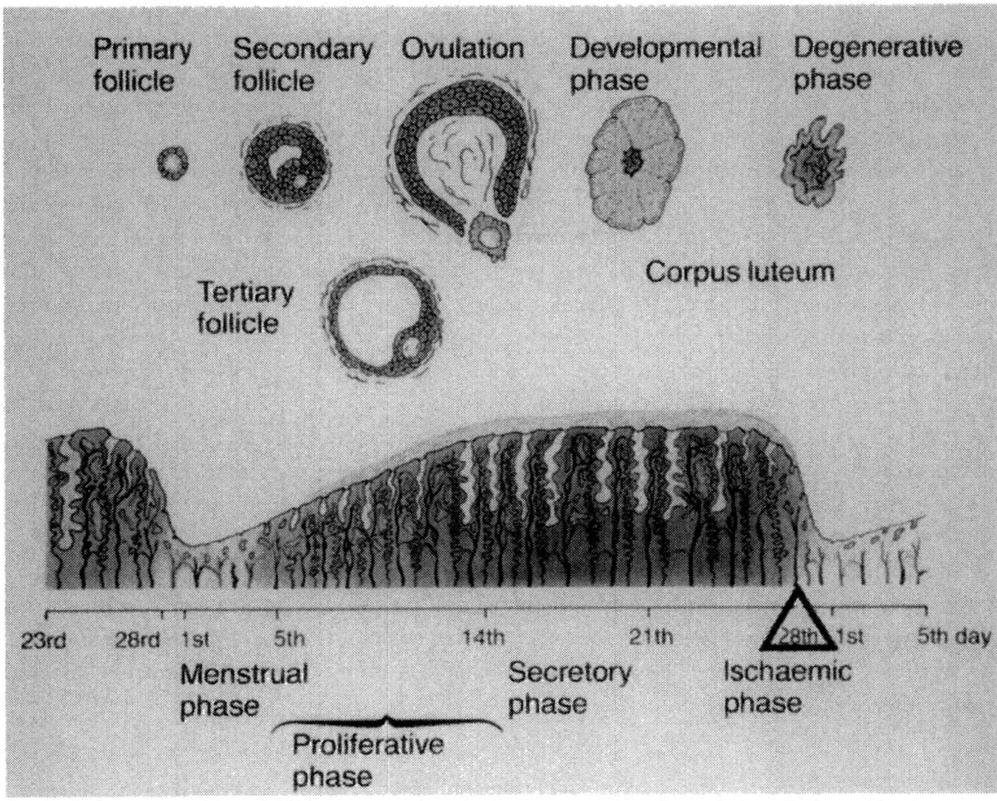

Fig. 20.1 Ovarian and endometrial changes during the menstrual cycle.

after the age of 40. These irregularities in cycle patterns are concomitant with hormonal changes, and they are considered to be characteristic of adolescence and the menopausal transition. We have studied the effect of chronological age on the length of the follicular and luteal phases in 325 Swedish and British women (Lenton *et al.* 1984*a*, *b*). The follicular phase was longest in the youngest women (18–24 years), and there was a small and steady decline in follicular phase length throughout reproductive life (45–50 years). A higher incidence of short luteal phases was found in the youngest (18–24 years) and oldest (45–50 years) women when compared to those aged 25–40 years. These changes in bleeding pattern throughout reproductive life are normal but could be a reason for fear and anxiety about possible underlying pathology.

Cycle abnormalities, including intermenstrual bleeding

It is important to put this problem in perspective, and to distinguish irregular cycles from intermenstrual bleeding. Different patterns of abnormal bleeding may often overlap, and this may provide clues to the underlying cause.

The menstrual cycles during the first 1–2 years following menarche are usually anovulatory and the regulation of the cycle shows a wide range. In a study by Apter and Vihko (1985) the pattern of ovulation in early cycles was studied using progesterone levels as an indicator of ovulation. More than 75 per cent of abnormal uterine bleeding in adolescent patients is due to immaturity of the hypothalamic–pituitary axis (Apter and Vihko 1985). The positive feedback mechanism that triggers the luteinizing hormone (LH) surge may not be established for up to five years after the onset of menarche (Hertweck 1992). Until this mechanism is in place there is continuous oestrogen stimulation of the endometrium without development of the progesterone-dominated secretory phase. As a result, the endometrial lining becomes quite thick and vascular. Oestrogen levels eventually fall spontaneously, resulting in heavy and prolonged bleeding. In some patients the endometrium will break down intermittently causing irregular spotting. Most adolescents who experience dysfunctional bleeding eventually begin ovulating regularly. Some adolescents with dysfunctional uterine bleeding may have persistent irregular bleeding and also decreased fertility as adult women (Southam and Richart 1966). In girls with persistent anovulation (5 per cent) there is a risk of endometrial hyperplasia and endometrial carcinoma later in life (Altchek 1977; Kurman *et al.* 1985). In a study by Claesson and Cowell (1981) the underlying diagnosis in 83 young girls admitted to a children's hospital for acute menorrhagia was dysfunctional uterine bleeding in 59 (74 per cent) and a coagulation disorder in 11 (19 per cent). These findings were well in agreement with those of Fraser and Baird (1972).

Anovulatory cycles with complete lack of luteinization, characterized by follicular activity only, also occur in women with the polycystic ovarian syndrome (Gusberg 1967; Ferenczy *et al.* 1982). Amenorrhoea or oligomenorrhoea are common symptoms in these patients but some may have dysfunctional uterine bleeding with episodes mimicking intermenstrual bleeding (Goldzieher and Green 1962).

Luteal insufficiency

Luteal insufficiency has been reported to be the cause of bleeding irregularities, and in particular short cycles due to early sloughing of the endometrium (Cook *et al.* 1983; Laatikainen *et al.* 1983). Menstrual disturbances after tubal sterilization (22–27 per cent) could also be due to luteal insufficiency (De Stefano *et al.* 1985). In a study by Radwanska *et al.* (1982) the oestrogen and progesterone levels were significantly lower in sterilized women with menstrual disturbances, when compared to a non-sterilized group and a group of sterilized women with normal menstrual bleeding patterns. These findings are in agreement with those of Hargrove and Abraham (1981 and Wilcox *et al.* (1992)). Thus in some cases bleeding irregularities could be caused by corpus luteum insufficiency. The treatment of choice would then be to replace or supplement progesterone exposure with combined oral contraceptives, continuous low-dose progestogen, or cyclic progestogen treatment on cycle days 16–26 to induce progestogen-withdrawal bleeding. Treatment with prostaglandin inhibitors has also been suggested for these women (Anderson *et al.* 1976).

Dysfunctional uterine bleeding in the perimenopausal period

After the age of 40 the functional capacity of the ovary begins to diminish (Sherman and Korenman 1975; Metcalf 1988). As the ovary ages, it becomes less sensitive and produces less oestrogen and progesterone despite elevated levels of gonadotrophins. With increasing age the number of short cycles due to reduced length of the follicular phase increases. As time passes the cycles become increasingly irregular and the production of progesterone disappears entirely, while oestrogen production still persists without the controlling influence of progesterone (Seltzer *et al.* 1990). Endometrial proliferation might then develop into different stages of hyperplasia. The result will be a structural instability and increased fragility that may lead to abnormal bleeding such as oligomenorrhoea, polymenorrhoea, intermittent short episodes, or prolonged anovulatory bleeding (Jutras and Cowan 1990). Increased production of prostaglandins in the endometrium (Smith *et al.* 1982) has been suggested to cause heavy bleeding in women with anovulatory cycles.

Intermenstrual bleeding in women using hormonal contraceptives

This problem is often called 'breakthrough bleeding'. The bleeding pattern in users of hormonal contraceptives is due to the effects of both exogenous and endogenous hormones on the endometrium, and particularly the effect of prolonged endometrial exposure to the progestogen component.

Combined oral contraceptive pills

Combined oral contraceptive pills inhibit ovulation. The bleeding occurring during the pill-free interval of seven days is a result of the withdrawal of exogenous oestrogen and progestogen. Erratic bleeding commonly occurs when pills are forgotten. Sometimes breakthrough bleeding and spotting occur even during regular pill intake. Gray (1980) reported that breakthrough bleeding occurred more often in pill users of low dose (2–20 per cent) ethinylestradiol than in those women using higher doses. Women using triphasic pills did experience fewer episodes of breakthrough bleeding when compared to monophasic pill users. Bleeding disturbances do not usually cause discontinuation of use in pill users (Belsey *et al.* 1988).

Progestogen-only oral contraceptives

There is a wide range of individual ovarian reactions in progestogen-only pill users. In a study by Landgren and Diczfalusy (1981), 40 per cent of women using a 0.3 mg norethisterone minipill seemed to ovulate while 20 per cent presented with a complete suppression of ovarian function. Another 20 per cent reacted to minipill use by follicular activity only while 20 per cent presented with follicular activity followed by luteal insufficiency. The frequency of irregular bleeding in women using minipills has been reported to vary between 50 per cent and 70 per cent (Belsey *et al.* 1988).

Long-acting progestogen-only contraceptive methods

In women using 150 mg depot medroxyprogesterone acetate every 90 days, bleeding abnormalities occur in approximately 90 per cent (Bassol *et al.* 1984). The most common disturbance is amenorrhoea but breakthrough bleeding sometimes occurs. In users of Norplant® with a daily release of between 0.05 and 0.08 mg levonorgestrel per day, inter-menstrual breakthrough bleeding is most frequent during the first year of use (Robertson *et al.* 1983). This is probably explained by the fact that ovulation is suppressed in a majority of women. During years 2–5 half to two thirds of Norplant® users seemed to ovulate (Brache *et al.* 1990). Due to this, the bleeding patterns improve with increased duration of use.

Other possible causes of intermenstrual bleeding

These include cervical and endometrial malignancies, and occur because of spontaneous bleeding from large, thin-walled and fragile vessels on the surface of the tumours.

Post-coital bleeding

Post-coital or contact bleeding is an important symptom which should never be ignored. It can be caused by a variety of conditions of which the most serious is cervical cancer. All women presenting with irregular or intermenstrual bleeding disturbances should also be asked specifically about the presence of post-coital bleeding. The mechanism is either by direct contact with minor trauma or indirect as in 'effort bleeding' where the uterus is forced downwards and a vulnerable external cervic covered with fragile columnar epithelium (e.g. ectropion) is rubbed towards the posterial vaginal wall during heavy lifting, bicycling, defecation, etc. Coitus is the most common cause of contact bleeding but this may also occur with the use of tampons, vaginal pessaries, or at application of vaginal medication. While cervical cancer is a cause of concern and should always be excluded, other reasons for the easily bleeding cervix are more common.

Causes of post-coital bleeding (Table 20.1)

Cervical ectopy

This term is used to describe the situation where the fragile but normal columnar cervical epithelium has advanced on to the surface of the ectocervix with a bright red velvety appearance. Ectopic columnar epithelium is a normal finding especially in parous women, and in some women using combined oral contraceptives a considerable endocervical eversion is induced. At menopause the exposed area of the transformation zone shrinks and may disappear completely into the endocervix. Cervical ectopy is asymptomatic in most cases but it may sometimes cause leukorrhoea or post-coital bleeding. Contact bleeding may occur spontaneously or with mild infectious cervical conditions (low grade chronic cervicitis). Infections with chlamydia appear to be more likely to occur in the presence of a large ectropion.

Cervical polyps

At inspection of the cervix a polyp is identified as a bright red vascular growth. It is pedunculated, originating from the endocervix, covered with endocervical epithelium and with a central fibrous tissue core. As a rule, cervical polyps are completely benign, but they are vascular and may sometimes cause post-coital or inter-menstrual bleeding. A polyp is easily removed by avulsion, or by ligation of the pedicle and excision.

Atrophic vaginitis

In elderly women, vaginal atrophy with low grade epithelial infection may be an alternative mechanism for contact bleeding. However, the most common cause is an inflammatory reaction of the cervix (atrophic cervicitis). This mechanism may also occur in pre-menopausal women who are hypo-oestrogenic for other reasons.

Genital infections

Inflammatory reactions in the vagina and cervix cause neovascularization, vascular dilatation, vascular fragility, and fluid exudation. Vaginal mucosal infections like *Candida* and *Trichomonas vaginalis* may cause minor bleeding from the vaginal walls and a bloody or red/brownish discharge. Human papilloma virus infection may be the cause of post-coital bleeding especially when exophytic polypoid condylomata are located around the vaginal introitus. Ulcerative lesions such as the manifestation of active vulval herpes virus infection are another cause. Chronic cervicitis is the most frequent cause of post-coital bleeding and chlamydial infection is the most common pathology. Non-specific and polymicrobial infection as well as *Neisseria gonorrhoea* can also cause contact cervicitis and post-coital bleeding.

Cancer of the cervix

Cervical cancer is a disease of the sexually active woman and most cases occur within the age span of 35–55 years with a peak incidence around 45 years. Rarely it can occur in very young women under 20 years. Intermenstrual bleeding, spotting, and often post-coital bleeding are cardinal symptoms during the early stages of this often curable cancer. The bleeding is caused by a vascular ulcer or polypoidal breakthrough of the epithelium in the cervical canal or at the os. As the tumour grows, 'effort' bleeding or spontaneous intermittent bleeding caused by tumour erosion of blood vessels may occur. Other forms of bleeding abnormality may occur such as metrorrhagia or menorrhagia.

Practical guidelines/management

Inter-menstrual and post-coital bleeding are common. As discussed above, the causes vary considerably and range from social stress to malignant disease. It is important, therefore, that the principles for management of these patients are known not only to gynaecologists but also to the general practitioner (Table 20.2). Investigation should be considered after one bleeding episode, depending on the circumstances. In many cases, investigation may be deferred unless episodes are repeated, prolonged, heavy, or accompanied by other symptoms or signs (Fraser and Petrucco 1996).

History

The age and bleeding pattern of the patient are key factors for the further investigation. In young women it is essential to exclude pregnancy and in older women a possible malignancy should

Table 20.2 Investigation of inter-menstrual bleeding and post-coital bleeding

All women	History Gynaecological examination Inspection (Pap smear test plus endocervical culture) Bimanual palpation Vaginal ultrasound including uterine size, endometrial thickness, and visualization of the ovaries; consider fluid distension sonography Consider colposcopy with cervical biopsy (and possible cervical curettage) Consider hysteroscopy and endometrial sampling Bleeding diary card
Fertile women < 45 years of age	Pregnancy test
Women > 45 years of age and post-menopausal women	Hysteroscopy with endometrial sampling

always be considered. Simple diary notations are valuable aids in order to get a structured picture of the bleeding pattern. Pregnancy and especially ectopic pregnancy should be ruled out in fertile women and pregnancy testing is recommended. The woman's life style is important, sexual history and recent changes in weight, exercise, concomitant medication, and current contraceptive use should be recorded. Available information from previous gynaecological examinations and surgical procedures should be obtained.

Gynaecological examination and investigations

All women with bleeding disturbances should be subject to vaginal examination including vaginal and cervical inspection and bimanual pelvic examination. All women with contact bleeding should undergo a full gynaecological examination and appropriate follow-up. A Pap smear test is indicated in all cases.

Even if the Pap smear test is normal, repeated contact bleeding is a strong indication for colposcopy and biopsies of the cervix. It should be recalled that the Pap smear test is a good method of screening for cervical atypia, dysplasia, and cervical intraepithelial neoplasia, i.e. the asymptomatic precursor stages generally not connected with bleeding disturbances. However, the Pap smear test is not a reliable method for the diagnosis of invasive cancer because necrotic surface cells may not show up as abnormal in the stained smear, or inflammatory cells may obscure the picture. The sensitivity is too low and some 10 per cent false-negative smears have been reported (Kolstad 1986).

Vaginal ultrasound offers a valuable complement to pelvic examination to diagnose changes in uterine size, myomata, polyps, and endometrial thickness, and to exclude pathological adnexal masses. After these initial measures further handling of the problem is dependent on the woman's age and the clinical history.

Since genital infections are common causes of irregular bleeding they should always be considered and excluded in sexually active women of fertile age. Swabs or scraping should be taken from the cervix and from the urethra for the laboratory diagnosis of *Chlamydia trachomatis* using the most appropriate local technology. Since the chlamydia organism is located within epithelial cells, the collection of a satisfactory amount of cellular material is essential. Cultures for *Neisseria gonorrhoeae* are often indicated. In cases where there is a clear clinical suspicion of genital infection, treatment with antibiotics such as doxycycline/tetracycline or erythromycin should be initiated immediately and before the laboratory reports are obtained. Further invasive investigations of the uterine cavity such as hysteroscopy and endometrial biopsies or curettage should not be performed until the microbiological results are obtained and infection is excluded. Otherwise, there is a small risk of the cervical infection being spread to the tubes.

Cancer of the cervix is more common than endometrial cancer in women under the age of 45 years. When there is a clinical suspicion both cervical biopsies from the suspicious tissue and a Pap smear test are indicated. Cervical biopsies should always be obtained in women with repeated contact bleeding even in the presence of normal smear. Cervical biopsies should be taken by a physician with appropriate experience and guided by colposcopy. An endocervical plus an endometrial curettage should be performed in many cases.

Indications for endometrial diagnostic measures

The most important single purpose of this investigation is to exclude endometrial cancer in its early stages. Careful patient selection will reduce the number of unnecessary D&Cs (dilatation and curettage) and hysteroscopies. It is important to remember that D&C alone misses a moderate amount of pathology.

An active approach is indicated for the following groups.

- Women with intermenstrual bleeding resistant to hormonal therapy and prolonged bleeding for more than 10 days (polyps and hyperplasia are frequent in this category and diagnosis with D&C, ultrasound, and hysteroscopy may also be of therapeutic value).
- Women with post-coital bleeding.
- Post-menopausal women (most women with endometrial cancer are found in this group).

A more conservative approach is recommended in women below the age of 45 years. The diagnostic information from histopathological examination alone in this category is low, while abnormal findings on hysteroscopy and ultrasound are more common.

References

Altchek, A. (1977). Persistent dysfunctional bleeding, endometrial hyperplasia, and polycystic ovarian disease. *Clinical Obstetrics and Gynecology*, **20**, 647–50.

Anderson, A.B.M., Haynes, P.J., Guillebaud, J., and Turnbull, A.C. (1976). Reduction of menstrual blood loss by prostaglandin synthetase inhibition. *Lancet*, **i**, 774–8.

Apter, D. and Vihko, R. (1985). Hormonal patterns of the first menstrual cycles. In *Adolescence in females* (ed. S. Venturoli, S. Flamingni, and J.R. Givens), pp. 216–38. Yearbook Medical, Chicago.

Bassol, S., Garza-Flores, J., Cravioto, M.C., Diaz-Sanchez, V., Fotherby, K., Lichtenberg, R., and Perez-Palacios, G. (1984). Ovarian function following a single administration of depomedroxyprogesterone acetate (DMPA) at different doses. *Fertility and Sterility*, **42**, 216–22.

Belsey, E.M. and World Health Organization (1988). Task force on long-acting systemic agents for fertility regulation. Vaginal bleeding patterns among women using one natural and eight hormonal methods of contraception. *Contraception*, **38**, 181–206.

Brache, V., Alvarez-Sanchez, F., Faundes, A., Tejada, A.S., and Cochon, L. (1990). Ovarian endocrine function through five years of continuous treatment with Norplant subdermal contraceptive implants. *Contraception*, **41**, 169–78.

Claesson, E.A. and Cowell, C.A. (1981). Acute adolescent menorrhagia. *American Journal of Obstetrics and Gynecology*, **139**, 277–80.

Cook, C.L., Rao, Ch.V., and Yussman, M.A. (1983). Plasma gonadotropin and sex steroid hormone levels during early, midfollicular, and midluteal phases of women with luteal phase defects. *Fertility and Sterility*, **40**, 45–8.

Daly, D.C., Tohen, N., Doney, T.J., Maslor, I.A., and Riddich, D.H. (1982). The significance of lymphocytic–leucocytic infiltrates in interpreting late luteal phase endometrial biopsies. *Fertility and Sterility*, **37**, 786–91.

De Stefano, T., Perlman, J.A., Peterson, H.B., and Diamond, E.L. (1985). Long-term risk of menstrual disturbances after tubal sterilization. *American Journal of Obstetrics and Gynecology*, **150**, 835–41.

Ferenczy, A., Bertrand, G., and Geland, M.M. (1979). Proliferation kinetics of human endometrium during the normal menstrual cycle. *American Journal of Obstetrics and Gynecology*, **133**, 859–67.

Ferenczy, A., Geland, M.M., and Tzipris, F. (1982). The cytodynamics of endometrial hyperplasia and carcinoma. A review. *Annual Pathology*, **3**, 189–202.

Flowers, D. and Wilborn, W.H. (1982). Observations on the physiology of menstruation. *Obstetrics and Gynecology*, **51**, 16–24.

Fraser, I.S. and Baird, D.T. (1972). Endometrial cystic glandular hyperplasia in adolescent girls. *Journal of Obstetrics and Gynaecology of the British Commonwealth*, **79**, 1009–15.

Fraser, I.S. and Petrucco, O.M. (1996). Management of intermenstrual and postcoital bleeding, and an appreciation of the issues arising out of the recent case of O'Shea versus Sullivan and Macquarie pathology. *Australian and New Zealand Journal of Obstetrics and Gynaecology*, **36**, 67–73.

Genz, T., Eiletz, J., Kreuzer, G., Pollow, K., and Schmidt-Gollwitzer, M. (1980). Untersuchungen zur endokrine Regulation des Endometriums während des menstruellen Zyklus. *Geburtshilfe Frauenheilkunde*, **40**, 990–9.

Goldzieher, J.W. and Green, J.A. (1962). The polycystic ovary. I. Clinical and histologic features. *Journal of Clinical Endocrinology and Metabolism*, **22**, 325–38.

Gray, R.W. (1980). Patterns of bleeding associated with the use of steroidal contraception. In *Endometrial bleeding and steroidal contraception* (ed. E. Diczfalusy, I.S. Fraser, and F.T.G. Webb), pp. 14–49. Pitman Press, Bath, UK.

Gusberg, S.B. (1967). Hormone dependence of endometrial cancer. *Obstetrics and Gynecology*, **30**, 287–93.

Hargrove, J.T. and Abraham, G.E. (1981). Endocrine profile of patients with post-tubal ligation syndrome. *Journal of Reproductive Medicine*, **26**, 359–62.

Hertweck, S.P. (1992). Dysfunctional uterine bleeding. *Obstetric and Gynecologic Clinics of North America*, **19**, 129–48.

Jutras, M.L. and Cowan, B.D. (1990). Abnormal bleeding in the climacteric. *Obstetric and Gynecologic Clinics of North America*, **17**, 409.

Kolstad, P. (1986). *Clinical gynecological oncology. The Norwegian experience*. Norwegian University Press, Oslo.

Kurman, R.J., Kaminski, P.F., and Norris, H.J. (1985). The behaviour of endometrial hyperplasia. A long-term study of 'untreated' hyperplasia in 170 patients. *Cancer*, **56**, 403–12.

Laatikainen, T., Andersson, B., Karkunen, J., and Wahlström, T. (1983). Progestin receptor levels in endometria with delayed or incomplete secretory changes. *Obstetrics and Gynecology*, **62**, 592–5.

Landgren, B.-M. and Diczfalusy, E. (1981). Hormonal effects of the 300 μg norethistosterone (NET) minipill. *Contraception*, **21**, 87–113.

Lenton, E.A., Landgren, B.-M., and Sexton, L.W. (1984*a*). Normal variation in the length of the luteal phase of the menstrual cycle; identification of the short luteal phase. *British Journal of Obstetrics and Gynaecology*, **91**, 685–9.

Lenton, E.A., Landgren, B.-M., Sexton, L., and Harper, R.-M. (1984*b*). Normal variations in the length of the follicular phase of the menstrual cycle: effects of chronological age. *British Journal of Obstetrics and Gynaecology*, **91**, 681–4.

Metcalf, M.G. (1988). The approach of menopause: a New Zealand study. *New Zealand Medical Journal*, **101**, 103–6.

Noyes, R.W., Hertig, A.T., and Rock, Y. (1950). Dating the endometrial biopsy. *Fertility and Sterility*, **1**, 3.

Radwanska, E., Headley, S.K., and Dmowski, P. (1982). Evaluation of ovarian function after tubal sterilization. *Journal of Reproductive Medicine*, **27**, 376–84.

Robertson, D.N, Sivin, I., Nash, H.A., Braun, J., and Dinh, J. (1983). Release rates of levonorgestrel from silastic capsules, homogenous rods and covered rods in humans. *Contraception*, **27**, 483–5.

Seltzer, V.L., Benjamin, F., and Deutsch, S. (1990). Perimenopausal bleeding patterns and pathological findings. *Journal of the American Medical Women's Association*, **45**, 132.

Sherman, B.M. and Korenman, S.G. (1975). Hormonal characteristics of the human menstrual cycle throughout reproductive life. *Journal of Clinical Investigation*, **55**, 699–706.

Smith, S.U., Abel, M.H., Kelly, R.W., and Baird, D.T. (1982). The synthesis of prostaglandins from persistent proliferative endometrium. *Journal of Clinical Endocrinology and Metabolism*, **55**, 284–9.

Southam, A.L. and Richart, R.M. (1966). The prognosis for adolescents with menstrual abnormalities. *American Journal of Obstetrics and Gynecology*, **94**, 637–45.

Treloar, A.E., Baynton, R.E., Benn, B.G., and Burn, B.W. (1967). Variation of the human menstrual cycle through reproductive life. *International Journal of Fertility*, **12**, 77–125.

Vollman, R.F. (1977). *The menstrual cycle*. Saunders, Philadephia.

Wilcox, L.S., Martinez-Schnell, B., Peterson, H.B., Ware, J.H., and Hughes, J.M. (1992). Menstrual function after tubal sterilization. *American Journal of Epidemiology*, **135**, 1368–72.

Zimmermann, R. (1988). Dysfunctional uterine bleeding. *Obstetric and Gynecologic Clinics of North America*, **15**, 107–10.

21 Post-menopausal bleeding

Christine Bain and Henry C. Kitchener

Introduction

The definition of post-menopausal bleeding (PMB) varies, but is usually defined as vaginal bleeding that occurs one year or more after the menopause. It is a clinical sign that causes alarm and anxiety in women and is of concern to the clinician, because of its association with malignant disease. Around 10 per cent of women presenting with this problem will have underlying cancer, with the likelihood increasing with the length of duration from menopause. The bleeding may vary from only a few spots of blood to several days of bleeding, or rarely a profuse haemorrhage. However small the amount, every case must be investigated thoroughly and sensitively. This chapter will be concerned only with bleeding from the genital tract and will outline the causes and modern management of this problem which can be divided into three groups dependent on the location of bleeding (Table 21.1). Bleeding from the urinary or gastrointestinal tract should be referred to the relevant specialist. However, it is important to note that haematuria and rectal bleeding may be confused with vaginal bleeding and if there is uncertainty it is best to investigate both possible sources. Previous studies (Brewer and Miller 1954; Keirse 1973; Caspi *et al.* 1977) have tried to identify the incidence of each cause of post-menopausal bleeding, but this is difficult due to exclusion criteria. In our centre in Aberdeen, which serves a female population of 300 000 we see 500–600 cases of PMB annually, a rate of around 1 per 500 women per year.

Table 21.1 The causes of post-menopausal bleeding

Location	Pathology	Causes to note
Vulva	Dermatitis/fissures	
	Cancer	
	Trauma	
Vaginal/cervix	Atrophic changes	
	Trauma	
	Cancer	
Endometrium	Atrophic changes	
	Hyperplasia ± atypia	HRT; tamoxifen; hormone-secreting ovarian tumours
	Cancer	

Aetiology

Atrophic changes

The menopause produces hypo-oestrogenic changes affecting both the uterine corpus and the lower genital tract. Tissue atrophy occurs with thinning of the epithelium which may lead to spontaneous bleeding. Blood loss is usually minimal, often reported as 'spotting', and may occur post-coitally especially when the vaginal mucosa is involved. Clinically, small areas of petechiae are seen due to superficial vessel rupture in the thin mucosa. The endometrium may be involved simultaneously or on its own, and atrophic endometritis may be diagnosed histopathologically or by hysteroscopy. Atrophic vaginitis and cervicitis are diagnosed clinically and can be treated with either topical oestrogen, or systemic hormone replacement which is more suitable in the presence of other menopausal symptoms.

Endometrial hyperplasia

This may occur by idiopathic means or because of exogenous stimulation such as estrogen or tamoxifen. Prolonged stimulation by either endogenous or exogenous estrogen, in the absence of progestogen, may lead to endometrial hyperplasia in both pre and post-menopausal women. Unopposed estrogen produces an increased risk of developing endometrial cancer after prolonged use (Ziel and Finkle 1975) which is why combining estrogen and progestogen in HRT formulations is mandatory for women who have not had a hysterectomy. Endometrial hyperplasia is classified according to the degree of architectural and cytological atypia as follows: simple hyperplasia – glandular and stromal hyperplasia and highly vascular; complex hyperplasia – similar to simple but less stroma; and, atypical hyperplasia – glandular abnormality, both at cellular level and structurally (Fig. 21.1). Cytological atypia is regarded as having significantly more malignant potential than architectural atypia alone.

Progression to endometrial carcinoma appears to be concentrated in those patients with cytological atypia. Hyperplasia and neoplasia are regarded by some as two quite distinct entities, unlike the continuum of change thought by many to be exemplified by cervical intraepithelial neoplasia (Ferenczy and Bergeron 1992). High grade atypical hyperplasia may be difficult to distinguish from endometrial cancer on histopathological assessment of curettings, and with progression to cancer reported as high as 20 per cent over 10 years, this is generally managed by hysterectomy. Most cases of endometrial hyperplasia are of unknown aetiology although conversion of androstenedione to estrogen in obese women may be responsible. Two significant causes identified in recent years are estrogen replacement and the use of tamoxifen for the treatment of breast cancer. A rare source of endogenous oestrogen production, but one that should be borne in mind particularly if a pelvic mass is present, is a granulosa cell tumour of the ovary.

Hormone replacement therapy (HRT)

This is now widely prescribed for osteoporosis prophylaxis as well as for relief of vasomotor symptoms associated with the menopause. Administration can be transdermal, subcutaneous, topical, and oral. Choice is determined by patient preference and clinical considerations. Patients who have not had a hysterectomy require careful counselling particularly with regard to the prescription of cyclical progestogen to prevent endometrial hyperplasia. Compliance can be

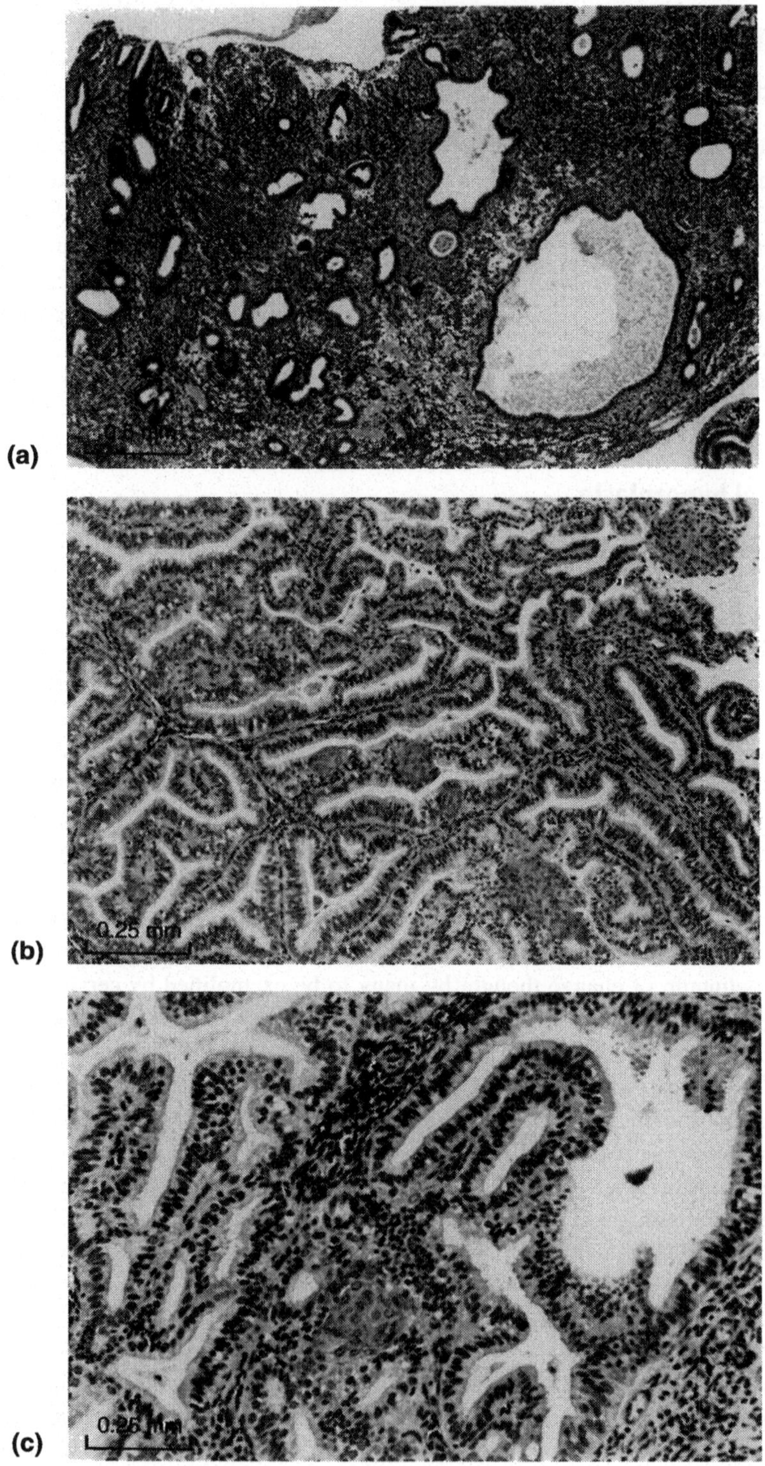

Fig. 21.1 (a) Simple hyperplasia of endometrium (photo: Dr I.D. Miller); **(b)** complex hyperplasia (photo: Dr I.D. Miller); and **(c)** atypical hyperplasia (photo: Dr I.D. Miller).

increased with a three-monthly withdrawal bleed which does not appear to increase the risk of hyperplasia. However, despite patient compliance of the progestogenic component, irregular bleeding can occur on combined hormone replacement therapy and may require investigation. These patients are still at risk of endometrial cancer though the incidence appears to be equal to that of the general population (Studd and Than 1981).

Tamoxifen

Tamoxifen is a synthetic, non-steroidal anti-oestrogenic drug, structurally similar to diethylstilbestrol. It is widely used for adjuvant therapy in post-menopausal patients with breast cancer where it has been found to be effective and safe with few side-effects. Twenty per cent of women on tamoxifen report vaginal dryness, hot flushes, and vulvovaginal irritation. However, recent reports have suggested that tamoxifen may be associated with a variety of endometrial abnormalities, including decidual reaction of the endometrial stroma (Nasri *et al.* 1991; Cohen 1992; Corley *et al.* 1992), endometrial hyperplasia (Neven *et al.* 1989; Cross and Ismail 1990), endometrial polyps (Neven *et al.* 1989; Nuovo *et al.* 1989), and of more concern, endometrial carcinoma (Killackey *et al.* 1985; Hardell 1988; Fornander *et al.* 1989; Antlante *et al.* 1990; Malfetano 1990; Mathew *et al.* 1990). The frequency of endometrial abnormalities appears to be related to the cumulative dose of the tamoxifen (De Muybler *et al.* 1991) and possibly the daily dose of the drug. In Sweden, 1846 post-menopausal patients were included in the uncontrolled randomized study conducted by Fornander *et al.* (1989). The group taking 40 mg of tamoxifen daily were found to have an increased risk of endometrial cancer as opposed to the control group, linking the drug with endometrial cancer. However, a subsequent Scottish study from a 10 year analysis of 1070 post-menopausal women with operable breast cancer showed no increase in the incidence of endometrial cancer after adjuvant tamoxifen at a dose of 20 mg per day for five years (Stewart 1992). This was confirmed by Lahti *et al.* (1993) who found that endometrial polyps occurred more frequently than endometrial cancer in their tamoxifen group compared with controls in a study of 103 asymptomatic post-menopausal breast cancer patients.

These data demonstrate the paradoxical effect of tamoxifen in an oestrogen-deficient environment and emphasize the need for thorough investigation of any patient on tamoxifen with post-menopausal bleeding. Furthermore, tamoxifen-associated cancers seem to be well differentiated with superficial invasion and are usually easily cured by hysterectomy. There is certainly a case for screening women who have been taking tamoxifen for three years or more for endometrial abnormalities because it is impossible to predict which post-menopausal women may develop endometrial pathology with tamoxifen (Cohen *et al.* 1993). Many women who have vaginal bleeding on tamoxifen have no associated pathology and the bleeding is an isolated event. In some, however, the bleeding is persistent and unless the tamoxifen can be stopped, a hysterectomy may be required.

Cancer

Post-menopausal bleeding is often the presenting symptom in gynaecological cancer. Many women who develop PMB will assume that they have developed cancer and become frightened. Furthermore, many older women will be embarrassed at having to undergo a gynaecological examination. These factors emphasize the need for sensitivity as well as thoroughness in dealing with this problem. There is no place for complacency in managing PMB which should be investigated promptly. This must include a careful history and as thorough an examination as is possible. Unless a malignant lesion from the vulva, vagina, or cervix is present, endometrial assessment is mandatory. Careful inspection of the vulva, vagina, and cervix excludes tumour in those organs but endocervical tumours may only be discovered by curettage. Almost all women with endometrial cancer present with abnormal bleeding and in the absence of another malignancy this tumour needs to be excluded as described in the following section.

The investigation of post-menopausal bleeding

Dilatation and curettage (D&C)

Until recently this has been the conventional method of diagnosing endometrial pathology. The procedure was also required for the staging of endometrial cancer until the revised classification was adopted in 1988. D&C requires general anaesthesia which is disadvantageous in the medically unfit and there is also the risk of uterine perforation which may result in having to abandon the procedure without obtaining a diagnosis.

Curettage alone may miss lesions, such as polyps and localized cancers, in up to 25 per cent of cases (Gimpelson and Rappold 1988). Although still in widespread use, the advent of endometrial sampling and vaginal ultrasound has reduced the need for D&C. Nevertheless in some women a satisfactory examination will not be possible without general anaesthesia. Under these circumstances curettage should be performed, as it should in cases where a negative endometrial biopsy has been followed by recurrent bleeding.

There are cases where normal proliferative endometrium is obtained, particularly in women close to the menopause. This need not routinely prompt a search for an estrogen-producing tumour which is both rare and would normally produce hyperplasia rather than simple proliferative changes.

Endometrial biopsy

This term is used for the outpatient procedure of obtaining endometrium. There are a wide variety of devices for doing this, with most consisting of a disposable plastic sheath with a blunt rounded distal tip and a diameter of around 3 mm. The device is introduced into the uterine cavity and a central plunger is withdrawn to create a vacuum within the sheath. The sample of endometrium is aspirated via a port at the distal end as it is moved across the endometrial surface. The most common instrument currently used is the pipelle device.

Stovall *et al.* (1991) have shown that endometrial biopsy has good histopathological reproducibility with no false negatives. More recently, Fothergill *et al.* (1992) compared formal curettage with pipelle sampling. In their study of 187 women, aged 35–84 years, 88 per cent showed similar results with both techniques and no case of atypia or carcinoma was missed by the pipelle in 62 post-menopausal women. However, Ferry *et al.* (1993) found that pipelle sampling provided the correct diagnosis in only 67 per cent of cases. The most difficult cancers to diagnose by endometrial biopsy were well differentiated, low volume, or minimally invasive tumours.

Rodriguez *et al.* (1993) reported that the pipelle device sampled only 4 per cent of the endometrial surface area compared with the Vabra aspirator which sampled 40 per cent, when the denudation produced was assessed in hysterectomy specimens. In patients with post-menopausal bleeding in whom it is important not to miss a lesion, as much of the cavity must be sampled as possible. In this regard a Karman type curette may be more appropriate as currently used in our post-menopausal bleeding clinic. In pre-menopausal women where endometrial tissue is always present, the pipelle may be expected to produce a sample, but for post-menopausal bleeding, a sampling device which involves more powerful suction may be better. At a practical level, a histopathological report saying 'inadequate tissue for analysis' need not prompt further investigation for the post-menopausal patient provided the cavity was satisfactorily cannulated; it merely reflects a lack of tissue. If appearances of cervical intraepithelial neoplasia (CIN) are reported, the cervix should be visualized by colposcopy and if this is unsatisfactory, a cone biopsy should be performed in order to exclude endocervical cancer.

Previous operations on the cervix, an intact hymen, severe vaginal irritation, and cervical stenosis due to atrophic change can all make endometrial biopsy difficult, but with care and patience, around 80 per cent of post-menopausal patients tolerate this procedure with ease (Shaker *et al.* 1991). Endometrial sampling is an effective method of diagnosing endometrial cancer and in general can be substituted for dilatation and curettage. Furthermore it is an easily learnt procedure and carries little risk of morbidity.

A further dimension to endometrial sampling is endometrial cytology. Considerable cytological experience is required to master the normal features of endometrial cells with their appearance changing in response to both hormonal stimulation and site of origin within the uterus (superficial or deep). The cytological features of adenocarcinoma are characteristic (Fig. 21.2), but endometrial hyperplasia is more difficult to distinguish from normality. This technique may be useful especially when the aspirate is not adequate for histological diagnosis (Roberts *et al.* 1994). Widespread application of this technique will require further research. At present endometrial cytology should not be considered as a definitive investigation for post-menopausal bleeding.

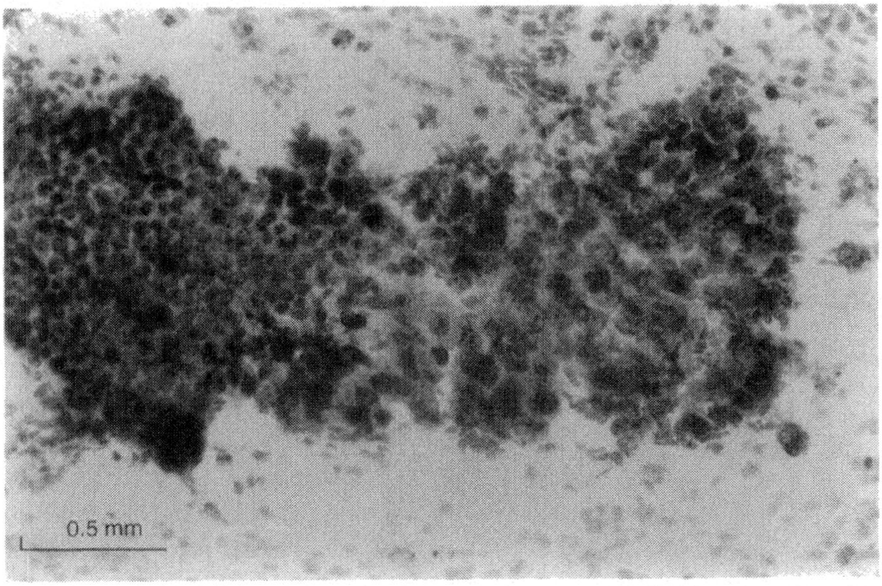

Fig. 21.2 Cytological appearance of papillary serous adenocarcinoma (photo: Dr E. Mann).

Hysteroscopy

Both D&C and endometrial biopsy are blind endometrial sampling techniques which can result in unrepresentative biopsies (Gimpelson and Rappold 1988). Hysteroscopy, which provides direct vision of the uterine cavity, enables directed biopsies to be taken from any suspicious areas (Fig. 21.3). Hysteroscopy used to be performed routinely under general anaesthesia, but although it is increasingly used with local anaesthesia even in post-menopausal patients (De Jong *et al.* 1990; Downes and Al-Azzawi 1993*a*) it can be rather uncomfortable. Although this obviously reduces the need for hospital admission and can provide early investigation for patients, it requires a higher level of expertise and more sophisticated facilities than performing an outpatient endometrial biopsy. Carbon dioxide gas is used to distend the uterus under local anaesthesia. This type of insufflation is contraindicated in patients with cardiopulmonary disease, because of the rare occurrence of carbon dioxide embolus, thereby reducing the proportion of post-menopausal patients who would be eligible for this investigation.

Despite these problems, hysteroscopy is considered useful by some for the management of post-menopausal bleeding. We do not advocate its use routinely, but hysteroscopy may identify intrauterine pathology such as polyps which may be missed at both D&C and endometrial sampling. As the number of reports about the effect of tamoxifen on the endometrium increases, consideration should be given to performing three-yearly hysteroscopy with directed biopsies for patients taking this drug. Hysteroscopy has also been reported to be of value in post-menopausal patients on HRT with abnormal bleeding, with 48 per cent of women in one study having a structural abnormality within the uterus (Downes and Al-Azzawi 1993*b*).

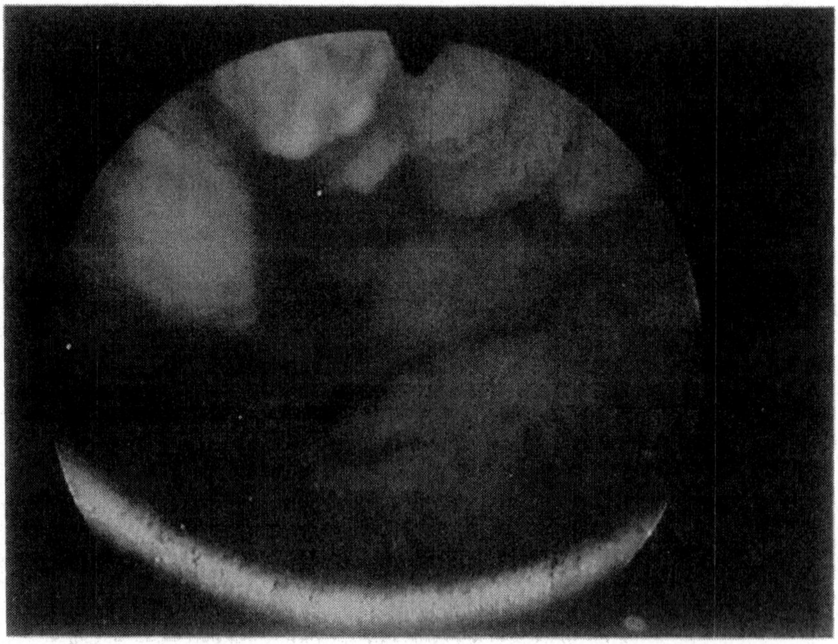

Fig. 21.3 Hysteroscopic view of adenocarcinoma of the endometrium (photo: Dr D.E. Parkin).

Hysteroscopy may increase the sensitivity of investigation, but its specificity depends very much on an expert operator. At the other end of the spectrum, hysteroscopy can readily confirm an atrophic endometrium without the need for biopsy.

Ultrasound

Ultrasound has become widely used in all fields of medicine, including obstetrics and gynaecology, because of its non-invasiveness and patient acceptability. Transvaginal scanning has been increasingly favoured for assessment of pelvic pathology due to its higher resolution. Despite the need for a vaginal probe, post-menopausal women find it very acceptable. It is much preferred to either endometrial sampling or hysteroscopy, both of which can be avoided by using this investigation. The normally smooth post-menopausal endometrial cavity produces a very narrow echo compared with the variation in endometrial thickness influenced by the hormonal changes in the menstrual cycle of pre-menopausal women.

There are several types of vaginal probe, but the slim line probes are more acceptable for the post-menopausal patient. All use higher frequency transducers than the transabdominal probes at frequencies normally between 5.0 MHz and 7.5 MHz. It is important to scan coronal views of the uterus as well as the sagittal plane, to determine the endometrial regularity section by section. Endometrial thickness is then measured in the longitudinal axis to avoid oblique semicoronal views which may increase the measurements. The correlation of the sonographic appearance of the endometrium with histopathological findings was found to be reliably assessed within 1 mm in 33 out of 38 cases (Fleischer *et al.* 1986). When the transvaginal scan is performed correctly, the negative predictive value of endometrial cancer is 100 per cent when the antero-posterior endometrial thickness is less than or equal to 5 mm (Fleischer *et al.* 1986; Goldstein *et al.* 1990). The positive predictive value is around 35 per cent (Goldstein *et al.* 1990), due to the inability to differentiate between proliferative endometrium, hyperplastic endometrium, endometrial polyps, and pre-invasive endometrial cancer. Sheth *et al.* (1993) have tried to classify the ultrasonic findings but ultrasound lacks this exactitude.

Loss of the subendothelial halo which consists of compact myometrium due to myometrial invasion is a reliable indication of endometrial cancer (Fig. 21.4). Although abnormal appearances are not specific for endometrial neoplasia when there is an intact subendothelial halo, ultrasound provides a sensitive screening method and indicates the need for endometrial biopsy reliably. However, the need for biopsy can be avoided in many women when the mid-line echo is narrow (Fig. 21.5).

Ultrasonography can also detect ovarian pathology along with the endometrial assessment and can be very helpful in obese women when vaginal examination is unhelpful. Ovarian volumes in post-menopausal women are half those of pre-menopausal women, and are affected by parity, weight, previous breast cancer, and age at menopause. As the ovaries can be much smaller and situated higher in the pelvis after menopause, gentle lower abdominal pressure may be required to visualize them with the vaginal probe. The bowel can also make visualization difficult, but fasting patients can reduce this problem. Even with optimum views, it can be extremely difficult to assess the ovary due to its high anatomical situation (or previous hysterectomy when the landmarks are absent) and transabdominal ultrasound may be required. Wolf *et al.* (1991) positively identified the ovaries in 68 per cent of post-menopausal women using both transabdominal and transvaginal scanning. It is important to emphasize the need for adequate training in ultrasound.

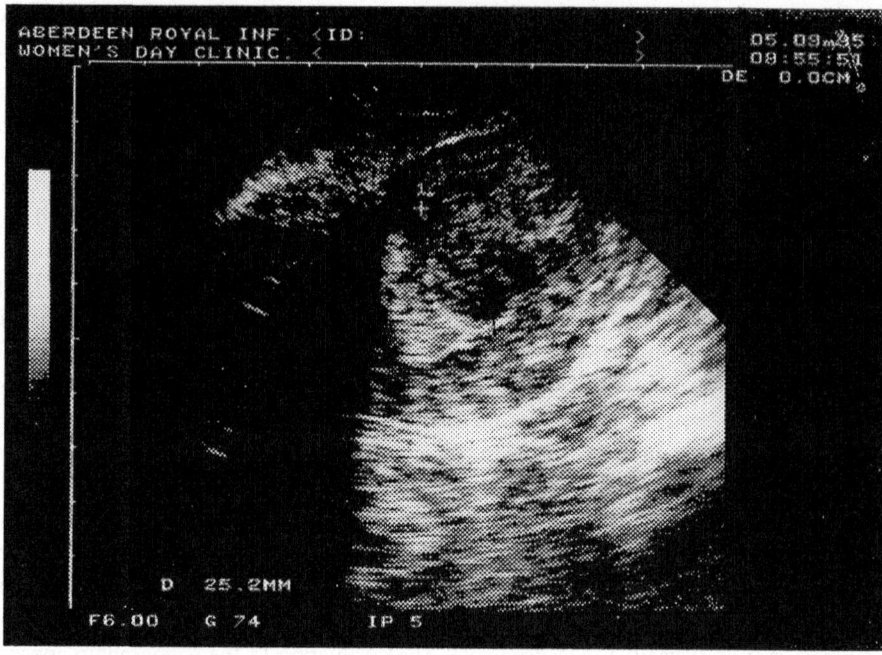

Fig. 21.4 The ultrasound scan appearance of endometrial cancer.

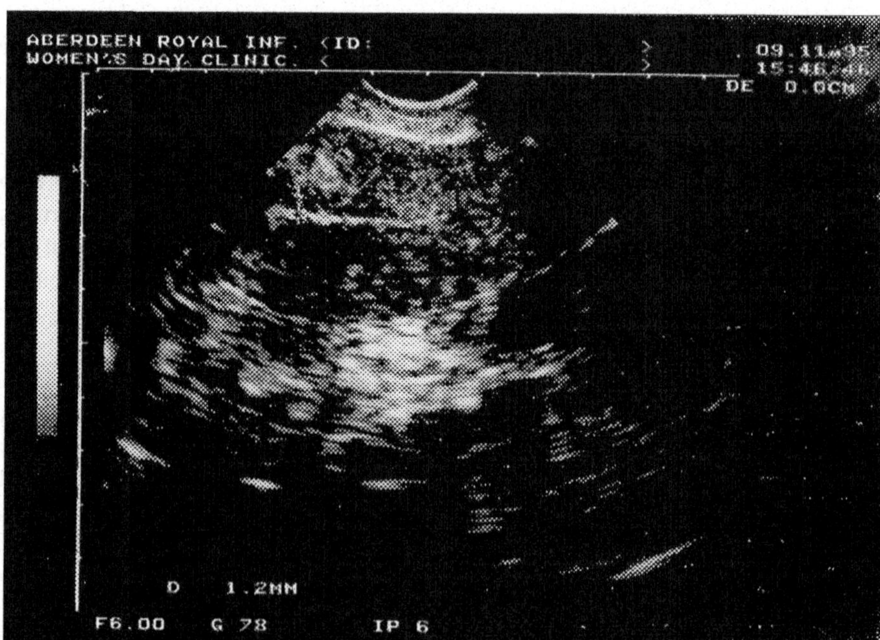

Fig. 21.5 Normal post-menopausal mid-line echo as seen by ultrasound scanning.

The technique is not difficult to master but there is a significant learning curve of perhaps 50 cases.

Transvaginal colour Doppler

A combination of high quality B-made images, pulsed wave Doppler, and colour Doppler in the same vaginal probe allows simultaneous structural investigation as well as the measurement of endometrial thickness. This has been extremely promising for the detection of adnexal masses (Kurjak *et al.* 1990; Fleischer *et al.* 1995) and is now being introduced into assessment of thickened endometrium (Bourne *et al.* 1991). Bourne *et al.* studied 138 post-menopausal women with end-points of both endometrial thickness and pulsability index derived from the flow velocity wave-forms recorded from both uterine outline and from within the tumour. The detection rate of endometrial cancer was 100 per cent, but the false-positive rate was 1 per cent in patients not receiving HRT and 11 per cent in those who were receiving HRT. These authors could not show that malignant tumours had an altered vascularization, but in conjunction with ultrasound trans-vaginal colour Doppler did not preclude further investigation especially in those receiving hormone replacement therapy. Doppler may be of more use in localized lesions within the endometrial cavity than it is for general endometrial changes. Further studies are awaited to see whether this form of imaging provides significantly greater diagnostic precision over conventional vaginal ultrasound.

The PMB clinic

Since 1989 in Aberdeen we have run a dedicated clinic for the management of PMB. This has the principal advantage of providing an optimal setting for streamlining the management of this common condition in which serious pathology is only found in around 10 per cent of women. The other 90 per cent can be managed in a 'one step' fashion which reduces delay and provides immediate reassurance in most cases. Our first protocol involved the use of endometrial biopsy which proved to be both effective and acceptable. Over 80 per cent of women tolerated the procedure satisfactorily and no cancers were missed (Shaker *et al.* 1991). We then changed the protocol in order to compare vaginal ultrasound assessment of the endometrium with an endometrial biopsy. This corroborated other reports which suggested that ultrasound was 100 per cent sensitive in detecting endometrial cancer. We determined that using vaginal scanning as a first screen would restrict the need for endometrial biopsy to less than 50 per cent of women (Campbell-Brown and Kitchener, unpublished data). Currently we continue to use ultrasound as a first line examination using endometrial biopsy only where ultrasound is abnormal. The clinic is well equipped, with a dedicated nurse and clerical infrastructure which enables around 300 patients per year to be evaluated (six to eight women per session). The PMB clinic is a very effective model of care for this important problem.

Summary

The successful management of PMB depends ultimately on making an accurate diagnosis which will dictate subsequent therapy. The principal advances that have been made are not so much in relation to treatment, but in methods of endometrial evaluation which have greatly reduced the need for hospital admission and general anaesthesia. Endometrial biopsy, which is very safe and quickly mastered, will be able to define the underlying pathology in the large majority of cases, but about 20 per cent of women still require general anaesthesia to enable a satisfactory exploration of the uterine cavity. Vaginal sonography is a less invasive technique and has been shown to be an effective first line investigation, negating the need for even endometrial sampling in well over 50 per cent of women. However, this requires expensive equipment and considerable expertise.

These outpatient techniques should be used as first line investigations, restricting the use of D&C for when these investigations are inconclusive, abnormal, or not tolerated. Women taking tamoxifen who develop PMB should be evaluated very carefully because of the increased risk of endometrial cancer and the possible presence of endometrial polyps. Recurrent PMB should be managed with equal care and hysteroscopy, which we do not routinely advocate, has a role in this setting. A dedicated clinic has the advantage of being able to provide reassurance at one visit to the 90 per cent of patients with PMB who have no significant pathology.

References

Antlante, G., Pozzi, M.F., Vincenzoni, C., and Vocaturo, G. (1990). Four case reports presenting new acquisition on the association of breast and endometrial cancer. *Gynecological Oncology*, **37**, 378–80.

Bourne, E., Campbell, S., Steer, C.V., Royston, P., Whitehead, M.I., and Collins, W.P. (1991). Detection of endometrial cancer by transvaginal ultrasonography with colour flow imaging and blood flow analysis: a preliminary report. *Gynaecology Oncology*, **40**, 253–9.

Brewer, J.I. and Miller, W.H. (1954). Post-menopausal uterine bleeding. *American Journal of Obstetrics and Gynecology*, **67**, 988.

Caspi, E., Perpinial, S., and Reif, A. (1977). Incidence of malignancy in Jewish females with post-menopausal bleeding. *Israel Journal of Medical Science*, **13**, 299.

Cohen, I. (1992). Endometrial decidual changes in a post-menopausal women treated with tamoxifen and megestol acetate. *British Journal of Obstetrics and Gynaecology*, **99**, 773–4.

Cohen, I., Rosen, D.J.D., Shapira, J., Cordoba, M., Gilboa, S., Altaras, M.M., *et al.* (1993). Endometrial changes in post-menopausal women treated with tamoxifen for breast cancer. *British Journal of Obstetrics and Gynaecology*, **100**, 567–70.

Corley, D., Rowe, J., Curtis, M.T., Hogan, W.M., Novmoff, J.S., and Livolsi, V.A. (1992). Post-menopausal bleeding from unusual endometrial polyps in women on chronic tamoxifen therapy. *Obstetrics and Gynecology*, **79**, 111–16.

Cross, S.S. and Ismail, S.M. (1990). Endometrial hyperplasia in an oophorectomised woman receiving tamoxifen therapy – case report. *British Journal of Obstetrics and Gynaecology*, **97**, 190–2.

De Jong, P., Doel, F., and Falconer, A. (1990). Outpatient diagnostic hysteroscopy. *British Journal of Obstetrics and Gynaecology*, **97**, 299–303.

De Muybler, X., Neven, P., De Somer, M., Van Belle, Y., Vanderick, G., and De Muylder, E. (1991). Endometrial lesions in patients undergoing tamoxifen therapy. *International Journal of Obstetrics and Gynaecology*, **36**, 127–30.

Downes, E. and Al-Azzawi, F. (1993*a*). How well do perimenopausal patients accept outpatient hysteroscopy? Visual analogue scoring of acceptability and pain in 100 women. *European Journal of Obstetrics and Gynaecology and Reproductive Biology*, **48**, 37–41.

Downes, E. and Al-Azzawi, F. (1993*b*). The predictive value of outpatient hysteroscopy in a menopause clinic. *British Journal of Obstetrics and Gynaecology*, **100**, 1148–9.

Ferenczy, A. and Bergeron, C. (1992). Endometrial hyperplasia. In *Advances in gynaecological pathology* (ed. D. Lowe and H. Fox), Ch. 11. Churchill Livingstone, Edinburgh.

Ferry, J., Farnsworth, M., Webster, M., and Wren, B. (1993). The efficacy of the pipelle endometrial biopsy in detecting carcinoma. *Australia and New Zealand Journal of Obstetrics and Gynaecology*, **33**, 76–8.

Fleischer, A.C., Kalemeris, G.C., Machin, J.E., Entman, S.S., and James, A.E. (1986). Sonographic depiction of normal and abnormal endometrium with histpathologic correlation. *Journal of Ultrasound Medicine*, **5**, 445–52.

Fleischer, A.C., Cullinan, J.A., Jones III, H.W., Peery, C.V., Bluth, R.F., and Kepple, D. (1995). Serial assessment of adnexal masses with transvaginal colour Doppler sonography. *Ultrasound in Medicine and Biology*, **21**, 435–41.

Fornander, T., Cedermartk, B., Mattsson, A., Skoog, L., Thieve, T., Askergren, J., *et al.* (1989). Adjuvant tamoxifen in early breast cancer. Occurrence of new primary cancer. *Lancet*, **21**, 117–20.

Fothergill, N.J., Brown, V.A., and Hill, S. (1992). Histological sampling of the endometrium – a comparison between formal curettage and the pipelle sampler. *British Journal of Obstetrics and Gynaecology*, **99**, 779–80.

Gimpelson, R.J. and Rappold, H.O. (1988). A comparative study between panoramic hysteroscopy and directed biopsies and dilatation and curettage: a review of 276 cases. *American Journal of Obstetrics and Gynecology*, **158**, 489–92.

Goldstein, S.R., Nachtigall, M., Snyder, J.R., and Nachtigall, L. (1990). Endometrial assessment by vaginal ultrasonography before endometrial sampling in patients with postmenopausal bleeding. *American Journal of Obstetrics and Gynecology*, **163**, 119–23.

Hardell, L. (1988). Tamoxifen as a risk factor for carcinoma of corpus uteri. *Lancet*, **ii**, 563.

Keirse, M.J.N.C. (1973). Aetiology of post-menopausal bleeding. *Postgraduate Medical Journal*, **49**, 344.

Killackey, M.A., Hakes, T.B., and Pierce, V.K. (1985). Endometrial adenocarcinoma in breast cancer patients receiving antiestrogen. *Cancer Treatment Report*, **69**, 237–8.

Kurjak, A., Ivica, Z., Zarko, A., and Davor, J. (1990). The assessment of abnormal pelvic blood flow by transvaginal colour and pulsed Doppler. *Ultrasound in Medicine and Biology*, **16**, 437–42.

Lahti, E., Blanco, G., Kauppila, A., Apaja-Sarkkinen, M., Taskinen, P.J., and Laatikainen T. (1993). Endometrial changes in postmenopausal breast cancer patients receiving Tamoxifen. *Obstetrics and Gynecology*, **81**, 660–4.

Malfetano, J.M. (1990). Tamoxifen: associated endometrial carcinoma in post-menopausal breast cancer patients. *Gynecological Oncology*, **39**, 82–4.

Mathew, A., Chabon, A.B., Kabakow, B., Drucker, M., and Hirschman, R.J. (1990). Endometrial carcinoma in five patients with breast cancer on tamoxifen therapy. *New York State Journal of Medicine*, **90**, 207–8.

Nasri, M.N., Shepherd, J.H., Stetchell, M.E., Lowe, D.G., and Chard, T. (1991). The role of vaginal scan in measurement of endometrial thickness in post-menopausal women. *British Journal of Obstetrics and Gynaecology*, **98**, 470–5.

Neven, P., De Muylder, X., Van Belle, Y., Vanderick, G., and De Mylder, E. (1989). Tamoxifen and the uterus. *Lancet*, **i**, 375–6.

Nuovo, M.A., Nuovo, G.J., McCaffray, R.M., Levine, R.V., Barron, B., and Winkler, B. (1989). Endometrial polyps in post-menopausal patients receiving tamoxifen. *International Journal of Gynecology and Pathology*, **8**, 125–31.

Roberts, M., Rodgers, A.D., Johri, S., and Case, B.D. (1994). Endometrial cytology: evaluation of samples obtained by outpatient aspiration. *British Journal of Obstetrics and Gynaecology*, **101**, 628–9.

Rodriguez, G.C., Yaqub, N., and King, M.E. (1993). A comparison of the pipelle device and the Vabra aspirator as measured by endometrial denudation in hysterectomy specimens. The pipelle device samples significantly less of the endometrial surface than the Vabra aspirator. *American Journal of Obstetrics and Gynecology*, **168**, 55–9.

Shaker, A.G., Anderson, and M., Kitchener, H.C. (1991). An outpatient approach to the management of post-menopausal bleeding. *British Journal of Obstetrics and Gynaecology*, **98**, 488–90.

Sheth, S., Hamper, V.M., and Kurman, R.J. (1993). Thickened endometrium in the post-menopausal woman: sonographic pathologic correlation. *Radiology*, **187**, 135–9.

Stewart, H.J. (1992). The Scottish trial of adjuvant tamoxifen in node-negative breast cancer. *Monographs National Cancer Institute*, **11**, 117–20.

Stovall, T.G., Photopulos, G., Poston, W.M., Ling, F.W., and Sandles, L. (1991). Pipelle endometrial sampling in patients with known endometrial carcinoma. *Obstetrics and Gynecology* **77**, 954–6.

Studd, J.W.W. and Than, M. (1981). Estrogen and endometrial cancer. In *Progress in obstetrics and gynaecology* (ed. J.W.W. Studd), Vol. 1. pp. 182–98. Churchill Livingstone, London.

Wolf, S.I., Gosink, B.B., Feldesman, M.R., Lin, M.C., Stuenkel, C.A., Braly, P.S., *et al.* (1991). Prevalence of simple adnexal cysts in postmenopausal women. *Radiology*, **180**, 65–71.

Ziel, H.K. and Finkle, W.D. (1975). Increased risk of endometrial carcinoma among users of conjugated estrogens. *New England Journal of Medicine*, **293**, 1167–70.

IV Dysmenorrhoea

22 The pathophysiology of dysmenorrhoea

Mats Åkerlund

Introduction

Painful menstruation is a common gynaecological problem. Different Scandinavian studies have shown that about 50 per cent of nulliparous women suffer from menstrual pain and that 10–20 per cent have to be absent from work 1–2 days each or every second menstruation (Bergsjö *et al.* 1975; Andersch and Milsom 1982). Although dysmenorrhoea tends to disappear after the first birth, a Norwegian study showed that more than 30 per cent of 30–40 year old women still had menstrual pain (Bergsjö *et al.* 1975).

From an aetiological point of view dysmenorrhoea is usually considered as primary or secondary. In primary dysmenorrhoea no underlying anatomical cause can be established, but the disturbance is functional. The most important causes of secondary dysmenorrhoea are endometriosis, adenomyosis, myomas, adhesions after pelvic inflammatory disease, and the presence of an intrauterine contraceptive device. A stenotic cervix, i.e. after conisation or other types of surgery, can also be the reason for secondary dysmenorrhoea. In this chapter the emphasis will be on the pathophysiology of primary dysmenorrhoea, although secondary dysmenorrhoea will also be covered to some extent.

Primary dysmenorrhoea

Uterine contractions, blood flow, and pain

A representative recording of uterine contractions and blood flow in a woman with painful menstruation is shown in Fig. 22.1. In most women suffering from primary dysmenorrhoea, myometrial hyperactivity can be demonstrated by intrauterine pressure recording (Åkerlund *et al.* 1976; Lundström *et al.* 1976; Andersson and Ulmsten 1978). The pattern varies between individuals so that contractions of increased amplitude, very frequent contractions with no period of complete

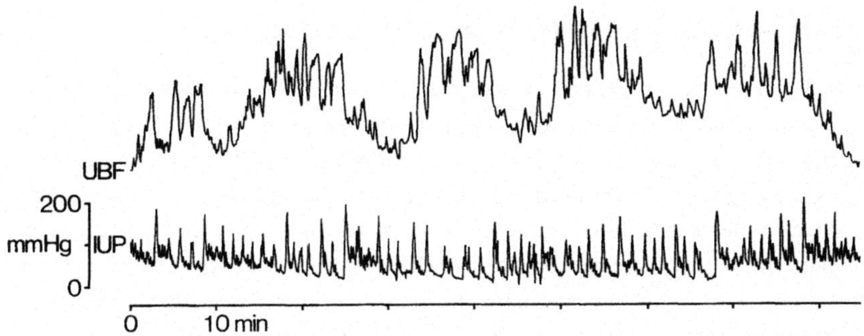

Fig. 22.1 Local endometrial blood flow (UBF) and intrauterine pressure (IUP) on the first day of menstruation in a woman with severe dysmenorrhoea (from Åkerlund *et al.* 1976).

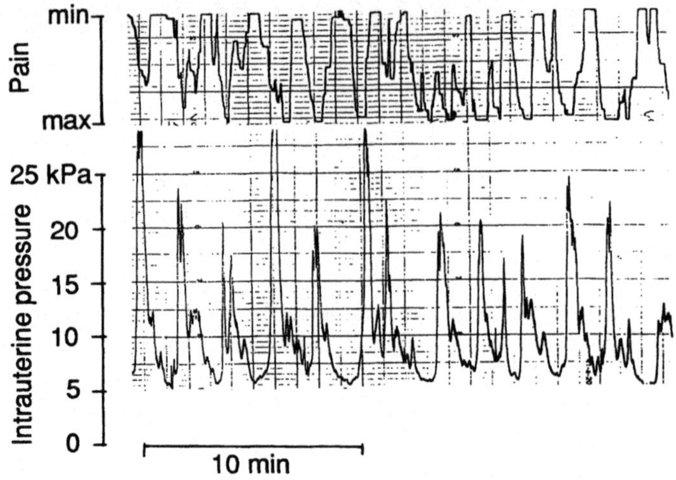

Fig. 22.2 Record of pain experienced (reversed visual analogue scale) and intrauterine pressure in a woman with severe primary dysmenorrhoea (from Ekström *et al.* 1990).

uterine relaxation in between, and/or a high basal tone can be found, and as a whole the contractile pattern is chaotic in comparison to that in healthy women at the onset of menstruation (Åkerlund *et al.* 1976). In parallel with this increased contractile activity the uterine blood flow is decreased (Fig. 22.1) and forceful contractions cause particularly well demarked reductions in flow locally in the endometrium (Åkerlund *et al.* 1976).

The perception of pain in primary dysmenorrhoea in relation to uterine activity was studied by recordings on a visual analogue scale performed by the women themselves in parallel to intrauterine pressure recordings (Ekström *et al.* 1990). An example is shown in Fig. 22.2. Due to the pronounced short-time variation in intrauterine blood flow in the condition, any correlation between uterine contractions and the degree of pain over 10 minute periods could not be demonstrated (Ekström *et al.* 1990). There was also frequently a time lag between individual peaks in pressure and maximal pain. This suggests that the important mechanism by which intensive uterine contractions cause pain is not the force *per se*, but a factor in between, namely the reducing effect that these contractions may have on the blood flow (Åkerlund *et al.* 1976). Uterine ischemia resulting from intensive contractions would lead to accumulation of acid metabolates, which then cause pain.

Vasopressin and other peptides in dysmenorrhoea

Women with primary dysmenorrhoea have an increased plasma concentration of vasopressin (Åkerlund *et al.* 1979; Strömberg *et al.* 1984; Hauksson *et al.* 1989; Ekström *et al.* 1992), and administration of this hormone causes the same pattern of myometrial hyperactivity and uterine ischemia as can be seen in the condition (Åkerlund and Andersson 1976). As shown in Fig. 22.3, even a moderate increase in the circulating level of vasopressin, which can be induced by infusion of hypertonic saline, increases uterine activity (Ekström *et al.* 1992). The hormone has a pronounced effect not only on the myometrium, but also on the smooth muscle of arterial walls, particularly the resistance arteries of the uterus (Ekström *et al.* 1991). Other peptides, such as oxytocin, endothelin, and noradrenaline may also contribute at least to the vasospasm of uterine arteries in dysmenorrhoea (Ekström *et al.* 1991).

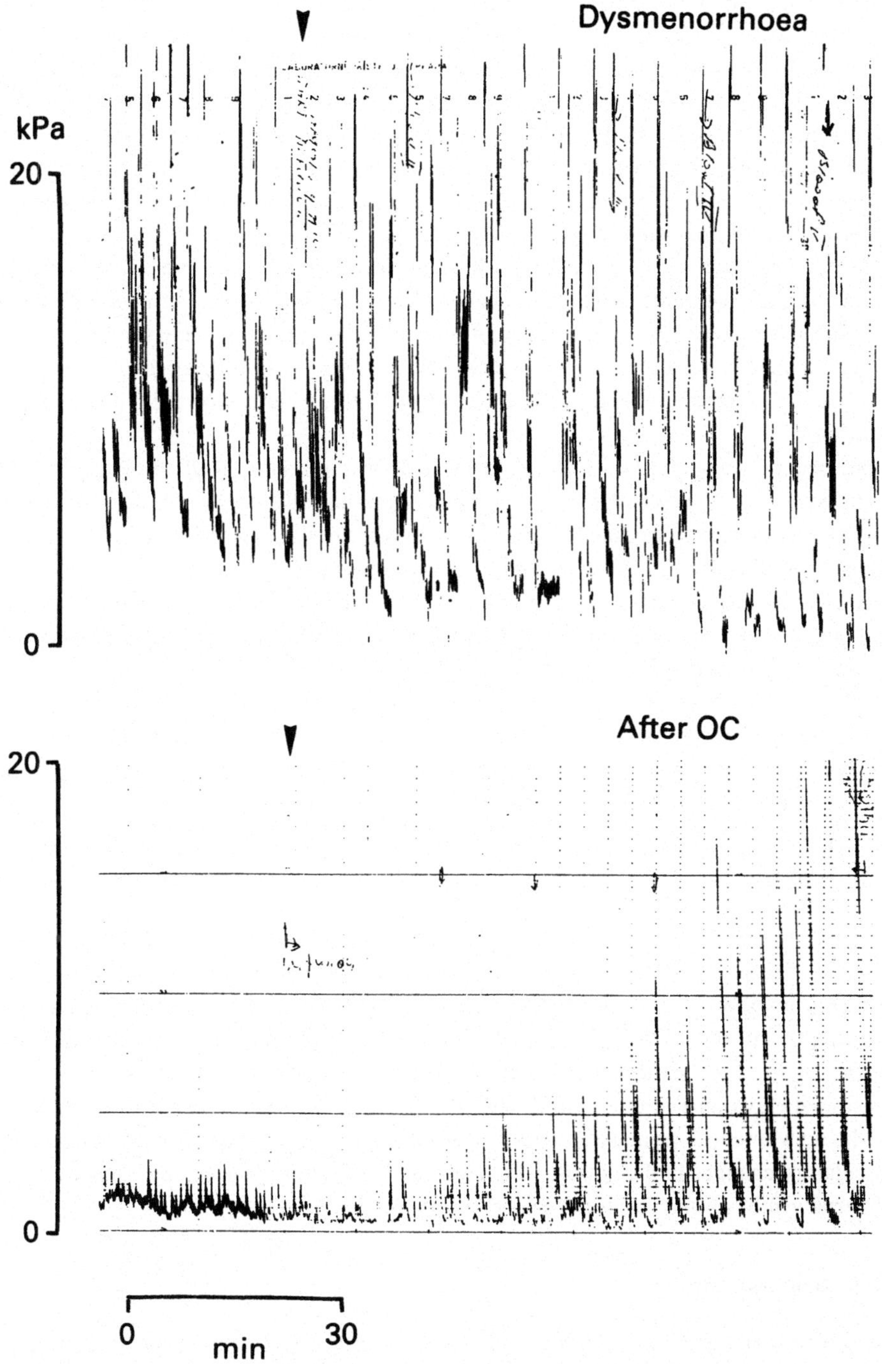

Fig. 22.3 Intrauterine pressure recordings in a woman on the first day of menstruation with intense dysmenorrhoeic pain (upper panel) and during withdrawal bleeding after three weeks of oral contraceptive (OC) treatment (lower panel). On both occasions infusion of hypertonic saline was started at the arrows. Plasma levels of vasopressin and oxytocin increased about three times and in parallel the uterine activity increased. The plasma level of vasopressin before infusion in women with dysmenorrhoea was 2.5 times higher than that after OC treatment. The concentrations of oxytocin and of the prostaglandin metabolite 15-keto-13,14-dihydro-PGF$_{2\alpha}$ were 20 per cent and 15 per cent higher in the women with dysmenorrhoea (from Ekström *et al.* 1992).

In the experiments with infusion of hypertonic saline (Ekström *et al.* 1992) not only vasopressin but also oxytocin levels increased, and furthermore, both type VIa vasopressin and oxytocin receptors have been demonstrated in myometrium from non-pregnant women (Maggi *et al.* 1992). On the basis of these results we have recently compared the effect of vasopressin and oxytocin on uterine activity *in vivo* in women in different ovarian hormonal states who were due to undergo hysterectomy (Bossmar *et al.* 1995*a*). We also studied the *in vitro* myometrial effects of the peptides after operation and measured myometrial concentrations of vasopressin VIa and oxytocin receptors. The density of vasopressin receptors was about five times higher than that of oxytocin (216 versus 54 fmol/mg protein). The effect of vasopressin on the uterus was five times more pronounced *in vivo*. The myometrial effects of oxytocin correlated with the concentration of its receptor, but such correlation was not seen for vasopressin. This may indicate that in parallel to the situation in pregnancy vasopressin acts on both vasopressin VIa and oxytocin receptors (Bossmar *et al.* 1994), whereas oxytocin only influences its own receptor.

The release of vasopressin is influenced by ovarian hormones. Thus, a cyclical variation is observed with peak values at the time of ovulation and usually the lowest concentrations at the onset of menstruation (Forsling *et al.* 1981). Furthermore, experiments in post-climacteric women showed that the release of vasopressin was stimulated by estrogen, an effect which was counteracted by progestogen (Forsling *et al.* 1982; Bossmar *et al.* 1995*b*). For oxytocin, progestogen does not seem to inhibit estrogen-induced release. Instead a further increase in the circulating level of oxytocin was observed (Bossmar *et al.* 1995*b*).

The uterine sensitivity to vasopressin is also affected by ovarian hormonal influence, as a markedly reduced response was observed after oral contraceptive treatment (Ekström *et al.* 1989). This is in agreement with the lower receptor concentration found in women taking oral contraceptive pills (Bossmar *et al.* 1995*a*).

Prostaglandins

Prostaglandins (PG) which stimulate contractions, mainly $PGF_{2\alpha}$, are also involved in the mechanism of dysmenorrhoea. Increased endometrial synthesis of $PGF_{2\alpha}$ has been demonstrated in dysmenorrhoeic women (Lundström and Gréen 1978). Lumsden *et al.* (1983) found that the concentrations of both $PGF_2\alpha$ and PGE_2 in menstrual blood were significantly increased compared to those in healthy controls on days 1 and 2 of the cycle and Nigam *et al.* (1991) demonstrated elevations of eicosanoids and platelet activating factor in menstrual blood of dysmenorrhoeic women. In primary dysmenorrhoea the myometrial hyperactivity, with accompanying circulatory changes in the uterus, which are caused by other factors, may lead to a secondary endometrial synthesis and release of PGs (Strömberg *et al.* 1983).

Therapeutic aspects

In the clinical management of both primary and secondary dysmenorrhoea, non-steroidal anti-inflammatory drugs which inhibit PG synthesis and release offer a basic treatment (Schwartz *et al.* 1974; Lundström *et al.* 1976). Ketoprofen is probably superior to naproxen, because of a more rapid uptake and action after oral administration (Åkerlund and Strömberg 1989). A combined oral contraceptive is the treatment of choice when women also require fertility control. In primary dysmenorrhoea such treatment decreases both the release of vasopressin from the posterior pituitary and the production of prostaglandins in the endometrium (Hauksson *et al.* 1987). As illustrated in Fig. 22.3, spontaneous uterine activity and the responsiveness of the uterus to vasopressin is also reduced in dysmenorrhoeic women treated by oral contraceptives (Ekström *et al.* 1989). A reduced uterine sensitivity to vasopressin and oxytocin is probably the effect of a lowered myometrial concentration of vasopressin VIa and oxytocin receptors (Bossmar *et al.* 1995*a,b*). The response to $PGF_{2}\alpha$ in dysmenorrhoeic women is also decreased by oral contraceptive treatment (Ekström *et al.* 1989).

In secondary dysmenorrhoea, the levonorgestrel-releasing intrauterine contraceptive device (Mirena®) may also be of benefit, by reducing prostaglandin synthesis in the endometrium (Sivin and Stern 1994). Other pharmacological methods that may be tried in difficult-to-treat cases besides non-steroidal anti-inflammatory drugs and oral contraceptives are calcium channel blocking agents (Andersson and Ulmsten 1978) and β_2-adrenoceptor stimulating drugs (Åkerlund *et al.* 1976), which act by reducing myometrial contractility.

Vasopressin VIa and oxytocin antagonists may also have a therapeutic potential in primary dysmenorrhoea. In collaboration with the Ferring Research Institute in Malmö, Sweden we have developed a series of oxytocin analogues which inhibit the effect of vasopressin on the uterus (Åkerlund *et al.* 1986; Melin *et al.* 1986; Hauksson *et al.* 1988). An illustration of the inhibitory effect of 1-deamino-2-D-Tyr(OEt)-4-Thr-8-Orn-oxytocin on vasopressin-induced contractile activity and uterine ischemia is shown in Fig. 22.4. The compound blocks both the oxytocin and the vasopressin VIa receptor and is effective in inhibiting both dysmenorrhoea (Åkerlund 1987) and preterm labor (Åkerlund *et al.* 1987). Other analogues, peptide and non-peptide, are also under development (Yamamura *et al.* 1991; Serradeil-le-Gal *et al.* 1993; Bossmar *et al.* 1997).

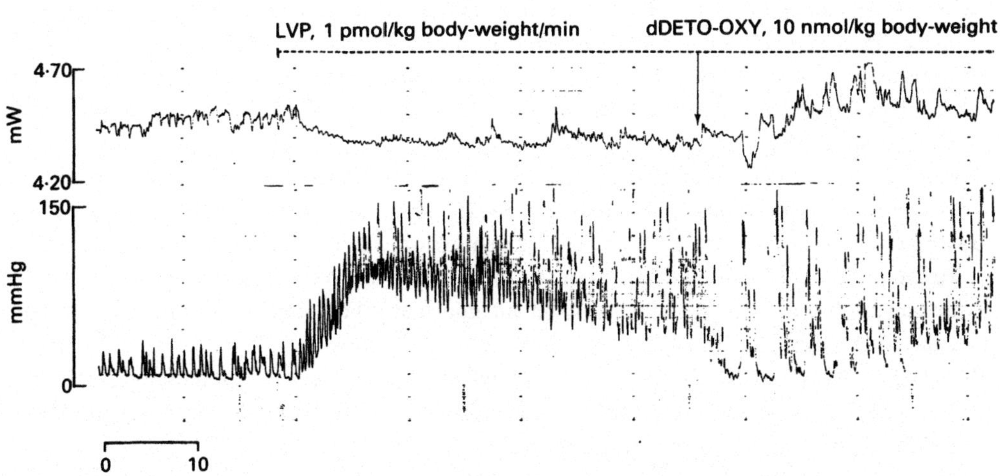

Fig. 22.4 Recording of uterine blood flow measured as added power and intrauterine pressure in a non-pregnant woman on day one of menstruation. Infusion of lysine vasopressin (LVP) and bolus injection over 1 min of the vasopressin and oxytocin antagonist 1-deamino-2-D-Tyr(Oet)4-Thr-8-Orn-oxytocin (dDETO-Oxy) are indicated. The LVP infusion induced dysmenorrhoea-like pain in all subjects, which was completely relieved for about 15 min after antagonist injection (from Hauksson *et al.* 1988).

Acknowledgements

This work has been supported by the Swedish Medical Research Council (B 95-17-X6571–13) and the University of Lund, Sweden.

References

Åkerlund, M. (1987). Can primary dysmenorrhoea be alleviated by a vasopressin antagonist? *Acta Obstetrica et Gynecologica Scandinavica*, **66**, 459–61.

Åkerlund, M. and Andersson, K.-E. (1976). Vasopressin response and terbutaline inhibition of the uterus. *Obstetrics and Gynecology*, **47**, 484–7.

Åkerlund, M., Strömberg, P., and Forsling, M.-L. (1979). Primary dysmenorrhoea and vasopressin. *British Journal of Obstetrics and Gynaecology*, **86**, 484–7.

Åkerlund, M., Andersson, K.-E., and Ingemarsson, I. (1976). Effect of terbutaline on myometrial acivity, endometrial blood flow, and lower abdominal pain in women with primary dysmenorrhoea. *British Journal of Obstetrics and Gynaecology*, **83**, 673–8.

Åkerlund, M. and Strömberg, P. (1989). Comparison of Ketoprofen and Naproxen in the treatment of dysmenorrhoea, with special regard to the time of onset of pain relief. *Current Medical Research Opinion*, **11**, 485–90.

Åkerlund, M., Hauksson, A., Lundin, S., Melin, P., and Trojnar, J. (1986). Vasotocin analogues which competetively inhibit vasopressin stimulated uterine activity in healthy women. *British Journal of Obstetrics and Gynaecology*, **93**, 22–7.

Åkerlund, M., Strömberg, P., Hauksson, A., Andersen, L.F., Lyndrup, J., Trojnar, J., and Melin, P. (1987). Inhibition of uterine contractions of premature labour with an oxtocin analogue. *British Journal of Obstetrics and Gynaecology*, **94**, 1040–4.

Andersch, B. and Milsom, I. (1982). An epidemiologic study of young women with dysmenorrhoea. *American Journal of Obstetrics and Gynaecology*, **144**, 655–60.

Andersson, K.-E. and Ulmsten, U. (1978). Effects of nifedipine on myometrial activity and lower abdominal pain in women with primary dysmenorrhoea. *British Journal of Obstetrics and Gynaecology*, **85**, 142–8.

Bergsjö, P., Jenssen, H., and Vellar, O.D. (1975). Dysmenorrhoea in industrial workers. *Acta Obstetrica et Gynecologica Scandinavica*, **54**, 255–9.

Bossmar, T., Åkerlund, M., Fantoni, G., Szamatowicz, J., Melin, P., and Maggi, M. (1994). Receptors for and myometrial responses to oxytocin and vasopressin in preterm and term human pregnancy: effects of the oxytocin antagonist atosiban. *American Journal of Obstetrics and Gynecology*, **171**, 1634–42.

Bossmar, T., Åkerlund, M., Szamatowicz, J., Laudanski, T., Fantoni, G., and Maggi, M. (1995a). Receptor-mediated uterine effects of vasopressin and oxytocin in non-pregnant women. *British Journal of Obstetrics and Gynaecology*, **102**, 907–12.

Bossmar, T., Forsling, M., and Åkerlund, M. (1995b). Circulating oxytocin and vasopressin is influenced by ovarian steroid replacement in women. *Acta Obstetrica et Gynecologica Scandinavica*, **74**, 544–8.

Bossmar, T., Brouard, R., Döberl, A., and Åkerlund, M. (1997). Effects of SR49059, an orally active V1a vasopressin receptor antagonist, on vasopressin-induced uterine contractions. *British Journal of Obstetrics and Gynaecology*, **104**, 471–7.

Ekström, P., Juchnicka, E., Laudanski, T., and Åkerlund, M. (1989). Effect of an oral contraceptive in primary dysmenorrhoea – changes in uterine activity and reactivity to agonists. *Contraception*, **49**, 39–47.

Ekström, P., Forsling, M., Kindahl, H., and Åkerlund, M. (1990). Perception of pain in primary dysmenorrhoea in relation to uterine activity and plasma concentrations of vasopressin and $PGF_{2\alpha}$ metabolite. *Proceedings of the Fourth International Conference on the Neurohypophysis. Journal of Neuroendocrinology*, Special Issue, 168–71.

Ekström, P., Alm, P., and Åkerlund, M. (1991). Differences in vasomotor responses between main stem and smaller branches of the human artery. *Acta Obstetrica et Gynecologica Scandinavica*, **70**, 429–33.

Ekström, P., Åkerlund, M. Forsling, M., Kindahl, H., Laudanski, T., and Mrugacz, G. (1992). Stimulation of vasopressin release in women with primary dysmenorrhoea and after oral contraceptive treatment – effect on uterine contractility. *British Journal of Obstetrics and Gynaecology*, **99**, 680–4.

Forsling, M.L., Åkerlund, M., and Strömberg, P. (1981). Variations in plasma concentrations of vasopressin during the menstrual cycle. *Journal of Endocrinology*, **89**, 263–6.

Forsling, M.L., Strömberg, P., and Åkerlund, M. (1982). Effect of ovarian steroids on vasopressin secretion. *Journal of Endocrinology*, **95**, 147–51.

Hauksson, A., Åkerlund, M., Forsling, M.L., and Kindahl, H. (1987). Plasma concentrations of vasopressin and a prostaglandin $F_{2\alpha}$ metabolite in women with primary dysmenorrhoea before and during treatment with a combined oral contraceptive. *Journal of Endocrinology*, **115**, 355–61.

Hauksson, A., Åkerlund M., and Melin P. (1988). Uterine blood-flow and myometrial activity at menstruation, and the influence of vasopressin and a synthetic antagonist. *British Journal of Obstetrics and Gynaecology*, **95**, 898–904.

Hauksson, A., Strömberg, P., Juchnicka, E., Laudanski, T., and Åkerlund, M. (1989). The influence of a combined oral contraceptive on uterine activity and reactivity to antagonists in primary dysmenorrhoea. *Acta Obstetrica et Gynecologica Scandinavica*, **68**, 31–4.

Lumsden, M.A., Kelly, R.W., and Baird, D.T. (1983). Primary dysmenorrhoea: the importance of both prostaglandins E_2 and $F_{2\alpha}$. *British Journal of Obstetrics Gynaecology*, **90**, 1135–40.

Lundström, V. and Green, K. (1978). Endogenous levels of prostaglandins $F_{2\alpha}$ and its main metabolites in plasma and the endometrium of normal and dysmenorrhoeic women. *American Journal of Obstetrics and Gynecology*, **130**, 640–6.

Lundström, V., Green, K., and Viqvist, N. (1976). Prostaglandins, indomethacin and dysmenorrhoea. *Prostaglandins*, **11**, 893–904.

Maggi, M., Magini, A., Fiscella, A., Giannini, S., Fantoni, G., Toffoletti, F., *et al.* (1992). Sex steroid modulation of neurohypophysial hormone receptors in human non-pregnant myometrium. *Journal of Clinical Endocrinology and Metabolism*, **74**, 385–92.

Melin, P., Trojnar, J., Johansson, B., Wilhardt, H., and Åkerlund M. (1986). Synthetic antagonists of the myometrial response to oxytocin and vasopressin. *Journal of Endocrinology*, **111**, 125–31.

Nigam, S., Benedetto, C., Zonca, M., Leo-Rossberg, I., Lübbert, H., and Hammerstein, J. (1991). Increased concentration of eicosanoids and platelet-activating factor in menstrual blood from women with primary dysmenorrhoea. *Eicosanoids*, **4**, 137–41.

Serradeil-Le-Gal, C., Bagnon, J., Garcia, C., Lacour, C., Guiraodou, P., Christophe, B., *et al.* (1993). Biochemical and pharmacological properties of SR49059, a new, potent, non-peptide antagonist of rat and human vasopressin VIa receptors. *Journal of Clinical Investigation*, **92**, 224–31.

Sivin, I. and Stern, J. (1994). Health during prolonged use of levonorgestrel 20 micrograms/d and the copper TCu 380Ag intrauterine contraceptive devices: a multicenter study. International Committee for Contraception Research (ICOR). *Fertility and Sterility*, **61**, 70–7.

Schwartz, A., Zor, U., Lindner, H.R., and Naor, S. (1974). Primary dysmenorrhoea. Alleviation by an inhibitor of prostaglandin synthesis and action. *Obstetrics and Gynecology*, **44**, 709–12.

Strömberg, P., Åkerlund, M., Forsling, M.L., Granström, E., and Kindahl, H. (1984). Vasopressin and prostaglandins in premenstrual pain and primary dysmenorrhoea. *Acta Obstetrics Gynecologica Scandinavica*, **63**, 533–8.

Strömberg, P., Åkerlund, M., Forsling, M.L., and Kindahl, H. (1983). Involvement of prostaglandins in vasopressin stimulation of the human uterus. *British Journal of Obstetrics Gynaecology*, **93**, 332–7.

Yamamura, Y., Ogawa, W.A., and Chihara, T. (1991). OPC-21268, an orally effective, non peptide vasopressin VIa receptor antagonist. *Science*, **252**, 572–4.

23 The clinical treatment of dysmenorrhoea

Mary Ann Lumsden

Introduction

Dysmenorrhoea is a significant clinical problem. Twenty-one per cent of women referred to gynaecological outpatient clinics with menstrual complaints have severe dysmenorrhoea without associated menorrhagia and in many of the remainder the complaint is associated with heavy menstrual blood loss (Warner 1995). Since women now experience up to 400 menstrual bleeds during their reproductive life the significance of the problem cannot be overstated and knowledge of the effective treatments available is essential.

The aetiology of dysmenorrhoea has already been discussed (Chapter 22). This review will focus on the clinical treatment of both primary and secondary dysmenorrhoea.

Primary dysmenorrhoea

Medical treatment

Primary dysmenorrhoea is amenable to treatment and a successful result should be obtained in 80 per cent of patients. The drugs most commonly used are described below. Acceptability of drug treatment is dependent upon the balance between efficacy and side-effects. The recommended drugs have a wide margin of safety with a low incidence of side-effects and are thus highly acceptable (Wenzloff and Shimp 1984).

Non-steroidal anti-inflammatory drugs (NSAIDs)

The non-steroidal anti-inflammatory agents (NSAIDs) revolutionized the treatment of dysmenorrhoea during the 1970s (Dingfelder 1981). These highly effective drugs work by the inhibition of prostaglandin synthesis. The analgesic effects are similar to those of paracetamol but the drugs also have anti-inflammatory effects and bind to receptors present in uterine tissues. There are a large number of members of this group of drugs and it is likely that most will be effective for the treatment of dysmenorrhoea. The drugs which are used most often are mefenamic acid and naproxen sodium, the latter being more commonly used in Scandinavia. In double-blind, placebo controlled, crossover studies, up to 94 per cent of women report a significant improvement or complete relief of their dysmenorrhoea with fenamates. The maximum recommended dose of mefenamic acid is 500 mg three times a day. As with all NSAIDs for the treatment of dysmenorrhoea, medication need only be given during menstruation itself. It should be stressed that the medication should be commenced at the onset of the period, or the pain, whichever comes first, and should be taken continuously. Treatment is less effective if it is delayed until the pain is more severe (Anderson 1981; Owen 1984).

Side-effects are rare when NSAIDs are given for only one or two days each month. However, these drugs should be used with caution in women with asthma and allergic disorders, or those with peptic ulceration.

Aspirin is a widely used drug with a low reported incidence of side-effects which is often used in the self medication for dysmenorrhoea. It is not as effective as other NSAIDs and is not the treatment of choice.

Combined oral contraceptive pill

This is the preferred treatment for young women who have dysmenorrhoea and also require effective contraception. Studies have demonstrated that the pill reduces uterine contractility as well as producing endometrial atrophy and reducing endometrial prostaglandin concentrations (Ekström *et al.* 1989). Contraindications for the use of the combined contraceptive pill have been extensively documented elsewhere. Furthermore, the potential adverse effects of long term use, including the risk of breast carcinoma, continue to be debated (UK National Case–Control Study Group 1989).

The efficacy and acceptability of NSAIDs and the combined oral contraceptive pill is so high that it is likely that the majority of young women will be effectively treated. If both of these treatments are unsuccessful then the patient should be investigated further to be certain that there is no underlying organic pathology. However, if investigations fail to yield pathology then the following treatments are available.

Progestogens

If a progestogen is prescribed in the second part of the menstrual cycle after ovulation then it may be helpful in treating dysmenorrhoea by promoting myometrial relaxation or inhibiting prostaglandin release. If prescribed prior to ovulation (for example from days 5 to 25 of the cycle) then it is likely to inhibit ovulation. Suggested regimens include dydrogesterone 10 mg twice a day, or norethisterone 5 mg three times a day. These drugs may be useful for women for whom estrogen is contraindicated or for those who do not wish to take the oral contraceptive pill. Side-effects are usually mild with nausea, headache, and bloating being the most common.

Nifedipine

The calcium antagonist nifedipine has been used widely in Scandinavia to treat dysmenorrhoea. It is an effective agent for inhibition of uterine contractility and can be given in doses of 20–40 mg with associated reduction in pain within 10–30 minutes (Ulmsten *et al.* 1978; Andersson and Ulmsten 1978). Side-effects including headache, flushing, and hypotension are common when the drug is used at high doses. These may preclude the therapy becoming widely accepted.

Beta adrenoceptor agonists

Beta$_2$ adrenoceptor agonists (β_2 sympathomimetics) relax uterine muscle and have been used widely in attempts to interrupt preterm labour. These agents have also been found to be effective in relieving spasmodic dysmenorrhoea (Akerlund *et al.* 1976). However, the use of these drugs is limited by their systemic side-effects which include tachycardia, palpitations, and hypotension. Beta adrenoceptor agonists are now rarely used in the modern management of dysmenorrhoea.

Danazol

Since dysmenorrhoea is a problem associated with menstruation any treatment causing amenorrhoea is likely to be effective. The agents most widely used in this context are danazol and the gonadotrophin-releasing hormone (GnRH) agonists.

Danazol is an androgenic steroid which produces endometrial atrophy and inhibits gonadotrophin output. At a daily dose of 400–800 mg, danazol induces amenorrhoea in the majority of women. Side-effects are common and have been extensively documented. They include weight gain, hirsutism, muscle cramps, headaches, and in severe cases, breast atrophy. However, it should be stressed that these effects are dose dependent and are much less common when doses of either 200 mg or 400 mg a day are given. A dose of 200 mg a day will often be accompanied by light bleeding which may be irregular in nature but which is rarely painful unless ovulation occurs.

The duration of administration of danazol is limited by side-effects which might also include adverse affects on lipid biochemistry. The manufacturers recommend that use of the drug should be restricted to three months.

Gonadotrophin-releasing hormone agonists

Two depot preparations are currently widely available in the United Kingdom, goserelin and leuprorelin acetate. Goserelin is given by monthly subcutaneous implant into the anterior abdominal wall whilst leuprorelin acetate is administered as an intramuscular injection. The efficacy and side-effects of the agonists are similar. Hypo-oestrogenic side-effects include hot flushes, night sweats, vaginal dryness, and bone mineral loss. Ten per cent of patients have breakthrough bleeding. The duration of administration is limited by the bone mineral loss (up to 10 per cent of bone mineral can be lost in six months) which can be attenuated by the concomitant administration of oestrogen/progestogen replacement therapy or tibolone.

In summary, the limiting factor for agents which induce amenorrhoea is that they can only be given for short periods of time. However, this may be useful to treat women with severe problems prior to definitive surgical treatment or to provide relief over a particularly difficult time in a patient's life.

Novel treatments

Oxytocin antagonists

Oxytocin antagonists are being developed for the treatment of pre-term labour and preliminary evidence suggests that they are effective in the treatment of dysmenorrhoea (see Chapter 22). The results of large-scale randomized controlled studies are awaited.

The levonorgestrel-intrauterine system (LNG-IUS)

It is possible that this new system will revolutionize the treatment of menstrual disorders (see Chapter 13). The preparation releases 20 μg of levonorgestrel daily which induces endometrial atrophy. In many patients, this is followed by a highly significant decrease in menstrual blood loss, which results in amenorrhoea in many patients, and a marked decrease in the complaint of dysmenorrhoea. The LNG-IUS is an effective contraceptive and also protects against pelvic infection. Side-effects are uncommon, the most troublesome being breakthrough bleeding which usually resolves within a few months. The system can be used long term and only requires replacement after five years (I-Cheng Chi 1991).

Transcutaneous nerve stimulation (TENS)

TENS is a good method of achieving pain relief without side-effects (Milsom *et al.* 1994; Kaplan *et al.* 1994). Though widely used as a means of analgesia in labour, TENS has not yet been used extensively to treat dysmenorrhoea.

Division of utero-sacral ligaments

This is easily performed using laser or electrocautery at the time of laparoscopy. The aim of the operation is to divide the nerve supply to and from the uterus. This does not appear to interfere with uterine function, but may well relieve the pain of dysmenorrhoea (Lichten and Bombard 1987; Gurgan *et al.* 1992).

Presacral neurectomy

This operation was performed by laparotomy in the first half of this century and the results of early studies suggested that it was effective in 60 per cent of women with intractable dysmenorrhoea (Ingersoll and Meigs 1948). More recently, the operation has also been carried out laparoscopically. A major complication is troublesome bleeding from presacral venous plexuses. The results of randomized studies assessing the effects of these procedures for the relief of dysmenorrhoea are awaited.

Secondary dysmenorrhoea

The causes of secondary dysmenorrhoea are shown in Table 1. In general, medical treatment is less successful in secondary dysmenorrhoea than primary dysmenorrhoea and involves either

Table 23.1 Causes of secondary dysmenorrhoea

Outflow obstruction	Müllerian duct abnormalties
	Cervical stenosis (e.g. after cone biopsy)
Intrauterine pathology	Fibroids
	Intrauterine contraceptive device
	Adenomyosis
	Endometrial polyps
Extrauterine pathology	Endometriosis
	Pelvic inflammatory disease
	Previous surgery
	Pelvic venous congestion

treatment of the associated condition or the induction of amenorrhoea. Surgery ranges from treatment of a specific underlying cause (such as the ablation of endometriotic deposits) to total abdominal hysterectomy and bilateral salpingo-oophorectomy (with the judicious prescription of estrogen replacement for younger women).

Endometriosis

Endometriosis is commonly associated with severe dysmenorrhoea, dysparunia, and pelvic pain. It is said that the dysmenorrhoea characteristically gets worse as menstruation proceeds, possibly due to bleeding from the ectopic endometrium. The dysmenorrhoea can be severe despite minimal disease. Effective symptomatic relief can be obtained using drugs such as progestogens, danazol, or GnRH analogues, which arrest growth of the endometriotic deposit. The choice of medication depends on the patient's tolerance of the side-effects. Relief of symptoms has been reported in many studies but the pain often recurs after discontinuation of therapy although the duration of the symptom-free interval is variable between patients and most do experience continuing relief for months after cessation of treatment.

Recent studies have addressed the use of laparoscopic laser ablation of endometriotic deposits along with the division of the utero-sacral ligaments for the treatment of endometriosis-associated pain (Sutton *et al.* 1994). Laparoscopic treatment was more effective than expectant management at the six-month follow-up visit. However, of five women in whom laparoscopic laser treatment failed, second-look laparoscopy after six to twelve months showed that three had pain in the absence of endometriosis whereas in two, the pain was not associated with the recurrence of treated endometriotic lesions, but with the development of new disease.

Pelvic infection

Active pelvic infection should always be treated by antibiotics, preferably after microbiological assessment. However, in situations where the problem becomes chronic then treatment may require induction of amenorrhoea. This may be achieved by either medical or surgical means.

Adenomyosis

This is a diagnosis usually made at hysterectomy and often accounts for treatment failures with either medical or ablative techniques. The diagnosis and treatment of adenomyosis is discussed in detail in Chapter 24.

Leiomyomata (fibroids)

Fibroids may cause dysmenorrhoea by affecting uterine contractility. Treatment is generally surgical (hysterectomy or myomectomy). Temporary relief from pain (and reduction in size of the fibroids) can be achieved using GnRH analogues, but the fibroids tend to grow again when the treatment is stopped (see Chapters 16 and 17). Alternatively, GnRH analogues can be used as preoperative adjuncts to shrink fibroids prior to hysterectomy or myomectomy (Lumsden *et al.* 1994).

Uterine abnormality

Several reports have described partial resolution of dysmenorrhoea following surgery to correct uterine abnormalities. However, the studies have been uncontrolled and the management of women with such uterine abnormalities must take other factors into account such as plans for future fertility (Fedele *et al.* 1994).

Surgical management

Surgery can be helpful in the treatment of dysmenorrhoea, although it is usual to try medical treatments first. In women with other menstrual problems for whom continuing fertility is not an issue, dysmenorrhoea may be an indication for hysterectomy. Other options are endometrial ablation, presacral neurectomy, and division of the utero-sacral ligaments.

Hysterectomy

Hysterectomy is an effective, definitive treatment for menstrual problems of all types. It may be performed abdominally or vaginally (with or without laparoscopic assistance). It is suitable for women who have completed their family and who wish to have an effective treatment resulting in amenorrhoea. The operation is associated with a high incidence of complications although most of these are minor. Wound or urinary tract infections occur in 10 per cent of cases. It has been suggested that vaginal hysterectomy is associated with a lower complication rate and a shorter recovery time after operation as a result of avoiding a large abdominal incision, though comparisons should be interpreted with caution due to selection bias (Dicker *et al.* 1982). Recently it has become possible to convert an abdominal hysterectomy to a vaginal procedure by completing part of the operation laparoscopically (Reich *et al.* 1989). This allows pelvic pathology to be dealt with and ovaries to be removed at vaginal hysterectomy in women where there is little uterine descent. There is much controversy over the place of this particular operation which is currently being evaluated.

Endometrial ablation

Endometrial ablation is a good surgical treatment for menorrhagia. However, it appears less successful for the treatment of dysmenorrhoea. In an audit of 1000 cases of endometrial ablation performed in Scotland over a two-year period it was found that 40 per cent of women had relief of their dysmenorrhoea as a result of an effective ablation. However, 12 per cent reported pain that was more severe or pain that started for the first time post-operatively. It is possible that pain arising after the operation is due to the formation of haematometra, particularly at the cornua. It was concluded that if dysmenorrhoea is the predominant symptom then endometrial ablation is not the treatment of choice (Scottish Hysteroscopy Audit Group 1995).

Summary

Dysmenorrhoea is a common clinical problem which can usually be treated effectively and safely. Its importance lies in the large number of women who are regularly affected by its social and economic sequelae. In young women, dysmenorrhoea is normally primary in nature and is due to over-production within the endometrium of agents, such as prostaglandin $F_{2\alpha}$, which contract both vascular and myometrial smooth muscle to cause ischaemic pain. This type of dysmenorrhoea should be treated using non-steroidal anti-inflammatory agents or the oral contraceptive pill. The existence of underlying organic pathology, such as leiomyomata, endometriosis/adenomyosis, or pelvic adhesions, is more likely in older women where treatment should be directed towards the specific cause.

References

Akerlund, M., Andersson, K.E., and Ingemarsson, I. (1976). Effects of terbutaline on myometrial activity, uterine blood flow, and lower abdominal pain in women with primary dysmenorrhoea. *British Journal of Obstetrics and Gynaecology*, **83**, 673–8.

Anderson, A. (1981). The role of prostaglandin synthetase inhibitors in gynaecology. *Practitioner*, **225**, 1460–70.

Andersson, K.-E. and Ulmsten, U. (1978). Effects of nifedipine of myometrial activity and lower abdominal pain in women with primary dysmenorrhoea. *British Journal of Obstetrics and Gynaecology*, **85**, 142–8.

Dicker, R.C., Greenspan, J.R., Strauss, L.T., Cowart, M.R., Scally, M.J., Peterson, H.B. *et al.* (1982). Complications of abdominal and vaginal hysterectomy among women of reproductive age in the United States. *American Journal of Obstetrics and Gynecology*, **144**, 841–8.

Dingfelder, J.R. (1981). Primary dysmenorrhoea treatment with prostaglandin inhibitors. *American Journal of Obstetrics and Gynaecology*, **140**, 874–9.

Ekström, P., Junicka, E., Laudanski, T., and Akerlund, M. (1989). Effect of an oral contraceptive in primary dysmenorrhoea – changes in uterine activity and reactivity to agonists. *Contraception*, **40**, 39–47.

Fedele, L., Bianchi, S., Bocciolone, L., Di Nola, G., Arcaini, L., and Franchi, D. (1994). Relief of dysmenorrhoea associated with septate uteri after abdominal or hysteroscopic metroplasty. *Acta Obstetrics Gynecology Scandinavica*, **73**, 56–8.

Gurgan, T., Urman, B., Aksu, T., Develioglu, O., Zeyneloglu, H., and Kisnisci, H.A. (1992). Laparoscopic CO_2 laser uterine nerve ablation for treatment of drug resistant primary dysmenorrhea. *Fertility and Sterility*, **58**, 422–4.

I-Cheng Chi, P.H. (1991). An evaluation of the levonorgestrel-releasing IUD: its advantages and disadvantages when compared to the copper-releasing IUDs. *Contraception*, **44**, 573–87.

Ingersoll, F.M. and Meigs, J.V. (1948). Presacral neurectomy for dysmenorrhea. *New England Journal of Medicine*, **238**, 357–60.

Kaplan, B., Peled, Y., Pardo, J., Raberinson, D., Hirsch, M., Ovadia, J., and Neri, A. (1994). Transcutanous electrical nerve stimulation (TENS) as a relief for dysmenorrhoea. *Clinical and Experimental Obstetrics and Gynaecology*, **21**, 87–90.

Lichten, E.M. and Bombard, J. (1987). Surgical treatment of primary dysmenorrhea with laparoscopic uterine nerve ablation. *Journal of Reproductive Medicine*, **32**, 37–41.

Lumsden, M.A., West, C.P., Thomas, E., Coutts, J., Hillier, H., Thomas, N., and Baird, D.T. (1994). Treatment with the gonadotrophin releasing hormone-agonist goserelin before hysterectomy for uterine fibroids. *British Journal of Obstetrics and Gynaecology*, **101**, 438–42.

Milsom, I., Hedner, N., and Mannheimer, C. (1994). A comparative study of the effect of high-intensity transcutaneous nerve stimulation and oral naproxen on intrauterine pressure and menstrual pain in patients with primary dysmenorrhea. *American Journal of Obstetrics and Gynaecology*, **170**, 123–9.

Owen, P.R. (1984). Prostaglandin synethetase inhibitors in the treatment of primary dysmenorrhea. *American Journal of Obstetrics and Gynaecology*, **148**, 96–103.

Reich, H.J., De Caprio, J, and McGlynn, F. (1989). Laparoscopic hysterectomy. *Journal of Gynecological Surgery*, **5**, 213–16.

Scottish Hysteroscopy Audit Group (1995). A Scottish audit of hysteroscopic surgery for menorrhagia: complications and follow up. *British Journal of Obstetrics and Gynaecology*, **102**, 249–54.

Sutton, C.J., Ewen, S.P., Whitelaw, N., and Haynes, P. (1994). Prospective randomised double-blind controlled trial of laser laparoscopy in the treatment of pelvic pain associated with minimal, mild and moderate endometriosis. *Fertility and Sterility*, **62**, 696–700.

UK National Case–Control Study Group (1989). Oral contraceptive use and breast cancer risk in young women. *Lancet*, **i**, 973–82.

Ulmsten, U., Andersson, K.-E., and Forman, A. (1978). Relaxing effects of nifedipine in the non-pregnant human uterus *in vitro* and *in vivo*. *Obstetrics and Gynaecology*, **52**, 436–41.

Warner, P. (1995). Characteristics of women referred for menstrual problems. In *Psychosomatic obstetrics and gynaecology* (ed. J. Bitzer and M. Stauber), pp. 335–42. Monduzze, Bologna, Italy.

Wenzloff, N.J. and Shimp, L. (1984). Therapeutic management of primary dysmenorrhoea. *Drug Intelligence and Clinical Pharmacology*, **18**, 22–6.

24 Adenomyosis uteri

Jan J. Brosens and Ivo A. Brosens

Introduction

Traditionally, the term adenomyosis denotes the presence of endometrial glands and stroma deep within the myometrium. Until recently, the diagnosis could only be made after hysterectomy by which time its clinical relevance was merely academic. This is not the only reason why adenomyosis has been neglected in the last few decades. The wide range of pathological criteria used to define adenomyosis, and differences in myometrial sampling, have hindered many attempts to correlate the presence of these ectopic endometrial foci with a specific clinical syndrome. Although adenomyosis is apparently associated with menorrhagia and dysmenorrhoea, current confusion is so profound that some even doubt its clinical relevance.

With new imaging and biopsy techniques, the ability to diagnose adenomyosis *in vivo* has generated renewed clinical and scientific interest. Recent studies using molecular and cellular markers have provided new insights into the pathophysiology of adenomyosis and although our understanding is still limited, it is clear that adenomyosis can no longer be regarded as merely the presence of ectopic endometrium. It is also a myoproliferative disease of the inner myometrium and is further characterized by an altered local paracrine and immune microenvironment.

Pathology

The definition of adenomyosis, namely the presence of endometrial foci in the myometrium, appears straightforward but the precise histopathological criteria have been the subject of considerable controversy. Lesions in the outer two-thirds of the myometrium will pose no diagnostic difficulties, but glands and stroma within the inner layer of the myometrium can sometimes be indistinguishable from normal indentations of the basal endometrial layer. The common approach to this problem is to insist on a minimum depth of myometrial invasion and current criteria range widely from the presence of glands and stroma 1 mm below the endometrial–myometrial junction to as deep as one third of the total myometrial thickness (Fig. 24.1), (Azziz 1989). Others have suggested that the diagnosis can be made confidently if the superficial implant is surrounded by myometrium showing some degree of hyperplasia (Hendrickson *et al.* 1987). These myoproliferative changes, characterized by dense and poorly orientated myocytes, are often difficult to delineate with routine light-optical microscopy and appear absent from post-menopausal uteri and during pregnancy (Sandberg and Cohn 1962; Hendrickson *et al.* 1987).

Many pathologists do not consider superficial adenomyosis a significant clinico-pathological entity and consequently do not report it (Hendrickson *et al.* 1987). There are several reasons for this. First, superficial implants are not always easy to distinguish from tangential sectioning of an

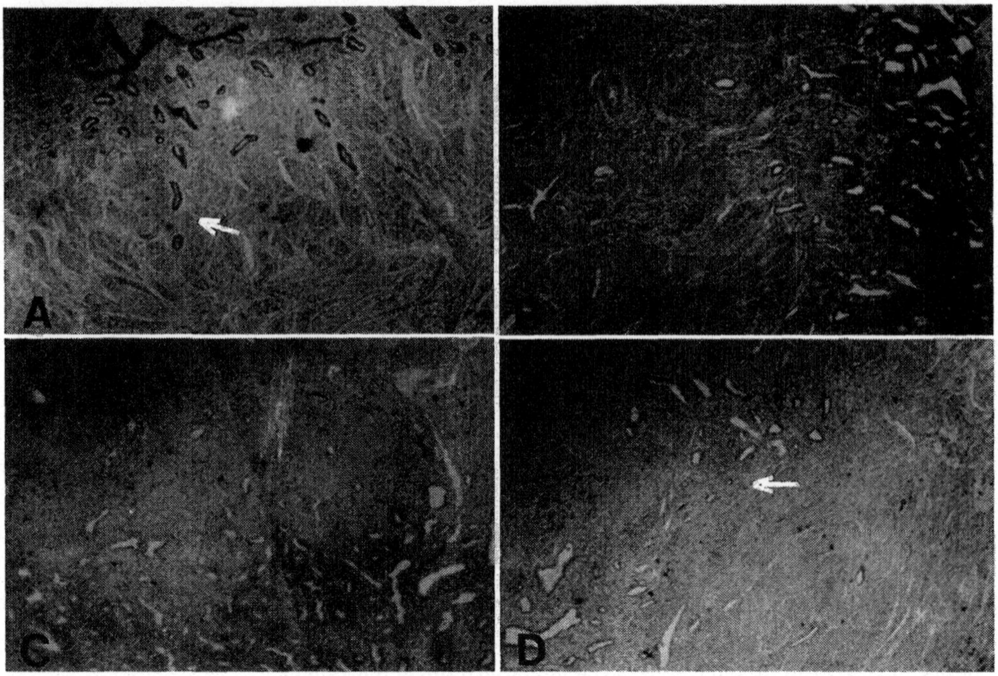

Fig. 24.1 Adenomyosis or not? (a) Normal irregular endometrial–myometrial interface with some glands penetrating into the subendometrial myometrium (arrow). (b), (c) Although the endometrial penetration into the myometrium remains very superficial, the underlying myometrium appears more compact and hyperplastic. The pre-operative MR appearance of hysterectomy specimen (c) showed extensive changes of the junctional zone. Only superficial adenomyosis was present on histology. (d) Large adenomyotic implant (arrow) deep in the myometrium. Haematoxylin and eosin stain, magnification was × 75.

irregular endometrial–myometrial junction. Second, islets in the subendometrial myometrium are invariably basal and largely unresponsive to cyclical changes in ovarian steroids. Unlike deep adenomyosis, focal haemorrhage in these superficial implants is rare and the myometrium is often not grossly distorted. Consequently, the apparent lack of a link between these superficial implants and symptoms like menorrhagia and dysmenorrhea has cast doubt on their significance. Finally, additional pelvic pathology is often found with adenomyotic uteri. For instance, uterine fibroids are present in 20 to 55 per cent of the cases and these additional findings often provide a more ready explanation for the symptomatology (Azziz 1989).

The hormonal responsiveness of eutopic endometrium increases from the basal layer to the functional zone and, to a certain extent, the response of ectopic glandular epitheliums also depends on its location. Inner myometrial implants are almost always basal but in the outer myometrium, partially secretory glands can sometimes be identified, often lying side by side with unresponsive glands. A full secretory response to endogenous or exogenous hormones is rarely seen. In the gravid uterus, decidualization is common in deep but rare in superficial implants (Sandberg and Cohn 1962). Furthermore, the density of the implants is greater in deep lesions suggesting higher proliferative activity. Coinciding with this is an increased tendency for focal haemorrhage in these deep lesions.

Adenomyosis is often classified into a diffuse and focal form. Focal adenomyosis, also termed adenomyoma, refers to isolated implants surrounded by often extensive but focal smooth muscle changes. It is less common than diffuse adenomyosis and not accompanied by a characteristic distortion of the inner myometrium (de Souza *et al.* 1995). It remains to be determined whether these lesions are really related to diffuse adenomyosis or represent a different pathological process such as Müllerian rests. Almost a hundred years ago, von Recklinghausen observed that ectopic mucosal implants were more commonly found in the posterior wall of the uterus and this has been confirmed by several other studies (Rokitansky 1860; Halvorsen and Moen 1993).

Prevalence

It is generally accepted that adenomyosis is a disease that mainly affects multiparous women in late reproductive life and the perimenopause. Seventy to 80 per cent of pathologically confirmed cases are indeed found in women in their fourth and fifth decades. Conversely, only 5 to 25 per cent of cases are reported in patients younger than 39 years, and 5 to 10 per cent occur in women older than 60 years. Eighty to 90 per cent of adenomyotic uteri are found in multiparous women (Azziz 1989; Vercellini *et al.* 1993). However, it is important to remember that these data are derived from pathological examination of extirpated uteri. Therefore it is not unexpected that the demographic trends in hysterectomy are similar to those mentioned for the prevalence of adenomyosis, namely with a peak incidence in multiparous patients in their late forties. Only one published study can be regarded as free of this bias. In 1931 Lewinski carried out a post-mortem study on 54 women who died from non-gynaecological causes (Lewinski 1931). Their ages ranged from less than 20 to more than 70 years old. Adenomyosis was found in 29 cases (54 per cent) and re-analysing the original data of this small study, Vercellini *et al.* found no difference in the incidence between various age groups (Vercellini *et al.* 1993).

Selection bias is not the only reason why it has been difficult to determine the true incidence of adenomyosis. Differences in myometrial sampling and the wide range of diagnostic criteria used to define adenomyosis are also important confounding factors. The first point is elegantly illustrated by the experience of Bird and co-workers, (Bird *et al.* 1972). After examining routine histological sections of 200 consecutive hysterectomy specimens, they found that 31 per cent of them harboured adenomyosis. However, if six extra blocks of myometrium were examined from six predetermined sites, the incidence rose sharply to 61 per cent. In most series, however, the reported incidence in unselected hysterectomy specimens ranges from 8 to 27 per cent (Azziz 1989). The introduction of new diagnostic techniques in daily practice will not only make a more systematic study possible but is also likely to challenge the concept of adenomyosis as a disease of the older, multiparous woman. For instance, the average age of women with magnetic resonance (MR) characteristics of adenomyosis in the limited study of de Souza *et al.* was only 34.4 years (SD ± 2.8 years) and 10 of 14 patients (71 per cent) were nulliparous (de Souza *et al.* 1995).

Signs and symptoms

Since the publication of Thomas Cullen's famous monograph in 1908, it has become axiomatic that a progressive, uniform enlargement of the uterus accompanied by menorrhagia and dysmenorrhoea is diagnostic of uterine adenomyosis (Cullen 1908). If the clinical picture were as uniform and simple as this statement implies then clinical diagnosis would pose few difficulties.

In reality, only 10 to 20 per cent of the cases are diagnosed pre-operatively. On the other hand, the pathological confirmation of clinically suspected cases is also low (10 to 38 per cent) and on the basis of this low verification rate, some have argued that the clinical diagnosis of adenomyosis can no longer be considered as a reliable pre-operative indication for hysterectomy (Azziz 1989; Vercellini *et al.* 1993; Gambone *et al.* 1990).

Several clinicopathological studies have suggested that the symptoms correlate with the depth of endometrial infiltration into the myometrium. Bird and co-workers found that superficial penetration was often the only significant finding in women who suffered from menorrhagia and they applied the term 'adenomyosis subbasalis' to this entity (Bird *et al.* 1972). Similar observations were made by McCausland and Fraser who reported separately a high incidence of superficial adenomyosis in women with dysfunctional uterine bleeding (60 and 40 per cent respectively) (McCausland 1991; Fraser 1994). Dysmenorrhoea is not associated with superficial implants and is therefore less common, affecting 20 to 30 per cent of patients with adenomyosis (Sandberg and Cohn 1962; Vercellini *et al.* 1993). Its incidence correlates with the depth and extent of endometrial penetration into the myometrium and it has been claimed that the onset of severe dysmenorrhoea requires a depth that exceeds 80 per cent of the total muscle thickness (Benson and Sneeden 1958; Nishida 1991).

Others have challenged the concept that adenomyosis is an important clinical entity. Kilkku *et al.* prospectively interviewed patients undergoing hysterectomy for benign pelvic disease (Kilkku and Erkolla 1984). They found no difference in frequency or severity of uterine bleeding, dysmenorrhoea, or pelvic pain between 28 women with histologically proven adenomyosis and 157 without, and concluded that symptoms attributed to adenomyosis were heterogeneous, non-specific, and probably related to coincidental pathology. Furthermore, not all adenomyotic uteri are thought to be symptomatic. In a retrospective review of the clinical notes of 701 cases of adenomyotic uteri, Benson and Sneeden reported that 16 per cent of the cases were 'incidental' (Benson and Sneeden 1958). A prospective study by Lee and co-workers appears to confirm this observation as adenomyosis was found in 20 per cent of uteri removed for prolapse (Lee *et al.* 1984). This study was, however, designed to correlate preoperative and pathological diagnoses and not to analyse symptomatology.

It is frequently stated that adenomyosis is a cause of infertility but there is as yet little objective evidence available to substantiate this claim. Using magnetic resonance imaging, de Souza and co-workers reported that 14 of 26 women (53.8 per cent) with infertility and symptoms of menorrhagia or dysmenorrhoea had lesions characteristic of adenomyosis (de Souza *et al.* 1995). This high incidence does not necessarily imply a causal relationship between adenomyosis and reproductive failure. In some cases, smooth muscle hyperplasia around implants in the cornua can cause proximal tubal obstruction and mimic salpingitis isthmica nodosa. Moreover, Ota and co-workers reported that high titres of antiphospholipid auto-antibodies are present in women with adenomyosis as often as in those with endometriosis, but the significance of these auto-antibodies in infertility remains unresolved (Ota *et al.* 1992). In a study of 151 uteri obtained at the time of Caesarean hysterectomy, mainly for the purpose of sterilization, adenomyotic implants were encountered in 27 specimens (17.2 per cent) (Sandberg and Cohn 1962). Its relatively high prevalence in pregnancy seems to be in conflict with claims that adenomyosis is an important cause of infertility. Except for a handful of case reports, there is no evidence that adenomyosis is associated with obstetrical problems (Azziz 1989).

Pathophysiology

The normal endometrial–myometrial interface

Microscopically, the normal endometrial–myometrial junction (EMJ) is irregular with tongues of endometrial glands and stroma interdigitating with the superficial myometrium. At the cellular level, the EMJ not only consists of smooth muscle, endometrial epithelial cells, and stromal fibroblasts but also of myofibroblasts and distinct aggregates of lymphoid cells (Fujii *et al.* 1989; Stewart *et al.* 1992). Myofibroblasts are ultrastucturally intermediate between smooth muscle cells and stromal fibroblasts. Electron microscopical studies of the developing fetal uterus suggest that myofibroblasts and endometrial stromal fibroblasts both originate from multipotent mesenchymal cells surrounding the fused paramesonephric ducts. Mature smooth muscle represents a stage of further differentiation. Unlike skeletal muscle cells, mature myocytes have the ability to re-enter the cell cycle *in vivo* and *in vitro*; a process which is associated with morphological dedifferentiation towards the phenotype of a fibroblast or myofibroblast (Draeger *et al.* 1993). At present the biological role of these smooth muscle-like cells at the normal EMJ remains unclear (Draeger *et al.* 1993).

Lymphoid aggregates in the endometrium are confined to the EMJ and consist mainly of activated CD3-positive T cells (Tabibzadeh *et al.* 1993). Recently, it has become clear that these cells play an important role in polarizing the endometrium. Not only the phenotypical responsiveness to sex steroids but also the proliferative activity of the endometrium is maximal in the functional layer and gradually diminishes towards the basalis. The low proliferative activity in the basal layer is associated with a markedly increased human leukocyte class II antigen (HLA-DR) expression by the glandular epithelium in this layer. Tabibzadeh and co-workers elegantly demonstrated *in vitro* that interferon–gamma (IFNγ) released by activated T cells can induce high HLA-DR expression in endometrial epithelial cells and dramatically inhibit their proliferative activity (Tabibzadeh *et al.* 1993). Furthermore, the effect of IFNγ gradually diminishes with increasing distance between the endometrial epithelial cells and the source of this cytokine.

Myometrial zonal anatomy

Evidence of a polarized microenvironment not only exists in the endometrium but also in the myometrium. Magnetic resonance studies of the uterus have revealed two distinct zones within the myometrium: the subendometrial myometrium or junctional zone (JZ) and the outer myometrium. Although there is no obvious histological zonal equivalent on light microscopy, morphometric studies have demonstrated that the JZ represents the innermost layer of the myometrium and, in comparison with the outer myometrium, there is a three-fold increase in nuclear area, a decreased extracellular matrix per unit volume, and a lower water content (McCarthy *et al.* 1989; Scoutt *et al.* 1991; Brown *et al.* 1991). The increased nuclear area reflects both an increased nucleo-cytoplasmatic ratio of the myocytes and an increased smooth muscle density.

The MR appearance of the uterine zonal anatomy is dependent on ovarian sex steroids. In premenarchal girls and post-menopausal women, the zonal anatomy is often indistinct, and in the reproductive years ovarian suppression with gonadotrophin-releasing hormone analogues leads to an MR appearance of the uterus mimicking that of a post-menopausal woman (Andreyko *et al.* 1988). Conversely, hormone replacement therapy in post-menopausal women results in a reappearance of the uterine zones. Although these observations seem to suggest a direct effect of sex steroids on the uterine zonal anatomy there is, to the best of our knowledge, no evidence for regional variation in oestrogen or progesterone receptor expression in myocytes. An alternative explantation is that the myometrial zonal polarization depends on juxtacrine interaction with the basal endometrial layer. Focal disruption of the JZ, observed with intrauterine but not ectopic pregnancy, provides some support for this hypothesis (Barton *et al.* 1993; Turnbull *et al.* 1995).

The subendometrial myometrium is not only structurally but also functionally different from the outer myometrium. In the non-gravid uterus, myometrial contractions emanate only from this layer and their orientation, amplitude, and frequency correlate with the phase of the menstrual cycle (de Vries *et al.* 1990). In the follicular and periovulatory phases retrograde propagated subendometrial contractions from the isthmus to the fundus can be observed, the amplitude and frequency of which increase as the cycle progresses towards ovulation. Dysrhythmic myometrial activity is present during the luteal phase, but during menstruation anterograde propagated subendometrial contractions from the fundus to the cervix can be seen.

The mechanisms coordinating these cycle-dependent contractions of the inner myometrium remain to be determined. Although very little focused research has been reported in this area, several cytokines have been identified which can potentially modulate the myometrial zonal differentiation and function. For instance, epidermal growth factor is not only a potent mitogen for myometrial smooth muscle cells but can also induce uterine contractions *in vitro*, both in intact tissue and in isolated myometrial cells (Gardner and Stancel 1989). Specific binding sites for endothelins have also been found in the myometrium and in tissue bath experiments endothelin-1 markedly increased contractility of myometrial strips (Bacon *et al.* 1995). Interestingly, the greatest density of endothelin binding sites is found on glandular epithelium in the EMJ and recent evidence suggests that endothelins in the endometrium can induce release of prostaglandin $F_{2\alpha}$ and further endothelins, in a paracrine and autocrine fashion. These factors are potent uterotonins in non-gravid uteri and may therefore mediate the contractions of the underlying myometrium in a juxtacrine fashion.

Pathogenesis

Adenomyosis is a disease characterized by disruption of the endometrial–myometrial interface with loss of normal uterine polarity, with smooth muscle proliferation and an altered local immune micro-environment. The traditional view that the smooth muscle proliferation is secondary to infiltration of endometrial elements has been challenged by the observations of Mori and co-workers who developed an animal model for adenomyosis (Mori *et al.* 1984, 1991). In this mouse model, intrauterine pituitary isografting was associated with a rapid induction of adenomyosis-like changes and ultrastructural studies revealed that the first step in the morphogenesis of adenomyosis is the dedifferentiation of myocytes with breakdown of the subendometrial smooth muscle layer, followed by migration of endometrial stromal cells and glandular elements.

Others, in the light of the close embryonic kinship between myocytes, myofibroblasts, and stromal fibroblasts, have suggested a metaplastic process in the pathogenesis of adenomyotic foci (Emge 1962).

Myoproliferative changes

In contrast to the patchy and focal infiltration of endometrial elements, the myoproliferative changes often affect the entire inner myometrium as demonstrated by diffuse thickening of the junctional zone on MR imaging. These smooth muscle changes are likely to compromise the cycle-dependent contractions of the inner myometrial layer. In support of this contention is the observation that, compared to non-pathological myometrium, the spontaneous motility of isolated myometrial strips from adenomyotic uteri is altered (Martinez-Mir *et al.* 1990). Some authors have postulated a role for the periovulatory retrograde subendometrial contractions in sperm transport through the genital tract (de Vries *et al.* 1990). The role of anterograde contractions in controlling menstrual flow and venous engorgement remains to be determined, but if important, then loss of normal subendometrial motility may contribute to excessive menstrual loss.

A recent study reported on the direction of the inner myometrial contraction waves during menstruation in women with and without endometriosis (Salamanca and Beltrán 1995). Interestingly, retrograde contractions were observed in almost 90 per cent of the patients with endometriosis but in only in 5 per cent of the controls. Conversely, anterograde waves were present in 85 per cent of the normal women but absent in all women with endometriosis. If confirmed, then these observations would strongly imply that inner myometrial dysfunction may result in excessive retrograde menstruation and in endometriosis.

Immunological factors

There are several lines of evidence that support a role for the immune system in the pathogenesis of adenomyosis. Ota and co-workers have demonstrated that adenomyosis is associated with increased numbers of myometrial macrophages, elevated antiphospolipid auto-antibodies and CA 125 levels in peripheral blood, and deposition of IgG, C3, and C4 in ectopic foci (Ota *et al.* 1992). Peripheral CA 125 (carcinogen antigen 125) levels are potentially useful as a serum marker for adenomyosis. Kobayashi and co-workers found that CA 125 antigens present on adenomyotic epithelial cells have a different molecular mass from those present on eutopic endometrium (Kobayashi *et al.* 1993). The antibody (OC 125) binding site is, however, the same. If an antibody unique to adenomyosis could be isolated and purified then a highly specific serum screening test could be developed. Adenomyotic uteri are also characterized by increased HLA-DR antigen expression in both eutopic and ectopic glandular cells, an observation that provides circumstantial evidence for a role for the T-cell lymphoid aggregates in the pathogenesis of the disease (Ota and Igarashi 1993).

Receptors and local hormonal environment

Few studies have focused on receptor expression in ectopic foci. Using a radio-ligand binding assay, Tamaya *et al.* reported differences in oestrogen and progesterone receptor expression in adenomyotic tissue samples (Tamaya *et al.* 1979). Oestrogen receptors were found in all samples examined but progesterone receptors were detected in only some, and when detected their concentration was lower than that of oestrogen receptors. Horie and co-workers demonstrated positive nuclear immunostaining for androgen receptor in eutopic and ectopic glandular and stromal cells but not in the myometrium (Horie *et al.* 1992). Interestingly, Lei *et al.* reported that adenomyotic glands express more immunoreactive hCG/LH receptor protein and mRNA than corresponding eutopic glands (Lei *et al.* 1993). The functional significance of this pattern of receptor expression is unknown but it may imply that certain hormonal conditions, such as those found during pregnancy, may promote endometrial infiltration. The expression of cell adhesion molecules has not yet been studied systematically but Lei and co-workers found no difference in immunostaining for cadherin, a cell adhesion receptor, between infiltrating and non-infiltrating glands (Lei *et al.* 1993).

Adenomyosis is further characterized by an altered local hormonal microenvironment. Compared to eutopic endometrium from normal uteri, adenomyotic tissues demonstrate increased aromatase and oestrone sulphatase activities, and elevated oestradiol levels in menstrual but not in peripheral blood of women with adenomyosis have been found (Takahashi *et al.* 1989; Yamamoto *et al.* 1993). The lymphoid cells in the EMJ also express oestrogen receptor and oestrogen has been shown to increase potently the activity of the IFNγ promoter in these cells (Fox *et al.* 1991). These lines of evidence are pertinent as they suggest that adenomyosis may be the result of a breakdown in the cross-talk between the local paracrine and immune microenvironments.

Prostaglandins

Adenomyotic foci are capable of prostaglandin (PG) synthesis as demonstrated by the intense immunostaining for cyclo-oxygenase, the rate-limiting enzyme in the PG pathway, in ectopic glandular epithelium (Van Voorhis *et al.* 1990). Excessive production of $PGF_{2\alpha}$ can cause uterine spasms and ischaemic pain and may explain why the incidence of dysmenorrhoea increases with increasing depth and density of endometrial implants in the myometrium.

Conversely, Koike and co-workers demonstrated that 6-keto-prostaglandin $F_{1\alpha}$ production in myometrial implants is significantly higher than that in endometrium, myometrium, or fibroids, especially during menstruation (Koike *et al.* 1992). $PGF_{1\alpha}$ is the inactive, stable metabolite of prostacyclin (PGI_2), a potent vasodilator and inhibitor of platelet aggregation which may contribute to the increased haemorrhagic potential of deeper lesions. Moreover, the eutopic endometrial production of the vasodilator prostaglandins PGE_2 and PGI_2 is also increased in the presence of adenomyosis and may further impair the mechanisms governing normal menstrual flow (Cameron *et al.* 1987).

Diagnosis

Adenomyosis will escape recognition if it is not considered. But because of the low precision of the clinical diagnosis, it is important to confirm the presumptive diagnosis prior to intervention. Historically, repeated bimanual examinations over a period of months, and from time to time just before and after a menstruation were recommended. In this way fluctuating changes in contour, size, and consistency of the uterus which typify extensive adenomyosis could be detected. In 1933, Halban further suggested administration of large doses of oestrogen during the second half of the menstrual cycle (Emge 1962). These not only aggravate menorrhagia and intensify fluctuations in the size of the uterus but also emphasize the presence of small knob-like elevations detectable in the outer layer of the myometrium.

The gross myometrial distortion which may accompany adenomyosis sometimes allows the diagnosis to be suspected at the time of laparoscopy or hysteroscopy. Mild and moderate adeno-

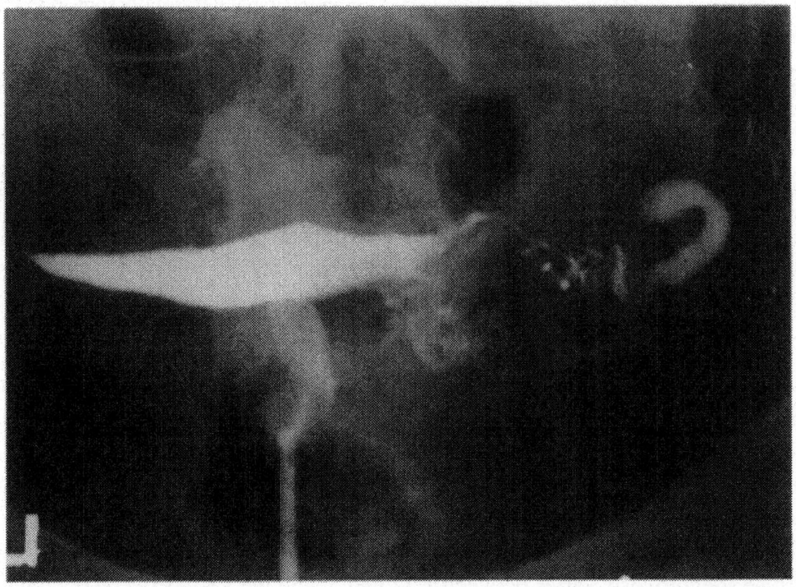

Fig. 24.2 Hysterosalpingogram in a patient with extensive adenomyosis. Contrast medium infiltrates the myometrium focally. Radiological signs of salpingitis isthmica nodosa and hydrosalpinx are present in the right Fallopian tube.

myosis cannot be diagnosed visually, and even extensive adenomyosis can be difficult to differentiate from multiple small fibroids.

Hysterography has been used in the diagnosis of adenomyosis. The most striking diagnostic feature is the demonstration of short, spicule-like structures extending perpendicularly from the borders of the uterine cavity (Fig. 24.2). However, the sensitivity of this technique is low as demonstrated by the study of Marshak and Eliasoph who could establish the diagnosis in only 38 of 150 cases with histologically proven adenomyosis (Marshak and Eliasoph 1955).

Ultrasonography

In recent years, ultrasound has been increasingly used to diagnose adenomyosis and the transvaginal approach is superior to abdominal sonography. Although adenomyotic uteri tend to be larger with asymmetrical thickening of the anterior and posterior walls, uterine morphometry alone is insufficient for the diagnosis (Brosens *et al.* 1995). Disease is best predicted on the basis of ill-defined myometrial areas with a heterogeneous echotexture. In extensive disease, small anechoic lakes of 1–3 mm diameter are sometimes detected. Lakes of this size are at the limit of ultrasonographic resolution and may represent larger cystic implants or, more likely, focal intramyometrial haemorrhage. Detecting areas of heterogeneous echogenicity within the myometrium is often complicated by the presence of various artefactual echogenic shadows and compounded by the presence of leiomyomata.

Three studies have compared endovaginal ultrasonography with light microscopy or MR imaging and the results are summarized in Table 24.1 (Brosens *et al.* 1995; Fedele *et al.* 1992; Ascher *et al.* 1994; Mark *et al.* 1987; Togashi *et al.* 1989). The prevalence of adenomyosis in these studies was high, probably reflecting the strict selection criteria. We have therefore

Table 24.1 Specificity, sensitivity, and likelihood ratios of endovaginal ultrasonography in the diagnosis of adenomyosis

	Prevalence (%)	Sensitivity (%)	Specificity (%)	LR+	LR–
Fedele *et al.* (1992)	22/43 (51)	80	74	5	0.27
Brosens *et al.* (1995)	28/56 (50)	53	75	2.12	0.63
Ascher *et al.* (1994)	17/20 (85)	86	50	1.72	0.28

The likelihood ratio of a positive test (LR+) is calculated as [sensitivity/(1 – specificity)' and the likelihood ratio of a negative test (LR-) as [)1 – sensitivity)/specificity].

re-analysed the data and calculated the likelihood ratios (LR). Likelihood ratios, in contrast to the more conventially used positive and negative predictive values, are not affected by the prevalence of the disease in the population studied. Calculation of LRs yields a score that allows categorization of test results: a LR+ between 2 and 5 indicates a fair clinical test, between 5 and 10 is good, and greater than 10 is excellent. An LR– between 0.5 and 0.2 indicates a fair clinical test, between 0.2 and 0.1 is good, and less than 0.1 is excellent. The LR+ of endovaginal ultrasonography in diffuse adenomyosis varies between 1.72 and 5, and the LR– between 0.27 and 0.63. So at present, endovaginal ultrasound can be regarded as a useful tool in trained hands when the clinical suspicion is high, but insufficiently accurate to be used as a screening device.

Magnetic resonance imaging

Magnetic resonance (MR) imaging has proved to be an excellent non-invasive imaging modality for evaluating the female pelvis and because of its ability to provide accurate soft tissue contrast, it is now the preferred technique for the non-invasive diagnosis of both focal and diffuse adenomyosis. Mark *et al.*, using MR imaging before surgery, correctly identified all eight cases in 21 patients with a strong clinical suggestion of adenomyosis (Mark *et al.* 1987). Togashi *et al.* assessed the potential of MR imaging in the differentiation of adenomyosis from leiomyoma in 93 patients who had a palpable, enlarged uterus (Togashi *et al.* 1989). Pathological examination showed that 71 enlarged uteri contained smooth muscle tumours, including one leiomyosarcoma, and 16 were enlarged due to adenomyosis. The cause of uterine enlargement was correctly diagnosed with MR imaging in 92 of the 93 cases. In a recent study, T2-weighted images provided accurate lesion detection in 17 of 19 cases with histologically proven adenomyosis (Hricak *et al.* 1992). Both cases not detected had the diffuse form of adenomyosis with an apparently normal junctional zone. The likelihood ratios calculated from these data (LR+ > 10 and LR– < 0.1 in all three studies) indicate that MR imaging is an excellent diagnostic test.

Adenomyosis is best demonstrated on T2-weighted images and the MR criterion for diffuse adenomyosis is an irregular thickening of the junctional zone (Fig. 24.3). There is, however, no consensus on the maximum width of a 'normal' junctional zone. Some authors have claimed that the diagnosis can be made confidently if the width of the junctional zone exceeds 5 mm (Ascher *et al.* 1994). Others have pointed out that the ratio of junctional zone width to the width of the outer myometrium or cervical stroma may be more meaningful criteria than absolute values (de Souza *et al.* 1995). Despite its excellent resolving power, MR imaging cannot yet reveal small glandular and stromal deposits in the myometrium. Togashi *et al.* demonstrated that the extent of the myoproliferative changes with adenomyosis correlates well with the extent of the diffusely

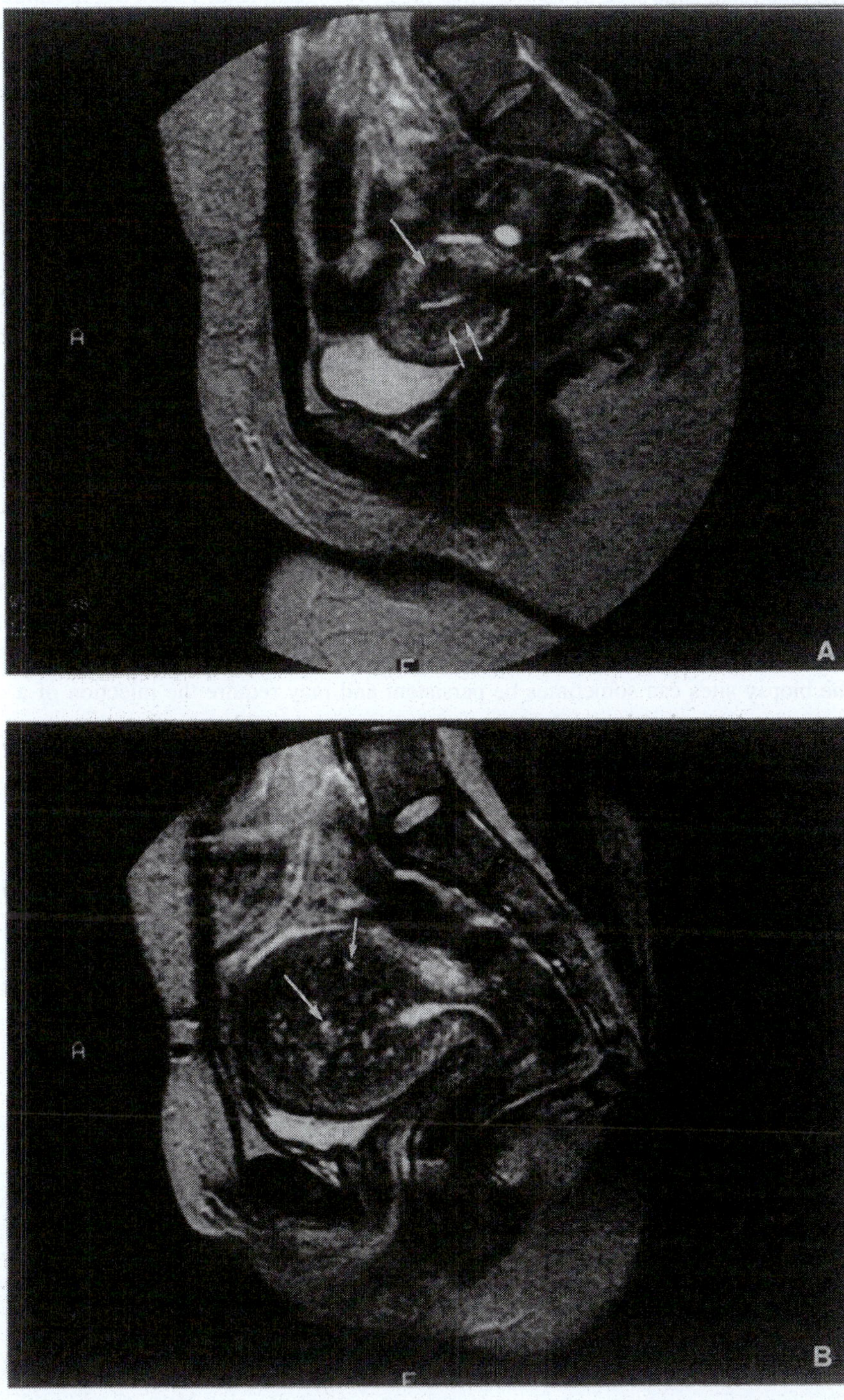

Fig. 24.3 T2-weighted spin-echo sagittal section through the uterus. (a) Diffuse adenomyosis: thickening and irregularity of the low signal band of junctional zone (short arrows). An irregular focal lesion characteristic of an adenomyoma is also seen in the posterior uterine wall (long arrow). (b) Extensive adenomyosis with complete loss of the normal myometrial zonal anatomy. The high signal spots throughout the myometrium (arrows) represent larger implants and focal intra-myometrial haemorrhage.

thickened junctional zone seen in T2-weighted images (Togashi *et al.* 1989). So, in contrast to the conventional microscopical diagnosis, the MR diagnosis is based on the distortion of the myometrial architecture and not on ectopic mucosal foci. Larger implants and focal haemorrhage are, however, sometimes seen as high signal-intensity spots in the myometrium.

Biopsy

McCausland advocated hysteroscopic resection of a myometrial strip of the posterior uterine wall for the histological confirmation of the diagnosis (McCausland 1991). After thorough curettage of the endometrial cavity, a single 1.5–3 cm myometrial biopsy specimen was taken with a 5 mm loop electrode. The myometrial surface of the biopsy was stained with a marking dye and care was taken to avoid tangential sectioning of the specimen. Of the 50 patients with heavy periods and normal uterine cavity, 33 had significant adenomyosis defined in this study as more than 1 mm of endometrial penetration. The accuracy of this technique has not yet been compared to conventional histological assessment of hysterectomy specimens. Furthermore, this procedure is not acceptable for patients who still have a desire for childbearing.

Alternatively, myometrial needle biopsies can be taken transabdominally, at the time of laparoscopy, or transcervically under ultrasound guidance (Popp *et al.* 1993). Needle biopsies are unlikely to impair fertility and their accuracy has recently been assessed *in vitro* (Table 24.2), (Brosens and Barker 1995). Although a highly specific technique, its sensitivity is low and dependent on the number of biopsies and the depth and extent of mucosal infiltration. Bleeding from the biopsy sites can sometimes be persistent and may require the injection of a vasoconstrictor, such as vasopressin, into the biopsy site (Popp *et al.* 1993).

Treatment

The two cardinal symptoms of adenomyosis are excessive menstrual loss and dysmenorrhoea. Symptomatic relief can be achieved with convential treatment such as mefenamic acid or danazol (Fraser *et al.* 1986). There is as yet no evidence that any form of medical therapy is specifically effective as the diagnostic elusiveness of adenomyosis has precluded controlled clinical trials.

Table 24.2 Sensitivity of 8, 4, and 2 myometrial needle biopsies, taken at random, in diagnosing adenomyosis

Number of biopsies	Adenomyosis		
	Grade I (n = 11)	Grade II (n = 11)	Grade III (n = 5)
8	9%	64%	100%
4	4.5%	38%	79%
2	2.3%	20%	56%

Adenomyosis was graded on the basis of the depth of glandular and stromal infiltration into the myometrium: grade I, adenomyosis within the inner third of the myometrium but at least 2 mm below the basal layer of the endometrium; grade II, penetration limited to the inner two thirds of the myometrium; and grade III, infiltration into the outer third of the myometrium. (Adapted from Brosens and Barker 1995.)

MR imaging has now resolved this impasse and has already been employed to monitor regression of adenomyotic implants in a pigtailed monkey treated with the pure anti-oestrogen, ICI 182, 780 (Waterton *et al.* 1993). Effective treatment of adenomyosis should not only cause involution of the endometrial implants but also aim to restore the myometrial zonal architecture and function. Spontaneous and induced adenomyosis in animals may be useful models to test novel approaches. For instance, keishi-bukuryo-gan, a traditional Chinese herbal remedy, was shown to inhibit the development of spontaneous adenomyosis in mice of SHN strain (Mori *et al.* 1993).

At present, the most common treatment for patients unresponsive to medical treatment is hysterectomy. Radical surgery is indicated in the older woman who has completed her family. More conservative techniques are currently being investigated as an alternative for women who wish to avoid hysterectomy. Endometrial ablation, either by coagulation or resection, will destroy the inner myometrium up to a depth of 3 mm. This may be effective treatment for those patients with predominantly subendometrial smooth muscle changes but minimal endometrial penetration. Wood *et al.* reported a 70 per cent cure rate in 30 women with adenomyosis treated either by endometrial resection, myometrial resection, or myometrial reduction by electrocoagulation (Wood *et al.* 1994). However, in patients with dysmenorrhea only three out of eight were cured. The higher density of implants, the increased incidence of intramyometrial haemorrhage, and the significant ectopic PG production contribute to the high failure rate of conservative surgery in deep adenomyosis. Function-preserving surgery has been attempted in patients who have not yet completed their families. Resection or destruction by laparoscopic myometrial needle electrocoagulation of deep focal lesions is feasible but requires accurate localization of the adenomyomata by MR imaging or transvaginal ultrasound.

References

Andreyko, J.L., Blumenfeld, Z., Marshall, L.A., Monroe, S.E., Hricak, H., and Jaffe, R.B. (1988). Use of an agonistic analog of GnRH (NAFARELIN) to treat leiomyomata: assessment by magnetic resonance imaging. *American Journal of Obstetrics and Gynecology*, **158**, 903–10.

Ascher, S.M., Arnold, L.L., Patt, R.H., Schruefer, J.J., Bagley, A.S., Semelka, R.C.R., *et al.* (1994). Adenomyosis: prospective comparison of MR imaging and transvaginal sonography. *Radiology*, **190**, 803–6.

Azziz, R. (1989). Adenomyosis: current perspectives. *Obstetric and Gynecologic Clinics of North America*, **16**, 221–35.

Bacon, C.R., Morrison, J.J., O'Reilly, G., Cameron, I.T., and Davenport, A.P. (1995). ET_A and ET_B endothelin receptors in human myometrium characterized by the subtype selective ligands BQ123, BQ3020, FR139317 and PD151242. *Journal of Endocrinology*, **144**, 127–34.

Barton, J.W., McCarthy, S.M., Kohorn, E.I., Scoutt, L.M., and Lange, R.C. (1993). Pelvic MR imaging findings in gestational trophoblastic disease, incomplete abortion and ectopic pregnancy: are they specific? *Radiology*, **186**, 163–8.

Benson, R.C. and Sneeden, V.D. (1958). Adenomyosis: a reappraisal of symptomatology. *American Journal of Obstetrics and Gynecology*, **76**, 1044–61.

Bird, C.C., McElin, T.W., and Manalo-Estrella, P. (1972). The elusive adenomyosis of the uterus. *American Journal of Obstetrics and Gynecology*, **112**, 583–93.

Brosens, J.J. and Barker, F.G. (1995). The role of myometrial needle biopsies in the diagnosis of adenomyosis. *Fertility and Sterility*, **63**, 1347–9.

Brosens, J.J., de Souza, N.M., Barker, F.G., Paraschos, T., and Winston, R.M.L. (1995). Endovaginal ultrasonography in the diagnosis of adenomyosis uteri: identifying the predictive characteristics. *British Journal of Obstetrics and Gynaecology*, **102**, 471–4.

Brown, H.K., Stoll, B.S., Nicosia, S.V., Fiorica, J.M., Hambley, P.S., Clarke, L.P., and Silbiger, M.L. (1991). Uterine junctional zone: correlation between histologic findings and MRI. *Radiology*, **179**, 409–13.

Cameron, I.T., Leask, R., Kelly, R.W., and Baird, D.T. (1987). Endometrial prostaglandins in women with abnormal menstrual bleeding. *Prostaglandins, Leukotrienes and Medicine*, **29**, 249–57.

Cullen, T.S. (1908). *Adenomyoma of the uterus*. W.B. Saunders, Philadelphia.

de Souza, N.M., Brosens, J.J., Schwieso, J.E., Paraschos, T., and Winston, R.M.L. (1995). The potential value of magnetic resonance imaging in infertility. *Clinical Radiology*, **50**, 75–9.

de Vries, K., Lyons, E.A., Ballard, G., Levi, C.S., and Lindsay, D.J. (1990). Contractions of the inner third of the myometrium. *American Journal of Obstetrics and Gynecology*, **162**, 679–82.

Draeger, A., Graf, A.H., Staudach, A., North, A.J., and Small, J.V. (1993). Smooth muscle differentiation in human myometrium and uterine leiomyoma. *Virchows Archiv B: Cell Pathology*, **64**, 21–7.

Emge, L.A. (1962). The elusive adenomyosis. *American Journal of Obstetrics and Gynecology*, **82**, 1541–62.

Fedele, L., Bianchi, S., Dorta, M., Arcaini, I., Zanotti, F., and Carinelli, S. (1994). Transvaginal ultrasonography in the diagnosis of diffuse adenomyosis. *Fertility and Sterility*, **58**, 94–7.

Fox, H.S., Bond, B.L., and Parslow, T.G. (1991). Estrogen regulates the IFNγ promotor. *Journal of Immunology*, **146**, 4362–7.

Fraser, I.S. (1994). Menorrhagia – a pragmatic approach to the understanding of causes and the need for investigations. *British Journal of Obstetrics and Gynaecology*, **101**, 3–7.

Fraser, I.S., McCarron, G., Markham, R., Resta, T., and Watts, A. (1986). Measured menstrual blood loss in women with menorrhagia associated with pelvic disease or coagulation disorder. *Obstetrics and Gynecology*, **68**, 630–3.

Fujii, S., Konishi, I., and Mori, T. (1989). Smooth muscle differentiation at endometrio-myometrial junction. An ultrastructural study. *Virchows Archiv A: Pathological Anatomy and Histopathology*, **414**, 105–12.

Gambone, J.C., Reiter, R.C., Lerich, J.B., *et al.* (1990). The impact of a quality assurance process on the frequency and confirmation rate of hysterectomy. *American Journal of Obstetrics and Gynecology*, **163**, 545.

Gardner, R.M., and Stancel, G.M. (1989). Blockade of epidermal growth factor-induced uterine contractions by indomethacin and nordihydroguaritic acid. *Journal of Pharmacological and Experimental Therapeutics*, **258**, 882–6.

Halvorsen, T.B. and Moen, M.H. (1993). The extent and clinical significance of adenomyotic lesions in the uterine wall. *Acta Pathologica, Microbiologica et Immunologica Seodinarica*, **101**, 907–13.

Hendrickson, M.R. and Kempson, R.L. (1987). Non-neoplastic conditions of the myometrium and uterine serosa. In *Obstetrical and gynaecological pathology* (3rd edn) (ed. H. Fox), Vol. 1 pp. 405–7. Churchill Livingstone, London.

Horie, K., Takakura, K., Imai, K., Liao, S., and Mori, T. (1992). Immunohistochemical localization of androgen receptor in the human endometrium, decidua, placenta and pathological conditions of the endometrium. *Human Reproduction*, **10**, 1461–6.

Hricak, H., Finck, S., Honda, G., and Göranson, H. (1992). MR imaging in the evaluation of benign uterine masses: value of gadopentetate dimeglumine-enhanced T1-weighted images. *American Journal of Radiology*, **158**, 1043–50.

Kilkku, P., Erkolla, R., and Grönroos, M. (1984). Nonspecificity of symptoms related to adenomyosis: a prospective comparative survey. *Acta Obstetrica et Gynecologica Scandinavica*, **63**, 229–31.

Kobayashi, H., Ida, W., Terao, T., and Kawashima, Y. (1993). Molecular characteristics of the CA 125 antigen produced by human endometrial epithelial cells: comparison between eutopic and heterotopic epithelial cells. *American Journal of Obstetrics Gynecology*, **169**, 725–30.

Koike, H., Egawa, H., Ohtsuka, T., Yamaguchi, M., Ikenoue, T., and Mori, N. (1992). Eicosanoids production in endometriosis. *Prostaglandins Leukotrienes and Essential Fatty Acids*, **45**, 313–17.

Lee, N.C., Dicker, R.C., Rubin, G.L., and Ory, H.W. (1984). Confirmation of the preoperative diagnosis for hysterectomy. *American Journal of Obstetrics Gynecology*, **150**, 283–7.

Lei, Z.M., Rao, ChV., Lincoln, S.R., and Ackermann, D.M. (1993). Increased expression of human chorionic gonadotrophin/human luteinizing hormone receptors in adenomyosis. *Journal of Clinical Endocrinology and Metabolism*, **76**, 763–8.

Lewinski, H. (1931). Beitrag zur Frage der Adenomiosis. *Zentralblatt fur Gynakologie*, **55**, 2163–16.

McCarthy, S., Scott, G., Majumdar, S., Shapiro, B., Thompson, S., Lange, R., and Gore, J. (1989). Uterine junctional zone: MR study of water content and relaxation properties. *Radiology*, **171**, 241–3.

McCausland, A.M. (1991). Hysteroscopic myometrial biopsy: its use in diagnosing adenomyosis and its clinical application. *American Journal of Obstetrics and Gynecology*, **166**, 1619–28.

Mark, S.A., Hricak, H., Heinrichs, L.W., Hendrickson, M.R., Winkler, M.L., Bachica, J.A., and Stickler, J.E. (1987). Adenomyosis and leiomyoma: differential diagnosis with MR imaging. *American Journal of Radiology*, **163**, 527–9.

Marshak, R.H. and Eliasoph, J. (1955). The roentgen findings in adenomyosis. *Radiology*, **64**, 846–51.

Martinez-Mir, I., Estän, L., Morales-Olivas, F., and Rubio, E. (1990). Studies of the spontaneous motility and the effect of histamine on isolated myometrial strips of the nonpregnant human uterus: the influence of various uterine abnormalities. *American Journal of Obstetrics and Gynecology*, **163**, 189–95.

Mori, T., Ohta, Y., and Nagasawa, H. (1984). Ultrastructural changes in uterine myometrium of mice with experimentally induced adenomyosis. *Experientia*, **40**, 1385–7.

Mori, T., Singtripop, T., and Kawahima, S. (1991). Animal model of uterine adenomyosis: is prolactin a potent inducer of adenomyosis in mice? *American Journal of Obstetrics and Gynecology*, **165**, 232–4.

Mori, T., Sakamoto, S., Matsuda, M., Kyokuma, M., Namiki, H., Kuwa, K. *et al.* (1993). Suppression of spontaneous development of uterine adenomyosis and mammary hyperplastic alveolar nodules by chinese herbal medicine in mice. *American Journal of Chinese Medicine*, **21**, 263–8.

Nishida, M. (1991). Relationship between the onset of dysmenorrhea and histologic findings in adenomyosis. *American Journal of Obstetrics and Gynecology*, **165**, 229–31.

Ota, H. and Igarashi, S. (1993). Expression of major histocompatibility complex class II antigen in endometriotic tissue in patients with endometriosis and adenomyosis. *Fertility and Sterility*, **60**, 834–8.

Ota, H., Maki, M., Shidara, Y., Kodama, H., Takahashi, H., Hayakawa, M. *et al.* (1992). Effects of danazol at the immunologic level in patients with adenomyosis, with special reference to autoantibodies: a multicenter cooperative study. *American Journal of Obstetrics and Gynecology*, **167**, 481–6.

Popp, L.W., Schwiedessen, J.P., and Gaetje, R. (1993). Myometrial biopsy in the diagnosis of adenomyosis uteri. *American Journal of Obstetrics and Gynecology*, **169**, 546–9.

Rokitansky, C. (1860). Über Uterusdrusen-Neubildung in Uterus- and Ovarial-sarcomen. *Zeitschrift der Kaiserlich-Königlicht Gesellschaft Ärzte zu Wien*. **16**, 577–81.

Salamanca, A. and Beltrán, E. (1995). Subendometrial contractility in menstrual phase visualized by transvaginal sonography in patients with endometriosis. *Fertility and Sterility*, **64**, 193–5.

Sandberg, E.G., and Cohn, F. (1962). Adenomyosis in the gravid uterus at term. *American Journal of Obstetrics and Gynecology*, **84**, 1457–65.

Scoutt, L.M., Flynn, S.D., Luthringer, D.J., McCauley, T.R., and McCarthy, S.M. (1991). Junctional zone of the uterus: correlation of MRI and histologic examination of hysterectomy specimen. *Radiology*, **179**, 403–7.

Stewart, C.J.R., Farquharson, M.A., and Foulis, A.K. (1992). The distribution and possible function of gamma interferon-immunoreactive cells in normal endometrium and myometrium. *Virchows Archiv A: Pathological Anatomy and Histopathology*, **420**, 419–24.

Tabibzadeh, S., Sun, X.Z., Kong, Q.F., Kasnic, G., Miller, J., and Satyaswaroop, P.G. (1993). Induction of a polarized micro-environment by human T cells and interferon-gamma in three-dimensional spheroid cultures of human endometrial epithelial cells. *Human Reproduction*, **8**, 182–92.

Takahashi, K., Nagata, H., and Kitao, M. (1989). Clinical usefulness of determination of estradiol level in menstrual blood for patients with endometriosis. *Acta Obstetrica et Gynecologica Japan*, **41**, 1849–50.

Tamaya, T., Motoyama, T., Ohono, Y., Ide, N., Tsurusaki, T., and Okada, H. (1979). Steroid receptor levels and histology of endometriosis and adenomyosis. *Fertility and Sterility*, **31**, 396–400.

Togashi, K., Ozasa, H., Konishi, I., Itoh, H., Nishimura, K., Fujisawa, T. *et al.* (1989). Enlarged uterus: differentiation between adenomyosis and leiomyoma with MRI. *Radiology*, **171**, 531–4.

Turnbull, L.W., Manton, D.J., Horsman, A., and Killick, S.R. (1995). Magnetic resonance imaging changes in uterine zonal anatomy during a conception cycle. *British Journal of Obstetrics and Gynaecology*, **102**, 330–1.

Van Voorhis, B.J., Huettner, P.C., Clark, M.R., and Hill, J.A. (1990). Immunohistochemical localization of prostaglandin H synthase in the female reproductive tract and endometriosis. *American Journal of Obstetrics and Gynecology*, **163**, 57–62.

Vercellini, P., Ragni, G., Trespidi, L., Oldani, S., Panazza, S., and Crosignani, P.G. (1993). Adenomyosis: a déjà vu? *Obstetric and Gynecological Survey*, **12**, 789–94.

Waterton, J.C., Breen, S.A., Dukes, M., Horrocks, M., and Wadsworth, P.F. (1993). A case of adenomyosis in a pigtailed monkey diagnosed by magnetic resonance imaging and treated with the novel pure antiestrogen, ICI 182780. *Laboratory and Animal Science*, **43**, 247–51.

Wood, C., Maher, P., and Hill, D. (1994). Biopsy diagnosis and conservative surgical treatment of adenomyosis. *Journal of the American Association of Gynecologic Laparoscopists*, **141**, 313–16.

Yamamoto, T., Noguchi, T., Tamura, T., Kitawaki, J., and Okada, H. (1993). Evidence for estrogen synthesis in adenomyotic tissues. *American Journal of Obstetrics and Gynecology*, **169**, 734–8.

25 Endometriosis and its influence on dysmenorrhoea and menstrual disturbances

R. William Stones and Eric J. Thomas

Introduction

Endometriosis is defined as the presence of endometrium-like glands and stroma outside the uterine cavity and myometrium. Adenomyosis, where such tissue is present within the myometrium, is reviewed in Chapter 24. Current opinion regarding the pathogenesis of endometriosis favours the concept of implantation of endometrial tissue shed during menstruation and passed via the Fallopian tubes into the peritoneal cavity, in contrast to the alternative hypothesis of coelomic metaplasia. The retrograde menstruation theory is consistent with the epidemiology of the condition, which is essentially more common in women who have experienced more episodes of menstruation. Interest presently centres on genetic, environmental, or local factors which might render endometrial tissue more likely to adhere to and invade the pelvic peritoneum and deeper tissues.

The clinical problems associated with endometriosis are those of pelvic pain, including dysmenorrhoea and dyspareunia, and infertility. The present review will focus on dysmenorrhoea and menstrual disturbance associated with endometriosis.

Endometriosis: causal or coincidental?

Endometriosis may present with pain, infertility, or both, and the causal role of endometriosis in an individual case is by no means always clear. A number of studies have tried to quantify the clinical impression that the extent of disease evident at laparoscopy correlates poorly with symptoms. In one study 160 women with newly diagnosed endometriosis were reviewed (Fedele *et al.* 1990). Of these women, 75 per cent were nulliparous, and the presenting symptoms were infertility (41 per cent), pelvic pain (26 per cent), and a pelvic mass (34 per cent). No statistical relationships were identified between pain symptoms and the stage or localization of endometriotic deposits. The same authors went on to report on a further group of infertility patients and noted more pelvic pain and dyspareunia, but not dysmenorrhoea, in those with stages I–II compared to stages III–IV endometriosis (Fedele *et al.* 1992).

Asymptomatic endometriosis may be identified at laparoscopy for another indication, such as sterilization. Taking an epidemiological approach, the presence of endometriosis among multiparous women undergoing laparoscopic sterilization was recorded (Sangi-Haghpeykar and

Table 25.1 Risk factors for endometriosis. Adapted from Sangi-Haghpeykar and Poindexter (1995)

Risk factor	Odds ratio	95% Confidence intervals
Advanced age	2.0	1.1–3.7
Asian race	8.6	1.4–20.1
Long cycle length	1.8	1.8–2.7
Single live birth	2.2	1.1–4.3
Long IUCD use	3.0	1.1–8.1
Uninterrupted cycle	2.9	1.3–6.4
Oral contraceptive use	0.5	0.2–0.9

Poindexter 1995). The disease was present in 126 out of 3384 (3.7 per cent) of women although where present, endometriosis was usually minimal. Five hundred and four negative controls were randomly selected for a case–control analysis from the sterilization group in order to determine associated risk factors for endometriosis. Factors with significant odds ratios are presented in Table 25.1. The conclusion from this study of fertile and essentially asymptomatic women is that endometriosis even at this level is associated with specific clinical features and probably represents the least severe end of a spectrum of disease, rather than simply a physiological variation within normality. This view suggests that a disease process which may not lead to morbidity in the vast majority of cases can in other cases lead to symptomatic disease. Another case–control study used 522 women admitted as acute emergencies and compared them to 129 women with various stages of endometriosis (Parazzini *et al.* 1995). Odds ratios did not vary greatly with the stage of endometriosis and these are listed in Table 25.2 for factors apparently protective against endometriosis. Assuming the revised American Fertility Society classification is a valid way of assessing endometriosis (see below) this study suggests that there is an epidemiological divide between those who have or do not have endometriosis, and that among those who do have endometriosis other factors determine the extent of symptoms and disease. This apparent complexity might be explained by considering retrograde menstruation as a necessary precondition, but requiring a pathological process such as disordered endometrial cell adhesion and implantation into ectopic sites to give rise to tissue damage and symptoms. A basis for understanding has started to emerge with the description of adhesion molecule ligands in normal endometrium and in endometriotic deposits (Bridges *et al.* 1994) but specific patterns of expression associated with endometriotic invasion have not yet been identified.

Table 25.2 Factors protective against endometriosis. Adapted from Parazzini *et al.* (1995)

Risk factor	Odds ratios: Endometriosis stage			
	I	II	III	IV
Two or more births	0.1	0.1	0.2	0.2
One or more induced abortion	0.4	0.5	0.2	0.2
Irregular cycle	0.3	0.5	0.5	0.3

Endometriosis and cancer

Some of the properties of endometriosis have led to comparisons with cancer. Although 'benign', endometriosis manifests many of the features of malignancy, with invasion of normal tissues, the establishment of a neovasculature, and metastases to distant sites as a result of haematogenous or lymphatic spread. In particular, an association between malignant ovarian tumours of the endometrioid type and endometriosis has been reported (Vercellini *et al.* 1993).

A recent study investigated the genotype of endometriotic tissue (Jiang *et al.* 1996). Monoclonality was conclusively established in 14 out of 17 cases, suggesting that, as in most cancers, the pathological tissue is derived from a single deranged cell. In addition, in two cases of endometriosis, loss of heterozygosity studies established that chromosomal deletions were present on the short arms of chromosome 9 and 22 in regions which are thought to harbour tumour suppressor genes. Progressive deletions of such regions are an important part of cellular progress towards malignancy, and this study demonstrated for the first time a possible genetic link between the mechanisms leading to endometriosis and malignant disease. Another recent *in vitro* study has reported the ability of cultured endometriotic cells to invade a collagen gel, a property shared by a human cancer cell line but not by cells from normal endometrial biopsies (Gaetje *et al.* 1995).

Superficial and deep endometriosis: different diseases, different stages?

Cornillie *et al.* (1990) carried out a systematic investigation of the relationship between symptoms in endometriosis and the depth of implantation, the activity of implants, and whether implanted endometriosis was in phase with the endometrium. Deep implantation of ⩾5 mm was seen on the uterosacral ligaments and in the pouch of Douglas but was not seen in the ovarian fossae. Deep and superficial implants tended to be active and in phase with the endometrium (58 per cent and 68 per cent respectively), whereas implants of intermediate depth (2–4 mm) tended to be inactive or only focally active, with only 38 per cent of implants in phase. Specific histological features in deeply invading lesions were infiltration along connective tissue septa into fibromuscular tissue (Figure 25.1) with penetration arrested at the border with underlying fatty tissue. Nerve fibres could usually be identified in specimens of deeply invading endometriosis which might explain the preponderance of patients presenting with pain among those with this type of lesion. Pain was present in 17 per cent of those with < 2 mm deposits, 53 per cent of those with 2–4 mm deposits, 37 per cent of those with 5–10 mm deposits, and all six women with very deep deposits of > 10 mm.

A second study of histological findings in relation to symptoms showed that depth of infiltration of endometriosis was the clearest discriminator for pelvic pain compared to other variables describing the lesions that could be included in staging schemes (Koninckx *et al.* 1991). Depth of infiltration is not a factor in the revised American Fertility Society scoring system, highlighting the limitations of this system where pain is the main complaint. This larger study again showed a preponderance of pain symptoms in women from whom specimens showed deeply infiltrating endometriosis, but the relationship was not total in that the majority of women with pain alone or both pain and infertility had lesions invading for 6 mm or less (Fig. 25.2). Further studies are needed to elucidate the possible significance for pain generation of the anatomical proximity of endometriotic deposits and nerve fibres.

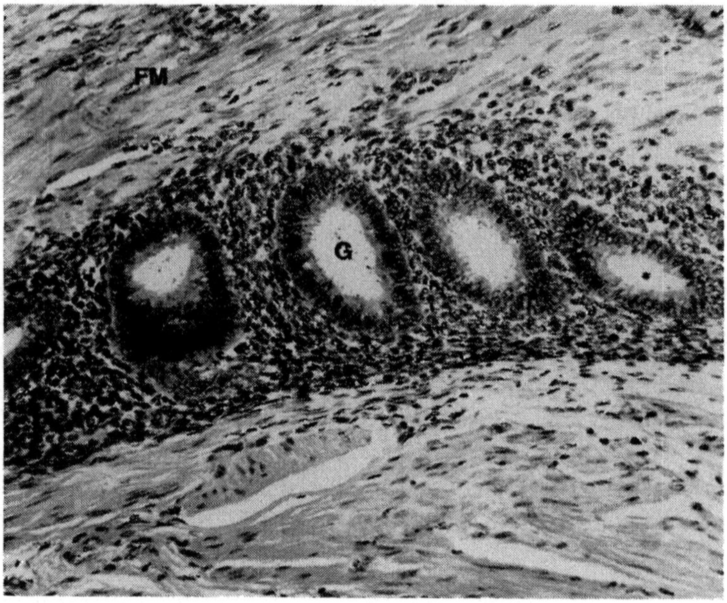

Fig. 25.1 Deep infiltration of endometriotic glands (G) and stroma (S) into the fibromuscular (FM) tissue. The loose connective tissue septum is completely replaced by endometriosis × 100. From Cornillie *et al.* (1990). Reproduced with permission of the publisher, the American Society for Reproductive Medicine (The American Fertility Society).

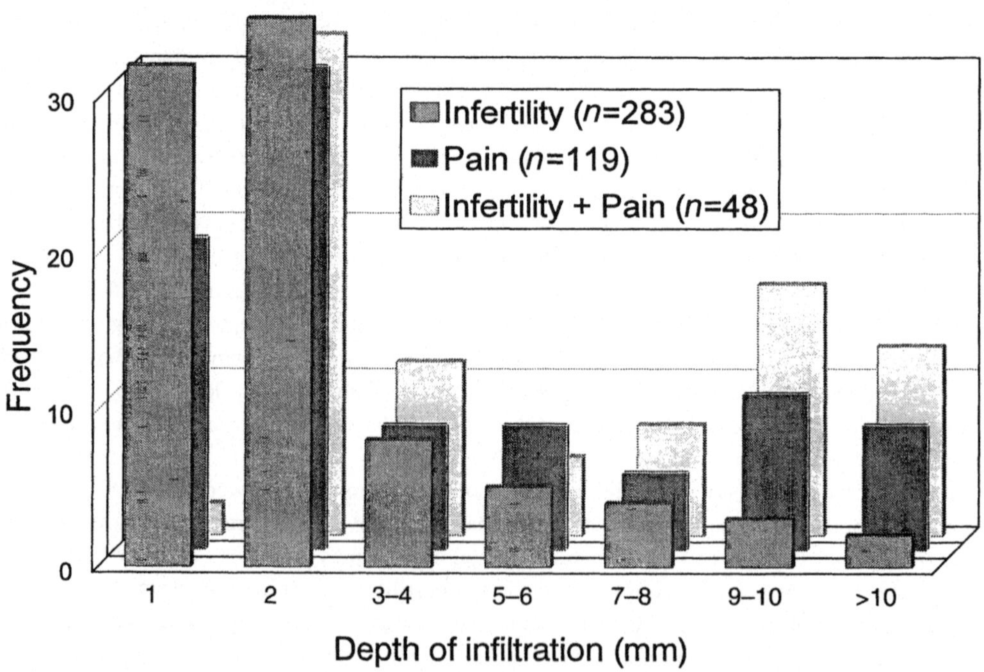

Fig. 25.2 Frequency distributions of depth of infiltration of pelvic endometriosis in women with infertility, pain, or infertility and pain. Adapted from Koninckx *et al.* (1991). Reproduced with permission of the publisher, the American Society for Reproductive Medicine (The American Fertility Society).

Endometriosis-associated dysmenorrhoea

Darrow *et al.* (1993) compared menstrual symptoms in 104 women with laparoscopically proven endometriosis with symptoms in two different control groups using a case–control format. The odds ratios for dysmenorrhoea using the two control groups were 2.5 (95 per cent confidence intervals (CI) 1.2 to 6.0) and 2.3 (95 per cent CI 1.1 to 5.3). This type of study is slightly circular in nature as the presenting symptom of dysmenorrhoea might well prompt investigation for endometriosis, and the lower confidence intervals almost reached unity. However, a very large study including 598 women undergoing laparoscopic sterilization, and those undergoing diagnostic laparoscopy for pain (156), or infertility (312), or hysterectomy (134) reported dysmenorrhoea to be the most common reported symptom in those with endometriosis (Mahmood *et al.* 1991). This symptom may be especially prominent in young women presenting with endometriosis: in a series of 73 patients aged 25 or younger, including 7 under 20, menstrual disturbance was rare (Punnonen and Nikkanen 1980), and in this age group a clear clinical distinction between primary and secondary dysmenorrhoea may not be apparent.

Primary or spasmodic dysmenorrhoea, as seen in 10–15 per cent of women as the extreme of the spectrum of normal, and in the absence of gross pathology, has an underlying basis in excessive local secretion of vasopressin and prostaglandins (see Chapter 22). Frequent tonic myometrial contractions cause local hypoxia and evoke pain in a manner similar to that of uterine contractions in labour. Three possible mechanisms whereby pelvic endometriosis might generate or exacerbate dysmenorrhoea need to be considered. Firstly there may be an increased quantity of endometrial tissue, albeit in inappropriate locations, acting on physiological mechanisms associated with dysmenorrhoea. Secondly, agents released from endometriotic tissue may have direct effects on sensory nerves. Thirdly, the distortion and restriction of normal mobility caused by adhesion formation, especially around the tubes and ovaries, may cause pain through traction and kinking.

Endometriotic lesions contain architecturally and biochemically functional tissue with many of the properties of endometrium. A range of endometrial products have algesic properties. These include prostaglandins of the E and F series, and production of the prostacyclin metabolite 6-keto-$PGF_{1\alpha}$ was shown to be increased in adenomyosis and ovarian endometriosis (Koike *et al.* 1992). More recently, a number of other locally active agents have been identified in endometrial tissue. Endothelins are synthesized in the glandular and stromal endometrial cells in a cycle-dependent manner (Economos *et al.* 1992) and act locally to release prostaglandin $F_{2\alpha}$ (Cameron *et al.* 1991). Binding sites identified by autoradiography were more numerous in the endometrium than in the myometrium although myometrial contractility is potently stimulated by endothelin-1 (Word *et al.* 1990). Thus, by increasing the quantity of active endometrial tissue, endometriosis would be expected to exacerbate dysmenorrhoea through the physiological mechanisms discussed above. However, endothelins-1, -2, and -3 evoke pain directly in a mouse model (Raffa and Jacoby 1991) and the release of endothelins and other algesic agents in extrauterine sites of implantation, stimulating local sensory nerves, may account for the more congestive or secondary type of dysmenorrhoea, as well as more diverse symptoms of pelvic pain which fall outside the scope of the present review.

The perception of pain involves far more complex processes than the generation of a noxious stimulus as part of a pathological process. Visceral sensation is mediated through unmyelinated C fibres without specialized endings which synapse in the dorsal horn of the spinal cord. Pain sensation arising from the stimulation of visceral afferents of this type is characterized by its diffuse nature, relatively poor localization to a site of origin, referral to a cutaneous dermatome, and modulation at the level of the spinal cord and higher centres. Studies in experimental animals have illuminated the visceral sensory mechanisms present in the urogenital tract, some of which may well be relevant in humans. In the rat vagina and uterus, visceral afferent nerve endings are grouped into single or multiple units with a maximal innervation density at the vaginal fornices and cervix (Berkley *et al.* 1988). These sensory units can be activated by mechanical stimulation, with impulses proceeding via the pelvic or hypogastric nerves, and their functional properties are influenced by the hormonal changes of the oestrous cycle (Robbins *et al.* 1992). Subpopulations of visceral sensory units are activated at different thresholds of mechanical or noxious chemical stimulation (Jänig and Koltzenburg 1993) and these thresholds are modified after chronic irritation. Thus, sensory units normally having a high threshold and not active under physiological conditions become sensitized so as to be active during stimulation at a low intensity. This provides an end-organ mechanism whereby pain may persist following the resolution of an acute inflammatory insult.

The influence of ovarian hormones on neurotransmission has been alluded to above. In addition, the uterus in a number of species manifests plasticity in respect of the pattern of innervation by autonomic and sensory nerves. For example, pregnancy is associated with a relative loss of uterine artery noradrenergic sympathetic nerves, while neuropeptide Y-containing nerves are preserved (Mione *et al.* 1990). 'Sensory–motor' nerves containing substance P and calcitonin gene-related peptide are present in the rat uterus (Papka *et al.* 1985). In contrast to sympathetic nerves, these proliferated at puberty to maintain the pre-pubertal innervation density and could also be depleted by neonatal capsaicin treatment (Brauer *et al.* 1994*a*). The density of parametrial but not myometrial calcitonin gene-related peptide-containing nerves was increased following chemical sympathectomy with guanethidine (Brauer *et al.* 1994*b*). Thus, complex developmental and hormonal factors influence the relative composition and innervation density of the uterine tissues. Species differences are also important: reflex ovulator species tend to have a more prominent vaginal and uterine sensory apparatus with a parasympathetic ovarian innervation not seen in humans.

At the level of the dorsal horn visceral sensation is modulated by nerves expressing substance P and the NMDA glutamate receptor (McMahon and Koltzenburg 1994). Excitatory and inhibitory influences reflecting local and distant central nervous arousal mechanisms determine the extent to which transmission to higher centres occurs. An example of analgesia acting at this level is transcutaneous electrical nerve stimulation, which is based on the stimulation of cutaneous small myelinated A fibres which act in the dorsal horn to inhibit the transmission of impulses from viscera travelling in C fibres. This modality is a logical therapeutic choice in dysmenorrhoea as well as for pain associated with labour, although its effectiveness is less well established in the latter indication. Finally, peripheral nerve injury may provoke central sprouting of myelinated afferents, leading to permanent modification of sensory pathways (Woolf *et al.* 1992).

Endometriosis-associated menstrual disturbance

Women with irregular or infrequent menstrual cycles had a reduced risk of endometriosis in a case–control study, with an odds ratio of 0.3 (95 per cent CI 0.2 to 0.5) (Candiani *et al.* 1991).

This relationship would be expected from the likelihood that endometriosis originates from the implantation of endometrium shed during menstruation. Also using the case–control approach, Darrow *et al.* (1993) reported a greater impact of endometriosis on the menstrual cycle in younger women. In those under the age of 30 the odds ratio for a menstrual flow of six or more days per month was 2.5 (95 per cent CI 1.1 to 5.9) and for a heavy menstrual flow was 2.5 (95 per cent CI 1.1 to 6.3), whereas these associations were less prominent in older women. However, the *lack* of menstrual symptoms in very young women with endometriosis has been noted above (Punnonen and Nikkanen 1980). This discrepancy may reflect different methodological approaches in the studies cited; patient self-selection could also explain some age-related phenomena in that those women with severe menstrual disturbance might seek surgical treatment at an earlier stage, removing themselves from the population eligible for epidemiological studies of endometriosis. Alternatively, there may be an 'age window' between the mid-third and fourth decades where menstrual disturbance features more prominently as a symptom of endometriosis. If this is correct, one might hypothesize a relationship with the natural history of the disease. The biochemical activity of endometriotic implants might change in parallel with the age of the lesions: an evolution of the visual appearances of lesions has been suggested (Redwine 1987) and there is no reason why this should not be associated with changing metabolic activity. Nisolle *et al.* (1993) reported morphological differences between lesions of different visual appearance, especially in the extent of stromal vascularization. Red lesions were more vascularized, and the authors considered these to represent early and active lesions, in contrast to white lesions which were thought to arise in the quiescent phase of the disease.

In considering the relationship between endometriosis and menstrual disturbance it would be naïve to think of endometriotic deposits as being directly equivalent to endometrium, and thus likely to undergo menstrual shedding under the influence of ovarian hormones. In fact, endometriotic deposits are often out of phase with the endometrium (Cornillie *et al.* 1990). Furthermore, menstruation depends on the architecture of the uterine spiral arteries feeding the endometrial capillary bed, and complex local mechanisms for vasomotor control and haemostasis. While one might envisage mechanisms whereby endometriotic implants might influence myometrial contractility and hence exacerbate dysmenorrhoea, as discussed above, it is unlikely that peritoneal deposits would have a corresponding influence on menstrual flow. A plausible mechanism for such an effect might be the antidromic release of vasodilator agents such as substance P and calcitonin gene-related peptide from perivascular nerve terminals in the uterine vasculature in response to activation of peritoneal visceral afferents; but nerves containing these transmitters are relatively sparsely represented in the human uterus.

A more obvious and satisfactory explanation for the relationship between menstrual disturbance and endometriosis is that the causality is the other way round: just as infrequent or irregular cycles protect from endometriosis, so regular but heavy periods would predispose to it by exposing the pelvic peritoneum to a heavier load of endometrial tissue via retrograde menstruation. Thus endometriosis is the result of heavy menstrual shedding rather than its cause.

Diagnosis of endometriosis

The presence of various symptoms in women with endometriosis has now been objectively reported in the case–control studies discussed above. Unfortunately, efforts to identify a symptom complex that would accurately enable the diagnosis to be made from the history alone have so far proved unsuccessful. For example, in 104 infertility patients undergoing laparoscopy, severe dysmenorrhoea was the only symptom predictive of endometriosis, which turned out to be present in 40 per cent (Forman *et al.* 1993).

The role of physical examination perhaps merits re-evaluation in the light of current thinking about the nature of the disease process in endometriosis. Pelvic examination is often unremarkable in women who turn out to have early stage endometriosis at laparoscopy, without extensive deposits, adhesion formation, or tissue damage. It is in this type of patient that endometriosis might well be considered coincidental rather than causal with respect to symptoms of pain. Pelvic tenderness without restriction of mobility or nodularity, and especially adnexal rather than uterine tenderness, may suggest pelvic congestion syndrome rather than endometriosis (Beard *et al.* 1988). On the other hand, it is precisely in those women with deeply invading endometriosis, extensive lesions, or adhesion formation leading to uterine or ovarian immobility that the causal role of endometriosis in generating pain is most convincing. In such individuals nodularity, restricted uterine mobility, and/ or a mass are likely to be detectable on bimanual examination, giving a strong indication as to the diagnosis.

Ultrasound has a role in the evaluation of adnexal masses and it may be possible to use sonographic criteria to identify likely ovarian endometriomas as distinct from other pathologies (Kurjak and Kupesic 1994). This would have the practical advantage of allowing surgery to be planned in the foreknowledge of the diagnosis, for example planning a definitive 'first look' laparoscopic procedure for smaller ovarian endometriomas, but aiming to drain larger chocolate cysts initially, followed by definitive surgery after an interval of ovarian suppression with a GnRH analogue (Donnez *et al.* 1993). With regard to the uterus itself in endometriosis, a fascinating recent report described the use of transvaginal ultrasound to observe subendometrial contractility in the menstrual phase in women with and without the disease (Salamanca and Beltran 1995). The direction of propagation of contraction waves was noted to be predominantly from the cervix to the fundus in those with endometriosis, in contrast to normal volunteers. If confirmed, a link is evident with the aetiological theory of implantation of endometrium via retrograde menstruation. It might also be possible to use this phenomenon as an aid to diagnosis.

Another modality which might enable non-invasive diagnosis is magnetic resonance imaging. This mainly has a role in identifying adenomyosis (see Chapter 22) but was shown to provide useful modification of the preoperative diagnosis in the work-up of gynaecological patients (Schwartz *et al.* 1994). Biochemical markers such as CA 125 are too non-specific to be of practical use.

In the absence of definitive non-invasive investigations, the diagnosis of endometriosis still rests on laparoscopy. The timing of laparoscopy will be influenced by the nature and severity of symptoms and signs, and by the patient's attitude to her condition. Some will welcome symptomatic treatment without a positive diagnosis involving surgery, whereas others can only derive reassurance from the definite information provided by laparoscopy.

Treatment

The choice of therapy of endometriosis depends on the presenting symptoms and the patient's reproductive status. Economic issues are also relevant as some licensed treatments for endometriosis are expensive, yet not curative. Increasingly, laparoscopic surgery is emerging as a preferred option (Stones and Thomas 1996).

First line treatment

Where dysmenorrhoea is the prominent presenting symptom, initial therapy will be symptomatic. Even where endometriosis has been identified as an associated factor, not all women will wish to take pharmacological agents as a first choice. The efficacy of another modality, transcutaneous electrical nerve stimulation (TENS), has been established in small but controlled studies, for example those of Mannheimer and Whalen (1985) and Lundeberg *et al.* (1985). Unfortunately, no studies have included subgroups identified as having endometriosis and the available data are confined to studies including women with primary dysmenorrhoea. However, the interaction between non-steroidal anti-inflammatory drugs and electrical stimulation has been investigated. In a four-way randomized cross-over study involving 32 women, real or sham electrical stimulation was used in combination with ibruprofen 400 mg four times daily or placebo (Dawood and Ramos 1990). During the TENS phase, subjects were allowed ibruprofen 'rescue' if necessary. The results showed a significant effect of TENS in reducing the need for additional analgesia. An interesting recent controlled study compared high and low frequency TENS with acupuncture seven and three days prior to the expected onset of menstruation, rather than during the menses (Thomas *et al.* 1995). This pre-emptive approach showed a benefit for low frequency TENS and acupuncture but not for high frequency TENS, effective during menstruation in the studies cited above.

In the field of psychological interventions for dysmenorrhoea, once again the emphasis has been on primary dysmenorrhoea. However, one study contrasted the good results of a behaviour therapy intervention in women with 'spasmodic' dysmenorrhoea, with poor outcome in those with 'congestive' dysmenorrhoea where endometriosis may have been a feature (Amodei *et al.* 1987). More studies of these alternative approaches to symptomatic relief are needed for those women with endometriosis who wish to avoid either drug treatment or surgical intervention.

While a number of controlled studies have reported on the efficacy of non-steroidal anti-inflammatory agents (NSAID) for primary dysmenorrhoea, there is a dearth of data relating to endometriosis-associated dysmenorrhoea. In the absence of such studies one has to fall back on experience of women with primary dysmenorrhoea, in whom the beneficial effects of NSAID are well established to the point of over-the-counter licensed availability (Dawood 1988). In practice, these benefits do appear to extend to the alleviation of endometriosis-associated dysmenorrhoea, and will be an attractive therapeutic option to many, firstly because the medication only has to be taken while symptoms are present, and secondly because there is no known adverse effect on fertility.

The combined oral contraceptive pill, again notably effective in primary dysmenorrhoea, may have a role in endometriosis. The combined pill carries the additional advantages of ovarian suppression which may alleviate other symptoms associated with endometriosis, especially menorrhagia, and the potential to slow progression of the disease. However, while recognizing the lack of controlled studies, the combined pill is frequently insufficient to control endometriosis symptoms, perhaps because ovarian suppression is not total, and more aggressive hormonal therapy is often needed. Danazol remains very useful despite its reputation for androgenic side-effects, and may be especially good at a lower dose for dysmenorrhoea and menorrhagia. While long term use of this agent at traditional dose levels has significant side-effects and adverse metabolic consequences, a recent study showed a significant improvement in dysmenorrhoea and other endometriosis symptoms during nine months' treatment with danazol at the very low dose of 50 mg daily. Unfortunately, pain scores returned to baseline six months after the end of treatment, and during treatment some adverse effects on the lipid profile were detected.

Second line hormonal therapy

Progestogens and GnRH analogues are well established in the symptomatic treatment of endometriosis and the choice of drug will depend on cost and the patient's tolerance of side-effects. Current interest is in the use of add-back oestrogen and/or progestogen to mitigate the symptomatic and metabolic adverse effects of GnRH analogues. To date the evidence suggests that endometriosis is not reactivated by adding exogenous oestrogen although the dose of oestrogen used has been low in published reports, for example a 25 μg transdermal patch. At this level of oestrogen replacement bone loss was not completely prevented and many women were still symptomatic (Howell *et al.* 1995). Regimens using higher levels of oral oestrogen and progestogen given in a cyclical (Thomas *et al.* 1991) or continuous manner (Gangar *et al.* 1993) during GnRH analogue therapy can alleviate menopausal symptoms and control menstrual disturbance. Reassuringly, 2 mg oestradiol valerate with norethisterone did prevent bone loss during GnRH therapy (Leather *et al.* 1993). Following initial positive reports (Reid *et al.* 1992) these regimens have not as yet been fully evaluated as to whether the beneficial effect of the GnRH analogue-induced ovarian suppression on endometriosis is maintained. A simpler approach is to reduce the dose of GnRH analogue, so that adverse effects are less pronounced. A reduced dose of intranasal nafarelin was effective in an open study in relieving endometriosis symptoms without causing significant bone loss, although hot flushes were still reported (Jacobson *et al.* 1994).

Surgery

Cost remains the major barrier to the routine use of GnRH analogues and means that even if combination regimens of the type described above can be perfected, long term therapy is ruled out on economic grounds. This, together with the significant rate of recurrence of endometriosis symptoms after stopping treatment, and the development of minimal access surgery, has led to a move towards surgical rather than medical treatment of endometriosis, especially once the threshold of the first line drugs has been passed.

Even when dysmenorrhoea and/or menstrual disturbance are the main complaints, preservation or enhancement of fertility may also be a priority for the patient. Those who have completed their family may well opt for hysterectomy, and in the presence of endometriosis there is good evidence on which to advise oophorectomy rather than ovarian conservation. In a series of 138 women, 29 had one or both ovaries preserved at hysterectomy for endometriosis. Of these, 18 (62 per cent) had recurrent symptoms and half of these went on to further surgery. In contrast, those whose ovaries had been removed had a 10.1 per cent rate of recurrence of symptoms, and 3.7 per cent required further surgery. The relative risk for pain recurrence in those with ovarian conservation was 6.1 (95 per cent CI 2.5 to 14.6) and that for reoperation was 8.1 (95 per cent CI 2.1 to 31.2) (Namnoum *et al.* 1995). In general the experience of oestrogen replacement therapy following oophorectomy is good, and the risk of stimulating remaining endometriotic deposits seems to be low. However, a subgroup of patients do go on to manifest persistent endometriosis whether or not they receive oestrogen replacement therapy (Redwine 1994). These cases fell into an older age group and there may have been more frequent involvement of the bowel. The prognosis in this series was good following surgical excision of remaining deposits.

The surgical approach for pelvic clearance will depend on the extent of the disease and will increasingly involve a laparoscopic or laparoscopically assisted vaginal approach, having due regard for the technical problems posed by extensive deeply infiltrating endometriosis (Magos

1993). Endometriosis may now be treated by conservative laparoscopic surgery, with deposits vapourized using a laser or excised with significant pain relief compared to controls undergoing diagnostic laparoscopy at six months (Sutton *et al.* 1994). Increasing skills in laparoscopic surgery have led to a revival of interest in surgical procedures for the relief of dysmenorrhoea which had fallen into disfavour as excessively invasive. Destruction of the uterosacral ligaments is considered to interrupt the sensory nerve supply to the uterus, and presacral neurectomy is directed at more proximal afferent fibres converging in the hypogastric plexus. The rationale for these procedures in a context of non-terminal disease may be questioned as the destruction of nerve axons is followed by their regrowth and reinnervation of end organs. On the other hand, presacral neurectomy does result in division of the appropriate nerves and published results, especially from uncontrolled studies, are supportive. For example, in a series of 85 women with endometriosis-associated dysmenorrhoea treated by laparoscopic presacral neurectomy, 94 per cent were improved a minimum of one year later (Nezhat and Nezhat 1992). Another positive report of an uncontrolled series concluded rather alarmingly that 'laparoscopic presacral neurectomy is safe and effective as an initial surgical intervention for treating midline dysmenorrhoea...' (Biggerstaff and Foster 1994). However, when women were randomized to standard conservative surgery alone ($n = 36$) or in combination with pre-sacral neurectomy ($n = 35$) there was no difference in endometriosis symptoms at long-term follow-up (Candiani *et al.* 1992).

Division of the uterosacral ligaments in order to relieve dysmenorrhoea has a less robust anatomical basis, as the nerve supply to the uterus is by no means confined to the ligament. Unfortunately, no randomized studies of laparoscopic division of the uterosacral ligaments have been reported and the procedure is frequently carried out at the time of treatment of endometriosis, which makes its relative contribution to symptom relief hard to assess. As further randomized controlled studies of laparoscopic procedures are reported, the place of conservative surgery in the management of endometriosis-associated dysmenorrhoea will become clearer.

Conclusions

Traditional concepts of the aetiology and pathogenesis of endometriosis are beginning to be modified as an understanding of the underlying molecular mechanisms emerges, and similarities with aspects of cancer biology are becoming apparent. An appreciation is emerging of the importance of individualizing therapy so as to optimize symptom control while minimizing side-effects and adverse metabolic consequences. Minimal access surgery has an increasing role in reducing the morbidity of radical curative procedures, and in providing a wider range of conservative surgical options.

References

Amodei, N., Nelson, R.O., Jarret, R.B., and Sigmin, S. (1987). Psychological treatments of dysmenorrhea: differential effectiveness for spasmodics and congestives. *Journal of Behaviour Therapy and Experimental Psychiatry*, **18**, 95–103.

Beard, R.W., Reginald, P.W., and Wadsworth, J. (1988). Clinical features of women with chronic lower abdominal pain and pelvic congestion. *British Journal of Obstetrics and Gynaecology*, **95**, 153–61.

Berkley, K.J., Robbins, A., and Sato, Y. (1988). Afferent fibres supplying the uterus in the rat. *Journal of Neurophysiology*, **59**, 142–63.

Biggerstaff, E.D. III and Foster, S.N. (1994). Laparoscopic presacral neurectomy for treatment of midline pelvic pain. *Journal of the American Association of Gynecological Lapasoscopists*, **2**, 31–5.

Brauer, M.M., Lincoln, J., Sarner, S., Blundell, D., Milner, P., Passaro M., and Burnstock, G. (1994*a*). Maturational changes in sympathetic and sensory innervation of the rat uterus: effects of neonatal capsaicin treatment. *International Journal of Developmental Neuroscience*, **12**, 157–71.

Brauer, M.M., Lincoln, J., Milner, P., Sarner, S., Blundell, D., Passaro, M., *et al.* (1994*b*). Plasticity of autonomic nerves: differential effects of longterm guanethidine sympathectomy on the sensory innervation of the rat uterus during maturation. *International Journal of Developmental Neuroscience*, **12**, 579–86.

Bridges, J.E., Prentice, A., Roche, W., Englefield, P., and Thomas, E.J. (1994). Expression of integrin adhesion molecules in endometrium and endometriosis. *British Journal of Obstetrics and Gynaecology*, **101**, 696–700.

Cameron, I.T., Davenport, A.P., Brown, M.J., and Smith, S.K. (1991). Endothelin-1 stimulates prostaglandin F_2 alpha release from human endometrium. *Prostaglandins, Leukotrienes and Essential Fatty Acids*, **42**, 155–7.

Candiani, G.B., Danesino, V., Gastaldi, A., Parazzini, F., and Ferraroni, M. (1991). Reproductive and menstrual factors and risk of peritoneal and ovarian endometriosis. *Fertility and Sterility*, **56**, 230–4.

Candiani, G.B., Fedele, L., Vercellini, P., Bianchi, S., and di Nola, G. (1992). Presacral neurectomy for the treatment of pelvic pain associated with endometriosis: a controlled study. *American Journal of Obstetrics Gynecology*, **167**, 100–3.

Cornillie, F.J., Oosterlynck, D., Lauweryns, J.M., and Koninckx P.R. (1990). Deeply infiltrating pelvic endometriosis: histology and clinical significance. *Fertility and Sterility*, **53**, 978–83.

Darrow, S.L., Vena, J.E., Batt, R.E., Zielezny, M.A., Michalek, A.M., and Selman, S. (1993). Menstrual cycle characteristics and the risk of endometriosis. *Epidemiology*, **4**, 135–42.

Dawood, M.Y. (1988). Nonsteroidal anti-inflammatory drugs and changing attitudes toward dysmenorrhea. *American Medicine*, **84**, 23–9.

Dawood, M.Y. and Ramos, J. (1990). Transcutaneous electrical nerve stimulation (TENS) for the treatment of primary dysmenorrhea: a randomized crossover comparison with placebo TENS and ibuprofen. *Obstetrics and Gynaecology*, **75**, 656–60.

Donnez, J., Nisolle, M., and Casanas, F. (1993). Endoscopic surgery. *Baillière's Clinical Obstetrics and Gynaecology*, **7**, 839–48.

Economos, K., MacDonald, P.C., and Casey, M.L. (1992). Endothelin-1 gene expression and protein biosynthesis in human endometrium: potential modulator of endometrial blood flow. *Journal of Clinical Endocrinology and Metabolism*, **74**, 14–9.

Fedele, L., Parazzini, F., Bianchi, S., Arcaini, L., and Candiani, G.B., (1990). Stage and localization of pelvic endometriosis and pain. *Fertility and Sterility*, **53**, 155–8.

Fedele, L., Bianchi, S., Bocciolone, L., di Nola, G., and Parazzini, F. (1992). Pain symptoms associated with endometriosis. *Obstetrics and Gynecology*, **79**, 767–9.

Forman, R.G., Robinson, J.N., Mehta, Z., and Barlow, D.H. (1993). Patient history as a simple predictor of pelvic pathology in subfertile women. *Human Reproduction*, **8**, 53–5.

Gaetje, R., Kotzian, S., Herrmann, G., Baumann, R., and Starzinski-Powitz, A. (1995). Invasiveness of endometriotic cells in vitro. *Lancet*, **346**, 1463–4.

Gangar, K.F., Stones, R.W., Saunders, D., Rogers, V., Rae, T., Cooper, S., and Beard, R.W. (1993). An alternative to hysterectomy? GnRH analogue combined with hormone replacement therapy. *British Journal of Obstetrics and Gynaecology*, **100**, 360–4.

Howell, R., Edmonds, D.K., Dowsett, M., Crook, D., Lees, B., and Stevenson, J.C. (1995). Gonadotropin-releasing hormone analogue (goserelin) plus hormone replacement therapy for the treatment of endometriosis: a randomized controlled trial. *Fertility and Sterility*, **64**, 474–81.

Jacobson, J., Harris, S.R., and Bullingham, R.E.S. (1994). Low dose intranasal nafarelin for the treatment of endometriosis. *Acta Obstetrica et Gynecologica Scandinavica*, **73**, 144–50.

Jänig, W. and Koltzenburg, M. (1993). Pain arising from the urogenital tract. In *Nervous control of the urogenital system*, (ed. C.A., Maggi), pp. 525–78. Harwood Academic Publishers, Chur, Switzerland.

Jiang, X., Hitchcock, A., Bryan, E.J., Watson, R.H., Englefield, P., Thomas, E.J., and Campbell, I.G. (1996). Microsatellite analysis of endometriosis reveals loss of heterozygosity at candidate ovarian tumor suppressor gene loci. *Cancer Research*, **56**, 3534–9.

Koike, H., Egawa, H., Ohtsuka, T., Yamaguchi, M., Ikenoue, T., and Mori, N. (1992). Correlation between dysmenorrheic severity and prostaglandin production in women with endometriosis. *Prostaglandins, Leukotrienes and Essential Fatty Acids*, **46**, 133–7.

Koninckx, P.R., Meuleman, C., Demeyere, S., Lesaffre, E., and Cornillie, F.J. (1991). Suggestive evidence that pelvic endometriosis is a progressive disease, whereas deeply infiltrating endometriosis is associated with pelvic pain. *Fertility and Sterility*, **55**, 759–65.

Kurjak, A. and Kupesic, S. (1994). Scoring system for prediction of ovarian endometriosis based on transvaginal color and pulsed Doppler sonography. *Fertility and Sterility*, **62**, 81–8.

Leather, A.T., Studd, J.W.W., Watson, N.R., and Holland E.F.N. (1993). The prevention of bone loss in young women treated with GnRH analogues with 'add-back' estrogen therapy. *Obstetrics and Gynecology*, **81**, 104–7.

Lundeberg, T., Bondesson, L., and Lundstrom, V. (1985). Relief of primary dysmenorrhea by transcutaneous electrical nerve stimulation. *Acta Obstetricia et Gynecologica Scandinavica*, **64**, 491–7.

McMahon, S.B. and Koltzenburg, M. (1994). Silent afferents and visceral pain. In *Progress in pain research and management*, Vol. 1, (ed. H.L., Fields, and J.C., Liebeskind), pp. 11–29. IASP Press, Seattle.

Magos, A. (1993). Endometriosis: radical surgery. *Baillière's Clinical Obstetrics and Gynaecology*, **7**, 849–64.

Mahmood, T.A., Templeton, A.A., Thomson, L., and Fraser, C. (1991). Menstrual symptoms in women with pelvic endometriosis. *British Journal of Obstetrics and Gynaecology*, **98**, 558–63.

Mannheimer, J.S. and Whalen, E.C. (1985). The efficacy of transcutaneous electrical nerve stimulation in dysmenorrhea. *Clinical Journal of Pain*, **1**, 75–83.

Mione, M.C., Cavanagh, J.F.R., Lincoln, J., Milner, P., and Burnstock G. (1990). Pregnancy reduces noradrenaline but not neuropeptide levels in the uterine artery of the guinea-pig. *Cell and Tissue Research*, **259**, 503–9.

Namnoum, A.B., Hickman, T.N., Goodman, S.B., Gehlbach, D.L., and Rock, J.A. (1995). Incidence of symptom recurrence after hysterectomy for endometriosis. *Fertility and Sterility*, **64**, 898–902.

Nezhat, C. and Nezhat, F. (1992). A simplified method of laparoscopic presacral neurectomy for the treatment of central pelvic pain due to endometriosis. *British Journal of Obstetrics and Gynaecology*, **99**, 659–63.

Nisolle, M., Casanas-Roux, F., Anaf, V., Mine, J.M., and Donnez, J. (1993). Morphometric study of the stromal vascularization in peritoneal endometriosis. *Fertility and Sterility*, **59**, 681–4.

Papka, R.E., Cotton, J.P., and Traurig, H.H. (1985). Comparative distribution of neuropeptide tyrosine-, vasoactive intestinal polypeptide-, substance P-immunoreactive, acetylcholinesterase-positive and noradrenergic nerves in the reproductive tract of the female rat. *Cell and Tissue Research*, **242**, 475–90.

Parazzini, F., Ferraroni, M., Fedele, L., Bocciolone, L., Rubessa, S., and Riccardi, A. (1995). Pelvic endometriosis: reproductive and menstrual risk factors at different stages in Lombardy, northern Italy. *Journal of Epidemiology and Community Health*, **49**, 61–4.

Punnonen, R.H. and Nikkanen, V.P. (1980). Endometriosis in young women. *Infertility*, **3**, 1–10.

Raffa, R.B. and Jacoby, H.I. (1991). Endothelin-1, -2 and -3 directly and big-endothelin-1 indirectly elicit an abdominal constriction response in mice. *Life Science*, **48**, PL-85–PL-90.

Redwine, D.B. (1987). The distribution of endometriosis in the pelvis by age groups and fertility. *Fertility and Sterility*, **47**, 173–5.

Redwine, D.B. (1994). Endometriosis persisting after castration: clinical characteristics and results of surgical management. *Obstetrics and Gynecology*, **83**, 405–13.

Reid, B.A., Gangar, K.F., and Beard, R.W. (1992). Severe endometriosis treated with gonadotrophin releasing hormone agonist and continuous combined hormone replacement therapy. *British Journal of Obstetrics Gynaecology*, **99**, 344–8.

Robbins, A., Berkley, K.J., and Sato, Y. (1992). Estrous cycle variation of afferent fibers supplying reproductive organs in the female rat. *Brain Research*, **596**, 353–6.

Salamanca, A. and Beltran E. (1995). Subendometrial contractility in menstrual phase visualized by transvaginal sonography in patients with endometriosis. *Fertility and Sterility*, **64**, 193–5.

Sangi-Haghpeykar, H. and Poindexter, A.N., III (1995). Epidemiology of endometriosis among parous women. *Obstetrics and Gynecology*, **85**, 983–92.

Schwartz, L.B., Panageas, E., Lange, R., Rizzo, J., Comite, F., and McCarthy, S. (1994). Female pelvis: impact of M.R., imaging on treatment decisions and net cost analysis. *Radiology*, **192**, 55–60.

Stones, R.W. and Thomas, E.J. (1996). Cost-effective medical treatment of endometriosis. In *Recent advances in obstetrics and gynaecology*, No 19 (ed. Journal Bonnar). Churchill Livingstone, Edinburgh.

Sutton, J.G., Ewen, S.P., Whitelaw, N., and Haines, P. (1994). Prospective, randomized, double-blind, controlled trial of laser laparoscopy in the treatment of pelvic pain associated with minimal, mild and moderate endometriosis. *Fertility and Sterility*, **62**, 696–700.

Thomas, E.J., Okuda, K.J., and Thomas, N.M. (1991). The combination of a depot gonadotrophin releasing hormone agonist and cyclical hormone replacement therapy for dysfunctional uterine bleeding. *British Journal of Obstetrics and Gynaecology*, **98**, 1155–9.

Thomas, M., Lundeberg, T., Bjork, G., and Lundstrom-Lindstedt, V. (1995). Pain and discomfort in primary dysmenorrhea is reduced by preemptive acupuncture or low frequency TENS. *European Journal of Physical Medicine and Rehabilitation*, **5**, 71–6.

Vercellini, P., Parazzini, F., Bolis, G., Carinelli, S., Dindelli, M., Vendola, N., *et al.* (1993). Endometriosis and ovarian cancer. *American Journal of Obstetrics and Gynecology*, **169**, 181–2.

Woolf, C.J., Shortland, P., and Coggeshall, R.E. (1992). Peripheral nerve injury triggers central sprouting of myelinated afferents. *Nature*, **355**, 75–8.

Word, R.A., Kamm, K.E., Stull, J.T., and Casey, M.L. (1990). Endothelin increases cytoplasmic calcium and myosin phosphorylation in human myometrium. *American Journal of Obstetrics and Gynecology*, **162**, 1103–8.

V Psychosomatic considerations and pre-menstrual syndrome

26 Psychosomatic and other influences on complaints of menstrual bleeding and pain

Pamela Warner

Introduction

For many health complaints there has been a relatively recent realization of the potential importance of psychosomatic aetiology. However, in women's health, particularly menstrual complaints, there is a history of ready attribution to psychological factors. It might be expected that this would have resulted in psychologically focused research, an enhanced understanding of the aetiology of menstrual complaints, and to the development of psychologically based treatment strategies. Regrettably this is not the case, as may be seen in current major reviews (Effective Health Care Bulletin 1995).

While there has been continuing endeavour and considerable success with regard to organic aetiology, there has been far less progress in psychosomatic understanding of menstrual complaints. Medical and surgical treatments have improved steadily, but there has been minimal formal integration of psychosocial factors into assessment and treatment. Perhaps this reflects the tendency for psychosomatic factors to have been invoked most readily when the validity of complaint is doubted, when no organic cause can be found, or when it is felt that the symptoms really are not severe enough to warrant complaint.

Contemporary thinking is that the 'mind–body' separation implicit in such an approach is overly simplistic, and unhelpful in understanding health complaints, which are rarely solely 'mental' or purely 'physical' (Sharpe *et al.* 1995). Instead an integrated approach is required, considering the contribution of both biological and psychosocial factors. This chapter will examine beliefs regarding psychosomatic influences in menorrhagia and pain, and the validity of the evidence on which they are based. Consideration will be given to how these beliefs have arisen, and the evidence will be related to current conceptualization of psychosomatic aetiology.

Psychosomatic aetiology in menorrhagia and pain

Professional beliefs regarding psychosomatic aetiology

For menorrhagia and pain the generally dismissive tone of a number of the attributions to psychosomatic aetiology has provoked counter-claims of sexual prejudice. This was held to be the only possible explanation for such ready acceptance of psychogenic causes for exclusively female complaints, without evidence and despite the potential organic causes already established (Lennane and Lennane 1973). More recently, a striking observation was not so much the preponderance of psychosomatic causes mooted in contemporary gynaecological textbooks, but how seldom any evidence was advanced to support them (Laws 1992).

In the gynaecological literature prior to the early 70s strong causal attributions have been made to psychological factors: describing menstrual complaint as a 'psychic conflict sailing under a gynaecological flag' (Rogers 1950); claiming that 'an unwholesome attitude to periods may be involved in the aetiology of menstrual complaints' (Levitt and Lubin 1967); or that 'pain is always secondary to an emotional problem' (Benson 1972); and hypothesizing 'faulty outlook ... leading to an exaggeration of minor discomfort' (Jeffcoate 1967). In 1973 Lennane countered that disorders such as dysmenorrhoea have been 'characterised by an unscientific recourse to psychogenesis and a correspondingly inadequate, even derisory approach to their management' (Lennane and Lennane 1973). Nearly twenty years later similar concerns were expressed, for a broader range of complaints (e.g. migraine and diseases such as pneumonia, cancer and hyperthyroidism), i.e. that exaggeration of the aetiological role of psychological factors has an adverse impact on the accuracy of diagnosis and the quality of care, and that this 'psychologization' of illness is more common in the case of female patients (Goudsmit and Gadd 1991).

In the intervening years psychosomatic attributions continued: that the majority of those complaining of menorrhagia were 'women for whom the complaint of menorrhagia appears to be an expression of psychosocial disturbance' (Greenberg 1983); and that 'If a woman presents in the surgery with menstrual complaint it is advisable to look for any associated psychiatric disorder' (Gath *et al.* 1987*a*). A more recent study of life events and menorrhagia '... suggested a causal chain running from provoking agent to onset of menorrhagia and mediated by an intervening depressive condition' (Harris 1989).

Similar statements are found in textbooks published between 1975 and 1990, the range of psychosomatic explanations for menstrual pain including avoidance of, or boredom with, unappealing tasks; anxious personality; emotional disturbance; failure to conform to the sex role; maternal influence; pressures of modern life; lack of fresh air; delayed childbearing; and low threshold for pain (Laws 1992). It is noted that this last attribution involves a pre-existing conviction that the pain really is not as bad as reported, since the pain is not objectively assessed.

Despite the range of psychosocial *causes* of dysmenorrhoea advanced by the textbooks, they all recommended the oral contraceptive pill as an effective treatment. Laws comments on the contrary logic implicit in this, unless a hormonal medication can 'remedy' psychological risk factors (Laws 1992). The contrast between psychosomatic aetiologies advanced and management advised is even more stark in the case of menorrhagia: despite at least three decades of reports suggesting psychosomatic aetiology for menstrual problems, a very recent review of menorrhagia was unable to recommend a single psychologically based treatment (Effective Health Care Bulletin 1995).

Evidence

The validity of any aetiological mechanisms proposed should be evaluated in the light of the research design and the findings. In the case of menorrhagia and pain almost all such reports are based on cross-sectional designs, a common approach being to examine the association between complaining and menstrual attitudes or measures of psychological distress. However, causal inference is problematic in such studies, since they run the risk of 'correlational bias' (Sackett 1979). Severe pain is an unpleasant experience with marked consequences for mood, especially if further bouts are anticipated (Sharpe *et al.* 1995). The finding of high anxiety levels in a patient with severe dysmenorrhoea or, indeed, enduring the disruption caused by menorrhagia, does not inform as to the direction of any causal association, since both cause and effect are plausible.

Indeed, association does not necessarily imply a causal link, at all, since the observed association may be due to confounding factors. An example might be the association that was found in a retrospective case–control study, between subjective complaint of menorrhagia and prior life event (e.g. the 'loss' of an important other or cherished goal) (Harris 1989). Over 20 per cent of the women sampled had to be excluded because the duration of menorrhagia exceeded five years (a prior criterion, set to ensure accurate recall of events/symptoms). It follows that for many subjects studied, with duration of problem up to four years, attendance at the clinic was not precipitated by a new complaint, but instead, perhaps, by a change in tolerance to an existing problem. This could result in confounding, an illusory association of menorrhagia with life event, if those who have suffered such an event have increased motivation to seek treatment, perhaps to compensate themselves for the adverse life event by eliminating the burden of excessive periods. The confounder would be treatment-seeking behaviour, and since the study involves referral to a hospital clinic the confounding could arise at the individual or family doctor level. All that is required is that ultimate referral is more likely because of the life event that has occurred. This is a variant of 'admission-rate bias', a common pitfall in clinical research (Sackett 1979).

In contrast to the majority of disorders that are believed to have psychosomatic aetiology, menorrhagia is unique in having the potential for objective assessment. Laboratory measurement of menstrual loss is possible, and when such assessment is undertaken the common finding is of normal blood loss in a substantial proportion of women referred for menorrhagia (Fraser *et al.* 1984). There were similar findings in a population study, that is, low to normal measured loss among many (67 per cent) of the 149 women categorizing their periods as 'heavy' (Hallberg *et al.* 1966). This has fuelled attribution to psychological factors, but more or less on the rebound, often without proper consideration of alternative explanations. Sackett terms this 'under-exhaustion bias' and notes that a failure to explore the range of hypothetical possibilities 'may lead to an authoritarian rather than authoritative interpretation' (Sackett 1979). Alternative explanations for some of the discordance in the clinical data might be referral error or regression to the mean. In the population data the explanation might be the crudeness of the subjective rating scale, distinguishing only light, moderate, and heavy periods. In either setting an explanation could be discrepant definitions, or variability in loss. Paradoxically, if a non-parametric correlation is calculated from the published data (Hallberg *et al.* 1966), it is revealed that despite the crudeness of the rating scale there is a statistically highly significant association between women's subjective ratings of loss and measured loss (r corrected for ties = 0.34, n = 474, $p < 0.00001$).

Reports vary in the extent to which their conceptual basis is explained, and this uncertainty adds to the difficulty of appraising the research design and the validity of the interpretation of findings. It is perhaps salient that the expert committee responsible for the Effective Health Care report on menorrhagia did not cite a single publication with findings of psychological aetiology in menorrhagia (Effective Health Care Bulletin 1995). In the case of dysmenorrhoea, there has been similar appraisal, that 'dysmenorrhoea seems to have attracted a disproportionate amount of psychological speculation when compared to other painful medical conditions' (Cox and Santirocco 1981).

Terminology and concepts in psychosomatic medicine

Background

Over the years there have been successive changes in the terms used to describe symptoms for which no simple organic cause can be found. Most of the older terms were coined originally to indicate some hypothesized *organic mechanism*, such as: hysteria (migrating uterus); hypochondriasis, neurosis, neuraesthenia (Sharpe *et al.* 1995). With usage the original meaning has been lost, so that they now denote psychological aetiology.

Of the terms intended from the outset to denote a *psychogenic mechanism*, 'psychosomatic' refers properly to physiological disorder that is caused by psychological stress; whereas 'somatization' is the experience of physical symptoms as a substitute for the real (but denied) psychological problem. Both models have been found wanting when applied to many non-specific medically unexplained symptoms, in that the symptoms occur in many cases in the absence of psychological distress, and both maintain a mind–body division that is unhelpful to our understanding and treatment of complaints (Sharpe *et al.* 1995). Furthermore, they imply to the patient that their physical symptoms are 'all in (or of) the mind', provoking fear of psychiatric illness, or resentment at the suggestion of 'imaginary' complaint (Sharpe *et al.* 1995).

Alternatively, it may be that *physiological disorder/discomfort causes psychological problems.* This 'disability hypothesis' could apply to any disorder that has distressing symptoms, and where organic cause is difficult to pin-point. Marked improvement in psychological well-being has been reported in women who have undergone hysterectomy for excessive (and often also painful) periods, so elimination of symptoms, albeit via major abdominal surgery, has resulted in improvement in psychological well-being (Gath *et al.* 1982).

Current thinking

The term now adopted is 'functional somatic symptoms', to imply an abnormality in the physiological functioning of the organism that is not associated with marked structural changes. This has the virtue of being a parsimonious description of the complaint, and, for the time being at least, is free of any implication as to mechanism (Sharpe *et al.* 1995). The contemporary view is that an understanding of medically unexplained symptoms requires a 'multicausal, interactive aetiological model which takes account of a number of relevant physical, psychological, and social factors' (Mayou *et al.* 1995). In many cases complaint will be the result of an interaction between physiological processes, psychological/personality factors, and feedback from others, including the reactions of health care professionals (Mayou *et al.* 1995).

The numerous aetiological factors that have been established may be categorized as predisposing (e.g. prior illness experience, personality); precipitating (e.g. normal/abnormal physiological processes, stressful events, psychiatric illness); or perpetuating (e.g. lack of psychosocial support, iatrogenic medicine, continuing physical symptoms) (Mayou *et al.* 1995). With so many factors to be considered, when in reality only a few are likely to be operating in any individual patient, it is inevitable that across the patient group no very strong associations are obtained.

Whatever the clinical aptness and philosophical appeal of this broad view of medically unexplained illness, it has profound consequences for research design. The complexity of the models envisaged make for unrealistic demands on study design, most seriously on sample size, but also in terms of the number of variables that need to be assessed. Perhaps this explains some of the lack of progress in psychosomatic understanding and management of complaints such as dysmenorrhoea and menorrhagia.

Applicability of model to menorrhagia and pain

The classification proposed for functional somatic symptoms focuses on the constellation of symptoms experienced, and duration or chronicity (Mayou *et al.* 1995), but virtually ignores the *severity* of the somatic symptoms. In contrast, dysmenorrhoea and menorrhagia are each characterized by a single specific symptom. Both 'symptoms' are experienced by the entire female population, intermittently for a time-span of about forty years, and over a continuum of severity, from minimal through to extreme. So it is the *severity* of symptoms rather than the occurrence that is pertinent. In the case of menorrhagia a further unique distinction is that an objective evaluation of menstrual blood loss (Hallberg and Nilsson 1964), and total fluid loss (Fraser *et al.* 1985), is possible. There is thus potential for substantially more powerful testing of the association of explanatory factors with subjective severity of symptoms, and in the case of menorrhagia, with measured menstrual loss.

Refinement of the psychosomatic model in the case of dysmenorrhoea and pain

Taking account of severity of symptoms

In menorrhagia and dysmenorrhoea it is the severity of symptoms that transforms what would otherwise be commonplace into an intolerable burden. However, in a recent study of patients referred for menorrhagia, dysmenorrhoea, or pre-menstrual syndrome, one of the most striking findings was that over half of menorrhagia referrals (57 per cent) did not rate their periods as 'very heavy'. (Bancroft *et al.* 1993). So whatever the basis for complaint it could not have been a subjective estimation of *excessive* periods. The proportion of dysmenorrhoea referrals failing to achieve a 'severe' categorization (severe pain that in nearly all periods affects daily activities) was only 16 per cent, suggesting a much more stringent treatment-seeking/referral criterion for this condition (Bancroft *et al.* 1993). Of even greater importance, within each referral group there were differences in patient characteristics between those reporting the complaint 'symptom' as subjectively severe, or not (Warner 1995).

Figure 26.1 hypothesizes the contribution to treatment seeking of factors over and above symptom severity: women with very severe symptoms tend to seek treatment more or less regardless of other factors (dark grey segment of figure), whereas women with moderate symptom severity may nevertheless seek treatment, if other factors contribute (light grey segment), e.g. financial concern at loss of earnings if work days are missed on account of symptoms; anxious personality; family history of gynaecological cancer, etc.

For example, menorrhagia referrals reporting 'very heavy' periods were more likely to be women over 40 years of age and to have high scores on the Anxiety subscale of the General Health Questionnaire (GHQ), whereas those reporting only 'heavy' periods were more likely to be in the 30 to 40 years age range, to report dysmenorrhoea in addition to heavy periods, and to have high scores on the Depression subscale of GHQ (Warner 1995). It is clearly essential to take

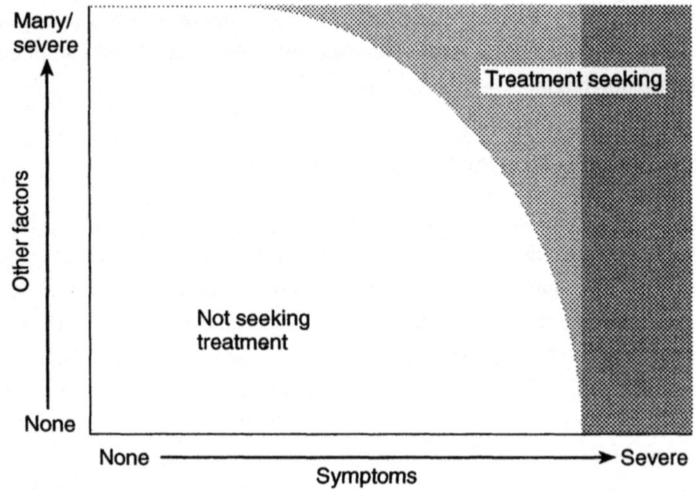

Fig. 26.1 Treatment seeking, symptom severity and other precipitating factors.

account of differences among patients in their own subjective evaluation of their symptoms, if wishing to understand factors influencing treatment seeking.

Specification of point of influence

A 'symptom' is a change in the body or its function that is perceived as evidence of disease. Therefore a patient presenting with menorrhagia or dysmenorrhoea must have both perceived a change and interpreted this as symptom of disease, but in addition must have completed a third stage, i.e. made a decision to seek medical help. If the patients being considered are referrals to a specialist outpatient clinic then a fourth stage is also necessary – the family doctor must judge that referral is necessary (Fig. 26.2).

The various aetiological factors may be operating at any or all the above stages, so any association with the status 'referred patient' may arise because of effects on: perception of symptoms; disease belief; treatment seeking; referral; or some combination of these. Clinic-based research may thus detect, as characteristic of the condition under study, factors that are related merely to treatment-seeking behaviour or referral, *in general*. Factors readily envisaged as exerting influence in this way are anxiety, personality, stressful events, and past experience of illness.

Indeed it is usual to find high levels of psychological symptoms or minor psychiatric illness in most clinical populations. Even for medical complaints it has been found that those seeking help are more likely to be experiencing psychological distress (Stoeckle *et al.* 1964), compared to

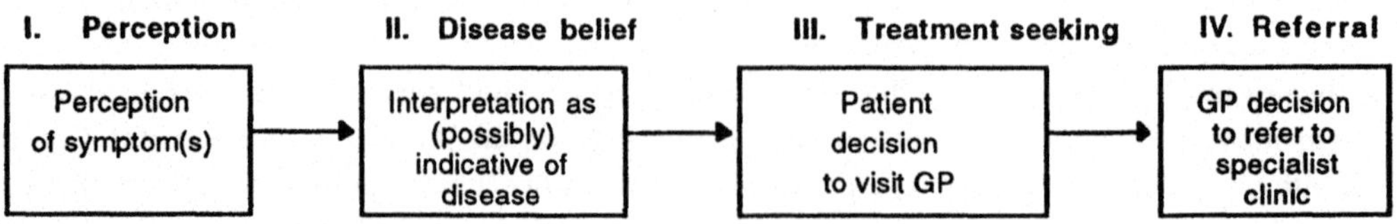

Fig. 26.2 Stages in becoming a patient referred for menorrhagia or dysmenorrhoea.

individuals with the same degree of symptoms but not seeking help. For menstrual problems specifically, those seeking help are more likely to have low self-esteem or to be depressed (Morse *et al.* 1988), whereas those not seeking help are more likely to have a low opinion of medical science or the medical profession (Scambler and Scambler 1985).

There are a number of factors influencing the decision process (Armstrong *et al.* 1991), including patient pressure on their family doctors to obtain referral (Kuh and Stirling 1995). The substantially increased admission rates that have been reported among women of lower socioeconomic status, both for D&C and for hysterectomy (Newton *et al.* 1991), may reflect the epidemiology of the conditions giving rise to these procedures. The alternative interpretation is that there are socioeconomic differences in the influences on treatment-seeking behaviour, referral, and treatment choice. In a study of referrals for menstrual disorders the best independent predictors of referral were: family doctor's belief that surgery would be necessary; patient preference for surgery; GP belief that patient wished surgery; number of previous surgical operations; older age of patient; and male GP (Coulter *et al.* 1994). While both subjective and GP-assessed symptom severity were associated with referral, they did not improve the predictive power of the multiple logistic regression model. Similar effects may account for the low substantiation of referral, by patients' subjective rating of symptoms, as reported above (Warner 1995).

Verifiability of complaint

The potential for understanding the complaint is substantially increased when objective verification is possible, as it is for menorrhagia (Hallberg and Nilsson 1964; Fraser *et al.* 1985). In practice, however, objective verification is rarely imposed, except in treatment trials. Furthermore, since clinical trials seldom include psychosocial assessments of patients they provide little chance of advancing our understanding of 'unjustified' complaint. One study has involved comprehensive psychological assessment and blood loss measurements on 143 women awaiting hysterectomy for menorrhagia (Hodges 1989). Subjective overestimation of bleeding was related neither to psychiatric vulnerability nor to factors such as menstrual attitudes, adverse life events, marital discord, illness behaviour, or chronic difficulties. However, overestimation *was* related to perceived adverse impact of periods (Hodges 1989). This study awaits replication in a less highly selected clinical group than women proceeding to hysterectomy.

Consideration of alternative explanations in menorrhagia and pain

Response bias

A number of studies are based on data obtained from symptom check lists, and a common finding is that women reporting menstrual symptoms also score highly on scales such as the General Health Questionnaire (GHQ), measuring psychiatric well-being, or the Eysenck Personality Inventory (EPI) neuroticism scale (Gath *et al.* 1987*a*). However, there is strong likelihood of confounding in such studies, as it has been found that subjective symptom reports are related to aspects of personality, i.e. individuals who score highly on dimensions such as 'negative affectivity' or neuroticism are also likely to score higher on self-report health scales than others with the same degree of symptoms (Watson and Pennebaker 1989).

Comorbidity

In the study mentioned above a substantial proportion (31 per cent) of clinic referrals with a subjectively severe menstrual problem reported *more than one* severe problem (Warner 1995), so for these women the clinical picture is confused. They are likely to make decisions about treatment seeking on the basis of the *accumulation* of menstrual symptoms experienced, but the choice of presenting symptom may be fairly arbitrary.

Despite dysmenorrhoea referrals being the smallest group, pain was the most frequently documented severe symptom, reported by 12 per cent of menorrhagia referrals in addition to excessive periods, and by 9 per cent *instead* of excessive periods (Warner 1994). Thus pain is not only a potential contributory factor to treatment seeking for excessive periods, but it would also appear to be the covert *main* reason in a number of cases. Laws has concluded that women 'experiencing menstrual pain confront strong pressure to be silent about it' (Laws 1992). Do some in desperation complain instead of their heavy periods?

The group with a combination of severe menstrual problems were markedly different to the women reporting severe menorrhagia or dysmenorrhoea alone (Warner 1995). Women with combined problems were strongly clustered in the 30 to 44 years age range (85 per cent of the group), had high neuroticism scores, and were highest for GHQ total score and all subscales except 'depression'. They were also more likely to favour radical surgical treatment (Warner 1994). In contrast, women reporting severe dysmenorrhoea alone were young (64 per cent less than 35 years), and scored high only on the EPI 'extroversion' scale and on the 'somatic and social dysfunction' scales of the GHQ, i.e. young women temperamentally bold enough to speak out about period pain and the associated discomfort and disruption to life. Of women reporting menorrhagia only, 63 per cent were 40 years or over, 86 per cent were parous, and about 50 per cent had been sterilized (the highest rates). In contrast to women with combined problems this group had notably high scores only for the 'anxiety' subscale of the GHQ (Warner 1995).

Where there is comorbidity between menstrual complaint and other disorders (such as diabetes, epilepsy, or depression), each complaint should be given equal prior weight, rather than one being presumed to invalidate another. The individuals thus afflicted may be well able to judge the disorder for which they require medical attention. For example, in a community survey women were asked about menstrual symptoms, whether they had consulted their GP in the last year, and why, and were also subjected to 'present state examination' (PSE) to assess psychiatric status (Gath *et al.* 1987*a*,*b*). Of 123 women who reported menstrual symptoms and had consulted their GP in the past year, those who had been identified as psychiatric cases comprised 17 per cent of those who said they had consulted for menstrual symptoms, but twice as many, 36 per cent, of those who had consulted for psychiatric problems. So on the whole, women experiencing comorbidity consult appropriately. The difficulty may rather be availability of acceptable and effective treatments.

Treatment aspirations

Alternatively, women may emphasize the complaint that they anticipate will achieve their treatment preference. The majority of women with menstrual complaint wish for a treatment that would make their periods 'normal' (89 per cent), but when asked about the perceived advantages of hysterectomy, the outcome most welcomed (by 74 per cent) was that it would mean 'no more pain with periods' (Warner 1994). There may also be a contraceptive agenda: 74 per cent of respondents favoured a hypothetical treatment with reversible contraceptive effect, and for 47 per cent even an irreversible contraceptive effect would be welcome (Warner 1994). In the circumstances, women with moderately heavy loss, severe pain, and wishing permanent contraception may anticipate more satisfactory outcome by emphasizing menstrual loss rather than dysmenorrhoea.

Patient–doctor communication

Given cultural constraints on complaining (Laws 1992), patient concerns may not be accurately communicated to the family or clinic doctor, particularly when there is comorbidity. Although 64 per cent of patients discussed treatment choice with their GP, in 45 per cent of consultations the GP was afterwards unaware of the patient's view (Coulter *et al.* 1994), and among patients with a strong treatment preference the GP was correct about this preference in only a third of cases (Coulter *et al.* 1994). Similarly, among women reporting at least one severe menstrual problem, 16 per cent were referred for a different, non-severe, menstrual problem (Warner 1995).

Inappropriate definition

The widely adopted definition of menorrhagia is blood loss in excess of 80 ml (Hallberg *et al.* 1966), a very stringent interpretation of 'normality' which, if applied to a single period, distinguishes the upper 3–4 per cent of the population, and exceeds the measured blood loss of many with a complaint of excessive periods. For example, 62 per cent of those with subjectively 'very heavy' periods had blood losses that failed to satisfy this criterion (Fraser *et al.* 1984). As commonly applied in clinical trials, to the average loss over two or more periods, it will be even more stringent. Doubts about women's ability to judge their own menstrual loss have arisen largely from such findings, based on this very stringent definition of menorrhagia.

It is of note that only 25 per cent of all women complaining of excessive bleeding were eligible for a recent treatment trial, on the basis of loss averaged over three periods (Bonnar and Sheppard 1996). Furthermore, the study groups had mean pre-treatment losses in excess of 163 ml, *twice* the criterion. Since losses of 80–100 ml are much more commonly found clinically than losses in excess of 100 ml, the conclusion must be that women with losses in the 'low menorrhagic' range do not maintain them consistently enough to achieve the criterion level averaged over three consecutive periods. They nevertheless have clinically defined complaint in one to two thirds of their periods. Diagnosis based on averaged losses is inappropriate, both because the substantial period-to-period variation in loss among women with heavy periods (Hodges 1989) results in underestimate of 'complaint', and also because it may be the unpredictability itself that is problematic.

A bizarre consequence of such a stringent criterion is that even where there is dramatic treatment effect (54 per cent reduction in blood loss in this study), the mean 'treated' blood loss remains as high as 75 ml (Bonnar and Sheppard 1996), suggesting that in about half the group, clinically defined menorrhagia persists despite 'effective' treatment. A further consequence is that the results of the trial findings are strictly applicable only to women with similar consistently heavy losses, and may not inform as to optimum treatment for the majority of clinic referrals, with intermittent or borderline menorrhagia.

Failure to satisfy the 80 ml criterion together with lack of identifiable cause does not necessarily imply 'unjustified' complaint: no unequivocal organic cause can be identified for many cases with menorrhagia confirmed by laboratory measurement. Of interest, reported impact of periods on daily life was found to be unrelated to measured blood loss (Hodges 1989), so an alternative interpretation is that blood loss volume is not a good indicator of menstrual complaint. This could be because periods include both blood and non-blood fluid, with the total fluid volume ranging from 1.2 to 9.0 times the blood volume (Fraser *et al.* 1985). Practically, it is 'containability' that is crucial (i.e. freedom from accidents), and this may depend more on pattern of flow, and physiology, than volume. Of referrals without subjectively extreme loss, 19 per cent instead report periods lasting 11 days or more (Warner 1994), on the face of it a reasonable interpretation of 'excessive periods'.

Treatment-seeking and referral decisions may reflect quality-of-life considerations, so that periods that are merely heavy may nevertheless be considered unacceptable for women in particular circumstances. The notional referral reason does not necessarily reflect the factor precipitating consultation with the family doctor, which could be a recent change in periods. Evidence from a pilot study of 43 women found that the problematic aspect of periods most commonly affirmed was 'periods different to how they were normally' (Warner and Crichley 1995), while reasons for the clinic visit were most often pain, blood loss, and tiredness. This study also supports the view that women do not think of heaviness in terms of volume of loss (Hodges 1989), since when asked to categorize the volume of their periods 41 per cent of women chose the response 'no idea', in preference to the offered volumes (Warner and Critchley 1995).

Contemporary expectations are that women should be able to conduct their lives largely free of disruption by menstrual problems. Complaint of 'heavy periods' involves a range of symptoms and concerns, a common one being simply change from 'normal' (Warner and Critchley 1995). Dysmenorrhoea seems to play a key role, though seldom itself the referral symptom, perhaps attributable to our cultural view of period pain. The existing definition of menorrhagia needs critical reevaluation so that it encompasses and distinguishes the spectrum of symptoms and adverse effects of 'heavy' periods.

Future research

Assessment

There is a corresponding requirement for a comprehensive assessment of menstrual complaint. Research is under way to develop such a clinical assessment, a questionnaire eliciting detailed subjective report of periods, symptoms, and their impact. This will be validated against objectively evaluated menstrual loss and standard measures of quality of life (Warner and Critchley 1995). Once standardized, this complaint profile should be a valuable tool in the clinical care of women referred for menorrhagia and dysmenorrhoea. It is important that patients *without* subjectively excessive menstrual loss are clearly distinguished, since a different diagnostic and perhaps management strategy is indicated. For them it will provide a profile of the real presenting symptoms and concerns, commonly including dysmenorrhoea.

Research design

Rigorous study of psychosomatic influences would require a substantial longitudinal population study. However, some of the influences detected may be irrelevant to the sequence of events leading to clinic appointment. Alternatively, they may be individual characteristics that are not amenable to change, and therefore unlikely to assist clinical management of patients. A more pragmatic approach would be to elucidate the factors that influence treatment seeking and referral, in relation to subjective severity of symptoms. This has the advantage that findings can be translated more readily into guidelines for primary care assessment and management, and could also lead to the development of patient education/support interventions that might, in a proportion of cases, obviate the need for specialist referral.

Conclusions

It is clear that our accumulated understanding of the association between menstrual complaints and psychosomatic factors needs to be critically reassessed. What is required is an understanding of the interplay of psychosocial and somatic factors in treatment-seeking behaviour in the individual patient. While this is probably undertaken in an unstructured way by many clinicians, the process needs to be formalized and recorded. To achieve this a comprehensive assessment of menstrual complaint is needed, allowing associations between factors to be examined, and treatment outcomes evaluated for differing complaint profiles. Only then can it be ascertained whether and in whom non-medical non-surgical interventions are effective.

Psychosomatic factors are of potential importance in many medical complaints, and it seems that in the past they have been most readily invoked in the area of menstrual complaints. Perhaps few such invocations have been valid, or helpful to women presenting with such complaints, but at least in menstrual problems there exists a tradition of acknowledging psychosomatic influences. This can be built on, and with appropriately focused and designed research there is a real chance of advancing our understanding of the multifactorial aetiology of clinical menorrhagia and dysmenorrhoea.

References

Armstrong, D., Fry, J., and Armstrong, P. (1991). Doctors' perceptions of pressure from patients for referral. *British Medical Journal*, **302**, 1186–8.

Bancroft, J., Williamson, L., Warner, P., Rennie, D., and Smith, S. (1993). Perimenstrual complaints in women complaining of PMS, menorrhagia and dysmenorrhoea; towards dismantling of the 'premenstrual syndrome'. *Psychosomatic Medicine*, **55**, 133–45.

Benson, R.C. (1972). *Gynecology and obstetrics. Current diagnosis and treatment.* (ed. M.A. Krupp and M.J. Chatton), pp. 377–434. Lange Medical Publications, Los Altos, California.

Bonnar, J. and Sheppard, B.L. (1996). Treatment of menorrhagia during menstruation: randomised controlled trial of ethamsylate, mefenamic acid, and tranexamic acid. *British Medical Journal*, **313** 579–82.

Coulter, A., Peto, V., and Doll, H. (1994). Patients' preferences and general practitioners' decisions in the treatment of menstrual disorders. *Family Practice*, **11**, 67–74.

Cox, D.J. and Santirocco, L.L. (1981). Psychological and behavioural factors in dysmenorrhoea. In *Dysmenorrhoea* (ed. M. Yusoff Dawood), pp. 75–93. Williams & Wilkins, Baltimore.

Effective Health Care Bulletin No 9 (1995). *The management of menorrhagia.* University of Leeds.

Fraser, I.S., McCarron, G., and Markham, R. (1984). A preliminary study of factors influencing perception of menstrual blood loss volume. *American Journal of Obstetrics and Gynecology*, **149**, 788–93.

Fraser, I.S., McCarron, G., Markham, R., and Resta, T. (1985). Blood and total fluid content of menstrual discharge. *Obstetrics and Gynecology*, **65**, 194–8.

Gath, D., Cooper, P., Bond, A., and Edmonds, G. (1982). Hysterectomy and psychiatric disorder II. Demographic and physical factors in relation to psychiatric outcome. *British Journal of Psychiatry*, **140**, 343–50.

Gath, D., Osborn, M., Bungay, G., Iles, S., Day, A., Bond, A., and Passingham, C. (1987*a*). Psychiatric disorder and gynaecological symptoms in middle-aged women: a community survey. *British Medical Journal*, **294**, 213–18.

Gath, D., Iles, S., and Day, A. (1987*b*). Psychiatric disorder and gynaecological symptoms in middle-aged women. *British Medical Journal*, **294**, 1033–4.

Goudsmit, E.M. and Gadd, R. (1991). All in the mind? The psychologisation of illness. *The Psychologist*, **4**, 56–60.

Greenberg, M. (1983). The meaning of menorrhagia: an investigation into the association between the complaint of menorrhagia and depression. *Journal of Psychosomatic Research*, **27**, 209–14.

Hallberg, L. and Nilsson, L. (1964). Determination of menstrual blood loss. *Scandinavian Journal of Clinical Laboratory Investigation*, **16**, 244–8.

Hallberg, L., Hogdahl, A.M., Nilsson, L., and Rybo, G. (1966). Menstrual blood loss – a population study. *Acta Obstetrica et Gynecologica Scandinavica*, **45**, 320–51.

Harris, T.O. (1989). Disorders of menstruation. In *Life events and physical illness* (ed. G.W. Brown and T.O. Harris), pp. 261–94. Hyman & Unwin, London.

Hodges, S. (1989). Psychological aspects of complaints of excessive menstrual bleeding. Ph.D. thesis, Oxford.

Jeffcoate, T.N.A. (1967). *Principles of gynaecology* (3rd edn), pp. 684–6. Butterworth, London.

Kuh, D. and Stirling, S. (1995). Socioeconomic variation in admission for diseases of the female genital system and breast in a national cohort aged 15–43. *British Medical Journal*, **311**, 840–3.

Laws, S. (1992) 'It's just the monthlies, she'll get over it': menstrual problems and men's attitudes. *Journal of Reproductive and Infant Psychology*, **10**, 117–28.

Lennane, K.J. and Lennane, R.J. (1973). Alleged psychogenic disorders in women – a possible manifestation of sexual prejudice. *New England Journal of Medicine*, **288**, 288–92.

Levitt, E.E. and Lubin, B. (1967). Some personality factors associated with menstrual complaints and menstrual attitudes. *Journal of Psychosomatic Research*, **11**, 267–70.

Mayou, R., Bass, C., and Sharpe, M. (1995). Overview of epidemiology, classification, and aetiology. In *Treatment of functional somatic symptoms* (ed. R. Mayou, C. Bass, and M. Sharpe), pp. 42–65. Oxford University Press.

Morse, C.A., Dennerstein, L., Varnavides, K., and Burrows, G.D. (1988). Menstrual cycle symptoms: comparison of a non-clinical sample with a patient group. *Journal of Affective Disorders*, **14**, 41–50.

Newton, J., Hayes. V., and Hutchinson, A. (1991). Factors influencing general practioners' referral decisions. *Family Practice*, **8**, 308–13.

Rogers, F.S. (1950). Emotional factors in gynecology. *American Journal of Obstetrics and Gynecology*, **59**, 321–7.

Sackett, D.L. (1979). Bias in analytical research. *Journal of Chronic Disease*, **32**, 51.

Scambler, A. and Scambler, G. (1985). Menstrual symptoms, attitudes and consulting behaviour. *Social Science and Medicine*, **20**, 1065–8.

Sharpe, M., Mayou, R., and Bass, C. (1995). Concepts, theories and terminology. In *Treatment of functional somatic symptoms* (ed. R. Mayou, C. Bass, and M. Sharpe), pp. 3–16. Oxford University Press.

Stoeckle, J.D., Zola, I.K., and Davidson, G.E. (1964). The quantity and significance of psychological distress in medical patients. *Journal of Chronic Disease*, **17**, 959–70.

Warner, P. (1994). Preferences regarding treatments for period problems: relationship to menstrual and demographic factors. *Journal of Psychosomatic Obstetrics and Gynaecology*, **15**, 93–110.

Warner, P. (1995). Characteristics of women referred for menstrual problems. In *Psychosomatic obstetrics and gynaecology*, (ed. J. Bitzer and M. Stauber), pp. 335–42. Monduzzi Editore, Bologna, Italy.

Warner, P. and Critchley, H.O.D (1995). Towards a new clinical assessment of menorrhagia. *Journal of Psychosomatic Obstetrics and Gynaecology*, **16** (Suppl. 1). 153.

Watson, D. and Pennebaker, J.W. (1989). Health complaints, stress, and distress: exploring the central role of negative affectivity. *Psychological Review*, **96**, 234–54.

27 Psychiatric morbidity and the menstrual cycle

Dennis Gath and Ann Day

This chapter begins with a review of associations between psychiatric disorders and menstrual disorders. This review is followed by descriptions of common psychiatric conditions such as anxiety disorders and depressive disorders. An account is then given of the causes of emotional disorders (precipitating, predisposing, and perpetuating factors). This account is followed by a review of some gynaecological syndromes including the premenstrual syndrome, dysmenorrhoea, amenorrhoea, menorrhagia (and its treatment with hysterectomy), and the menopause. Finally an account is given of methods of detecting and assessing psychiatric disorders in the gynaecology clinic.

In 1986 a psychiatric research team in Oxford carried out a survey of 521 women aged 35–59 years who were randomly selected from two group general practices. These women were interviewed in their homes by women research assistants, and were assessed by means of standardized psychiatric measures and detailed gynaecological enquiry (Gath *et al.* 1987). A salient finding was that psychiatric morbidity (predominantly emotional disorder) was significantly associated with various gynaecological symptoms, which included dysmenorrhoea, the pre-menstrual syndrome, excessive menstruation (clots and flooding), and flushes and sweats (but not the disappearance of menstruation for over six months).

High levels of emotional disorder have been found in women attending gynaecological outpatient clinics. For example, Byrne (1984) used a self-rated questionnaire, the General Health Questionnaire (GHQ) (Goldberg 1972), to measure psychiatric morbidity in 211 women aged 18–65 years who had been referred to a gynaecological clinic. Forty-six per cent of these women had high scores on the GHQ, indicating substantial morbidity. In a second phase of Byrne's study, a random sub-sample of the clinic population (35 women) was interviewed with the Present State Examination (PSE) (Wing *et al.* 1974), which is a standardized psychiatric interview. In this subgroup the overall prevalence rate for emotional disorders was 29 per cent (10/35), whereas in a comparison group of women from the general population (n = 140) the prevalence rate was significantly lower (17 per cent). It should be emphasized that high levels of psychiatric morbidity are found not only in gynaecological clinics but also in most medical and surgical clinics.

In the Oxford community survey cited above, the main psychiatric disorders were anxiety (30 per cent of women) and depression (66 per cent). These two disorders, anxiety and depression, are frequent amongst women both in the community and in gynaecological practice, and they are therefore described below.

Anxiety disorders

Anxiety disorders can be divided into generalized anxiety disorders (in which symptoms are persistent, varying little from one situation to another), and phobic disorders (in which symptoms are episodic and associated with defined circumstances).

The clinical features of anxiety disorders are characteristic. The face looks strained, the brow is furrowed, and the posture is tense. The patient is often pale and sweating, and may be restless and tremulous. The psychological symptoms of generalized anxiety disorder include feelings of fearful anticipation, irritability, sensitivity to noise, restlessness, and poor concentration which may lead to complaints of poor memory (although true memory disorder does not occur in anxiety disorder), and repetitive worrying thoughts.

The physical symptoms of generalized anxiety disorder can include menstrual discomfort, amenorrhoea, frequency and urgency of micturition, and lack of libido. There is a characteristic sleep disturbance – the patient goes to bed, lies awake worrying, falls asleep but wakes intermittently, often has unpleasant dreams, may have occasional night tremors, may waken suddenly feeling fearful, and often feels unrefreshed in the morning.

Patients with anxiety may hyperventilate, as shown by shallow breathing, dizziness, tinnitus, headache, precordial discomfort, weakness, faintness, numbness, tingling in the extremities, and sometimes carpopedal spasm.

Anxiety symptoms can occur with any psychiatric disorder, including depressive disorder. Hence, when a psychiatrist sees a patient with features of an anxiety disorder, the first steps are to exclude concomitant depressive disorder, to explain the nature and cause of the symptoms to the patient, and to reassure the patient about any specific concerns.

If an anxiety disorder is severe, short-term benzodiazepine treatment may be helpful (but benzodiazepines should not be prescribed long term because of the risk of habituation). The main aim of the psychiatrist is to help the patient to resolve stressful problems or to come to terms with them. Further treatment of anxiety may include relaxation training, respiratory control of hyperventilation, or a systematic course of a brief and practical psychological treatment known as problem solving (Catalan *et al.* 1991).

Patients with generalized anxiety disorder may worry about their symptoms in a way that prolongs their anxiety. Thus an anxious patient may worry that the symptoms portend a serious medical condition, or that other people notice the patient's anxiety, or that other members of the family have been distressed by the symptoms.

Depressive disorders

Depressive disorders are common in gynaecological patients, but often go undetected. If not recognized, a depressive disorder can cause much distress to the patient, and may aggravate gynaecological symptoms. Hence it is important that gynaecologists should be able to recognize depressive disorders.

Depressive syndromes may be classified as mild, moderate, or severe. The moderate syndrome will be described first, because it is particularly likely to present in gynaecological practice. The central features of the moderate depressive syndrome are low mood, loss of interests, lack of enjoyment, pessimistic thinking and reduced energy – all of which lead to impaired efficiency.

Often patients with the moderate syndrome have a sad appearance, and they may show slowness of movement and speech. Their sad mood is not relieved by other people's efforts to be cheering. Anxiety is often experienced, together with irritability and restlessness.

An important group of depressive symptoms is referred to as biological. Symptoms in this group include loss of appetite, loss of weight, constipation, reduced sexual drive, and amenorrhoea. A particularly distressing symptom is early morning waking, which occurs two or three hours before the usual time of waking; the patient lies awake and is beset with pessimistic thoughts about the past and the future.

The mood is often worse in the morning than in the evening (diurnal variation). Depressed patients may blame themselves disproportionately about minor issues. They also complain frequently about physical symptoms, such as constipation and aching discomfort in various parts of the body.

In mild depressive disorder, the symptoms described above are present, but are less intense than in the moderate syndrome. Mild depressive disorders have the usual depressive symptoms of low mood, lack of energy and lack of interest, together with irritability. The sleep disturbance is difficulty in falling asleep rather than early morning waking. Biological features (such as poor appetite and weight loss) are unusual. The mood is usually worse in the evening than in the morning.

In severe depressive disorder, the clinical features described above are particularly intense, and in addition there may be delusions and hallucinations. A brief account of anxiety and depressive disorders can be found in the *Concise Oxford textbook of psychiatry* (Gelder *et al.* 1994). A more detailed account can be found in the third edition of the *Oxford textbook of psychiatry* (Gelder *et al.* 1996).

Determinants of emotional disorders

The determinants of emotional disorders may be divided into precipitating factors, predisposing factors, and perpetuating factors.

Precipitating factors

In studies of psychiatric aspects of hysterectomy in Oxford, it was found that many women were significantly depressed before hysterectomy but not after the operation (Gath *et al.* 1982*a*; Osborn and Gath 1990). From detailed history taking, it was evident that the experience of menorrhagia over several months or years had been a major determinant of this depressive state before surgery.

Predisposing factors

In the Oxford studies it was frequently found that the risks of psychiatric disorder were increased by predisposing factors in the patient. By far the most important predisposing factor was psychiatric vulnerability, as defined by the personality dimension of neuroticism, a previous history of psychiatric problems, or a family history of psychiatric disorder. Neuroticism is the life-long tendency to experience symptoms such as anxiety or depression either spontaneously or in response to the ordinary challenges of day to day life. Neuroticism can be measured reliably with a standardized self-rated questionnaire (Eysenck and Eysenck 1963). Personality attributes such as neuroticism are important because they may influence the extent to which psychiatric morbidity is associated with the menstrual cycle. Thus, a woman's personality may influence her experience of the menstrual cycle, how she construes and evaluates it, and whether she accepts or rejects it. Personality factors may also influence her consultation and complaint behaviour.

When assessing personality, a psychiatrist combines information from the patient's past record – for example, education, work, and marriage – with further information elicited directly about social relationships, leisure activities, prevailing mood, character, attitudes, and habits (particularly use of alcohol and drugs).

Perpetuating factors

In assessing perpetuating factors as determinants of psychiatric disorder, the psychiatrist enquires about stressful circumstances that have been sustained over a long time – for example, relationship difficulties, financial problems, social isolation, poor housing, problems with neighbours, and job difficulties.

Following this account of psychiatric morbidity, some relevant gynaecological syndromes will be reviewed.

A review of some gynaecological syndromes

Pre-menstrual syndrome

In Oxford, a study was carried out to determine how far symptoms of the pre-menstrual syndrome (PMS) are determined by psychological factors as distinct from physical factors such as ovarian hormones (Osborn and Gath 1990). For this purpose, PMS symptoms were studied in a sample of 56 women awaiting hysterectomy for benign menorrhagia. The reason for choosing this patient group was that both psychological and physical factors could influence PMS symptoms before hysterectomy, but after the operation, in the absence of menstrual periods, only physical factors could induce cyclical symptoms like those of PMS. The patients were aged under 45 years and were having regular menstrual periods (and were therefore likely to have normal ovarian function). To avoid any effects due to awareness of the purpose of the study, the women were told that the study was concerned with hysterectomy and its relationship to mood and bodily symptoms, but PMS was not mentioned.

On entering the study, the women kept symptom-diaries daily for 12 weeks. The diaries provided a check-list on which to rate the severity of eight physical and eight psychological symptoms of PMS interspersed with irrelevant symptoms. Hysterectomy was then carried out. Starting six months after the operation, the symptom-diaries were again completed daily for 12 weeks. During these weeks, the 'premenstruum' was identified by means of twice weekly estimates of plasma progesterone. In this way it was possible for the investigator to discover whether there was any intensification of 'PMS' symptoms in the 'pre-menstrual' phase of the ovarian cycle. Psychiatric assessments were made both before and after the 12 week diary assessments.

Before hysterectomy, there was a substantial level of PMS amongst the patients as shown by pre-menstrual peaking of symptoms in the diary. After hysterectomy, there was a significant reduction in the number and severity of PMS symptoms rated in the diaries. When the 12 weeks of diary ratings were completed, the women were asked (amongst other questions) whether they recalled experiencing PMS symptoms. Before hysterectomy, a large number of women recalled PMS symptoms of considerable severity. After the operation, only a few women recalled post-operative cyclical symptoms like those of PMS, and severity ratings were lower.

Both sets of findings indicated that psychological factors (such as the expectation of having symptoms pre-menstrually) were likely to be important determinants of PMS symptoms. This was confirmed by the finding that, before hysterectomy, both neuroticism and psychiatric symptoms were correlated with retrospectively recalled PMS and (less strongly) with diary symptoms of PMS.

In Oxford a controlled clinical trial was recently carried out to evaluate a psychological treatment known as cognitive therapy for the pre-menstrual syndrome (by comparison with a waiting list control group) (Blake *et al.* 1995). In cognitive therapy, the therapist (usually a psychologist) aims to detect and correct any incorrect and maladaptive ideas which patients hold about themselves and their health. The aim of the trial was to help women to recognize and change such distorted views about themselves and their pre-menstrual symptoms. By comparison with the waiting list control group, the group receiving cognitive therapy had a significantly better outcome for emotional symptoms, physical symptoms, and general well-being, both pre-menstrually and during menstruation. These findings showed that cognitive therapy can be a valuable treatment for the pre-menstrual syndrome.

Dysmenorrhoea

Of the 521 women in the Oxford community survey detailed above, 265 were pre-menopausal women, of whom 152 (57 per cent) reported painful menstrual periods in the preceding six months. Within this sub-group 40 women (26 per cent) reported that period pains had interfered with their everyday life, and 96 (63 per cent) took medication for the pain.

On assessment with the Present State Examination (PSE), and with a self-rated questionnaire (the 60-item GHQ), psychological morbidity was found to be strongly associated with experiencing painful periods and with periods interfering with daily life, but associations were less strong with the use of medication for period pain. It should be emphasized that no firm inference can be drawn from this finding as to whether the psychological morbidity was a primary or secondary factor.

Amenorrhoea

There have been several reports that women may experience amenorrhoea when they have a significant change in their way of life. For example, sustained amenorrhoea has been reported amongst women entering the armed forces or being detained in prison.

In psychiatric patients, amenorrhoea may be induced by anti-psychotic drugs which block D-2 receptors. Examples of such drugs are chlorpromazine, sulpiride, and risperidone.

Amenorrhoea is a characteristic feature of anorexia nervosa. The main clinical features of this condition are obsessive concern with body shape and weight. Most of the patients are young women. The condition generally begins with dieting in a young woman who has been overweight and makes a determined effort to achieve an abnormally low body weight. For this purpose, she avoids carbohydrates, induces vomiting, exercises excessively, and purges herself.

In addition to amenorrhoea, these patients often have depressed mood and lack of interest in sex. If starvation is maintained, the consequences include a low blood pressure, slow pulse, and low temperature. Constipation is common. If vomiting and laxative use are maintained over a long time, alkalosis and hypokalaemia may result. The principles of treatment are to assess the severity of anorexia nervosa, to detect the presence of any depressive disorder, and to assess any family problems. Following this assessment, the next stages in treatment are to give advice about healthy eating and the hazards of extreme dieting; agree a target for weight gain and a plan for achieving it; treat a depressive disorder if present, and provide help with family problems. The patient should be followed up regularly.

Menorrhagia

In the community survey reported above four indices were used in the assessment of menorrhagia; these were the woman's report of flooding, clots, duration of periods, and the number of pads or tampons used. In addition two 'subjective' indices were used (estimated heaviness of the period and degree of interference with life). When asked about these indices in the past six months, 37 women (14 per cent) reported flooding on six or more days, whilst 84 women reported passing clots at the same frequency. There were significant associations between emotional state (measured with the GHQ and PSE) and (i) the woman's subjective assessment of very heavy menstrual periods, and (ii) the passing of menstrual clots. Nevertheless psychiatric state was less strongly associated with indices of menorrhagia than it was with dysmenorrhoea or the pre-menstrual syndrome.

Hysterectomy

Two recent studies (Osborn and Gath 1990; Gath *et al.* 1995) have examined psychological determinants of selection for hysterectomy in women complaining of excessive menstruation. These studies were a sequel to an earlier hysterectomy study (Gath *et al.* 1982*a*). In that study over half of the patients were psychiatric 'cases' (as determined by a standardized psychiatric examination, the Present State Examination (Wing *et al.* 1974) four weeks before the operation; in most of these patients psychiatric disorder was of long duration and not simply a reaction to the prospect of imminent surgery. After hysterectomy, just over half of these patients recovered psychiatrically within 3–4 months, whilst the rest were still psychiatrically unwell at 18 months. This finding suggested that two groups of patients can be identified. In the first group, pre-hysterectomy psychiatric disorder is secondary to 'true' menorrhagia; understandably, when the latter is relieved by hysterectomy, psychiatric health improves. In the second group, pre-hysterectomy psychiatric disorder arises from other causes, for example marital disharmony, and is primary in the sense that it leads to complaints about levels of menstruation which have previously been well tolerated. Understandably hysterectomy does not benefit the mental state.

A later study examined these issues in over 200 women awaiting hysterectomy for complaints of excessive menstruation. The research design was the same as in the original study but with two additions: (i) the women's menstrual loss was measured in the laboratory over 2–3 cycles; (ii) more detailed assessments were made of psychological factors that could influence complaints of excessive menstruation (Hodges *et al.* 1997).

Two examples can be given of the findings from this study. First, in 42 per cent of women the highest menstrual loss was less than 80 ml (the level used to indicate menorrhagia in clinical research). Second, in the whole group of women, levels of psychiatric morbidity were lower than in the first Oxford hysterectomy study (Gath *et al.* 1982*a*). Further analysis will show whether these findings reflected alleviation of menorrhagia by drugs, or improved selection of patients (for example, by exclusion of patients with 'primary' psychiatric disorder).

Recently, the findings from the three earlier Oxford studies of hysterectomy were compared (Gath *et al.* 1995). The studies were carried out in 1975–76, 1980–82, and 1985–86 and were concerned with different issues, but each study examined psychiatric morbidity among women undergoing hysterectomy for menorrhagia of benign origin. In all three studies levels of psychiatric morbidity were measured before the operation and six months after the operation. Psychiatric morbidity was measured with the Present State Examination and with established self-report questionnaires. Levels of psychiatric morbidity fell significantly across the three studies. In study 1, the proportions of psychiatric cases were 58 per cent before hysterectomy and 26 per cent after; in study 2 they were 28 per cent before and 7 per cent after; and in study 3 they were 3.9 per cent before and 4 per cent after. This decline in psychiatric morbidity was not associated with demographic and social characteristics, previous psychiatric history, family psychiatric history, the nature of the women's menstrual complaints, or the women's understanding and expectations of the operation.

An important finding was that the prescribing of psychotropic medication was significantly higher in study 1 than in study 2 or study 3. By contrast, in the subsequent study 3, anti-menorrhagic drugs were prescribed twice as frequently as in the two earlier studies.

Menopause

There has been considerable debate whether the menopause is associated with high rates of depression. It has been reported that rates of depression are high amongst women attending menopause clinics, but these findings are not surprising in so far as emotional symptoms are common in all hospital outpatients clinics (Mayou and Hawton 1986). There have been interview surveys of menopausal women in Sweden (Hallstrom and Samuelsson 1985), England (Gath *et al.* 1987), the USA (McKinlay *et al.* 1987), and Canada (Kaufert *et al.* 1988). These surveys used large random samples and precise definitions, and all agreed in finding no excess of depressive disorder at the menopause.

It has often been suggested that the menopause may lead to depression in women who regret the loss of their fertility or regard themselves as becoming less feminine. Research has shown, however, that such reactions are very uncommon in women undergoing an 'artificial menopause' as a result of hysterectomy with or without bilateral oophorectomy (Gath *et al.* 1982*a*, *b*).

It is important to stress that a perimenopausal woman may be depressed for psychological reasons unrelated to the menopause. For example there may be problems such as her parents being ill, the children leaving home, or her husband being less supportive. Indeed, research has shown that depression in middle-aged women is related less to the menopause than to the vicissitudes of life (Greene and Cooke 1980; McKinlay *et al.* 1987; Gath and Iles 1990).

Recently, researchers in Oxford carried out a search of the literature on Medline in relation to psychological symptoms amongst women who were either naturally or surgically menopausal, or who were receiving hormone replacement therapy for menopausal symptoms (Pearce *et al.* 1995).

The authors found evidence for a small increase in psychological morbidity, which did not usually amount to psychiatric disorder, before natural menopause and after surgical menopause. The authors commented that the response of psychosocial symptoms to hormone replacement therapy with oestrogens is variable and most marked in surgical menopause. In some studies hormone replacement therapy is little more effective than placebo. The authors concluded that the use of hormone replacement therapy to treat psychological symptoms at the menopause (but not necessarily due to the menopause) is questionable. It seems, however, that oestrogen therapy benefits psychological symptoms after surgery and menopause.

The detection and assessment of psychiatric disorder in the gynaecology clinic

During a gynaecological consultation in an outpatient clinic, a patient may appear significantly distressed. It is well worthwhile to determine whether this distress is a transient response to attending a clinic, or whether it is evidence of a significant and enduring emotional disorder.

In a gynaecological clinic pressure of time will seldom allow the clinician to undertake a detailed psychiatric history and examination. It is feasible, however, to carry out a brief psychiatric interview based on a few screening questions that can be informative. These questions can be grouped under three headings:

- **Lack of general well-being** – fatigue, irritability, poor concentration, poor sleep, and a feeling of being under pressure.
- **Anxiety** – tension, sweating, frequent palpitations, repeated anxious thoughts.
- **Depression** – persistent low mood, lack of energy, loss of interest, loss of confidence, pessimism.

If the answers to these questions suggest psychiatric problems, it can be informative and convenient to ask the patient to complete a brief standardized questionnaire, which detects the presence and severity of emotional symptoms in the present and the recent past. A suitable questionnaire is the 28-item General Health Questionnaire (GHQ) (Goldberg 1972), which has been very widely used and has proved valuable in medical, surgical, and gynaecological clinics. The GHQ can be easily administered and scored by a nurse or other member of staff.

The questionnaire detects and measures levels of anxiety, depression, somatic symptoms, and social functioning. High scores indicate that a psychiatric consultation would be appropriate.

Another useful self-rated questionnaire is the Profile of Mood States (POMS) (McNair and Lorr 1964) which has also been widely used in clinic populations. This questionnaire consists of 41 mood adjectives which are rated by the patient on a standard scale; the responses can be readily scored to indicate levels of anger, tension, depression, fatigue, and vigour.

If these methods of enquiry suggest significant emotional distress, it can be valuable to ask the patient whether she has recently experienced any adverse life events (such as marital breakdown, bereavement, loss of a job) which may be contributing to her psychiatric symptoms, or may be reducing her tolerance of her gynaecological symptoms.

An important determinant of emotional disorders is alcohol abuse. If there is any suspicion of such abuse, it can be helpful to ask four questions that are particularly likely to be informative:

1. Have you ever felt you might cut down your drinking?
2. Have people annoyed you by criticizing your drinking?
3. Have you ever felt guilty about your drinking?
4. Have you ever had a drink first thing in the morning as an eye-opener?

A mnemonic for these questions is CAGE, from the initial letters of Cut, Annoyed, Guilty, and eye-opener. Two or more affirmative replies identify problem drinkers.

In concluding this chapter, the last word on the menstrual cycle should be reserved for Soranus, a physician of Ephesus, who practised his profession first at Alexandria and afterwards at Rome, in the reigns of Trojan and Hadrian, AD 98–138. According to Soranus, 'The menses are about to occur when a woman feels somewhat uneasy in walking, when a feeling of heaviness appears in the loins. Some women develop a torpor, some yawning and pandiculation, while others develop nausea and loss of appetite.'

The *Oxford English Dictionary* defines pandiculation as an instinctive movement, comprising the extension of the legs, the raising and stretching of the arms, and the throwing back of the head and trunk, accompanied by yawning.

References

Blake, F., Gath, D., and Salkovskis, P.M. (1995). Psychological aspects of premenstrual syndrome: developing a cognitive approach. In *Treatment of functional somatic symptoms*, (ed. R. Mayou, C. Bass, and M. Sharpe). Oxford University Press.

Byrne, P. (1984). Psychiatric morbidity in a gynaecology clinic: an epidemiological survey. *British Journal of Psychiatry*, **144**, 28–34.

Catalan, J., Gath, D.H., Anastasiades, P., Bond, S.A.K., Day, A., and Hall, L. (1991). Evaluation of a brief psychological treatment for emotional disorders in primary care. *Psychological Medicine*, **21**, 1013–18.

Eysenck, H.J. and Eysenck, S.B.G. (1963). *The Eysenck personality inventory*, University of London Press.

Gath, D. and Iles, S. (1990). Depression and the menopause. Leading article. *British Medical Journal*, **300**, 1287–8.

Gath, D.H., Cooper, P., and Day, A. (1982*a*). Hysterectomy and psychiatric disorder: I. Levels of psychiatric morbidity before and after hysterectomy. *British Journal of Psychiatry*, **140**, 335–42.

Gath, D., Cooper, P., Bond, A., and Edmonds, G. (1982*b*). Hysterectomy and psychiatric disorder: II. Demographic and physical factors in relation to psychiatric outcome. *British Journal of Psychiatry*, **140**, 343–50.

Gath, D., Osborn, M., Bungary, G., Iles, S., Day, A., Bond, A., and Passingham, C. (1987). Psychiatric disorder and gynaecological symptoms in middle aged women: a community survey. *British Medical Journal*, **294**, 213–18.

Gath, D.H., Rose, N., Bond, A., Day, A., Garrod, A., and Hodges, S. (1995). Hysterectomy and psychiatric disorder: are the levels of psychiatric morbidity falling? *Psychological Medicine*, **25**, 277–83.

Gelder, M., Gath, D., and Mayou, R. (1996). *The Oxford textbook of psychiatry* (3rd edn), (1079 pages). Oxford University Press.

Gelder, M., Gath, D., and Mayou, R. (1994). *The concise Oxford textbook of psychiatry.* Oxford University Press.

Goldberg, D. (1972). *The detection of psychiatric illness by questionnaire*, Maudsley Monograph No 21. Oxford University Press, London.

Greene, J.S. and Cooke, D.J. (1980). Life stress and symptoms at the climacterium. *British Journal of Psychiatry*, **136**, 486–91.

Hallstrom, T. and Samuelsson, S. (1985). Mental health in the climacteric. The longitudinal study of women in Gothenburg. *Acta Obstetrica et Gynaecologica Scandinavica*, **130**, (Suppl.), 13–18.

Hodges, S., Gath, D., Bond, A., Day, A., and Garrod, A. (1997). Psychological factors influencing perception of menstrual blood loss in the context of hysterectomy for excessive menstrual bleeding. I: Psychiatric health. (Unpublished).

Kaufert, P.A., Gilbert, P., and Hassaret, T. (1988). Researching the symptoms of menopause: an exercise in methodology. *Maturitas*, **10**, 117–31.

McKinlay, J.B., McKinlay, S.M., and Brambila, D. (1987). The relative contributions of endocrine changes and social circumstances to depression in middle-aged women. *Journal of Health and Social Behaviour*, **28**, 345–63.

McNair, D.M. and Lorr, M. (1964). An analysis of mood in neurotics. *Journal of Abnormal and Social Psychology*, **69**, 620–7.

Mayou, R. and Hawton, K. (1986). Psychiatric disorder in the general hospital. *British Journal of Psychiatry*, **149**, 172–90.

Osborn, M. and Gath, D. (1990). Psychological and physical determinants of premenstrual symptoms before and after hysterectomy. *Psychological Medicine*, **20**, 565–72.

Pearce, J., Hawton, K., and Blake, F. (1995). Psychological and sexual symptoms associated with the menopause and the effects of hormone replacement therapy. *British Journal of Psychiatry*, **167**, 163–73.

Wing, J.K., Cooper, J.E., and Sartorius, N. (1974). *The measurement and classification of psychiatric symptoms*. Cambridge University Press, London.

28 Pre-menstrual syndrome: aetiology and clinical management

Changulanda Medappa Joshi, Abha Govind, and P.M. Shaughn O'Brien

Introduction

Since the first documentation of pre-menstrual syndrome (PMS) by Frank in 1931, numerous treatment methods have been advocated. The syndrome has no known aetiology and an uncertain and variable course. None the less a psychoneuroendocrine mechanism triggered by the normal endocrine events of the ovarian cycle seems the most plausible explanation. No single intervention will uniformly eradicate symptoms in all patients presenting with PMS. Logical approaches to treatment would therefore include modulations or elimination of the ovarian cycle or correction of a neurotransmitter metabolic abnormality. Women with PMS present with heterogeneous symptoms; therefore management approaches must be designed on an individual basis.

Definition and classification

Various definitions of pre-menstrual syndrome have been used by different researchers. This has contributed to contradictory findings of research into its epidemiology, aetiology and treatment. Definition of PMS must refer to the cyclical recurrence, in the luteal phase of the menstrual cycle, of any combination of distressing physical, psychological, and/or behavioural changes of sufficient severity to result in deterioration of interpersonal relationships and/or interference with normal activities (Reid and Yen 1981). Definitions along these lines are widely accepted.

The prevalence of PMS has been variously reported as ranging from 5 per cent to 95 per cent; this reflects the imprecision of diagnostic criteria rather than any biological factor. PMS is unusual in that women usually present themselves with the presumed diagnosis of PMS and it is the clinician's role to determine the validity of this. Many other disorders may be misdiagnosed as PMS. It is the timing and not the type of symptom which is important for the definition and diagnosis of pre-menstrual syndrome. Whether or not symptoms have to be completely relieved by menstruation poses another debate. Complete resolution of symptoms would clearly define the group of patients who were symptomatic in the luteal phase only, but unfortunately this does not take into account the large number of patients who have a continuous background of mild to severe psychological or physical symptoms which become significantly exaggerated pre-menstrually.

Women presenting with PMS may fall into four categories (O'Brien 1987):

1. **Physiological pre-menstrual symptoms.** Physiological symptoms have the appropriate character and timing but are not severe enough to disrupt normal functioning and thus do not

require specific treatment. Such women may need counselling and reassurance, particularly if they have been led by media or others to believe they have a syndrome.

2. **Primary PMS.** This is a disorder of physical, psychological, and/or behavioural symptoms recurring during the luteal phase of the menstrual cycle. The symptoms should resolve completely by the end of menstruation and women should be free of symptoms for a period of at least a week between menstruation and ovulation. The symptoms must be severe enough to interfere appreciably with normal functioning or interpersonal relationships. Symptoms must have occurred in at least four of the six previous menstrual cycles.

3. **Secondary PMS.** The definition is similar to that of primary PMS, but differs in that there is partial rather than complete resolution of symptoms after menstruation. These women have an underlying psychological disorder as well as a cyclical disorder. The symptoms of primary PMS, the cyclical component of the secondary PMS, and physiological premenstrual symptoms are presumed to be generated by the endocrine changes of the ovarian cycle.

4. **Psychiatric disorder wrongly attributed to PMS.** Many of the typical psychological symptoms found in PMS are common to other psychiatric illnesses, for instance the broad range of symptoms associated with depression. This group of women have continuous or non-cyclical psychological symptoms which are wrongly attributed (by patient and doctor) to PMS. It is imperative that such patients do not receive treatments designed for PMS; if the severity warrants they should undergo psychiatric evaluation and related treatment.

Many research groups have proposed their own definitions. Psychiatrists in America have recently devised the unsuccessful and limited term 'premenstrual dysphoric disorder' (PMDD), which refers only to the psychological disturbances of PMS. PMDD is a category that appears in the *Diagnostic and statistical manual of mental disorders* (American Psychiatric Association 1994), which is the standard nosology of psychiatric disorders. Pre-menstrual dysphoric disorder replaces the previous term 'late luteal phase dysphoric disorder' (LLPDD). This latter term is also limited as it excludes women who have symptoms throughout the luteal phase of the cycle and also those with predominantly somatic symptoms.

Symptoms

Symptoms of pre-menstrual syndrome are wide ranging. Over 150 symptoms have been recorded in the research literature (Table 28.1). There are, however, typical psychological symptoms which include irritability, aggression, depression, unexplained crying, anxiety, tension, loss of control, and poor concentration. Key physical symptoms include bloatedness, mastalgia, breast swelling, headache, migraine, clumsiness, and pelvic pain. Abdominal bloatedness and swelling usually occur in the absence of weight gain or water retention. There has also been a resurgence of interest in the phenonomen of pre-menstrual exacerbation of conditions such as epilepsy, heart failure, allergies, and asthma. It is estimated that 40 per cent of women experience significant pre-menstrual symptoms but only 5 per cent report some severe impairment of their work, lifestyle, or interpersonal relationship.

PMS may occur at any time after menarche or at the onset of ovulatory cycles; women most often seek treatment for their symptoms in their third or fourth decades. Symptoms may occur in the absence of menstrual bleeding when ovarian cyclicity exists such as following hysterectomy

Table 28.1 Symptoms of PMS (Common symptoms are marked with an asterisk)

Psychological	Physical
* Aggression	Accident-prone
Agitation	Acne
Anorexia	Asthma
* Anxiety	Bloatedness (actual)
Argumentative	Bloatedness (feeling of)
Confusion	Blurred vision
* Crying bouts	* Breast swelling
Decreased alertness	* Breast tenderness
Decreased libido	* Clumsiness
* Depression	Constipation
Diminished self-esteem	Diarrhoea
Drowsiness	Diminished activity
Emotional lability	Diminished efficiency
Energetic	Diminished performance
Fatigue	Dizziness
Food craving	Epilepsy
Hopelessness	Finger swelling
Housebound	Flushes
Hunger	Formication
Hypersomnia	*Headache
Impulsive behaviour	Joint pain
Increased libido	Mastodynia
Insomnia	Migraine
* Irritability	Muscle pain
Lack of inspiration	Nausea
Lack of volition	Oedema
Lethargy	Oliguria
Listlessness	Pain–iliac fossa
Loss of attention to appearance	Pain–lower abdomen
* Loss of concentration	Pain–pelvic
Loss of confidence	Polyuria
Loss of judgement	Poor coordination
Loss of self-control	*Pre-menstrual dysmenorrhoea
Malaise	Pruritus
Mood swings	Puffiness
Sadness	Sinusitis
Social isolation	Skin lesions
Suicidal tendency	Sore eyes
*Tension	Sweating
Thirst	Vaginal discharge
Violence	Vertigo
	Vomiting
	Weakness
	Weight increase (true)

with conservation of ovaries (Backstrom *et al.* 1981) and following endometrial ablation (Joshi and O'Brien, unpublished data). Women generally report that symptoms worsen with age until menopause. Pre-menstrual symptoms are thought to affect women equally regardless of socio-economic status or culture, but specific symptoms may be identified more frequently in one culture than in another (Hasin *et al.* 1988).

Aetiology

To date, no gynaecological or endocrine abnormality has been identified in the aetiology. Natural ovarian activity, however, appears to be a prerequisite as it is clear that PMS closely relates to the changes of the menstrual cycle. The syndrome does not occur when cyclical ovarian activity is absent, such as before puberty, during pregnancy, and after the menopause.

Current consensus points to the normal ovarian cycle as the trigger for events in the central nervous system and other target tissues. The symptoms are thought to be caused by increased responsiveness of the tissues to the hormonal changes of the normal cycle, particularly to the high concentration of progesterone in the luteal phase. This may be mediated through a deficiency of neurotransmitters such as serotonin or endorphins.

Ovarian hormones

Abnormality of ovarian hormone secretion is an appealing theory, as PMS symptoms, by definition, occur in the luteal phase of the menstrual cycle and disappear after the menopause or during periods of amenorrhoea. However, there is no consistent agreement that PMS symptoms correlate with specific changes or differences in oestrogen or progesterone levels (Backstrom and Mattsson 1975; O'Brien 1987; Hammarback *et al.*; 1989; Rubinow *et al.*, 1988).

Oestrogens

These steroids can have various stimulatory actions on the central nervous system. However, only a minority of women experience PMS symptoms at mid-cycle, when oestrogen levels peak. Oestrogens have a positive effect on the biosynthesis, uptake, and turnover of monoamines and opioids (Shoupe and Lobo 1985) in the central nervous system, which is consistent with an anti-depressant effect. Some women receiving the oestrogen receptor antagonist clomiphene citrate report lability of mood or depression (Reid 1988). These findings suggest that oestrogen with-drawal or deficiency may be involved in this syndrome.

Progesterone deficiency

This has been a popular theory as a cause for PMS. The symptoms appear to depend on ovulation and follow the pattern of progesterone produced by the corpus luteum. The best argument against the belief that low progesterone levels alone cause PMS symptoms is the fact that progesterone levels are lowest in the first half of the cycle, when symptoms are absent (Shoupe 1991). Moreover, there are no convincing studies to substantiate the role of progesterone replacement in the treatment of PMS.

Recent research shows that women with pre-menstrual syndrome who have had a hysterectomy and bilateral salpingo-oophorectomy do not redevelop symptoms when they receive continuous oestrogen therapy. They do, however, develop well defined symptoms when given progesterone

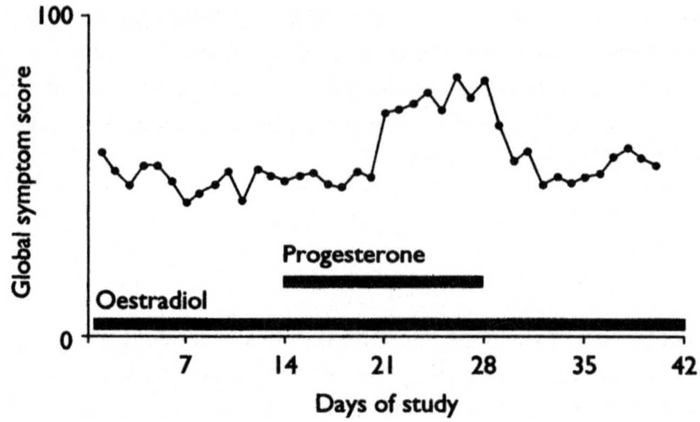

Fig. 28.1 Symptom scores for pre-menstrual syndrome in women who have had hysterectomy and bilateral oophorectomy and require HRT. During oestrogen-only therapy they have no symptoms. When progesterone is added experimentally for two weeks symptoms recur. (Reproduced with permission from O'Brien 1993.)

or progestogens (Henshaw *et al.* 1996) (Fig. 28.1). This suggests that progesterone is the key factor in the genesis of PMS.

Factors other than the differences in the levels of individual hormones must, therefore, be important; interactions with other endocrine or biochemical systems may operate or differences in receptor status may be relevant. The recurrence of symptoms in some women who take progestagens as part of HRT may be further evidence of a differential response to cyclical progesterone. Despite receiving identical doses of sex steroids only certain women develop PMS, again suggesting that PMS symptoms represent a differential response to the same level of ovarian steroids.

If normal ovarian function (rather than hormonal imbalance) is the cyclical trigger for the neuroendocrine events within the CNS, then the logical approach to treatment would include modulation or removal of the ovarian trigger or modulation of neurotransmitter metabolism. There is good evidence to suggest that this trigger can be eliminated or simulated with predictable outcome.

Abolishing ovarian cyclicity with drugs such as danazol and GnRH analogues or by bilateral oophorectomy reliably cures PMS by eliminating the ovarian trigger (Casson *et al.* 1990; Muse 1992). On the other hand serotonergic drugs reduce premenstrual symptoms by modulating the neuroendocrine relationship to the ovarian steroids (Rapkin 1992).

Neuroendocrine response

Recent research into the unexplained abnormal end-organ response to normal ovarian endocrine function has been directed towards neurotransmitter function. The most convincing neuroendocrine hypotheses relate to serotonergic and opioid mechanisms, but catecholamines, encephalins, monoamines, gamma amino-butyric acid, and prostaglandins could all be involved (Backstrom *et al.* 1992). Furthermore, if the explanation for PMS is neuroendocrine, it becomes much easier to explain why exogenous factors such as environment, dietary intake, and underlying psychological status can also influence the manifestation of PMS.

Abnormally low levels of β-endorphin have been shown in the luteal phase of women with PMS compared with asymptomatic controls (Chuong *et al.* 1985) and modulation of β-endorphin concentration by the endorphin inhibitor naltrexone reduces PMS-like symptoms (Chuong 1988).

Deficiency of vitamin B_6 (pyridoxine) may be important as it is a cofactor in the final step in the synthesis of serotonin and dopamine from tryptophan. No convincing data have yet demonstrated abnormalities either of brain amine synthesis or deficiency of cofactors like vitamin B6. Decreased serotonergic activity seems to be important in endogenous depression, and low serotonin levels have been demonstrated throughout the cycle in women with PMS in red blood cells and platelets (Rapkin 1992). Several therapeutic studies have reported effective treatment of PMS, particularly psychological symptoms, by serotonin re-uptake inhibitors (SSRIs) such as fluoxetine (Menkes *et al.* 1992).

Prolactin

The role of prolactin in PMS has been investigated perhaps because it is considered a stress hormone and it also stimulates the breast and promotes sodium, potassium, and water retention in animals. It has not been clearly demonstrated to undergo cyclical change in the normal menstrual cycle, nor do women with PMS demonstrate elevated blood levels of prolactin. Women with hyperprolactinaemia do not report PMS-like symptoms. Therapeutic studies of bromocriptine have failed to demonstrate any significant effect on symptoms, with the notable exception of cyclical mastalgia. Hence, the role of prolactin in PMS now seems doubtful (O'Brien and Symonds 1982).

Prostaglandins and essential fatty acids

Abnormalities in essential fatty acid synthesis have been demonstrated in a study by Brush and colleagues (1984) but these findings have not been replicated by others (O'Brien and Massil 1990). The ubiquitous nature of prostaglandins make them prime candidates to play an aetiological role in PMS. However, no precise explanation linking prostaglandin activity to PMS has yet been forthcoming. Both prostaglandin inhibitors and precursors have been claimed to relieve PMS. In *in vitro* studies, interactions at a cellular and receptor level have been demonstrated between polyunsaturated essential fatty acids and the activity of oestrogen, progesterone, angiotensin II, and β-endorphins. Interaction by angiotensin II and essential fatty acids and various prostaglandins has been shown *in vivo*. Hence, a defective prostaglandin metabolism may give rise to a breakdown in this balance, allowing exaggerated response to normal circulating levels of these different hormone systems.

Endocrine effects on fluid and electrolytes

Several research studies have addressed the role of sodium and water retention in PMS. Although many women develop abdominal distension and pre-menstrual bloatedness as a symptom they do so usually without increasing weight, total exchangeable body sodium, total body water, extracellular fluid volume, or plasma volume (Hussain 1993). This finding clearly questions the rationale for diuretic therapy in PMS. It now seems more likely that the symptoms of bloatedness exceed in severity any physical changes which occur and there may be a large perceived component. Alternatively, it is possible that these symptoms are related to gaseous gut distension, or hypotonia due to progesterone-induced relaxation of the smooth muscle in the small or large intestine, or both.

Diagnosis

PMS is a diagnosis of exclusion. Other physical and mental disorders must be ruled out before this diagnosis can be made. A careful physical and psychological history must be obtained. Physical examination including pelvic and breast examination is necessary if hormone therapy is likely to be considered. The role of blood tests is limited though in certain situations it may be appropriate to measure a full blood count, gonadotrophin concentrations, and thyroid function tests.

The use of retrospective histories of pre-menstrual symptoms alone leads to over-diagnosis of PMS (Rapkin *et al.* 1988). Prospective daily ratings of symptoms are required to substantiate the patient's history of pre-menstrual symptoms. To quantify PMS one would wish to measure

(1) the character, timing, and severity of the cyclical symptoms;

(2) the degree of underlying psychological dysfunction;

(3) the degree to which the patient's normal activities are disrupted.

In clinical practice the above three factors are determined from the history and by prospective self-documentation of symptoms using simple 'pre-menstrual calendars'. This provides limited information. However, in the near future computerized recording of symptoms on a linear visual analogue scale and symptom analysis will be possible using a simple patient hand-held device – PMS Symptometrics (O'Brien 1995).

The measurement of the cyclical component of PMS symptoms has been attempted using a wide variety of tools including Moos' menstrual distress questionnaire (Moos 1985); specific linear visual analogue scales (Faratian *et al.* 1984) or the 'calendar of premenstrual experiences' (COPE) developed by the University of California, San Diego; 'prospective record of the impact and severity of menstrual symptoms' (Reid 1988); and the 'premenstrual assessment form' (Halbreich 1982).

It is possible to quantify underlying psychopathology using established psychiatric questionnaires. The simplest one is the General Health Questionnaire (Goldberg and Hillier 1979) completed in the follicular phase of the menstrual cycle.

Based on the previous definition it can be seen that the following criteria must be fulfilled to diagnose PMS:

(1) symptoms must occur specifically in the luteal phase of the menstrual cycle;

(2) symptoms must disappear (primary PMS) or improve (secondary PMS) during menstruation;

(3) the character of symptoms need not be specific and the symptoms may be psychological or somatic;

(4) symptoms should be of sufficient severity to significantly disrupt the patient's life and interpersonal relationships;

(5) symptoms should have been present in at least four of the previous six cycles.

It often is difficult to categorize patients presenting with PMS. A gonadotrophin-releasing hormone analogue test is of value in such situations. The GnRH depot goserelin is given monthly for three months to eliminate cyclical ovarian function completely and the effect on prospectively recorded symptoms is determined. Complete elimination of symptoms is usual in correctly diagnosed PMS in which case there are symptoms demonstrated to be dependent on ovarian activity. If symptoms continue into the third month an underlying psychiatric diagnosis should be considered and investigated further.

Table 28.2 Differential diagnosis of PMS

Psychiatric disorders	May be confused because of the similarity of symptoms and because of the bipolar and periodic nature of some psychiatric disorders, for example manic depressive psychosis Many women prefer to 'label' their psychological inadequacies as gynaecological rather than psychiatric There are no objective tests but there are many structured interview techniques and questionnaires. Disappearance or improvement of symptoms following menstruation is critical
Intrafamilial and psychosexual problems	Distinguish between cause and effect
Other causes of breast symptoms	Cyclical breast pain may be considered part of PMS Can be distinguished from non-cyclical breast disease by history Non-cyclical disease includes several disorders requiring breast examination and investigations including mammography, ultrasonography, aspiration, and biopsy Breast cancer must, of course, be considered
Other causes of abdominal bloatedness and water retention	Only a few women exhibit significant water retention in PMS More women have idiopathic oedema which is also cyclical but only occasionally coincides by chance with the menstrual cycle Some women call progressive obesity 'PMS bloatedness' These can all be distinguished by twice daily weighing
Endometriosis, pelvic infection, and dysmenorrhoea	Primary dysmenorrhoea occurs with menses Secondary dysmenorrhoea is related to pelvic pathology and often occurs premenstrually Laparoscopy will exclude endometriosis or pelvic infection
Medical causes of lethargy and tiredness	Occasionally anaemia! – haemoglobin Rarely hypothyroidism or hyperthyroidism
Perimenopause	May be confused in patients over 40 years Flushes may uncommonly occur in PMS Usually distinguished from history Raised circulating FSH concentrations may assist diagnosis of the perimenopausal woman

Differential diagnosis

The majority of patients present to the gynaecologist with self-diagnosis of PMS. PMS is confirmed by excluding other disorders as many disorders have been wrongly attributed to PMS (Table 28.2). The essence of diagnosis in all of these disorders is the timing and cyclicity of symptoms. If the symptoms are not relieved by the end of menstruation then an alternative explanation must be sought.

Treatment

Numerous treatment regimens have been proposed (see Table 28.3). In the absence of a specific aetiological explanation most treatments offered have been empirical with little or no scientific

Table 28.3 Range of treatment approaches for PMS for which success has been claimed

Non-drug	Non-hormonal	Psychotropic agents	Hormonal
Acupuncture	Beta-blockers	Alprazolam	Bromocriptine
Bilateral oophorectomy	Diuretics	Buscrirone	Danazol
Cognitive therapy	Essential fatty acids	Clomipramine	GnRH analogues
Counselling	Magnesium	Clonidine	Oestradiol implants
Diet	Non-steroidal anti-inflammatory drugs	Fenfluramine	Oestrogen patches
Education	Nortriptyline	Fluoxetine	Oral contraception
Homeopathy	Pyridoxine	Lithium	Progestogens
Hypnosis	Spironolactone	Naltrexone	Progesterone
Hysterectomy	Vitamins	Nortriptyline	Testosterone
Intravaginal electrical stimulation	Zinc	Paroxetine	
Irradiation of ovaries		Serotonin agonists	
Isolation			
Music therapy			
Nutritional manipulation			
Psychotherapy			
Rest			
Salt restriction			
Self-help groups			
Stress management			
Yoga			

basis for their use. There are difficulties in interpreting the research literature on treatment of PMS. Attempts at meta-analysis of treatment methods have been thwarted by methodological issues such as inconsistencies in definition, diagnosis, subject selection, subject numbers, rating and quantification technique, and the large number of uncontrolled trials.

Treatment has been offered, based on unproven aetiologies. At times two treatments having opposite physiological effects have often been proposed. For example, both oestrogens (Magos *et al.* 1986) and synthetic androgens such as danazol (Sarno *et al.* 1987) have been proposed.

When considering claims for drug efficacy it must be remembered that placebo responses in excess of 90 per cent have been reported in some studies. The choice of placebo itself can present a problem. In a placebo-controlled trial of a diuretic and antidepressant for example, subjects could probably identify the period of treatment with the active drug because of its adverse effects. If they do, the blindness is broken and the study becomes open to bias.

Treatment of patients who may have PMS begins with a review of the results of the physical and psychological diagnostic work-up and daily symptom ratings. As with all medical disorders, the treatment depends on the establishment of the correct diagnosis and classification. It is surprising how often this is ignored in PMS. Completing the daily symptom questionnaire is important for various reasons. First the ratings define the pattern of symptoms. Secondly they are a visual adjunct which the doctor can show so that women can see their symptom profile, especially in instances where the pattern is not consistent with the diagnosis of PMS. Thirdly, it is an important step in management. As they chart their symptoms, many women gain a sense of control over their problems. Visualizing the type, severity, and timing of symptoms can make them seem more manageable. This sense of control may be enough to relieve distress in some women.

The specific approaches to treatment may be non-pharmacological and pharmacological. Women with minimal symptoms will benefit from counselling and reassurance. Indeed, all women will benefit from this. The management of women with severe pre-menstrual syndrome can also be relatively straightforward as it is easier to justify medical or surgical elimination of the menstrual cycle. Patients with serious but less severe symptoms are the most difficult to manage.

Non-pharmacological methods

For many women it is enough to have an understanding and sympathetic doctor, who is prepared to take their symptoms seriously, explain what is known of the biological basis of PMS, and reassure them. Some women benefit from a PMS support group that is time-linked and led by a professional (Pearlstein *et al.* 1992). Relaxation and stress management can be included in formalized psychotherapy or taught through acupuncture, hypnosis, or yoga to suit individual needs (Goodale *et al.* 1990). Structured cognitive therapy is effective. Prior and Vigna (1987) suggest that exercise can minimize some premenstrual symptoms related to fluid retention and it may also increase self-esteem. It is plausible that the elevation of endorphins as a result of exercise may be a mechanism involved. Women should be encouraged to participate in some kind of regular physical exercise throughout the month. It is the regularity rather than intensity of exercise that seems to be important.

The literature suggests that women who consume large amounts of caffeine or its equivalent (theophylline) in coffee, tea, or colas report more severe symptoms. It is advisable to recommend that women decrease caffeine pre-menstrually to minimize its potential contribution to irritability and insomnia. Many other specific dietary interventions have been proposed such as limited consumption of refined sugar, salt, red meat, alcohol, chocolate, and dairy products and increased intake of fish, whole grains, legumes, complex carbohydrates, green leafy vegetables, and *cis*-linoleic acid-containing foods (Lyon and Lyon 1984). Consuming a carbohydrate-rich, protein-poor diet was reported to improve luteal mood symptoms in patients with PMS (Wurtman *et al.* 1989). These authors suggested that the positive mood was due to increase in the synthesis of brain serotonin as a result of the dietary intervention. Dairy products interfere with magnesium absorption and refined sugar increases the urinary excretion of magnesium. Magnesium deficiency causes a specific depletion of brain dopamine. Decreased salt intake has been recommended as a way to minimize premenstrual bloating. It is advisable to minimize its potential contribution to irritability and insomnia. Reduction in alcohol intake pre-menstrually may improve symptoms.

Nutritional supplementation including pyridoxine (vitamin B_6), magnesium, and calcium has been widely advocated. The use of vitamin B_6, calcium, and magnesium has some logic as they are cofactors in neurotransmitter synthesis. However, there are studies to both support and refute their efficacy (Kleijnen *et al.* 1990; Johnson 1992).

If pyridoxine is used the dosage should be 50–100 mg daily. While using pyridoxine, women should be monitored closely for signs of neurotoxicity such as muscle weakness, numbness, clumsiness, and paraesthesia.

Evening primrose oil has been strongly promoted in recent years. The rationale for its use is that some women with PMS have reduced blood levels of essential fatty acids. Although there is good evidence that this treatment relieves breast symptoms, studies on general PMS show only trends in favour of its use compared with placebo, using doses of eight 500 mg capsules daily (Khoo *et al.* 1990; O'Brien and Massil 1990). None of the studies has been large enough to conclude that treatment is ineffective.

Pharmacological methods

Hormonal therapy

Progesterone and progestagens have been advocated on the unproven, theoretical basis that PMS might be caused by relative progesterone deficiency in the luteal phase of the menstrual cycle. Progesterone has been administered as pessaries, injections, and in oral micronized forms. Several well-controlled trials have shown no benefit from using high doses of progesterone suppositories/pessaries over placebo (Freeman *et al.* 1990). However, progesterone and progestogens continue to be prescribed because of the large number of anecdotal reports of efficacy (Dalton 1984).

If progestagens are effective and it is unlikely that progesterone deficiency is being corrected, it is possible that the steroids act via their mild central nervous sedative effect at high doses. Furthermore, in addition to the data already shown in Fig. 28.1, results from several studies of women receiving oestrogen replacement who were given cyclical progesterone demonstrated that symptoms *appeared* following progesterone administration (Moline 1993). Large doses of progesterone given rectally may cause local soreness, flatulence, and diarrhoea.

Pharmacological suppression of the ovarian cycle

If a woman does not respond to less invasive treatment, the next step is to consider elimination of the ovarian trigger. Several hormonal preparations have been used to achieve this including oral contraceptives, gonadotrophin-releasing hormone analogues (GnRH), danazol, oestradiol implants, and oestradiol patches.

Oral contraceptive pill

Combined oral contraception would seem a logical approach to the treatment of PMS (particularly in women who also need contraception), by suppressing ovulation. Both retrospective and prospective studies report that oral contraceptives may minimize symptoms of PMS (Andersch and Hahn 1981; Graham and Sherwin 1992). However, in other studies, oral contraceptives have been shown to be no more effective than placebo (Backstrom *et al.* 1992). Indeed some women report worsening of symptoms (Bancroft and Rennie 1993). Studies are needed to identify those patients who might benefit and the type of formulation that should be used. Continuous combined regimens ought to be effective but there have been no published studies.

GnRH analogues

Gonadotrophin-releasing hormone (GnRH) analogues act by creating a reversible pseudomenopause. These drugs can be given as nasal sprays, subcutaneous injections, or as a subcutaneous depot implant. Depot goserelin 3.6 mg per month reliably and predictably eradicates both physical and psychological symptoms (Brown *et al.* 1994). Initial temporary symptom exacerbation may occur in these women in the first month. The main concern with this treatment is the resultant hypo-oestrogenic state causing unpleasant symptoms but the associated hot flushes are better tolerated than the symptoms of pre-menstrual syndrome. Long-term treatment without the concomitant administration of ovarian steroids (see below) cannot be recommended because of the risk of osteoporosis. Symptoms usually return with the menstrual cycle or more precisely with the first ovulation.

The use of short courses of GnRH analogues has several important roles. Firstly, for women whose psychological health and interpersonal relationships are deteriorating, being free of symptoms for six months can be invaluable, saving jobs and marriages. Secondly, the freedom from symptoms in the absence of the ovarian endocrine cycle shows the woman and her family that her problem has a biological basis and that she does not have a personality disorder. Finally, in severely affected women who are to undergo hysterectomy for another gynaecological disorder, the potential benefit of performing bilateral oophorectomy during the same operative procedure can be demonstrated.

Recently there have been encouraging reports of attempts at using long-term GnRH analogue along with concurrent hormonal replacement therapy 'HRT add-back therapy' (Leather *et al.* 1993). In a prospective, placebo-controlled trial, Mezrow *et al.* (1994) showed that GnRH analogue depot leuprorelin with 'add-back' oestrogen and progestogen was effective in treating PMS symptoms with progressive improvement over a 12 month period. This therapy prevents changes in lipids and adequately protects the endometrium. There was some loss of bone density but it was not statistically significant.

Danazol

Menstrual cycles can be eliminated reversibly using danazol. In a double-blind study, danazol 100–400 mg per day was shown to be superior to placebo (Watts *et al.* 1987). In view of the higher incidence of adverse effects normally demonstrated with danazol, the lower dose would seem appropriate but such doses do not normally suppress ovarian cyclicity. In a small study in which danazol was administered at the onset of symptoms, PMS symptoms were reduced significantly (Sarno *et al.* 1987). In a much larger study of luteal-phase-only therapy (Abukhalil and O'Brien, unpublished data) no beneficial effect was seen for the general symptoms of PMS but breast symptoms were significantly reduced. Such intermittent therapy was associated with virtually no adverse effects. With all danazol regimens masculinization of a female fetus is a risk, hence appropriate barrier contraception should be advised. A study of the safety and efficacy of the long term use of this drug is warranted.

Oestrogen implants and transdermal patches

Oestradiol implants and patches have an important role in treating severely affected young women and also in women approaching the menopause. These implants have been used successfully by Magos *et al.* (1986) to treat PMS. Women with PMS received 100 mg implants of oestradiol and cyclical oral norethisterone. Overall symptoms were reduced in 87 per cent of cases. However, the addition of cyclical progestogen was associated with the return of mild PMS-like symptoms. Transdermal oestrogen with cyclical oral progestogen produced similar results (Watson *et al.* 1989). Oestrogen patches in doses of 200 μg or 100 μg effectively reduce symptoms. In future it may be possible to give continuous oestrogen (orally, or in the form of an implant or transdermal patches) and insert a levonorgestrel intrauterine contraceptive system (Mirena®) which provides endometrial protection, but the low blood level of progestagen avoids the return of PMS-like symptoms.

Oophorectomy

Bilateral oophorectomy will cure PMS. Symptoms persist after hysterectomy with conservation of ovaries although there are reports suggesting amelioration of PMS symptoms following hysterectomy (Metcalf *et al.* 1992). The hypo-oestrogenic side-effects of bilateral oophorectomy can be prevented by oestrogen replacement therapy without the need for cyclical progestogens. This is probably the only permanent cure for PMS but it is inappropriate for all but a few severely affected women. The assessment of PMS is an important component of the counselling in all women undergoing hysterectomy. In older women who are nearing the menopause, oophorectomy may be less questionable. However, in women less than 40 years of age, bilateral oophorectomy is rarely justifiable unless there are other indications for a hysterectomy such as fibroids or dysfunctional bleeding. In such women one should conduct a 'goserelin test' to determine the likely benefit of bilateral oophorectomy. Even then, if oophorectomy is performed in younger women it is crucial to ensure long-term compliance with oestrogen replacement therapy to prevent bone mineral loss and cardiovascular disease.

Specific symptom management

Women with predominantly psychological symptoms

Psychological symptoms are the principal concern of many women with PMS. Surprisingly there are few trials of psychotropic agents. The possible reasons for this could be reluctance on the part of clinicians to give continuous long-term medication to women to treat symptoms which occur for only one week each month. Most antidepressants take several weeks of daily doses to induce symptom improvement. In addition, women may not want to take antidepressants because of the perceived stigma of mental illness. Since the introduction of PMDD as a diagnostic entity representing the affective component of PMS, more treatment studies with psychotropic drugs have appeared in the literature. Selective serotonin reuptake inhibitors (SSRI) such as fluoxetine and paroxetine are being used more frequently. Double-blind studies have shown fluoxetine to be effective and safe for short-term use (Stone *et al.* 1991; Steiner *et al.* 1995). Pearlstein and Stone (1994) studied the efficacy and safety of long-term fluoxetine treatment of luteal phase dysphoric disorder. Sixty-four women with prospectively confirmed PMS were treated for a mean of 18.6 months. Half of those treated achieved complete remission of their symptoms, while the others achieved significant remission. The most common side-effect was sexual dysfunction, which occurred in 17 per cent of women. Symptoms recurred in most women following discontinuation of treatment. Treatment with fluoxetine at a dose of 20 mg per day reduces the potential for side-effects while maximizing the therapeutic efficacy. There is a case report that describes the success of fluoxetine during the symptomatic phase only (Daaman and Brown 1992). Paroxetine, 20 mg per day, is another SSRI currently under investigation.

Alprazolam, a benzodiazepine, has also been evaluated. It has been claimed to be effective given in a dose of 0.25 mg four times daily during the luteal phase at the onset of symptoms

(Smith *et al.* 1987; Freeman *et al.* 1995). The disadvantage of alprazolam is that some patients experience sedation and unreliable patients who do not restrict use to the luteal phase are at risk of dependence.

Women with predominantly physical symptoms

Fluid retention

As already discussed, the majority of women who experience bloating and a 'feeling of weight gain' have no objective demonstrable pre-menstrual weight gain or sodium and water retention (Hussain 1993). Hence there is a significant risk if diuretic therapy is used irrationally. There is, however, a small group of women who do have water retention. Diuretic therapy should be reserved for those with clearly demonstrable oedema or weight gain. A potassium-sparing diuretic such as spironolactone avoids the potential to develop secondary hyperaldosteronism (Vellacott and O'Brien 1987).

Cyclical mastalgia

Women with cyclical breast swelling or pain may try one of a variety of non-prescription remedies. Evening primrose oil (up to 8 capsules of 500 mg) can be used. Vitamin E (tocopherol) 500 units per day has also been claimed to be of use. For severe cases of mastalgia, danazol taken either continuously or during the luteal phase only can be tried. Bromocriptine has been used successfully but unpleasant side-effects can occur. It is better to start with a lower dose and gradually increase if necessary and to administer at night.

Suggested approach to management

As PMS patients present with heterogenous symptoms, the therapeutic approach must usually be designed on an individual basis. Management of patients who may have PMS begins with a thorough evaluation of symptoms. PMS should be distinguished from other psychological and medical illnesses. If necessary a GnRH analogue such as goserelin can be administered for three months in complex cases to distinguish between PMS and other psychological problems. Management of symptoms should begin with education and support.

Whilst treating a patient with PMS the following factors must be considered: age; type of symptoms; proximity of the menopause; previous treatment; severity of symptoms; other associated gynaecological conditions, particularly menorrhagia; the patient's desire for children; the patient's own view. In women with mild symptoms, counselling, stress management, and dietary modification should be tried. Women with moderate symptoms can be prescribed pyridoxine at a dose of 100 mg daily in addition to counselling. If psychological symptoms are predominant then SSRI drugs should be tried. In the younger age group oral contraceptive pills could be useful and a trial of combined continuous therapy should be considered. If danazol or GnRH analogues have to be used, adequate contraceptive measures should be advised.

For women over 40 years, oestradiol either in the form of patches or an implant, along with cyclical progestagen may be helpful. GnRH analogues should be reserved for women with severe symptoms with the addition of 'add back' oestrogen/progestogen if treatment is to exceed six months duration.

Before considering surgical intervention, continuous oestrogen plus a progestogen-containing IUCD might be considered. Bilateral oophorectomy should be the last resort in patients with severe symptoms affecting quality of life. There may also be a case for bilateral oophorectomy if there is a gynaecological indication for hysterectomy in women who also suffer from PMS.

Specific symptom management includes evening primrose oil, luteal phase danazol, and bromocriptine for breast tenderness and swelling. Spironolactone can be used during the luteal phase to relieve objectively documented fluid retention. Pre-menstrual migraine can be treated with Imigran®, Sanomigran®, Cafergot®, or Migarleve®, though hormone interventions may also be effective.

Summary

Until the aetiology of PMS, is understood it is unlikely that a single agent will be found that is effective for all patients. Presently, PMS is best treated based on specific symptoms and their severity, or by suppression of the menstrual cycle using a hierarchial approach. PMS patients need to be treated by sympathetic doctors or other health professionals. Adequate time should be allocated to listen to the patients and counsel them, preferably in a PMS clinic separate from a routine gynaecological outpatient clinic. The severity of impairment must be weighed against short term and possible long term adverse effects of treatment.

References

American Psychiatric Association (1994). *Diagnostic and statistical manual of mental disorders*, (4th edn). American Psychiatric Association, Washington DC, USA.

Andersch, B. and Hahn, L. (1981). Premenstrual complaints ii. Influence of oral contraceptive. *Acta Obstetrica et Gynecologica Scandinavica*, **60**, 579–83.

Backstrom, T. and Mattsson, B. (1975). Correlation of symptoms in premenstrual tension to oestrogen and progesterone concentrations in blood plasma. *Neuropsychobiology*, **1**, 80–6.

Backstrom, T., Boyle, H., and Baird, D.T. (1981). Persistence of symptoms of premenstrual tension in hysterectomized women. *British Journal of Obstetrics and Gynaecology*, **88**, 530–6.

Backstrom T., Hansson-Malmstrom, Y., and Lindhe, B.A. (1992). Oral contraceptives in premenstrual syndrome: a randomised comparison of triphasic and monophasic preparations. *Contraception*, **46**, 253–68.

Bancroft, J. and Rennie, D. (1993). The impact of oral contraceptives on the experience of perimenstrual mood, clumsiness, food craving and other symptoms. *Journal of Psychosomatic Research*, **37**, 195–202.

Brown, C.S., Ling F.W., Andersen, R.N., Farmer, R.G., and Arheart, K.L. (1994). Efficacy of depot leuprorelin in premenstrual syndrome: effect of symptom severity and type in a controlled trial. *Obstetrics and Gynecology*, **84**, 779–86.

Brush, M.G., Watson, S.J., Horrobin, D.F., and Manku, M.S. (1984). Abnormal essential fatty acid levels in plasma of women with premenstrual syndrome. *American Journal of Obstetrics and Gynecology*, **150**, 363–6.

Casson, P., Hahn, P.M., Van Vugt, D.A., and Reid, R.L. (1990). Lasting response to ovariectomy in severe intractable premenstrual syndrome. *American Journal of Obstetrics and Gynecology*, **162**, 99–105.

Chuong, C.J. (1988). Clinical trial of naltrexone in premenstrual syndrome. *Obstetrics and Gynecology*, **72**, 332–6.

Chuong, C.J., Coulam, C.B., Kao, P.C., and Bergstal, E.J. (1985). Neuropeptide levels in premenstrual syndrome. *Fertility and Sterility*, **44**, 760–5.

Daaman, M.J. and Brown, W.A. (1992). Single dose fluoxetine in the management of premenstrual syndrome. *Journal of Clinical Psychiatry*, **53**, 210–11.

Dalton, K. (1984). *The premenstrual syndrome and progesterone therapy* (2nd edn). William Heineman Medical Books Ltd, London.

Faratian, B., Gaspar, A., O'Brien, P.M.S., Filshie, G.M., Johnson, I.R., and Prescott, P. (1984). Premenstrual syndrome: weight, abdominal size and perceived body image. *American Journal of Obstetrics and Gynecology*, **150**, 200–4.

Frank, R.T. (1931). The hormonal causes of premenstrual tension. *Archives of Neurology and Psychiatry*, **26**, 1053–7.

Freeman, E., Rickel, K., Sondheimer, S.J., and Polansky, M. (1990). Ineffectiveness of progesterone suppository treatment for premenstrual syndrome. *Journal of the American Medical Association*, **264**, 349–53.

Freeman, E.W., Rickles, K., Sondheimer, S.J., and Polansky, M. (1995). A double-blind trial of oral progesterone, alprazolam, and placebo in treatment of severe premenstrual syndrome. *Journal of the American Medical Association*, **274**, 51–7.

Goldberg, D.P. and Hillier, V. (1979). A scaled version of the general health questionnaire. *Psychological Medicine*, **9**, 139–45.

Goodale, I.L., Domar, A.D., and Benson, H. (1990). Alleviation of premenstrual syndrome with relaxation response. *Obstetrics and Gynecology*, **75**, 649–55.

Graham, C.A. and Sherwin, B.B. (1992). A prospective treatment study of premenstrual symptoms using a triphasic oral contraceptive. *Journal of Psychosomatic Research*, **36**, 257–66.

Halbreich, U., Endicott, J., Schacht, S., and Nee, J. (1982). The diversity of premenstrual changes as reflected in the Premenstrual Assessment Form. *Acta Psychiatrica Scandinavica*, **65**, 46–65.

Hammarback, S., Damber, J.E., and Backstrom, T. (1989). Relationship between symptoms severity and hormone changes in women with premenstrual syndrome. *Journal of Clinical Endocrinology and Metabolism*, **68**, 125–30.

Hasin, M., Dennerstein, L., and Gotts, G. (1988). Menstrual cycle complaints: cross-cultured study. *Journal of Psychosomatics in Obstetrics and Gynecology*, **9**, 35–42.

Henshaw, C., Foreman, D., Belcher, J., Cox, J., and O'Brien, S. (1996). Can one induce premenstrual symptomatology in women with prior hysterectomy and bilateral oophorectomy? *Journal of Psychosomatics in Obstetrics and Gynecology*, **17**, 21–8.

Hussain, S.Y. (1993). The compartmental distribution of fluid and electrolytes in relation to the symptomatology of the ovarian cycle and premenstrual syndrome. Ph.D. Thesis, University of London.

Johnson, S. (1992). Clinician's approach to the diagnosis and management of premenstrual syndrome. *Clinical Obstetrics and Gynaecology*, **35**, 637–57.

Khoo, S.K., Munro, C., and Battistutta, D. (1990). Evening primrose oil and treatment of premenstrual syndrome. *Medical Journal of Australia*, **153**, 189–92.

Kleijnen, J., Riet, G.T., and Knipschild, P. (1990). Vitamin B6 in the treatment of the premenstrual syndrome – a review. *British Journal of Obstetrics and Gynaecology*, **97**, 847–52.

Leather, A.T., Studd, J.W.W., Watson, N.R., and Holland, E.F. (1993). The prevention of bone loss in young women treated with GnRH analogues with 'add-back' estrogen therapy. *Obstetrics and Gynecology*, **82**, 104–7.

Lyon, K.E., and Lyon, M.A. (1984). The premenstrual syndrome. *Journal of Reproductive Medicine*, **29**, 705–8.

Magos, A.L., Brincat, M., and Studd, J.W.W. (1986). Treatment of the premenstrual syndrome by subcutaneous oestradiol implants and cyclical oral norethisterone: placebo-controlled study. *British Medical Journal*, **292**, 1629–33.

Menkes, D.B., Ebrahim, T., Mason, P.A., Spears, G.F.S., and Howard, R.C. (1992). Fluoxetine treatment of severe premenstrual syndrome. *British Medical Journal*, **305**, 346–7.

Metcalf, M.G., Braiden, V., Livesley, J.H., and Wells, J.E. (1992). The premenstrual syndrome, amelioration of symptoms after hysterectomy. *Journal of Psychosomatic Research*, **36**, 569–84.

Mezrow, G., Sharpe, D. Spicer, D., Lobo, R., Leung, B., and Pike, M. (1994). Depot leuprolide acetate with estrogen and progestin add-back for long-term treatment of premenstrual syndrome. *Fertility and Sterility*, **62**, 932–7.

Moline, M.L. (1993). Pharmacologic strategies for managing premenstrual syndrome. *Clinical Pharmacology*, **12**, 181–96.

Moos, R. (1985). Premenstrual symptoms: a manual and overview of research with the menstrual distress questionnaire. Department of Psychiatry and Behavioural Sciences, Stanford University School of Medicine, Palo Alto, CA 94304, USA.

Muse, K. (1992). Hormonal manipulation in the treatment of premenstrual syndrome. *Clinical Obstetrics and Gynaecology*, **35**, 658–66.

O'Brien, P.M.S. (1993). Helping women with premenstrual syndrome. *British Medical Journal*, **307**, 1471–5.

O'Brien, P.M.S. (1987). Premenstrual syndrome. Blackwell Scientific, Oxford.

O'Brien, P.M.S. (1995). Symptometrics: quantification of premenstrual syndrome using a simple patient operated hand-held computer device. *Proceedings of the 27th British Congress of Obstetrics and Gynaecology*, Dublin. Abstract 181, Royal College of Obstetricians and Gynaecologists.

O'Brien, P.M.S. and Massil, H. (1990). Premenstrual syndrome clinical studies on essential fatty acids. In *Omega-6 essential fatty acids. Pathophysiology and roles in clinical medicine* (ed. D. Horrobin), pp. 523–45. Wiley-Liss, New York.

O'Brien, P.M.S. and Symonds, E.M. (1982). Prolactin levels in the premenstrual syndrome. *British Journal of Obstetrics and Gynaecology*, **89**, 306–8.

Pearlstien, T.B. and Stone, A.B. (1994). Long-term fluoxetine treatment of late luteal phase dysphoric disorder. *Journal of Clinical Psychiatry*, **55**, 332–5.

Pearlstein, T., River-Tovar, A., and Frank, E. (1992). Nonmedical management of late luteal phase dysphoric disorder: a preliminary report. *Journal of Psychotherapy Practice Research*, **1**, 49–55.

Prior, J.C. and Vigna, Y. (1987). Conditioning exercise and premenstrual symptoms. *Journal of Reproductive Medicine*, **32**, 423–8.

Rapkin, A.J. (1992). The role of serotonin in premenstrual syndrome. *Clinical Obstetrics and Gynaecology*, **35**, 629–36.

Rapkin, A.J., Buckman, T.C., Sutphin, M.S., Chang, L.C., and Reading, A.K. (1988). Platelet mono-amine oxidase B activity in women with premenstrual syndrome. *American Journal of Obstetrics and Gynecology*, **159**, 1536–40.

Reid, R.L. (1988). Etiology: medical theories. In *The premenstrual syndrome* (ed. W.R. Keye, Jr), pp. 66–93. W.B. Saunders, Philadelphia.

Reid, R.L. and Yen, S.S.C. (1981). Premenstrual syndrome. *American Journal of Obstetrics and Gynecology*, **139**, 85–104.

Rubinow, D.R., Hoban, C., Grover, G.N., Galloway, D.S., Roy-Byrne, P., Andersen, R., *et al.*, (1988). Changes in plasma hormone across the menstrual cycle in patients with menstrually related mood disorder and in control subjects. *American Journal of Obstetrics and Gynecology*, **158**, 5–11.

Sarno, A.P., Miller, E.J., and Lundbland, E.G. (1987). Premenstrual syndrome: beneficial effects of periodic, low-dose danazol. *Obstetrics and Gynecology*, **70**, 30–6.

Shoupe, D. (1991). The premenstrual syndrome. In *Infertility, contraception and reproductive endocrinology*, (3rd edn), (ed. D.R. Mishell Jr, V. Davajan, and R.A. Lobo), pp. 503–17. Blackwell Scientific, Boston.

Shoupe, D. and Lobo, R.A. (1985). The effects of estrogen and progestin on endrogenous opioid activity in oophorectomized women. *Journal of Clinical Endocrinology and Metabolism*, **60**, 178–83.

Smith, S., Rinehart, J.S., Ruddock, V.E., and Schiff, I. (1987). Treatment of premenstrual syndrome with alprazolam: results of a double blind, placebo-controlled randomized crossover clinical trial. *Obstetrics and Gynecology*, **70**, 37–42.

Steiner, M., Steinberg, S., Stewart, D., Carter, D., Berger, C., Reid, R., Douglas, G., and Streiner, D. (1995). Fluoxetine in the treatment of premenstrual dysphoria. *New England Journal of Medicine*, **332**, 1529–34.

Stone, A.B., Pearlstein, T.B., and Brown, W.A. (1991). Fluoxetine in the treatment of late luteal phase dysphoric disorder. *Journal of Clinical Psychiatry*, **52**, 290–3.

Vellacott, I.D. and O'Brien, P.M.S. (1987). Effects of spironolactone on premenstrual symptoms. *Journal of Reproductive Medicine*, **32**, 429–34.

Watson, N.R., Studd, J.W.W., Savvas, M., Garnett, T., and Baber, R.J. (1989). Treatment of severe premenstrual syndrome with oestradiol patches and cyclical oral norethisterone. *Lancet*, **ii**, 730–2.

Watts, J.F., Butt, W.R., and Edwards, R.L. (1987). A clinical trial using danazol for the treatment of premenstrual tension. *British Journal of Obstetrics and Gynaecology*, **94**, 30–4.

Wurtman, J., Brzezcnski, A., Wurtman, R.J., and Laferrera, B. (1989). Effect of nutrient intake on premenstrual tension. *American Journal of Obstetrics and Gynecology*, **161**, 2228–33.

VI Contraception and hormone replacement therapy

29 Contraceptive steroids and endometrial morphology

Moses A. Okon, T.C. Li, and Peter Dockery

Introduction

The response of the endometrium to contraceptive steroid treatment depends on a number of variables:

(1) which class of hormone or combination of hormone (e.g. oestrogen, progestogen, or oestrogen/progestogen combination) has been administered;

(2) if a particular class of hormone has been administered, which type has been used (e.g. whether natural or synthetic and if synthetic, which particular one and what potency);

(3) the dose; whether the hormone has been given in a single or multiple doses; if multiple, what was the daily dose and the duration of therapy;

(4) the time of the menstrual cycle at which the treatment was started often governs the state of the endometrium prior to the hormonal treatment;

(5) bioavailability, which depends on the route of administration; and finally,

(6) individual biological variation in response.

Combined oral contraceptive pill

The effect of the contraceptive pill on endometrial histology depends on the factors discussed above. The endometrium of women taking combined oral contraceptives may sometimes show early secretory activity in the glands but secretory changes typical of the mid and late luteal phase are lacking. During the last week of the cycle the glands become atrophic, small, and tubular with a lining of flattened cuboidal epithelium. Variable predecidual and vascular changes may be seen in the stroma. In subsequent treatment cycles the atrophic gland appearance and decidual change may be more marked (Haines and Taylor 1975). In this situation the glands and stroma fail to develop completely and mitoses are rare. There is premature appearance of persistently deficient secretory change in the glands, which remain uncoiled, and stromal oedema occurs and persists until a distinct predecidual or decidual reaction takes place (Fechner 1971; Dallenbach-Hellweg 1980). Prolonged administration of contraceptive steroids produces further arrest of secretory changes. The glands decrease in number and the endometrium generally becomes thin and atrophic. Patchy necrosis may occur and cause breakthrough bleeding (Ober 1966; Blaustein *et al.* 1968; Sarfati and Brux 1973; Maqueo 1980). The blood vessels become thinner and often dilated like sinusoids after prolonged therapy. Prolonged use also results in the disappearance of the minimal secretory changes leading to complete atrophy of the glands followed by stromal atrophy. The electron microscopic appearance is that of progressive disappearance of the cilia and rudimentary nucleolar channel system (Ober 1966).

Progestogens

The effect of progestogens on the endometrium depends on priming of the endometrium by oestrogen. The changes elicited by most progestogens on an oestrogen primed endometrium are similar, and consist of a variable degree of secretory response in the glands followed by suppression of glandular proliferation and secretion, and suppressed stromal proliferation, commonly followed by a decidual reaction (Abell 1975).

Continuous high-dose progestogen treatment may be used in conditions such as endometriosis and endometrial hyperplasia. It produces an initial suppression of glandular proliferation, followed by an incomplete glandular secretory response, and stromal oedema. Continued administration results in diffuse decidual change in the stroma (Abell 1975; Haines and Taylor 1975). The decidua may persist for weeks and may be shed as an endometrial decidual cast, as occurs in ectopic pregnancy.

Continuous low-dose progestogen administration is used as the oral 'minipill' for contraception. The endometrium becomes thin with sparse glands and a compact stroma with no oedema formation (Moghissi *et al.* 1973). Long-term, low-dose progestogen exposure is associated with varying histological endometrial appearances, including proliferation, secretion, suppressed or irregular secretion, decidualization, and even atrophy (Kim-Bjorklund *et al.* 1991). High-dose long-term progestogen treatment usually causes a more uniform atrophic change (Silverberg *et al.* 1986). Breakthrough bleeding has often been a major problem with the 'minipill' and has limited its use. The mechanism for this bleeding has not been fully clarified, although available evidence suggests that changes in the endometrial vasculature play an important part. The endometrial vascular response probably depends on the dose, duration, and type of progestogen used and the degree of interaction with endogenous ovarian hormones.

Furthermore, vascular changes are not always consistent with the degree of suppression of the non-vascular components of the endometrium (Hourihan *et al.* 1990; Rogers *et al.* 1993). The effect on endometrial blood vessels is especially prominent following levonorgestrel administration which causes well developed arterioles and dilated sinusoids, and which may account for the higher incidence of breakthrough bleeding with this progestogen (Graham and Fraser 1982). The most consistent vascular change observed with the progestogen pill is dilated venules and sinusoids (Hourihan *et al.* 1986; Song *et al.* 1995).

Cyclical administration of progestogen

The cyclical administration of high doses of progestogen is often used for the treatment of dysfunctional uterine bleeding. The effect of cyclical treatment with progestogens given from days 5 to 25 of the menstrual cycle has been studied by Borushek *et al.* (1963) and Flowers (1964). The initial response consisted of a lack of epithelial proliferation with glands which were hypoplastic and tubular. Between days 7 and 12, there was spotty, incomplete vacuolation of epithelium and marked stromal oedema. Some vessels were prominent and congested. Later changes depend on the dose of progestogen. Historically, when 19-*nor* steroid progestogen was initially used, the dose administered was high and the stroma underwent a diffuse decidual reaction not dissimilar to the changes which occur in pregnancy. When the dose of 19-*nor* steroids was considerably reduced, a decidual reaction was either not observed or was patchy or poorly formed. Progestogens with acetate radicals produce either no decidual response, or a patchy and ill-developed decidual reaction (Abell 1975).

Cyclical treatment with low-dose progestogen for contraceptive purposes is associated with a hypoplastic picture, similar to that of resting endometrium. These regimens were developed to mimic the natural cycle with a predominant oestrogenic effect in the follicular phase and a predominant progestogenic effect in the luteal phase. However, the cyclical or sequential use of progestogens is no longer a common practice because the endometrial protective effect is less than that afforded by continuous combined regimens (Kelly *et al.* 1976; Weis and Sayvetz 1980).

Progestogen implants

This method was developed to improve uptake and compliance with hormonal contraceptives by removing the need for daily tablets or frequent depot injections. Norplant® (Roussel Laboratories Ltd, UK) is a levonorgestrel (LNG) subdermal implant which achieves peak plasma LNG concentrations of between 1000 and 2000 pg/ml in the first week and this gradually declines to levels of 180–350 pg/ml by the end of five years. During the first year of use ovulation is suppressed in the majority of women. Approximately half of women have ovulatory cycles in subsequent years.

The endometrial response to implants depends to a large extent on whether or not ovarian activity is suppressed. As suppression of ovarian activity occurs to a variable degree, biopsy materials show changes ranging from proliferative to secretory, atrophic, suppressed, decidualized, or iatrogenic progestogenic effects (Kim-Borklund *et al.* 1991; Song *et al.* 1995).

As irregular bleeding is a common side-effect of progestogen use, a number of investigators have attempted to study the response of the vascular component of the endometrium to progestogen implants and the associated bleeding patterns (Johannisson *et al.* 1991; Fraser and Peek 1992; Rogers *et al.* 1993). Rogers *et al.* (1993) examined the effects of Norplant on the endometrial microvasculature and found no correlation between endometrial histology and bleeding pattern during the preceding three months. They observed that 54 per cent of Norplant users had atrophic endometrium, but the majority of these subjects had prolonged, frequent, or irregular bleeding problems which occurred despite the atrophy.

They also reported an increased microvascular density in Norplant subjects compared to the controls. The effect of the progestogen implant on endometrial vasculature appears to be somewhat different to that of oral progestogens. In a study of 19 patients using oral norethisterone (5–30 mg daily over 2 weeks to 6 months) or medroxyprogesterone acetate (MPA) (15–80 mg daily for 8 days to 5 months), Song *et al.* (1995) observed that progestogen exposure reduced the density of microvessels but increased the number of dilated venules in the endometrium.

Hourihan *et al.* (1986) examined the effect of oral progestogen (after norethisterone and levonorgestrel for 4 to 33 weeks), and similarly noted that there was an increase in the total number of veins and dilated veins in the functional layers of the endometrium. In addition, this study also found a decrease in the number of arterioles at the endometrial–myometrial junction.

It is uncertain whether the dilated venules or the altered microvascular density observed in these studies directly causes breakthrough and irregular bleeding. Maqueo (1980) found pronounced sinusoid formation in the endometria from women on higher dose combined oral contraceptives and depot MPA. These dilated vessels were associated with histologically suppressed or secretory endometrial patterns. However, the presence of dilated vessels did not correlate with the episodes of bleeding. This finding is also common in the endometrium of combined oral contraceptive pill users who do not normally experience as much breakthrough bleeding as those women taking progestogen-only pills.

Perhaps the functional integrity of the vessel wall is of greater importance in determining bleeding during continuous progestogen treatment. It may be that the vessels are breached by local necrosis in the progestogen-treated women (Irey *et al.* 1970; Irey and Norris 1973), or there may be defective desmosomal function induced by progestogens (Wilborn and Flowers 1984) thus allowing fluid and cells to leak through the endothelium of the endometrial microvasculature.

Levonorgestrel-releasing intrauterine devices

The levonorgestrel-releasing intrauterine device (IUD) has been developed as a means of providing contraception and of reducing menstrual blood loss. Its advantage over inert or copper-bearing IUDs is the significant reduction of menstrual blood loss, which falls by as much as 90 per cent (Anderson and Rybo 1990). Its advantage over injectable and oral progestogen is the minimal systemic absorption and therefore the absence of significant systemic side-effects. Moreover, in contrast to the variable endometrial morphology seen in oral, injectable, and implant users (Kim-Bjorklund *et al.* 1991), the endometrial morphology in women using a norgestrel-releasing IUD appears to be remarkably consistent. The local delivery of norgestrel directly downregulates the endometrial oestrogen receptor and consistently results in endometrial suppression (Nilsson *et al.* 1978; Silverberg *et al.* 1986; Barbosa *et al.* 1990).

Nilsson *et al.* (1978) studied the effect of a D-norgestrel-releasing IUD (releasing 20 μg and 40 μg D-norgestrel daily) in 12 regularly menstruating women. The histological appearance of the endometrial specimens of all 12 subjects was very uniform. There was no significant difference between specimens obtained during the 'luteal' phase and those obtained during the 'follicular' phase or those obtained from subjects not ovulating during treatment. The effect on the endometrium was not dose dependent. Histologically, the glands of the endometrium showed atrophy and the depth of the endometrium was 1–3 mm. The stroma was swollen and decidual changes were observed. Mitotic activity was suppressed. These changes were seen throughout the endometrium and were not limited to the superficial layers and neither were they influenced by the site of the biopsy in relation to the position of the IUD. An inflammatory reaction of leukocytic infiltration not dissimilar to that seen around inert IUDs was also observed. Similar findings have been reported by other workers (Perino *et al.* 1987). In addition, Zhu *et al.* (1989) observed that the arterial walls became thickened, the spiral arterioles were suppressed, and capillary thrombosis occurred. Sheppard and Bonnar (1983) observed a significantly lower density of small blood vessels in endometrial samples from patients with progesterone-releasing intrauterine devices compared to control samples. These changes may account for the reduction in menstrual flow.

Silverberg *et al.* (1986) examined 92 women who had used a levonorgestrel-releasing IUD. The endometrial morphology was similar regardless of the duration of IUD use (from three to seven years) or the stage of the menstrual cycle at which the biopsy was taken. The endometrial glands were atrophic and the stroma decidualized. The predominance of the stromal decidual change was generally greater in biopsies taken soon after insertion of the IUD.

Morphological changes in the endometrium in response to the levonorgestrel IUD also reflect the presence of a foreign body (i.e. the coil) and include an increase in endometrial neutrophils, lymphocytes, plasma cells, and macrophages (Zhu *et al.* 1989). Sometimes focal stromal necrosis and calcification may occur particularly after long-term use (Silverberg *et al.* 1986).

Progestogen-releasing vaginal rings

Johannisson (1990) examined the effects of different doses of progestogens released by vaginal rings on endometrial morphology. Two different dose levels of norethisterone (NET) (50 μg and 200 μg per 24 h) and three dose levels of levonorgestrel (10 μg, 20 μg, and 25 μg per 24 h) were examined. Endometrial biopsies were obtained after 6 and 10 months. While the release of 50 μg NET/24 h did not appear to have any significant effect on the number of glands per mm^2 nor on the size of the glands, the release of 200 μg/24 h significantly diminished the number of glands after 10 weeks and their size after only six weeks. With levonorgestrel, the release of 10 μg/24 h did not seem to have any significant effect on the number and size of glands. However, at a release of 20 μg/24 h the diameter of the glands was significantly smaller than in the control women after 6 weeks of use. After 6 and 10 weeks of use of a 25 μg/day-releasing ring the size of the glands was significantly smaller than the controls. Thus, in terms of its effects on the endometrium, the progestogen-releasing vaginal ring may have similar advantages to that of the progestogen-releasing IUD.

Post-coital contraception

Oestrogens

Administered in sufficient dose in the follicular phase, oestrogen abolishes the luteal phase of the endometrium. Proliferation of glands and stroma is stimulated. Relatively high doses of oestrogen given in the early luteal phase may act as a post-coital contraceptive. In a study of five healthy volunteers, Haspels *et al.* (1977) examined the effect of intramuscular administration of oestrogens (12.5 mg of oestradiol phenylpropionate) in the early luteal phase; if the oestrogens were given on day four after the luteneizing hormone surge (LH+4) or after, no change in endometrial histology was noted. However, if the oestrogens were given on days LH+1 to LH+3, the endometrium demonstrated dissociated secretory changes or secretory endometrium with pronounced epithelial proliferation.

Van Santen *et al.* (1988) examined the endometrial ultrastructural changes induced by high-dose ethinyl oestradiol in four women with regular menstrual cycles. A biopsy was performed during a cycle when no medication was given (control cycle). In a subsequent cycle another biopsy was performed after treatment with 5 mg ethinyl oestradiol daily for five days, given during the luteal phase. In the treatment cycles there was morphological evidence of retarded endometrial development, as reported by previous light microscopic studies. In addition, electron microscopy revealed that the nuclear channel system, which is normally present in the nucleus of epithelial cells in the secretory phase, was totally absent in the treatment group.

Oestrogen/progestogen

Yuzpe *et al.* (1974) examined the effect of a single dose of ethinyl oestradiol and DL-norgestrel (half the current standard Yuzpe regimen) on endometrial morphology. They observed a significant delay in the maturation of the glandular component of the endometrium. Ling *et al.* (1979) studied the effect of two doses of 0.1 mg of ethinyl oestradiol and 1 mg of DL-norgestrel administered 12 h apart around the predicted time of ovulation. They found significant asynchrony in the development of the glandular and stromal endometrial components: the glands appeared to lag behind the stroma by two to six days in maturation. A repeat study by the same group produced similar findings (Ling *et al.* 1983). These observed changes appear to reflect a significant disruption of function of the endometrial cell which renders the implantation site unsuitable for nidation.

Danazol

Danazol, 17α-pregnan-2-4-dien-20-yno[2,3-]-isoxazol-17-ol (a synthetic steroid derived from 17α-ethisterone) may also be used for post-coital contraception (Henderson and Tsang 1980; Rowlands *et al.* 1986). The drug is a weak androgen but has in addition anti-androgenic, progestogenic, anti-progestogenic, oestrogenic, and anti-oestrogenic properties. At a dose of 200 mg repeated after 12 h it has a high patient acceptability because of the absence of vomiting and other side-effects associated with oestrogen/progestogen combinations (Rowlands *et al.* 1983), but it appears to be less effective when compared with the Yuzpe regimen or mifepristone (Webb *et al.* 1992).

There are limited data on the short term effects of danazol on endometrial morphology. Tamaya *et al.* (1983) reported that danazol administration in the luteal phase to patients with in-phase endometrium decreased endometrial oestrogen and progesterone receptor levels, and reduced serum progesterone, LH, and FSH levels. Danazol, used as post-coital contraception, produced no consistent patterns of alteration in urinary ovarian steroids. This suggested a heterogeneous effect on ovarian function and that the main mechanism of action of danazol as a post-coital contraceptive is at the endometrial level (Rowlands *et al.* 1986). This has been confirmed by subsequent studies which showed that danazol has a direct suppressive effect on human endometrial cells (Rose *et al.* 1988).

When danazol is administered long term, the multiple effects produce a hypo-oestrogenic, hypo-progestogenic, and hyper-androgenic effect with induced endometrial atrophy and inhibition or delay of ovulation. Jeppsson *et al.* (1984) studied the effect of danazol (600 mg daily) on endometrial morphology in 10 women. Biopsies were obtained at four weeks in five patients and at eight weeks in the remaining five patients. Their results showed that danazol induced endometrial atrophy in three women and reduced secretory vacuoles in the remaining two cases as early as four weeks into therapy. The endometrial morphological changes observed included reduced glandular size and number, a flattened epithelium, and reduced mitotic activity. The stroma consisted of small or spindle-shaped cells, sometimes with slight oedema but with no decidual reaction. These effects were dose related. Ultrastructural changes included complete involution of the cytoplasmic organelles with cytoplasmic collapse in glandular cells (Marchini *et al.* 1992).

Mifepristone

Mifepristone (RU486) can block ovulation or retard endometrial development, dependent on whether it is given before or after ovulation. The drug appears to have a potential as an emergency contraceptive for the prevention of pregnancy. To examine this possibility the WHO supported two randomized trials to compare the efficacy and side-effects of a single dose of RU486 with those of the standard Yuzpe and Lancee (1977) regimen (0.1 mg ethinyl oestradiol plus 0.5 mg of levonorgestrel repeated after 12 h). The studies confirmed the potential value of mifepristone in emergency contraception (Glasier *et al.* 1992; Webb *et al.* 1992). In the two studies combined, 597 women were given RU486 and none of them became pregnant compared with nine pregnancies among 589 subjects in the Yuzpe regimen group. In general the women treated with RU486 experienced fewer side-effects than those treated with the Yuzpe method, although they were more likely to report a delayed onset of the next menstruation. The effect of RU486 on endometrial morphology is discussed in detail below.

Antiprogestogens

Antiprogestogens are synthetic steroids which block the effects of progesterone at the cellular level by binding to progesterone receptors in the endometrium. Through these effects, antiprogestogens are believed to prevent implantation, if given early in the luteal phase, and to induce abortion if given after successful implantation has taken place (Hermann *et al.* 1985; Shoupe *et al.* 1985; Schaison *et al.* 1985).

Although several compounds have been synthesized only three, namely, mifepristone (RU486), onapristone, and lilopristone have been given to humans. Like most steroids which cross-react with other steroid receptors, the antiprogestogens are not specific and also have antiglucocorticoid (Neef *et al.* 1984) and antiandrogen (Philibert *et al.* 1985) activities. The effect of an antiprogestogen on endometrial morphology depends on when and how the drug has been administered, as will be described below.

Early luteal phase as a once-a-month contraceptive

Li *et al.* (1988*a*) examined the morphological changes in the endometrium after a single oral dose (5 mg to 200 mg) of RU486 in the first half of the luteal phase of the cycle in 30 normal subjects. Quantitative histological techniques were employed and the results were compared with a normal fertile population. RU486 was found to have a number of effects:

(1) inhibition of glandular secretory activity;

(2) acceleration of degenerative changes, including a significant increase in the number of apoptotic bodies in the glandular epithelium;

(3) marked vascular changes which included an increase in venule diameter, reduction in the amount of stromal oedema, stromal extravasation, and decreased leukocytic infiltration in the stroma; and

(4) increased stromal but not glandular mitotic activity.

The above findings have been confirmed by other workers (Batista *et al.* 1992; Katkam *et al.* 1995). In addition Johannisson *et al.* (1989) reported that the administration of RU486 during the pre-ovulatory phase did not modify the vascular structure, but if administered in the post-ovulatory phase it resulted in necrosis of capillary endothelial cells and diminution in the capillary lumen and adventitia.

The ultrastructural changes in the glandular epithelium following the administration of mifepristone have been examined in biopsy materials reported in our earlier study (Li *et al.* 1988*a*/*b*). The appearance of the glandular epithelium three days after a single dose of mifepristone, whatever the day of administration between LH+2 and LH+6, appear remarkably similar. The cells lose much of their polarity and lysosome-like electron dense bodies are a common feature of the apical cytoplasm (Fig. 29.1). Nuclear channel systems and giant mitochondrial profiles are absent (Fig. 29.2). Basal deposits of glycogen-rich materials are seen in much reduced amounts.

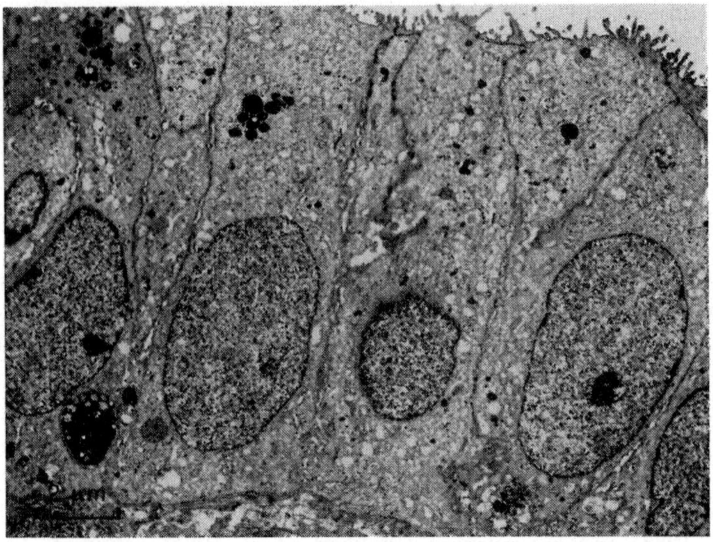

Fig. 29.1 Typical appearance of the glandular epithelium biopsied three days after early luteal administration of RU486. Note electron dense bodies in the apical cytoplasm (upper part of micrograph)

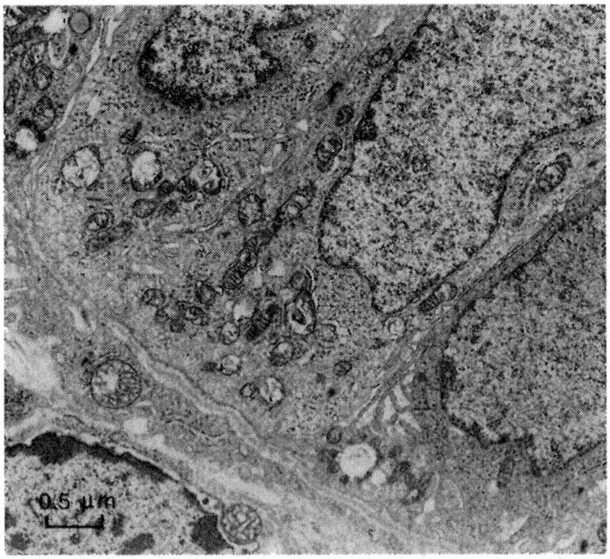

Fig. 29.2 Basal cytoplasm of a glandular epithelial cell treated with RU486 on day LH+3 and biopsied on LH+5. Note the lack of giant mitochondrial profiles.

Degenerating cells are encountered within the epithelium (Fig. 29.3), which would correspond to the degenerative changes described by Li *et al.* (1988 *a*/*b*).

The effect of mifepristone on endometrial glandular secretory activity was further examined by Graham *et al.* (1991) by using immunohistochemical techniques to assess the production and secretion of D9B1 epitope. When RU486 was given two days after the LH peak, it prevented the

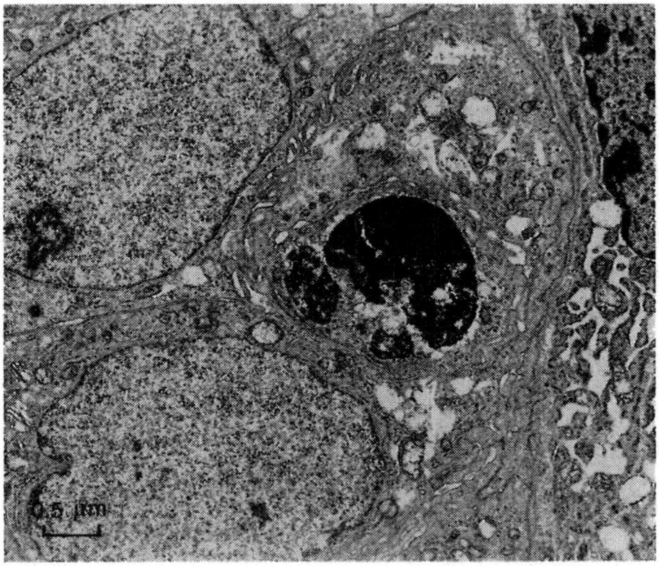

Fig. 29.3 A degenerating cell in the glandular epithelium, a characteristic feature of RU486-treated tissue.

appearance of the epitope. When it was given five days after the LH surge, epitope already present in the gland cells was subsequently secreted.

This observation is backed up by the morphometric electron-microscopical data shown in Fig. 29.4. A two-way analysis of variance of these data reveals a significant effect of treatment, day of biopsy, and interaction. The values for the control groups on days LH+5,6 were significantly larger than RU486-treated groups.

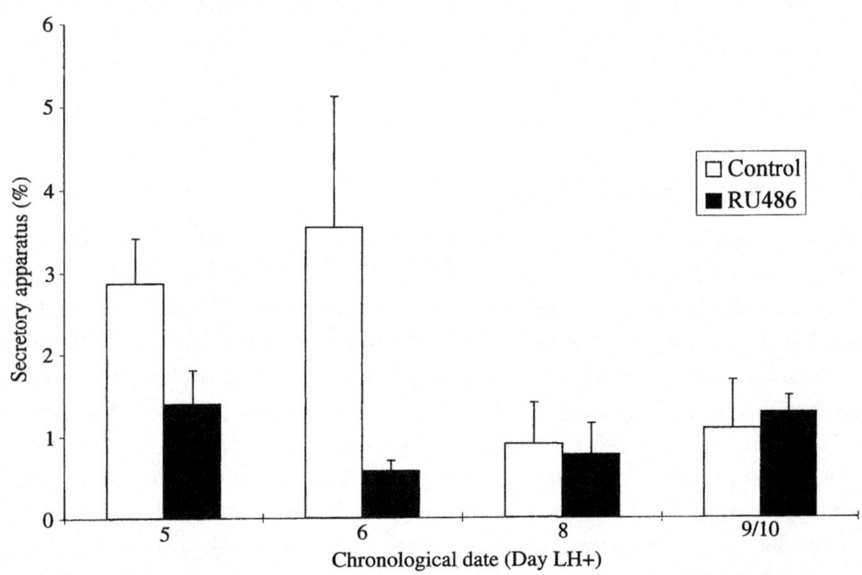

Fig. 29.4 Percentage of the glandular epithelial cell occupied by secretory apparatus, comparing RU486-treated tissue with controls. The columns represent the mean + SD for four or five women in each group.

The above results suggest that a single dose of mifepristone administered in the early luteal phase has a profound effect on endometrial morphology in the peri-implantation period. The contraceptive value of such a strategy has been examined by Gemzell-Danielsson *et al.* (1993), who reported one pregnancy during 157 cycles of treatment in 21 women who received a single dose of 200 mg mifepristone administered in the early luteal phased (timed by LH surge). While such an approach appears to produce encouraging results, there are a number of practical problems for its use as a once-a-month pill. The administration of the antiprogestogen needs to be timed precisely, for example by LH surge. If it is given too early, ovulation may be suppressed, leading to postponement of the next period and disruption of the regular cycle. If it is given too late it may induce endometrial bleeding but may not produce endometrial shedding or prevent implantation (Li *et al.* 1988 *a*, *b*). On the other hand its use as a one-off post-coital emergency contraception appears to have great potential.

Late luteal phase administration

A number of clinical trials have been published on the use of a single dose of mifepristone as a late luteal contraceptive (Van Look and von Hertzen 1995). Among the 236 subjects studied there were 76 pregnancies prior to treatment. The failure rate per treated pregnancy cycle was 11/76 (14.5 per cent) which suggests that the once-a-month late luteal phase administration of mifepristone is not a viable approach to fertility regulation. Endometrial morphology following late luteal phase administration has been less well studied because this regimen frequently results in menstruation. The administration of RU486 in the mid-luteal phase may also induce menstrual bleeding. When compared with spontaneous menstruation, RU486-induced menstruation was associated with a reduction in the amount of glandular secretory activity, predecidual reaction, and leukocytic infiltration (Li *et al.* 1990). This observation suggests that menstruation may occur independently of these morphological features. Predecidual reaction may, however, be closely related to endometrial shedding at the time of menstruation. Similarly, Garzo *et al.* (1988) reported that the leukocytic infiltration, local necrosis, and haemorrhage seen in the endometrium 2–3 days before the onset of spontaneous menstruation were not observed in endometrial biopsy specimens taken 12–24 h before the onset of bleeding in women treated with mifepristone during the mid luteal phase of the cycle.

Continuous daily administration

More recently, attention has turned to the effects of continuous, low-dose mifepristone starting on the first or second day of menstruation. Batista *et al.* (1992) examined 11 normally cycling women who were given a daily dose of 1 mg mifepristone. The follicular phase of the cycle was prolonged by an average of six days and the LH surge was delayed, but the length of the luteal phase was not altered. Endometrial morphology in the mid-luteal phase (days LH+7 to +9) showed that endometrial development was retarded by an average of two days. Peak levels of placental protein 14 were also reduced. The low dose of mifepristone did not disturb ovarian cyclicity, steroidogenesis, or ovulation. These abnormalities in endometrial morphology and function appear to be similar to those seen in subfertile women with a luteal phase defect. The authors concluded that a daily 1 mg dose of mifepristone significantly disturbs endometrial development. It is therefore possible for this regimen to be proposed as a new generation 'minipill' – a novel strategy for fertility control (Cameron *et al.* 1996).

The effect of long-term (six months) mifepristone administration at a significantly higher daily dose (50 mg) on endometrial morphology has been reported by Murphy *et al.* (1995). Basal endometrium appeared to be undisturbed or mildly thickened. The functional layers were mildly hyperplastic, especially obvious in the stromal compartment in which cellularity and mitotic activities were prominent. The glands were of variable sizes and shapes, consistent with a hyperplastic picture; with mitotic figures present in the epithelial cell. There was a mixture of secretory and proliferative activities in the gland, with proliferative changes predominating. This endometrial morphology is consistent with a chronic unopposed oestrogen effect. These findings call for caution in the use of antiprogestogens long term until more studies have been performed to determine the optimal dose and duration of administration.

Conclusion

There is clear evidence that contraceptive steroids significantly alter endometrial morphology and function. The progestogen-releasing IUDs and antiprogestogens represent important recent developments. The optimal regimen is one which effectively prevents implantation but produces little systemic side-effects and no unscheduled vaginal bleeding. A better understanding of endometrial physiology and the response of the endometrium to contraceptive steroids is an important prerequisite to achieving this goal.

References

Abell, M.R. (1975). Endometrial biopsy: normal and abnormal diagnostic characteristics. In: *Gynaecological endocrinology*, (ed. J.J. Gold), pp. 156–90. Harper and Row, New York.

Anderson, J.K. and Rybo, G. (1990). Levonorgestrel-releasing intrauterine device in the treatment of menorrhagia. *British Journal of Obstetrics and Gynaecology*, **97**, 690–4.

Barbosa, I., Bakos, O., Olsson, S.-E., Odlind, V., and Johannisson, E.D.B. (1990). Ovarian function during use of levonorgestrel-releasing IUD. *Contraception*, **42**, 51–66.

Batista, M.C., Cartledge, T.P., Zellmer, A.N., Merino, M.J., Axiotis, C., Loriaux, D.L., and Nieman, L.K. (1992). Delayed endometrial maturation induced by daily administration of antiprogestin RU 486: a potential new contraceptive strategy. *American Journal of Obstetrics and Gynecology*, **167**, 60–5.

Blaustein, A., Shenker, L., and Post, R.C. (1968). The effect of oral contraceptives on the endometrium. *International Journal of Fertility*, **13**, 466–78.

Borushek, S., Abell, M.R., Smith, L. and Gold, J.J. (1963). The effects of Provest on the endometrium. *International Journal of Fertility*, **8**, 605–18.

Cameron, S.T., Critchley, H.O.D., Thong, K.J., Buckley, C.H., Williams, A.R., and Baird, D.T. (1996). Effects of daily low dose mifepristone on endometrial maturation and proliferation. *Human Reproduction*, **11**, 2518–26.

Dallenbach-Hellweg, G. (1980). The influence of contraceptive steroids on the histological appearance of the endometrium. In *Endometrial bleeding and steroid contraception*, (ed. E. Diczfalusy, I.S. Fraser, and F.T.G. Webb), pp. 153–73. Pitman, Bath.

Fechner, R.E. (1971). The surgical pathology of the reproductive system and breast during oral contraceptive therapy. *Pathology Annual*, **6**, 299–319.

Flowers, C.E. Jr., (1964). Effects of a new low-dosage form of norethynodrel mestranol: clinical evaluation and endometrial study. *Journal of the American Medical Association*, **188**, 1115–20.

Fraser, I.S. and Peek, M.J. (1992). Effects of exogenous hormones on endometrial capillaries. In *Steroid hormones and uterine bleeding*, (ed. N.J. Alexander and N. d'Arcangues), pp. 67–79. American Association for the Advancement of Science Press, Washington DC, USA.

Garzo, V.G., Lui, J., Ulmann, A., Baulieu, E., and Yen, S.S.C. (1988). Effects of an antiprogesterone (RU486) on the hypothalamic–hypophyseal–ovarian–endometrial axis during the luteal phase of the menstrual cycle. *Journal of Clinical Endocrinology and Metabolism*, **66**, 508–17.

Gemzell-Danielsson, K., Swahn, M.-L. Svalander, P., and Bygdeman, M. (1993). Early luteal phase treatment with mifepristone (RU 486) for fertility regulation. *Human Reproduction*, **8**, 870–3.

Glasier, A., Thong, K.J., Mackie, M., and Baird, D.T. (1992). Mifepristone (RU486) compared with high-dose estrogen and progestogen for emergency postcoital contraception. *New England Journal of Medicine*, **327**, 1041–4.

Graham, S. and Fraser, I.S. (1982). The progestogen-only mini-pill. *Contraception*, **26**, 373–88.

Graham, R.A., Li, T.C., Seif, M.W., Aplin, J., and Cooke, I.D. (1991). The effects of the antiprogesterone RU486 (mifepristone) on an endometrial secretory glycan: an immunocytochemical study. *Fertility and Sterility*, **55**, 1132–6.

Haines, M. and Taylor, C.W. (1975). *Gynaecological pathology*, (2nd edn), pp. 130–57. Churchill Livingstone, Edinburgh.

Haspels, A.A., Linthorst, G.A., and Kicoric, P.M. (1977). Effect of postovulatory administration of a 'morning after' injection on corpus luteum function and endometrium. *Contraception*, **15**, 105–12.

Henderson, K.M. and Tsang, B.K. (1980). Danazol suppresses luteal function in vitro and in vivo. *Fertility and Sterility*, **33**, 550–6.

Hermann, W.L., Schindler, A.M., Wyss, R., and Bischof, P. (1985). Effects of the antiprogesterone RU 486 in early pregnancy and during the menstrual cycle. In *The antiprogestin steroid RU486 and human fertility control*, (ed. E.E. Baulieu and S.J. Segal), pp. 199–209. Plenum Press, New York.

Hourihan, H.M., Sheppard, B.L., and Bonnar, J. (1986). A morphometric study of the effects of oral norethisterone or levonorgestrel on endometrial blood vessels. *Contraception*, **34**, 603–12.

Hourihan, H.M., Sheppard, B.L. and Brosens, I.A. (1990). Endometrial haemostasis. In *Contraception and mechanisms of endometrial bleeding*. (ed. C. d'Arcangues, I.S. Fraser, J.R. Newton, and V. Odlind), pp. 363–79. Cambridge University Press.

Irey, N.S. and Norris, H.J. (1973). Intimal vascular lesions associated with female reproductive steroids. *Archives of Pathology*, **96**, 227–34.

Irey, N.S., Manion, W.C., and Taylor, H.B. (1970). Vascular lesions in women taking oral contraceptives. *Archives of Pathology*, **81**, 1–8.

Jeppsson, S., Mellquist, P., and Rannevik, G. (1984). Short-term effects of danazol on endometrial histology. *Acta Obstetrica et Gynecologica Scandinavica*, **123**, (Suppl.), 41–4.

Johannisson, E. (1990). Endometrial morphology during the normal cycle and under the influence of contraceptive steroids. In *Contraception and mechanisms of endometrial bleeding* (ed. C. d'Arcangues, I.S. Fraser, J.R. Newton, and V. Odlind), pp. 53–72. Cambridge University Press.

Johannisson, E., Oberholzer, M., Sawhn, M., and Bygdeman, M. (1989). Vascular changes in the human endometrium following administration of the progesterone antagonist RU486. *Contraception*, **39**, 103–17.

Johannisson, E., Brosens, I., Cornillie, F., Elder, M., White, J., Sheppard, B., *et al.* (1991). Morphometric study of the human endometrium following continuous exposure to levonorgestrel released from vaginal rings during 90 days. *Contraception*, **43**, 361–74.

Katkam, RR., Gopalkrishnan, K., Chwalisz, K., Schillinger, E., and Puri, C.P. (1995). Onapristone (ZK 98.299): a potential anti progestin for endometrial contraception. *American Journal of Obstetrics and Gynecology*, **173**, 779–87.

Kelly, H.W., Miles, P.A., Buster, J.E., and Scragg, W.H. (1976). Adenocarcinoma of the endometrium in women taking sequential oral contraceptives. *Obstetrics and Gynecology*, **47**, 200–2.

Kim-Bjorklund, T., Landgren, B.M., and Johannisson, E. (1991). Morphometric studies of the endometrium, fallopian tube and the corpus luteum during contraception with 300 μg norethisterone (NET) minipill. *Contraception*, **43**, 459–74.

Li, T.C., Lenton, E.A., Dockery, P., Rogers, A.W., and Cooke, I.D. (1988a). Why does RU486 fail to prevent implantation despite success in inducing menstruation? *Contraception*, **38**, 401–6.

Li, T.C., Rogers, A.W., Dockery, P., Lenton, E.A., Thomas, P., and Cooke, I.D. (1988b). The effects of progesterone receptor blockade in the luteal phase of normal fertile women. *Fertility and Sterility*, **50**, 732–42.

Li, T.C., Dockery, P., Rogers, A.W., and Cooke, I.D. (1990). Histological and clinical features of menstruation induced by the antiprogestogen mifepristone (RU486) as compared to menstruation occurring spontaneously. *Journal of Obstetrics and Gynaecology*, **10**, 1447–50.

Ling, W.Y., Robichaud, A., Zayid, I., Wrixton, W., and McLeod, S.C. (1979). Mode of action of DL-norgestrel and ethinylestradiol combination in postcoital contraception. *Fertility and Sterility*, **32**, 297–302.

Ling, W.Y., Wrixon, W., Zayid, I., Acorn, T., Popat, R., and Wilson, E. (1983). Mode of action of DL norgestrel and ethinylestradiol combination in postcoital contraception. II. Effect of post-ovulatory administration on ovarian function and endometrium. *Fertility and Sterility*, **39**, 292–7.

Marchini, M., Fedele, L., Bianchi, S., Di Nola, G., Nava, S., and Vercellini, P. (1992). Endometrial patterns during therapy with danazol or gestrinone for endometriosis: structural and ultrastructural study. *Human Pathology*, **23**, 51–6.

Maqueo, M. (1980). Vascular changes and perivascular changes in the endometrium of women using contraceptive steroids. In *Endometrial bleeding and steroid contraception*, (ed. E. Diczfalusy, I.S. Fraser, and F.T.G. Webb), pp. 138–52. Pitman, Bath.

Moghissi, K.S., Syner, F.N., and Mcbride, L.C. (1973). Contraceptive mechanism of microdose norethindrone. *Obstetrics and Gynecology*, **41**, 585–90.

Murphy, A.A., Roberts, V., Kettle, L.M., Parmley, T., Morales, A.J., and Yen, S.S.C. (1995). Endometrial effects of long-term low-dose administration of RU 486. *Fertility and Sterility*, **63**, 761–6.

Neef, G., Elger, W., Henderson, D., and Weichert, R. (1984). New steroids with antiprogestational and antiglucocorticoid activities. *Steroids*, **44**, 349–72.

Nilsson, C.G., Luukainen, T., and Arko, H. (1978). Endometrial morphology of women using a D-norgestrel-releasing intrauterine device. *Fertility and Sterility*, **29**, 397–401.

Ober, W.B. (1966). Synthetic progestogen-estrogen preparations and endometrial morphology. *Journal of Clinical Pathology*, **19**, 138–47.

Ober, W.B. (1977). Effects of oral and intrauterine administration of contraceptives on the uterus. *Human Pathology*, **8**, 513–27.

Perino, A., Quartararo, P., Catinella, E., Genova, G., and Cittadini, E. (1987). Treatment of endometrial hyperplasia with levonorgestrel-releasing intrauterine devices. *Acta Europia Fertilitatis*, **18**, 137–40.

Philibert, D., Moguilewsky, M., Mary, I., Leccaque, D., Tournemine, C., Secchi, J., and Deraedt, R. (1985). Pharmacological profile of RU 486 in animals. In *The antiprogestin steroid RU486 and human fertility control*, (ed. E.E. Baulieu and S.J. Segal), pp. 49–68. Plenum Press, New York.

Rogers, P.A.W., Au, C.L., and Affandi, B. (1993). Endometrial microvascular density during the normal menstrual cycle and following exposure to long-term levonorgestrel. *Human Reproduction*, **8**, 1396–404.

Rose, G.L., White, O.J., Dowsett, M., Jeffcoate, S.L., and Mudge, J.E. (1988). The inhibitory effects of danazol, danazol metabolites, gestrinone, and testosterone on the growth of human endometrial cells in vitro. *Fertility and Sterility*, **49**, 224–8.

Rowlands, S., Guillebaud, M.A., Bound, W., and Booth, M. (1983). Side effects of danazol compared with an ethinylestradiol/norgestrel combination used for postcoital contraception. *Contraception*, **27**, 39–49.

Rowlands, S., Kubba, A.A., Guillebaud, M.A., and Bound, W. (1986). Possible mechanism of action of danazol and an ethinylestradiol/norgestrel combination used as postcoital contraceptive agents. *Contraception*, **33**, 539–45.

Sarfati, R. and Brux, J. (1973). Vascular fragility of the endometrium under oestrogen–progestin treatment. Treatment by disodium flavonate. *European Journal of Obstetrics, Gynecology and Reproductive Biology*, **2**, 87–94

Schaison, G., George, M., Lestrat, N., and Baulieu, E.E. (1985). RU486 in women with normal or anovulatory cycles. In *The antiprogestin steroid RU486 and human fertility control* (ed. E.E. Baulieu and S.J. Segal), pp. 271–8. Plenum Press, New York.

Sheppard, B.L. and Bonnar, J. (1983). The effect of IUDs on the ultrastructure of the endometrium in relation to bleeding complications. *American Journal of Obstetrics and Gynecology*, **146**, 829–39.

Shoupe, D., Mishell, D.R., Lacarra, M., Gutierrez, E., Lahteenmaki, P., and Spitz, I.M. (1985). Endocrinologic effects of antiprogesterone RU486 in the luteal phase of normal women. In *The antiprogestin steroid RU486 and human fertility control*, (ed. E.E. Baulieu and S.J. Segal), pp. 285–93. Plenum Press, New York.

Silverberg, S.G., Haukkamaa, M., Arko, H., Nilsson, C.G., and Luukkainen, T. (1986). Endometrial morphology during long-term use of levonorgestrel-releasing intrauterine devices. *International Journal of Gynecological Pathology*, **5**, 235–41.

Song, J.Y., Markham, R., Russell, P., Wong, T., Young, L., and Fraser, I.S. (1995). The effect of high-dose medium- and long-term progestogen exposure on endometrial vessels. *Human Reproduction*, **10**, 797–800.

Tamaya, T., Murakami, T., Yamada, T., Wada, K., Fujimoto, J., and Okada, H. (1983). Serum hormone and steroid hormone receptor levels during luteal-phase and long-term treatment with danazol. *Fertility and Sterility*, **40**, 585–9.

Van Look, P.F.A. and von Hertzen, H. (1995). Clinical uses of antiprogestogens. *Human Reproduction Update*, **1**, 19–34.

Van Santen, M.R., Haspels, A.A., Heijnen, H.F., and Rademakers, L.H. (1988). Interfering with implantation by postcoital estrogen administration: endometrium epithelial cell ultrastructure. *Contraception*, **38**, 711–24.

Webb, M.C., Russell, J., and Elstein, M. (1992). Comparison of Yuzpe regimen, danazol, and mifepristone (RU486) in oral postcoital contraception. *British Medical Journal*, **305**, 927–31.

Weis, N.S. and Sayvetz, T.A. (1980). Incidence of endometrial cancer in relation to the use of oral contraceptives. *New England Journal of Medicine*, **302**, 551–4.

Wilborn, W.H. and Flowers, C.E. (1984). Endometrial conservation during menstruation. *Seminars in Reproductive Endocrinology*, **2**, 307–41.

Yuzpe, A.A. and Lancee, W.J. (1977). Ethinylestradiol and DL-norgestrel as a postcoital contraceptive. *Fertility and Sterility*, **28**, 932–6.

Yuzpe, A.A., Thurlow, H.J., Ramzy, I., and Leyshon, J.I. (1974). Postcoital contraception: a pilot study. *Journal of Reproductive Medicine*, **13**, 53–61.

Zhu, P.D., Luo, H.Z., Xu, R.H., Cheng, J., Wu, S.C., Chen, J.H., *et al.* (1989). The effect of intrauterine devices, the stainless steel ring, the copper T220, and releasing levonorgestrel, on the bleeding profile and morphological structure of the human endometrium – comparative studies of three IUDs. A morphometric analysis of 96 cases. *Contraception*, **40**, 425–38.

30 Disturbances of bleeding with intrauterine contraceptive devices and hormonal intrauterine systems

Viveca Odlind

Introduction

Menstrual bleeding disturbance is often reported as a side-effect in users of intrauterine devices (IUDs) for contraception and it is the most common reason for discontinuation of IUD use. Around 40–50 per cent of all terminations in IUD users occur as a consequence of perceived bleeding problems (Table 30.1). Termination rates for bleeding problems vary between studies and between centres, probably, in part, reflecting variations in attitudes and counselling among service providers (Table 30.2). The rates are similar for inert and copper IUDs and hormone releasing systems but the nature of the bleeding problems reported by the women is very different in users of inert or copper IUDs as compared with that in users of hormonal intrauterine contraception. The most common complaints with copper IUDs are increased menstrual blood loss, prolonged menstrual bleeding periods, and intermenstrual bleeding. The most common complaints with hormone-releasing intrauterine systems are intermenstrual bleeding, irregular bleeding, and amenorrhoea.

Development of modern IUDs

The first modern intrauterine devices (IUDs) made of polyethylene were introduced into family planning programmes during the late 1950s in many countries. Later, when intrauterine adminis-

Table 30.1 Terminations of IUD use per 100 women at 12 months for bleeding problems in relation to all reasons for termination in three selected randomized trials

Device	Termination for bleeding	Termination for all other	Bleeding/as a percentage of all other reasons	Reference
TCu 200Ag	12.2	11.1	52	Luukkainen *et al.* (1983)
Nova-T	11.9	12.0	50	
LNG-IUS	8.7	11.6	43	Luukkainen *et al.* (1986)
TCu 380Ag	7.0	13.2	35	Sivin *et al.* (1987)
LNG-IUS	10.9	15.6	41	

Table 30.2 Cumulative discontinuation rates per 100 woman–years after 60 months. Results from four randomized comparative studies

Device	Pregnancy	Expulsion	Bleeding	Reference
Nova-T	12.3	6.6	15.7	WHO (1990)
TCu 220C	6.6	7.5	15.7	
Nova-T	4.2	5.5	20.4	Andersson *et al.* (1994)
LNG-IUS	0.3	4.9	15.1	
TCu 220C	4.0	9.3	17.0	WHO (1990)
TCu 380A	1.4	8.2	18.5	
TCu 380Ag	1.4	7.4	23.3	Sivin *et al.* (1990)
LNG-IUS	1.1	11.8	15.4	

tration of copper was reported to increase contraceptive efficacy, IUDs medicated with copper were developed (Zipper *et al.* 1969). The early polyethylene IUDs were large and frequently caused side-effects, especially bleeding and pain. Modern IUDs medicated with copper are smaller and, therefore, cause less bleeding and pain and, since they also have lower pregnancy rates, the copper-bearing IUDs have gradually replaced the inert devices in many areas of the world.

Modern IUDs are highly effective, safe, long-acting, easy to administer, reversible, do not interfere with sexual life and they are inexpensive and could therefore be expected to be a highly acceptable contraceptive method to many women. However, use of the IUD varies considerably between countries in the world. In the People's Republic of China, IUDs are used by some 30 to 40 per cent of women, whereas in the USA, only 1–2 per cent of women using contraception use an IUD (Mauldin and Segal 1994). IUD use is also high in the Nordic countries and in Hungary, whereas relatively few women rely on IUDs in France and the UK (Mauldin and Segal 1994).

Besides the development and subsequent improvement of copper IUDs that has continued over the past 25 years, another line in intrauterine contraception was followed in the development of hormone-releasing intrauterine systems. In the late 1960s, when slow-release systems for drug delivery became available, devices fitted with a capsule releasing progesterone were tried. The initial purpose was to decrease the expulsion rate by administering uterine relaxing hormones into the uterine cavity. This theory proved wrong as the expulsion rate of the progesterone-releasing system did not differ from that of other IUDs, but it was found that intrauterine progesterone significantly reduced menstrual blood loss (Bergkvist and Rybo 1983). Subsequent research led to the development of an improved device releasing a synthetic progestogen, the levonorgestrel-releasing system (LNG-IUS). In order to distinguish the steroid-releasing intrauterine methods from inert or copper IUDs, which have a very different mechanism of action, the former devices are usually referred to as intrauterine systems (IUS).

Efficacy of modern IUDs

Copper IUDs

The copper surface area, which has been reported to be the determinant of the contraceptive efficacy, varies among currently used IUDs between 200 and 380 mm^2. There have been several recent large, randomized, comparative studies showing excellent efficacy of the modern high-load copper IUDs, i.e. TCu 380 and Multiload 375, with pregnancy rates similar to those following surgical sterilization (Table 30.2). In long-term randomized clinical trials the TCu 380 has been found to have significantly lower pregnancy rates than the TCu 200 (Sivin and Stern 1979; Chi *et al.* 1990), the Nova-T (World Health Organization 1990), and the TCu 220 (World Health Organization 1990). The pregnancy rate of the TCu 380 was slightly but not significantly lower than that of Multiload 250 (World Health Organization 1990; Chi *et al.* 1990) and the Multiload 375 in other randomized studies (Cole *et al.* 1985; Champion *et al.* 1988; Sastrawinata *et al.* 1991).

There is now evidence to support that the TCu 380 has an effective life-span of more than seven years, during which time the pregnancy rate remained low in several studies (Sivin *et al.* 1991; World Health Organization 1990). Also the Multiload 250 has been shown to remain effective for 8–10 years (Batar 1985). The Nova-T has shown an effective life span of five years in earlier studies, but in recent studies the performance of this device has tended to deteriorate with prolonged use compared to other IUDs (World Health Organization 1990; Andersson *et al.* 1994).

Hormone-releasing intrauterine systems

There are currently two different systems for intrauterine hormone release available on the market. The progesterone-releasing IUS (Progestasert®), releases 65 μg per 24 h from a total load of 38 mg progesterone (World Health Organization 1983). The Progestasert gives inadequate protection against ectopic pregnancy and has a lifetime of only one year, which are disadvantages and reasons for its limited use worldwide. The levonorgestrel-releasing IUS (LNG-IUS; Mirena®, or Levonova® in the Nordic countries, has the frame of a Nova-T on which a silastic capsule has been attached to the vertical arm, releasing 20 μg of levonorgestrel per 24 h from a total load of 52 mg (Allonen 1994). The LNG-IUS gives excellent protection against pregnancy, including ectopics, and has an active lifetime of at least five years, which has made it a very promising contraceptive method (Table 30.2). The LNG-IUS has been shown to have a significantly lower pregnancy rate than the Nova-T during five years in one study (Andersson *et al.* 1994). In another study over seven years, the pregnancy rate of the LNG-IUS was slightly but not significantly lower than that of TCu 380 (Sivin *et al.* 1991).

Bleeding disturbances with copper IUDs

Change in menstrual blood loss

All inert and copper-releasing IUDs increase menstrual blood loss (MBL). Although some studies suggest that the volume of MBL is highest during the first cycles after insertion and decreases gradually thereafter, other studies suggest that most of the increase in MBL will remain throughout the whole period of IUD use (Andrade and Orchard 1987; Liedholm *et al.* 1975). The magnitude of the increase in MBL is related to the size of the device. With larger types of IUDs, i.e. Lippes' loop and other plastic non-medicated devices, the MBL has been shown to increase by at least 100 per cent (Shaw *et al.* 1980). Smaller copper devices, i.e. CuT200, Nova-T, TCu 380, and Multiload®, generally cause an increase in MBL by 40–80 per cent (Andrade and Orchard 1987; Larsson *et al.* 1975*a*; Liedholm *et al.* 1975; Milsom *et al.* 1989). Although assessments of MBL and termination rates for bleeding vary considerably between studies, there is little evidence for a real difference between different copper IUDs.

The mechanism for the increased MBL is not fully understood (Fraser 1982). An IUD in the uterus produces a localized trauma in the endometrium with a foreign body response leading to a number of biochemical changes in the endometrium, reactions that are enhanced by the copper release. The result is an environment in the uterus that is toxic to sperm and to the embryo. The trauma and foreign body reaction in the endometrium adjacent to the device will result in increased vascularity and white cell influx as well as a local increase of the fibrinolytic activity and impaired haemostasis (Larsson *et al.* 1975*b*). Apart from having increased fibrinolytic activity in the endometrium, IUD users have also been reported to have increased endometrial plasminogen activator concentrations (Kasonde and Bonnar 1976). Studies of the endometrium of IUD users have demonstrated superficial erosion leading to microvascular bleeding into the cavity and increased vascular permeability leading to interstitial haemorrhage (Sheppard 1987). Another factor contributing to the increased blood loss may be alterations in the balance between the prostaglandins which regulate endometrial haemostasis, mainly prostacyclin, which inhibits haemostasis through vasodilatation and prevention of platelet aggregation, and thromboxane A_2, which has the opposite effects (Smith *et al.* 1981; Sheppard 1987).

Prolonged menstrual bleeding

Users of inert or copper IUDs often report a prolongation of their menstrual period by 1–2 days. In some studies this type of bleeding is referred to as intermenstrual spotting, but it is more probably directly related to the endocrine menstrual cycle changes. It has been demonstrated that in IUD users, the menstrual bleeding starts before progesterone levels have decreased to the low levels at which normal menstruation is usually precipitated (Nygren and Johansson 1973). The mechanism behind this premature precipitation of menstruation, resulting in prolongation of menstruation in IUD users, is probably related to the localized trauma in the endometrium. Use of a copper-IUD does not affect ovarian function (Nygren and Johansson 1973).

Intermenstrual bleeding

Intermenstrual bleeding in IUD users should be considered as potentially pathological until properly evaluated since it may be a symptom of an underlying pathology, which is unrelated to IUD use, i.e. infection or neoplasia (see Chapter 20). However, many IUD users report 1–3 days of spotting during the midcycle, a sign which may be explained by a drop in oestrogen levels subsequent to ovulation, precipitating bleeding in a predisposed endometrium. There are no recent studies to confirm whether this explanation is valid or not. The blood volumes lost as intermenstrual bleeding are usually quite insignificant for the health of the woman but the bleeding may affect acceptability and considerably reduce continuation of the method (Shaw *et al.* 1980).

Health impact of increased MBL

The amount of blood loss at normal menstruation without IUD varies between populations, the mean MBL in healthy women often reported at around 40 ml and slightly more in certain Asian countries, i.e. the People's Republic of China and Japan (World Health Organization 1987). With a MBL of 60–80 ml or more, most women will develop a negative iron balance, a depletion of iron stores, and subsequently iron-deficiency anaemia. Before recommending an IUD, it is therefore important to balance the benefit of effective contraception against the risk of developing severe anaemia in each individual woman. The increase in MBL subsequent to IUD insertion is clearly reflected in a reduction of serum ferritin levels (Andrade and Orchard 1987). The haemoglobin level is a less accurate early marker of increased MBL in IUD users, but haemoglobin levels will decrease if excessive MBL is allowed to continue. The health consequences even of a moderately increased MBL may be severe in women with pre-existing anaemia and/or low iron intake (Rybo and Andersson 1994). If there is already a confirmed or suspected iron deficiency already at the time of insertion it is wise to start iron supplementation.

Management of bleeding disturbances during copper IUD use

Although bleeding disturbances occur in users of IUDs, other causes of changes in the bleeding pattern, unrelated to IUD use, should always be ruled out. Perception of MBL is very subjective and it is difficult to obtain an adequate assessment of the volume of MBL by history (Fraser *et al.* 1984). However, women with an IUD who give a history of a pronounced increase in MBL compared to that before IUD use should be investigated for signs of anaemia and given iron supplementation. Treatment with antifibrinolytic drugs, i.e. tranexamic acid, will reduce MBL by around 50 per cent (Milsom *et al.* 1991). Mefenamic acid and other non-steroidal anti-inflammatory drugs (NSAIDs) will reduce MBL by around 25 per cent (Ylikorkala and Viinikka 1983). Therefore, such drugs can usually control a moderate increase in MBL in otherwise healthy women and IUD use could continue. In cases of intolerable bleeding and/or anaemia, or if there is a suspicion of underlying pathology, removal of the IUD should be considered. Removal should also be recommended if treatment with antifibrinolytic drugs or NSAIDs does not reduce the MBL. Women who cannot tolerate either the prolongation of the bleeding period by 1–2 days or a short episode of midcycle intermenstrual spotting should be advised to have the IUD removed, since the altered menstrual pattern is usually not possible to treat.

Endometrial and endocrine effects of LNG-IUS

The LNG-IUS exerts its contraceptive effect by a strong, local progestational action on the cervical mucus, which becomes thick and impermeable to sperm, and on the endometrium which is rendered thin and inactive. This endometrial effect is believed to be the main mechanism of contraceptive action (Nilsson *et al.* 1978). In addition, the LNG-IUS probably causes a foreign body reaction, similar to that of copper-IUDs. Although the levonorgestrel release is low (20 μg/24 h) and ovulation is not normally inhibited, minor effects on ovulatory function have been reported (Nilsson *et al.* 1980, 1984; Barbosa *et al.* 1990).

Effects on menstruation by LNG-IUS

Irregular and frequent bleeding

After insertion of the LNG-IUS there is often a period of frequent, irregular bleeding or spotting during the initial 2–3 months. During this time the number of bleeding/spotting days is usually increased but the volume of blood loss is reduced compared to the woman's normal menstruation (Nilsson 1977; Allonen 1994). After around six months of LNG-IUS use, frequent episodes of bleeding/spotting are rare and should *not* be regarded as 'normal' with this device.

Amenorrhoea

With prolonged use, the MBL is dramatically reduced and many women develop amenorrhoea or report extremely scanty regular bleeds (Andersson *et al.* 1994). This profound change in menstrual pattern is the result of the strong progestational effect on the endometrium, which becomes very thin (Nilsson *et al.* 1978). Few women develop amenorrhoea during the first months of use but at the end of the first year around 20 per cent of LNG-IUS users have amenorrhoea or extremely scanty bleeding (Andersson *et al.* 1994). There is no difference in ovulatory function between those women using the LNG-IUS who do and those who do not experience amenorrhoea (Nilsson *et al.* 1980, 1984). The amenorrhoea is uterine, i.e. the women usually remain ovulatory throughout LNG-IUS use. With long-term LNG-IUS use increasingly more women develop amenorrhoea and at the end of five years around 50 per cent report amenorrhoea. The remaining women report short irregular or regular episodes of spotting. Almost nobody reports menstrual-like bleeding after five years. When a new LNG-IUS is inserted immediately after removal of the old one, there is usually very little bleeding disturbance and most women continue to have exactly the bleeding pattern they have experienced during the latter phase of the first segment of LNG-IUS use.

Abnormal bleeding patterns during LNG-IUS use

If the expected period of frequent spotting does not improve and disappear within three to six months, or if a woman starts to have frequent spotting/bleeding after a period of normal pattern, this should be noted as a reason for further evaluation of other causes for prolonged bleeding. If the bleeding pattern changes during LNG-IUS use and menstruation suddenly returns to a pre-insertion nature and becomes heavier again, this could indicate an unnoticed expulsion of the LNG-IUS or other pathology which needs evaluation.

Management of bleeding disturbances with LNG-IUS

If the bleeding pattern is intolerable to the woman or if there is a suspicion of underlying pathology, the LNG-IUS should be removed. The most important factor to ensure acceptability of the LNG-IUS is careful pre-insertion counselling and good support and encouragement during the first months of use. As opposed to the situation with other long-acting progestogens for contraception, the changes in bleeding pattern with the LNG-IUS are extremely predictable, which makes counselling easy. The expected changes must be carefully explained, with, if necessary, a simple explanation for the reduced bleeding. Many women fear amenorrhoea as it is perceived as a sign of either pregnancy or ill health. Therefore, the gradual development of uterine amenorrhoea, despite normal endocrine cycles, must be explained. The use of a bleeding diary is highly recommended as it allows the woman to see the gradual improvement of the initial spotting period and also to see that there is usually some cyclicity in the pattern of scanty bleedings that follow. A bleeding card also allows the doctor to judge whether the individual pattern is normal for the LNG-IUS and to use the diary as a basis for counselling.

LNG-IUS as a treatment for menorrhagia

The LNG-IUS has been demonstrated to have profound effects on MBL in women with menorrhagia, reducing MBL by more than 90 per cent (Andersson and Rybo 1987; Scholten 1989). The studies have been performed in women with 'idiopathic' menorrhagia (ovulatory dysfunctional uterine bleeding), i.e. where it has not been possible to identify any specific cause for the heavy bleeding. The results are encouraging and should make the LNG-IUS an important, simple, inexpensive, and reversible alternative to endometrial resection (ablation), which, apart from being irreversible, may be more complicated and costly.

Conclusion

Whilst intrauterine contraception is one of the most important long-term family planning methods available, menstrual bleeding disturbance remains a common problem and a factor which can limit method acceptability among women in all societies. Therefore, from a reproductive health perspective it is important that careful counselling, medical follow-up, and removal facilities always accompany promotion and use of intrauterine contraceptive methods.

References

Allonen, H. (1994). The levonorgestrel IUD. In *Proceedings of the Fourth International Conference on IUDs*, (ed. C.W., Bardin, and D.R., Mishell, Jr), pp. 284–92. Butterworth-Heinemann Newton, MA, USA.

Andersson, K. and Rybo, G. (1987). Levonorgestrel-releasing intauterine device in the treatment of menorrhagia. *British Journal of Obstetrics and Gynaecology*, **97**, 690–4.

Andersson, K., Odlind, V., and Rybo, G. (1994). Levonorgestrel-releasing and copper-releasing (Nova T) IUDs during five years of use. *Contraception*, **49**, 56–72.

Andrade, A.T.L. and Orchard, E.P. (1987). Quantitative studies on menstrual blood flow in IUD users. *Contraception*, **36**, 129–44.

Barbosa, I., Bakos, O., Olsson, S.E., Odlind, V., and Johansson, E.D.B. (1990). Ovarian function during use of a levonorgestrel releasing IUD. *Contraception*, **42**, 247–59.

Batar, I. (1985). M.L., Cu 250 IUD: a decade of experience. *Advances in Contraception*, **1**, 329–35.

Bergkvist, A. and Rybo. G. (1983). Treatment of menorrhagia with intrauterine release of progesterone. *British Journal of Obstetrics and Gynaecology*, **90**, 255–8.

Champion, C.B., Behlilovic, B., Arosemena, J.M., Randic, L., Cole, L.P., and Wilkens, L.R. (1988). A three-year evaluation of the TCu 380Ag and Multiload 375 intrauterine device. *Contraception*, **38**, 631–9.

Chi, I.C., Farr, G., Thompson, K., Acosta, M., Alvarado, G., and Rivera, R., *et al.* (1990). Is the copper T 380A device associated with increased risk of removal due to bleeding and pain? – An analysis. *Contraception*, **42**, 159–69.

Cole, L.P., Potts, D.M., Aranda, C., Behlilovic, B., Etman, E.S., Moreno, J., and Randic, L. (1985). An evaluation of the TCu 380Ag and the Multiload Cu 375. *Fertility and Sterility*, **43**, 214–17.

Fraser, I.S. (1982). Abnormal uterine bleeding due to hormonal steroids and intauterine devices. In Recent advances in fertility regulation (ed. C.F., Chang, D., Griffin, and A., Woolman), pp. 265–300. Atar Press, Copenhagen.

Fraser, I.S., McCarron, G., and Markham, R. (1984). A preliminary study of factors influencing percptions of menstrual blood loss volume. *American Journal of Obstetrics and Gynecology*, **149**, 788–93.

Kasonde, J.M. and Bonnar, J. (1976). Aminocaproic acid and menstrual blood loss in women using intrauterine devices. *British Medical Journal*, **4**, 17–19.

Larsson, B., Hamberger, L., and Rybo, G. (1975*a*). Influence of copper intrauterine contraceptive device (Cu-7-IUD) on the menstrual blood loss. *Acta Obstetrica et Gynecologica Scandinavica*, **54**, 315–18.

Larsson, B., Liedholm, P., and Åstedt, B. (1975*b*). Increased fibrinolytic activity in the endometrium of patients using copper IUD. *International Journal of Fertility*, **20**, 77–80.

Liedholm, P., Rybo, G., Sjöberg NO., and Sölvell, L. (1975). Copper-IUD – influence on menstrual blood loss and iron deficiency. *Contraception*, **12**, 317–25.

Luukkainen, T., Allonen, H., Nielsen, N.C., Nygren, K.G., and Pyörälä, T. (1983). Five years experience of intrauterine contraception with the Nova-T and the Copper-T 200. *American Journal of Obstetrics and Gynecology*, **147**, 885–92.

Luukkainen, T., Allonen, H., Haukkamma, M., Lähteenmäki, P., Nilsson, C.G., and Toivonen, J. (1986). Five years experience with levonorgestrel-releasing IUDs. *Contraception*, **33**, 139–48.

Mauldin, W.P. and Segal, S.J. (1994). IUD use throughout the world: past, present and future. In *Proceedings of the Fourth International Conference on IUDs* (ed. C.W. Bardin and D.R. Mishell Jr), pp. 1–10. Butterworth-Heinemann/Newton, MA, USA.

Milsom, I., Rybo, G., and Lindstedt, G. (1989). The influence of copper surface area on menstrual blood loss and iron status in women fitted with an IUD. *Contraception*, **41**, 271–81.

Milson, I., Andersson, K., Andersch, B., and Rybo, G. (1991). A comparison of flurbiprofen, tranexamic acid and a levonorgestrel-releasing intrauterine contraceptive device in the treatment of idiapathic menorrhagia. *American Journal of Obstetrics and Gynecology*, **164**, 879–83.

Nilsson, C.G. (1977). Comparative quantitation of menstrual blood loss with a D-norgestrel-releasing IUD and a Nova-T-Copper device. *Contraception*, **15**, 379–87.

Nilsson, C.G., Luukkainen. T., and Arko, H. (1978). Endometrial morphology of women using a D-norgestrel-releasing intrauterine device. *Fertility and Sterility*, **29**, 397–401.

Nilsson, C.G., Läuhteenmäki, P., and Luukkainen, T. (1980). Patterns of ovulation and bleeding with a low levonorgestrel-releasing intrauterine device. *Contraception*, **21**, 155–64.

Nilsson, C.G., Lähteenmäki, P., and Luukkainen, T. (1984). Ovarian function in amenorrhoeic and menstruating users of levonorgestrel-releasing intrauterine device. *Fertility and Sterility*, **41**, 52–4.

Nygren, K.G. and Johansson, E.D.B. (1973). Premature onset of menstrual bleeding during ovulatory cycles in women with an intrauterine contraceptive device. *American Journal of Obstetrics and Gynecology*, **117**, 971–5.

Rybo, G. and Andersson, K. (1994). IUD use and endometrial bleedings. In *Proceedings of the Fourth International Conference on IUDs*, (ed. C.W. Bardin and D.R. Mishell Jr), pp. 210–18. Butterworth-Heinemann/Newton, MA, USA.

Sastrawinata, S., Farr, G., Prihadi, S.M., Hutapea, H., Anwar, M., Wahyudi, I., *et al.* (1991). A comparative clinical trial of the TCu 380A, Lippes' loop D, and Multiload Cu 375 IUDs in Indonesia. *Contraception*, **44**, 141–54.

Scholten, P.C. (1989). The levonorgestrel IUD, clinical performance and impact on menstruation. Dissertation, University of Utrecht, Holland.

Shaw, S.T., Andrade, A.T.L., Souza, J.P., Macauley, L.K., and Rowe, P.J. (1980). Quantitative menstrual and intermenstrual blood loss in women using Lippes' loop and copper T intrauterine devices. *Contraception*, **21**, 343–52.

Sheppard, B.L. (1987). Endometrial morphological changes in IUD users. A review. *Contraception*, **36**, 1–10.

Sivin, I. and Stern, J. (1979). Long-acting, more effective copper IUDs: a summary of US experience. *Studies in Family Planning*, **10**, 263–81.

Sivin, I., Stern, J., Diaz, M., Faundes, A., El, Mahgoub, S., *et al.* (1987). Two years of intrauterine contraception with levonorgestrel and with copper: a randomized comparison of the TCu 380Ag and levonorgestrel 20 mcg/day devices. *Contraception*, **35**, 245–55.

Sivin, I., El, Mahgoub, S., McCarthy, Mishell, D.R., Shoupe, D., Alvarez, F., *et al.* (1990). Long-term contraception with the levonorgestrel 20 mcg/day (LNg 20) and the Copper T380Ag intrauterine devices: a five-year randomized study. *Contraception*, **42**, 361–78.

Sivin, I., Stern, J., Coutinho, E., Mattos, C.E.R., El, Mahgoub, S., Diaz, S., *et al.* (1991). Prolonged intrauterine contraception: a seven-year randomized study of the levonorgestrel 20 mcg/day (LNG 20) and the copper T380Ag IUDs. *Contraception*, **44**, 473–80.

Smith, S.K., Abel, M.H., Kelly, R.W., and Baird, D.T. (1981). Prostaglandin synthesis in the endometrium of women with ovular dysfunctional uterine bleeding. *British Journal of Obstetrics and Gynaecology*, **88**, 434–42.

World Health Organization (WHO) Task Force on Intrauterine Devices for Ferility Regulation (1983). The Alza TIPCS52, a longer acting progesterone IUD: safety and efficacy compared to the Tcu 220C and Multiload 250 in two randomized multicentre trials. *Clinical Reproduction and Fertility*, **2**, 113–28.

World Health Organization (1987). Mechanism of action, safety and efficacy of intrauterine devices. Report of a WHO Scientific Group. *Technical Report Series*, **753**. World Health Organization, Geneva.

World Health Organization (WHO) (1990). The TCu 380A, TCu, 220C, Multioload 250 and Nova T IUDs at 3, 5 and 7 years of use – results from three randomized multicentre trials. *Contraception*, **42**, 141–58.

Ylikorkala, O. and Viinikka, L. (1983). Comparison between antifibrinolytic and antiprostaglandin treatment in the reduction of increased menstrual blood loss in women with intrauterine contraceptive device. *British Journal of Obstetrics and Gynaecology*, **90**, 78–83.

Zipper, J.A., Medel, M., and Prager, R. (1969). Experimental suppression of fertility by intrauterine copper and zinc in rabbits. *American Journal of Obstetrics and Gynecology*, **105**, 529–34.

31 Menstrual disturbance and contraceptive steroids: mechanisms and management

Martha Hickey and Ian S. Fraser

Introduction

Contraceptive steroids are used by an estimated 100 million women worldwide (Olive and Schlaff 1992), and provide safe, reliable, and affordable protection against unwanted pregnancy. All contraceptive steroids have the capacity to alter normal menstrual bleeding patterns, and the majority of women using these methods will notice some change in their regular menstrual cycle. For those contraceptive methods containing oestrogen and a progestogen, the change may be minor and quite acceptable to the user. For those using progestogen-only methods, the disruption of menstrual bleeding pattern may be profound, and dissuade the woman from utilizing these methods or from continuing with them (Odlind and Fraser 1990). As progestogen-only contraceptives have a number of distinct advantages over oestrogen and progestogen combinations – including safety, high efficacy, simplicity, flexibility of delivery systems, and cost – breakthrough bleeding constitutes a major problem for contraceptive providers.

Tolerance of menstrual disturbance with contraceptive steroids

During the normal menstrual cycle, major disturbances in the length, quantity, and timing of menstrual bleeding are relatively uncommon, and most women are attuned to their monthly cycle as an indicator of their general well-being and reproductive health (Snowden and Christiaen 1983). Amenorrhoea, particularly for women in developing countries who do not have access to rapid pregnancy testing, implies pregnancy, lactation, or ill health. Prolonged bleeding or spotting may indicate genital tract disease, and has major social implications in cultures where religious activities are forbidden during menstruation. When sexual contact is avoided during menstruation, prolonged and unpredictable bleeding may disrupt family life. For women who are aiming to take control of their fertility, the cooperation of family and society is vital in promoting acceptance of the widespread use of contraception.

Tolerance of any unwanted effects will depend on the individual woman, particularly her understanding of the contraceptive method and her expectations of bleeding patterns, the attitude and understanding of her contraceptive providers, and the alternative methods available to her. Tolerance will also depend on the consequence of an unwanted pregnancy, including the availability of termination of pregnancy. It is likely that tolerance varies greatly between women and may show profound cultural variation. Counselling by the health worker and his/her confidence in and understanding of the contraceptive method certainly seem to be important factors (Fraser 1983).

Menstrual disturbance is given by women as the reason for approximately half of all contraceptive method discontinuation for all progestogen-only contraceptives (Belsey 1988*a*). In contrast, women give menstrual disturbance as their reason for discontinuation of the combined oral contraceptive pill (OCP) in less than one-third of cases (d'Arcangues *et al.* 1990). With the widespread introduction of effective long-acting, low-dose progestogen contraceptive systems, such as Norplant, there has been increased interest in the mechanisms of bleeding disturbances, and the development of effective treatment methods. Menstrual disturbance is also the main reason stated for discontinuation of post-menopausal hormone therapy (Magos *et al.* 1985).

Mechanisms of bleeding disturbance with contraceptive steroids

Understanding of the mechanisms of normal menstrual bleeding is incomplete, and current knowledge still stems from the elegant experiments of Markee (1940) observing bleeding in a variety of spontaneous and hormonal cycles within endometrial explants placed in the anterior eye chamber of the rhesus monkey. Normal menstrual bleeding is characterized by its regular onset, loss of the majority of blood and endometrial tissue in the first 24 h (Ferenczy 1976*a*, *b*), cessation of bleeding within 4–6 days, and the absence of bleeding between menstrual periods. This bleeding is thought to arise predominantly from the spiral arterioles following profound vasoconstriction and dilatation (Markee 1940), and cease when normal flow resumes in these vessels.

Endogenous and exogenous sex steroids strongly influence and may indirectly control menstrual bleeding patterns. The sex steroid hormone environments in which endometrial bleeding may occur are listed in Table 31.1.

With oestrogen priming, progesterone leads to luteal changes and progesterone withdrawal will stimulate bleeding. Continued progesterone can prevent this bleeding but oestrogen alone cannot (Allen 1927). Without oestrogen, bleeding will not occur. Oestrogen fluctuations in the presence of progesterone are less likely to produce bleeding than oestrogen fluctuations alone.

Table 31.1 Endometrial bleeding may occur in a variety of sex steroid hormone environments (from Fraser 1990)

Sex steroid environment	Clinical application
Oestrogen and progesterone withdrawal from oestrogen-primed endometrium	Normal menstrual bleeding; combined OCP withdrawal
Withdrawal of unopposed oestrogen	Anovulatory dysfunctional uterine bleeding
High-dose continuous progestogens	For example, depot medroxyprogesterone acetate
Low-dose continuous progestogens	Contraceptive implants, e.g. Norplant

There is much individual variation in bleeding patterns in response to exogenous steroids and it is not known whether this variation exists at a hormonal, vascular, or endometrial level. The hypothesis that all women have the capacity to exhibit breakthrough bleeding given appropriate hormonal stimulation is attractive but remains unproven.

In general, oestrogen-containing contraceptives produce fewer bleeding complications than progestogen-only methods (Odlind and Fraser 1990), and women with anovulatory reactions to progestogen-only methods have more bleeding disturbance that those with luteal activity (Landgren *et al.* 1982). Frequent bleeding may occur in association with low oestrogen and progesterone levels in women using these contraceptive methods (Faundes *et al.* 1991). However, the impact on bleeding pattern will vary according to the progestogen used, as well as the dose and duration, and differs markedly between individuals. Bleeding patterns may alter in response to exogenous sex steroids and remain in this modified pattern, or may show change over time, such that the woman is quite unable to predict when she will bleed.

Steroid regimens that suppress ovarian activity produce regular bleeding if the endometrium is repeatedly oestrogen primed (OCP) or scant bleeding with spotting when there is no oestrogen priming (DMPA). Where ovarian activity is incompletely suppressed (e.g. with Norplant and the progestogen-only pill), the most troublesome irregular and frequent bleeding patterns are observed.

Effect of contraceptive steroids on endometrial stroma and glands

High-dose progestogens can lead to endometrial 'atrophy' with marked regression of stroma and glands. The number and size of endometrial glands is decreased, dependent on the type, dose, and delivery of the progestogen (Johannisson 1990). Stromal density is increased and predecidual changes are sometimes observed.

Sex steroid receptors located in the glandular epithelium in the endometrium are highly specific and self-regulate according to local sex steroid concentrations (Snijders *et al.* 1992). The interaction between receptors is complex, but oestrogen tends to increase oestrogen receptors (ER) and decrease progesterone receptors (PR); progesterone tends to decrease both ER and PR.

Sex steroid receptors have not been identified in endometrial vascular endothelial cells (Perrot-Applanat *et al.* 1988), but appear to be located in stromal cells around the spiral arterioles. Prolonged progestogen exposure may result in downregulation of PR to render the endometrium functionally hypo-progestogenic and hypo-oestrogenic (King and d'Arcangues 1992). It is possible that the poor or absent histological response to oestrogen treatment observed in women exposed to prolonged progestogens may be due to an inability of the endometrium to respond initially to oestrogens following progestogen-induced down-regulation of receptors. However, Lau *et al.* (1996) observed a decrease in PR in Norplant users, with the lowest receptor concentrations seen in those with prolonged or frequent bleeding, compared to non-bleeders. In contrast, Critchley *et al.* (1993) found a significant increase in PR staining of endometrial stroma in Norplant users at three to 12 months of exposure. Oestrogen receptor concentration was reduced, consistent with downregulation of ER by progestogens. It is unclear whether the increase in PR is a result of increased synthesis or decreased turnover, and whether increased PR immunoreactivity corresponds to an increase in the number of functional PR.

Levonorgestrel (LNG) is a 19 *nor*-testosterone derivative. Little is known about the action of androgen receptors in the endometrium, but it is possible that the actions of LNG may be mediated in part through these receptors. Clinically, androgenic action is minimal in most women taking levonorgestrel.

Effect of contraceptive steroids on the endometrial vasculature

In order that breakthrough bleeding may begin, there is likely to be some form of endometrial vascular damage (Fraser and Diczfalusy 1980). The role of endometrial blood vessel structure and function has recently received increased attention in the study of bleeding disturbances with contraceptive steroids. Ovarian steroids and exogenous steroids appear to influence vascular structure, growth, and blood flow in the human endometrium but accurate *in vivo* work is difficult given the physical location of the uterus and size of superficial endometrial vessels.

Blood vessels of the myometrium and the basal layer of the endometrium do not appear to be significantly influenced by changes in circulating ovarian steroid levels (Johannisson 1990). The vessels of the superficial 'functional' layer, including the distal part of the spiral arterioles, the capillaries, the venous lakes, and the veins, undergo profound cyclical changes (Johannisson 1990).

The spiral arterioles

Long-term, low-dose levonorgestrel via a contraceptive vaginal ring (CVR) leads to a reduction in endometrial arteriole number and size, and a change in vascular morphology, with a decrease in arteriole spiralling (Hourihan *et al.* 1990). Haemostatic plugs and endothelial gaps were increased. Similar findings have been observed following oral levonorgestrel exposure (Hourihan *et al.* 1991). Oral norethisterone (NET) produces contracted endothelial cells and an increase in plasmalemmal vesicles (Johannisson *et al.* 1982), which may imply a loss of integrity of microvascular structure.

Endometrial veins

Several authors (e.g. Maqueo 1980; Ludwig 1982; Hourihan *et al.* 1991) have observed dilatation in the subepithelial venules and superficial vessels after long-term progestogen-only exposure. Dilated vessels have also been noted in the normal menstrual cycle (Markee 1940), and following oestrogen and progestogen exposure, and high-dose progestogens (Ober 1970; Song *et al.* 1995). The clinical significance of these dilated vessels is unclear. It has been suggested that irregular bleeding following exogenous sex steroids may be from these dilated vessels (Ludwig 1982), but there is little evidence for this. It is difficult to assess vascular dilatation *in vitro* as the vessels rapidly collapse (Rogers *et al.* 1993).

The endometrial microvasculature

The nature as well as the pattern of bleeding in women taking sex steroids may differ from normal menstrual bleeding. The bleeding site in breakthrough bleeding (BTB) is unknown, but the intermittent, light, and prolonged bleeding observed in women using progestogen-only contraceptives may arise from a different source from that of normal menstrual bleeding. Rogers *et al.* (1993) noted that bleeding may occur from an 'atrophic' endometrium in Norplant users and suggested that the bleeding site may be the endometrial–myometrial vascular plexus. Others (Johannisson 1990; Hourihan *et al.* 1990) conclude that BTB occurs from superficial endometrial venules and capillaries. Identifying the precise break in the endothelium and epithelium that has led to bleeding is difficult using biopsy samples, and little has been reported from *in vivo* studies about the bleeding site in BTB. Limitation of the quantity and duration of normal menstrual bleeding is thought to be associated with the ability of the spiral arterioles to contract (Markee

1940). Bleeding from other endometrial vessels cannot be controlled in this manner, and this may account for the variable quantity and duration of BTB. There is preliminary evidence that endothelin expression is reduced in Norplant users (Marsh *et al.* 1995), and this may indicate defective haemostasis. Immunostaining for factor VIII-related antigen, an essential component of the haemostatic response, is considerably elevated in Norplant users, but this does not appear to be related to bleeding patterns (Au and Rogers 1993).

Microvascular fragility

The endothelium plays a major role in controlling the permeability of blood vessels, and changes in cell morphology and cell-to-cell contact may be important in BTB following contraceptive steroid exposure. The ultrastructure of endometrial cells is highly variable, even within vessels (Blackwell and Fraser 1988). This heterogenity may complicate investigations of endometrial endothelial cell function (Au and Rogers 1993).

Endometrial capillaries consist only of a thin layer of endothelial cells and their underlying basement membrane (BM). If these capillaries are fragile, there are a number of possible sites of weakness, as discussed below.

The endothelial cell cytoskeleton

The cytoskeleton is important in maintaining mechanical rigidity and cell adhesion (Tropey *et al.* 1992). A loss of cytokeratin elements in the epithelial cytoskeleton has been observed in Norplant users (Wonodiresko *et al.* 1993), but the epithelium has not been examined in further detail.

Endothelial cell junctions and intercellular adhesion

Endometrial endothelial cells are linked by tight junctions, and these junctions appear to be influenced by sex steroid hormones. Blackwell and Fraser (1988) and Sixma *et al.* (1980) observed a weakening of tight junctions in the late luteal phase. Separation of tight junctions may increase capillary permeability leading to fluid loss between endothelial cells. Exogenous progestogens produce contracted endothelial cells with gaps observed between cells (Shaw *et al.* 1981). The addition of oestrogen after progestogenic stimulation of endometrial blood vessels appears to 'stabilize' the vessels and to reverse the fragility associated with unopposed progestogen exposure (Fraser 1983). Similarly, the onset of regular cycles in women exposed to Norplant is generally associated with regulation of bleeding episodes (Sivin 1994).

As stated, Johannisson (1990) noted contracted endothelial cells and increased plasmalemmal vesicles after norethisterone treatment, and Hourihan (1985) observed gaps in the endothelium of endometrial blood vessels after progestogen exposure. These may represent a breakdown in endothelial cell integrity or in tight junctions between endothelial cells, perhaps facilitating breakthrough bleeding.

Tight junctions maintain cohesion between endometrial endothelial cells. Integrity of the junctions may influence the extravasation of red blood cells. Basement membrane forms a further 'barrier' maintaining vessel integrity. Disruption of endothelial cell junctions, or fragility of the basement membrane, may contribute to 'capillary fragility' (Fraser and Peek 1992). Capillary fragility is thought to increase in the premenstrual (and postovulatory) menstrual phase (Clemetson *et al.* 1962), and oestrogen is thought to increase capillary strength. Recently, vascular fragility has been demonstrated *in vivo* in women exposed to Norplant (Hickey *et al.* 1996), and the extent of fragility appears to be related to the bleeding patterns observed in this population.

Endothelial cell basement membranes (BM)

An alteration in the strength or integrity of the BM on endometrial capillaries could contribute to vascular fragility and BTB (Blackwell and Fraser 1988; Fraser and Peek 1992). Integral components of BM include collagen IV, laminin, and heparan sulphate proteoglycan (Martin *et al.* 1988). Disease processes can alter BM structure and function. In diabetes mellitus there is a characteristic thickening of the BM, but with a loss of functional capacity and 'leakiness' (Martin *et al.* 1988), and in some tumours and inflammatory conditions the BM is absent or disrupted (Barsky *et al.* 1983). During angiogenesis the BM is broken down and reconstructed in a regulated sequence, with laminin appearing first. It is possible that the rate of BM synthesis is correlated with angiogenesis and endothelial cell proliferation (Maragoudakis *et al.* 1993). Disruption of the basement membrane may influence the integrity of endometrial blood vessels and allow the extravasation of erythrocytes. In the late secretory phase of the normal menstrual cycle, increased fragmentation of the basement membrane and stromal degeneration are seen, before the onset of bleeding (Roberts *et al.* 1992).

Preliminary inspection of the endometrial endothelial cell basement membrane in Norplant users has failed to demonstrate any apparent abnormality in basement membrane morphology, but the functional characteristics of the BM have not been explored (Palmer *et al.* 1996).

Local or systemic changes in blood pressure

Sex steroid hormones are known to be vasoactive. Changes in pressure through the endometrial vasculature may induce vascular damage and even rupture, particularly in vessels that are already 'fragile'. Oestrogen causes a fall in uterine vascular resistance and an increase in uterine blood flow (Fraser *et al.* 1987; Alexander and d'Arcangues 1992). This effect is lost with the addition of progesterone.

Endometrial leukocyte populations and breakthrough bleeding

Endometrial changes preceding menstruation resemble inflammation in a number of key areas (Finn 1986). In particular, an influx of granulated leukocytes and the action of inflammatory mediators suggest that these migratory cells may contribute to the process of tissue breakdown that accompanies menstruation.

Migratory leukocytes in the endometrium are involved in phagocytosis, antigen processing, the release of cytotoxic mediators, and the release of growth factors (Clark and Daya 1990). Activated macrophages can make holes in endometrial epithelium and substances released by stimulated inflammatory cells such as platelet activating factor (PAF) increase vascular permeability (Harper 1990). The release of PAF is stimulated by progesterone (Harper 1990), and platelet and haemostatic plugs in endometrial vessel walls increase after exposure to progestogens. The white cells are chemotactic for vasoactive substances that may weaken vascular integrity and result in the outflow of red blood cells. High-dose progestogens such as DMPA are associated with an influx of migratory leukocytes (Song *et al.* 1995). Perivascular white cells may influence endometrial integrity and promote tissue breakdown and BTB.

Prostaglandins

Prostaglandin production is influenced by exogenous contraceptive steroids, with $PGF_{2\alpha}$ and epoxide levels increased by levonorgestrel exposure. Epoxides may influence bleeding patterns by inhibiting platelet aggregation and causing vasodilation (White *et al.* 1991).

Epithelial integrity

Normal menstrual bleeding is thought to involve subepithelial haemorrhage, with rupture of these areas producing frank bleeding. The role of the epithelium in BTB has received little attention. Epithelial cytokeratin deficiency has been observed in Norplant users (Wonodiresko *et al.* 1993). Fragility, or disruption of the epithelium, may control whether capillary bleeds present as vaginal bleeding or are contained in the endometrium. Subepithelial haemorrhages are frequently observed following exposure to danazol (Brooks *et al.* 1991), but this drug is less frequently associated with BTB.

Endometrial repair and regeneration

The cessation of menstrual bleeding is rapid and effective in normal menstrual cycles. Following exposure to contraceptive steroids, bleeding tends to be prolonged, suggesting that the normal endometrial repair mechanisms may be dysfunctional. During normal menstruation, bleeding from the spiral arterioles is controlled by profound vasoconstriction at the endometrial–myometrial junction, the main site of endothelin receptors (Cameron *et al.* 1992). Vasconstriction may be deficient when bleeding arises predominantly from veins and capillaries in the endometrium where endothelin action is reduced. Following vasoconstriction, endometrial repair and regeneration ensure that bleeding ceases and the endometrium is prepared for implantation. There is evidence that these mechanisms may be disrupted by contraceptive steroids.

Angiogenenesis

Angiogenesis describes the growth of new blood vessels from pre-existing vessels, and is an intrinsic part of the repair and regeneration process in the normal menstrual cycle. Potent growth factors such as vascular endothelial growth factor (VEGF), fibroblast growth factor (FGF), and the ambient endometrial oxygen tension are likely to be of importance. The endothelial cell growth factor VEGF has the potential to influence vascular permeability, and also to increase microvascular density. VEGF is stimulated by progesterone and inhibited by the progesterone antagonist, mifepristone (see Chapter 7).

In the normal menstrual cycle, mean endometrial microvascular density remains static despite cyclical neovascularization and major changes in growth, oedema, and regression of glandular and stromal tissues, suggesting that the mechanisms controlling endometrial vascularization are tightly regulated (Rogers *et al.* 1993). Exposure to long-term, low-dose levonorgestrel (as Norplant) results in atrophy of endometrial stromal and glandular elements in approximately one third of users after three months (Rogers *et al.* 1993), but with a 158 per cent increase in microvascular density. It is uncertain whether this represents a genuine increase in vessel numbers, retarded cell death (apoptosis), or a relative increase in vascular density due to comparatively greater regression of endometrial glands and stroma. Abnormally proliferating vessels may be structurally abnormal and may be more prone to BTB. Using proliferating cell nuclear antigen (PCNA) as a marker of endothelial cell proliferation and angiogenesis, Goodger *et al.* (1994) found that cell proliferation was reduced in these women with increased microvascular density by 3–12 months of exposure. Endothelial cell proliferation in the early months after Norplant insertion has not been explored.

Endometrial remodelling

Epithelial repair begins from peri-glandular tissue following endometrial shedding (Bartelmez 1937; Ludwig 1990) and is completed by day 4–5 of the menstrual cycle (Ferenczy *et al.* 1979). Repair is followed by extensive remodelling in preparation for characteristic cyclical changes. Disruption of this process could prolong bleeding and also diminish endometrial integrity, producing increased 'fragility' and bleeding tendency.

Lysosomes

Lysosomes are intracellular membrane-bound vacuoles containing destructive hydrolytic enzymes. They are vital to tissue remodelling and regeneration and are present in all animal tissues (De Duve and Waittaux 1966). Lysosomal activity is sex-steroid dependent. A marked rise in lysosomal enzyme activity occurs in the late secretory phase and during early menstruation (Henzl *et al.* 1972), in particular in the endometrial glands. Increased lysosomal activity may induce irregular endometrial breakdown and bleeding.

Matrix metalloproteinases

Matrix metalloproteinases (MMPs) are a highly regulated family of enzymes that together can degrade most components of the extracellular matrix. They are active in normal and pathological processes involving tissue remodelling. Produced in an inactive form, they are controlled by the balance of tissue inhibitors and activators, which in turn are controlled by sex steroid hormones, cytokines, and growth factors (Rogers *et al.* 1994). MMP activity is greatest on days 1–4 of the menstrual cycle, when bleeding is occurring (Hampton and Salamonsen 1994). MMPs are activated by progesterone withdrawal and by migratory leukocytes. Paracrine regulators of MMP activity include transforming growth factor β (TGFβ), tumour necrosis factor (TNF), PGE and $PGF_2\alpha$, endothelins and interleukin 1 (IL-1). Migratory leukocytes are observed before but not during normal menstrual bleeding (Clark and Daya 1990). Their role in promoting tissue breakdown may be indirect, via the activation of MMPs.

Adhesion molecules

Adhesion molecules are those molecules which permit cell adhesion to other cells and to the extracellular matrix, allowing cells to respond to endocrine and paracrine signals. In the endometrium, endothelial cell expression of adhesion molecules is cyclical. During the menstrual stage of the normal cycle, leukocytes are recruited to the endometrium by integrins (Tabibzadeh and Poubouridis 1990) and leukocyte binding to endothelial cells is increased (Tawia *et al.* 1993). Disturbances of adhesion molecule expression by contraceptive steroids may influence vascular integrity.

Cytokines

Cytokines are small peptides that affect the growth and differentiation of a wide variety of cells. Their action is local and via specific cell surface receptors. The endometrium is a main site of cytokine production and there is evidence that these proteins are actively involved in the regulation of endometrial function.

Cytokines such as interleukins, TNF and CSF, free oxygen radicals, and adhesion molecules are likely to be important in endometrial remodelling and repair. Cytokines are chemotactic for leukocytes; the chemokine interleukin-8 (IL-8), located in the perivascular endometrium (Critchley *et al.* 1994), can selectively induce neutrophil chemotaxis and activate white cells in the endometrium (Clark and Daya 1990).

Production of IL-8 is inhibited by progesterone (Kelly *et al.* 1994), thus sex steroids may act indirectly to control leukocyte changes in the endometrium. Cytokines also influence vasoconstriction, haemostatic plug formation, mitogenesis, and angiogenesis.

Despite the marked alterations in endometrial structure observed in women exposed to long-term progestogens, none of the parameters studied so far has shown any correlation with menstrual bleeding patterns (Rogers *et al.* 1993; Critchley *et al.* 1993; Wonodiresko *et al.* 1993). There may be a 'missing link' which causes these altered vessels to bleed, and this has not yet been explored. A possible factor is mechanical stress, for instance a myometrial contraction. A 'fragile' vessel may remain intact until it is unable to withstand the shearing stress of uterine wall movement. Further *in vivo* studies are needed to determine the nature of vascular fragility following progestogen exposure and the local mechanisms that control vascular integrity.

Treatment regimens

Whenever irregular bleeding is observed, genital tract pathology should be excluded. Breakthrough bleeding with oestrogen and progestogen contraceptives is more common with low-dose preparations, and may respond to increasing the dose of oestrogen or progestogen, or to changing the type of progestogen. There has been little attempt to explore systematically the benefits of various changes in OCP type to control BTB.

With progestogen-only contraceptives, there are no established methods of regulating bleeding episodes. The number of different preparations used for this purpose (Table 31.2) demonstrates the absence of a definitive approach to problematic bleeding following prolonged low-dose progestogen exposure.

Table 31.2 Treatments used to regulate bleeding episodes in women taking progestogen-only contraceptives

Sex steroid hormones	Low-dose oestrogen
	Combined oestrogen and progestogen
	Anti-progestogens
	Increased progestogen
Prostaglandin synthetase inhibitors	
Antifibrinolytics	
Antihistamines	
Vitamin E	
Placebo	
Counselling	

For all of these methods, those who are unable to tolerate bleeding disturbances will discontinue use of the contraceptive, leaving a cohort of those with either better bleeding patterns or greater tolerance of disrupted bleeding.

The aims of treatment have been varied and often poorly defined. The initial use of oestrogen in combination with progestogen-only contraception (as DMPA) was to terminate a prolonged bleeding episode, and to exert some 'control' over bleeding patterns in order to improve patient morale in the short term (Fraser 1983). In the long term, spontaneous improvement in bleeding patterns is expected to increase acceptability. Prolonged and repeated use of oestrogens defeats the aims of progestogen-only contraception, and is not a valid approach to treatment.

Whether oestrogen treatment regimens improve bleeding in the longer term remains unclear. There is some evidence that supplemental oestrogen may regulate bleeding patterns with progestogen-only contraceptives, at least for the duration of oestrogen use (Fraser 1983; Diaz *et al.* 1990), and even for 90 days after treatment (Witjaksono *et al.* 1996) but this requires further clarification.

There have been few large-scale studies of regimens to improve menstrual bleeding patterns in users of progestogen-only contraception, and comparisons between studies are hampered by varying regimens and preparations as well as the known cultural variation in bleeding patterns (Belsey 1988*b*). In a large prospective trial, Diaz *et al.* (1990) compared regimens of ethinyloestradiol, levonorgestrel, and ibuprofen with a placebo, and showed that all three regimens were effective, with the best results obtained with oestrogen. The mechanisms for oestrogen-induced cessation of bleeding may be via oestrogenic promotion of epithelial repair and regeneration.

The beneficial effects of oestrogen on the endometrium may be hindered by a progestogen-induced depletion of endometrial oestrogen receptors (Critchley *et al.* 1993). A recent major prospective trial comparing placebo, ethinyloestradiol (EE), and oestrone sulphate for prolonged bleeding with DMPA (Said *et al.* 1996) reported that frequent bleeding was the most common pattern associated with a request for treatment, and that ethinyloestradiol was effective in stopping bleeding by day 5 in 50 per cent of cases. Both placebo and oestrone sulphate were effective in stopping bleeding by day 9 in approximately the same number of cases. This marked placebo effect seems to be a constant feature in all trials of treatment regimens, and the reason for this is unclear. Similarly, in the WHO trial (Said *et al.* 1996) a range of treatment efficacy from 50 to 100 per cent was observed between centres. No long-term improvement in bleeding patterns was observed. A recent trial comparing ethinyloestradiol with the OCP (EE and LNG) and a placebo in Norplant users (Witjaksono *et al.* 1996) found that treatment significantly reduced the length, but not the number of bleeding episodes, and that EE and the OCP were more effective than placebo treatment.

The use of ethinyloestradiol in DMPA users increased the number of bleeding episodes, but the episodes were shortened (Said *et al.* 1996). This suggests that ethinyloestradiol is acting on the reparative or regenerative process to terminate a bleeding episode. In the Norplant users studied by Rogers *et al.* (1993), those women with higher levels of endogenous oestrogens had less increase in microvascular density and a more 'normal' vascular pattern.

The use of ethinyloestradiol for the treatment of prolonged bleeding episodes following progestogen exposure seems to conflict with the observation that those women with persistently higher endogenous oestradiol levels have more bleeding and spotting days than those with low oestrogen levels (Faundes *et al.* 1991). It is possible that endogenous oestradiol may exert different endometrial effects to exogenous ethinyloestradiol. Endogenous E2 is converted to oestrone (E1) by 17-oxidase reductase, but this does not occur with EE. The effect of supplemental oestrogen on the endometrium is likely to be temporary. Prolonged oestrogen combined with progestogens will eventually induce endometrial atrophy and amenorrhoea.

The role of treatment in improving patient tolerance and acceptance of progestogen-only contraceptives has not been explored. It cannot be assumed that more frequent but shorter bleeding episodes are more acceptable to all or most women, and this must be explored in different cultures before a clinical role for these treatment regimens can be established.

Conclusions

Modern contraceptive steroids offer women the option of safe and reliable protection against unwanted pregnancy, with a choice of delivery systems and hormonal combinations. The main disadvantage of these methods is the disruption of menstrual bleeding patterns. This is particularly marked in users of long-acting, low-dose progestogen-only contraceptives.

Bleeding patterns correlate poorly with circulating levels of endogenous and exogenous sex steroid hormones, and there is increasing evidence that local endometrial mechanisms are important in the initiation and control of normal and contraceptive-induced menstrual bleeding.

Oestrogen supplementation will often terminate a bleeding episode, but there is little evidence that this provides long-term benefit, and there are no well established long-term treatment regimens. Future development is likely to be in the understanding of local endometrial mechanisms controlling the initiation, protraction, and cessation of menstrual bleeding and the manipulation of these mechanisms by non-hormonal means.

Improvements in the education of women about their own reproductive system may increase patient tolerance of changes in menstrual bleeding patterns and utilization of contraceptive methods.

References

Alexander, N.J. and d'Arcangues, C (eds.) (1992). *Steroid hormones and uterine bleeding*, pp. 344. American Association for the Advancement of Science, Washington DC

Allen, E. (1927). Menstrual cycle of monkey, Macau rhesus: observations on normal animals, effects of removal of ovaries and effects of injection of ovarian and placental extracts into spayed animals. *Contributions to Embryology*, **19**, 1–44.

Au, C.L. and Rogers, P.A.W. (1993). Immunohistochemical staining of von Willebrand factor in human endometrium during the normal menstrual cycle. *Human Reproduction*, **8**, 17–23.

Barsky, S., Baker, A., Siegal, G.P., Togo, S., and Liotta, L.A. (1983). Use of anti-basement membrane antibody to distinguish blood vessels and capillaries from lymphatic capillaries. *American Journal of Surgery and Pathology*, **7**, 667–77.

Bartelmez, G.W. (1937). Menstruation. *Physiological Review*, **17**, 28–72.

Belsey, E.M. (1988*a*). Task force on long-acting systemic agents for fertility regulation. The association between vaginal bleeding patterns and reasons for discontinuation of contraceptive use. *Contraception*, **38**, 207–35.

Belsey, E.M. (1988*b*). Task force on long-acting-systemic agents for fertility regulation. The association between vaginal bleeding patterns among women using one natural and eight hormonal methods of contraception. *Contraception*, **38**, 181–206.

Blackwell, P.M. and Fraser, I.S. (1988). A morphometric and ultrastructural study of microvessels of the functional zone of normal human endometrium with some notions on possible secretory functions of the endothelial cells. *Asia-Oceania Journal of Obstetrics and Gynaecology*, **14**, 233–50.

Brooks, P.G., Serden, S.P., and Davos, I. (1991). Hormonal inhibition of the endometrium for resectoscopic endometrial ablation. *American Journal of Obstetrics and Gynecology*, **164**, 1601–8.

Cameron, I.T., Davenport, A.P., van Papendorp, C., Barker, P.J., Huskisson, N.S., Gilmour, R.S., *et al.* (1992). Endothelin-like immunoreactivity in human endometrium. *Journal of Reproduction and Fertility*, **95**, 623–8.

Clark, D.A. and Daya, S. (1990). Macrophages and other migratory white cells in the endometrium; relevance to endometrial bleeding. In *Contraception and mechanisms of endometrial bleeding* (ed. d'Arcangues C., Fraser, I.S., Newton, J.R., and Odlind V.), pp. 363–83. Cambridge University Press.

Clemetson, C.A.B., Blair, L., and Brown, A.B. (1962). Capillary strength and the menstrual cycle. *Annals of the New York Academy of Sciences*, **93**, 279–99.

Critchley, H.O.D., Bailey, D.A., Au, C.L., Affandi, B., and Rogers, P.A.W. (1993). Immunohistochemical sex steroid receptor distribution in endometrium from long-term subdermal levonorgestrel users and during the normal menstrual cycle. *Human Reproduction*, **8**, 1632–9.

Critchley, H.O.D., Kelly, R.W., and Kooy, J. (1994). Perivascular expression of chemokine interleukin-8 in human endometrium: a preliminary report. *Human Reproduction*, **9**, 1406–9.

d'Arcangues, C., Odlind, V., and Fraser, I.S. (1990). Dysfunctional uterine bleeding induced by exogenous hormones. In *Contraception and mechanisms of endometrial bleeding* (ed. C. d'Arcangues, I.S., Fraser, J.R., Newton, and V. Odlind), pp. 81–105. WHO/Cambridge University Press, Cambridge.

Diaz, S., Croxatto, H.B., Pavez, M., Belhadj, H., Stern, J., and Sivin, I. (1990). Clinical aspects of treatments for prolonged bleeding in users of Norplant implants. *Contraception*, **42**, 97–109.

De Duve and Waittaux, R. (1966). Functions of lysosomes. *Annual Review of Physiology*, **28**, 435–92.

Faundes, A., Brache, V., Tejeda, A.S., Cochon, M.T., and Alvarez-Sanches, F. (1991). Ovulatory dysfunction during continuous administration of low-dose levonorgestrel by subdermal implants. *Fertility and Sterility*, **56**, 27–31.

Ferenczy, A. (1976*a*). Studies on the cytodynamics of human endometrial regeneration. 1. Scanning electron microscopy. *American Journal of Obstetrics and Gynecology*, **124**, 64–74.

Ferenczy, A. (1976*b*). Studies on the cytodynamics of human endometrial regeneration. 11. Transmission electron microscopy and histochemistry. *American Journal of Obstetrics and Gynecology*, **124**, 582–95.

Ferenczy, A., Bertrand, G., and Gelfand, M.M. (1979). Proliferation kinetics of human endometrium during the normal menstrual cycle. *American Journal of Obstetrics and Gynecology*, **133**, 859–67.

Finn, C.A. (1986). Implantation, menstruation and inflammation. *Biological Review*, **61**, 313–28.

Fraser, I.S. (1983). A survey of different attitudes to the management of menstrual disturbance in women using injectable contraceptives. *Contraception*, **28**, 385–97.

Fraser, I.S. (1990). Treatment of dysfunctional uterine bleeding with oral, intramuscular or intrauterine progestogens. pp 139–148 In. *Advances in reproductive endocrinology. Vol. 2: Dysfunctional uterine bleeding*, (ed. R.W. Shaw), pp. 139–48. Parthenon, Lancs, UK.

Fraser, I.S. and Diczfalusy, E. (1980). A perspective of steroidal contraception and abnormal bleeding. What are the prospects for improvement? In *Endometrial bleeding and steroidal contraception* (ed. E. Diczfalusy, I.S. Fraser, and F.T.G. Webb), pp. 384–413. Pitman Press, Bath.

Fraser, I.S. and Peek, M.J. (1992). Effects of exogenous hormones on endometrial capillaries. In *Steroid hormones and uterine bleeding* (ed. Nancy, J. Alexander and Catherine d'Arcangues), pp. 67–79. American Association for the Advancement of Science, Washington DC.

Fraser, I.S., McCarron, G., Hutton, B., and Macey, D. (1987). Endometrial blood flow measured by ^{133}Xenon clearance in women with normal menstrual cycles and dysfunctional uterine bleeding. *American Journal of Obstetrics and Gynecology*, **156**, 158–66.

Fraser, I.S., Hickey, M., and Song, J.Y. (1996). A comparison of mechanisms underlying disturbances of bleeding due to spontaneous dysfunctional uterine bleeding or to hormonal contraception. *Human Reproduction*, **11**, Supplement 2, 165–78.

Goodger, A.M., Rogers, P.A.W., and Affandi, B. (1994). Endometrial endothelial cell proliferation in long-term users of subdermal levonorgestrel. *Human Reproduction*, **9**, 1647–51.

Hampton, A.L. and Salmonsen, L.A. (1994). Expression of messenger ribonucleic acid encoding matrix metalloproteinases and their tissue inhibitors is related to menstruation. *Journal of Endocrinology*, **141**, R1–3.

Harper, M.J.K. (1990). Platelet activating factor and the reproductive system. In *Contraception and mechanisms of endometrial bleeding* (ed. C.d'Arcangues, I.S., Fraser, J.R., Newton, and V., Odlind), pp. 289–305. WHO/Cambridge University Press, Cambridge.

Henzl, M.R., Smith, R.E., Boost, G., and Tyler, E.T. (1972). Lysosomal concept of menstrual bleeding in humans. *Journal of Clinical Endocrinology and Metabolism*, **34**, 860–75.

Hickey, M., Fraser, I.S., Dwarte, D. and Graham, S. (1996). The endometrium in Norplant users: an hysteroscopic study. *Human Reproduction*, **11**, Supplement 2, 35–44.

Hourihan, H.M. (1985). The human endometrial vasculature: the normal menstrual cycle, dysfunctional bleeding and the effect of norethisterone and levonorgestrel. PhD Thesis, University of Dublin.

Hourihan, H.M., Sheppard, B.L., and Brosens, I.A. (1990). Endometrial haemostasis. In *Contraception and mechanisms of endometrial bleeding* (ed. C. d'Arcangues, I.S. Fraser, J.R. Newton, and V. Odlind), pp. 95–116. WHO/Cambridge University Press, Cambridge.

Hourihan, H.M., Shephard, B.L., and Bonnar, J. (1991). The morphological response of blood vessels of the endometrium to low dose oral norethisterone and levonorgestrel. *Journal of Obstetrics and Gynaecology*, **11**, 47–54.

Johannisson, E. (1990). Endometrial morphology during the normal cycle and under the influence of contraceptive steroids. In *Contraception and mechanisms of endometrial bleeding*, (ed. C. d'Arcangues, I.S. Fraser, J.R. Newton, and V. Odlind), pp. 53–81. WHO/Cambridge University Press, Cambridge.

Johannisson, E., Landgren, B.M., and Diczfalusy, E. (1982). Endometrial morphology and peripheral steroid levels in women with and without intermenstrual bleeding during contraception with the 300 microgram norethisterone (NET) minipill. *Contraception*, **25**, 13–30.

Kelly, R.W., Illingworth, P., Baldie, G., Leask, R., Brouwer, S., and Calder, A.A. (1994). Progestogen control of interleukin 8 production in the endometrium and choriodecidual cells underlines the role of the neutrophil in menstruation and parturition. *Human Reproduction*, **9**, 253–8.

King, R.J.B. and d'Arcangues, C. (1992). Steroid hormone effects on uterine blood vessels. In *Steroid hormones and uterine bleeding*, (ed. Nancy, J. Alexander and Catherine d'Arcangues), Ch. 4, pp. 25–36. American Association for the Advancement of Science, Washington DC.

Landgren, B.M., Johannison, E., Masironi, B., and Diczfalusy, E. (1982). Pharmacokinetic and pharmacodynamic investigations with vaginal devices releasing levonorgestrel at a constant, zero order rate. *Contraception*, **26**, 567–85.

Lau, T. Witjaksono, J. and Rogers, P.A.W. (1996). Progesterone receptors in Norplant endometrium users and during the normal menstrual cycle. *Human Reproduction*, **11**, supplement 2, 90–4.

Ludwig, H. (1982). The morphological response of the endometrium to long-term treatment with progestational agents. *American Journal of Obstetrics and Gynecology*, **142**, 462–7.

Magos, A.L., Brincat, M., Studd, J.W.W., Wardle, P., Schlesinger, P., and O'Dowd, T. (1985). Amenorrhoea and endometrial atrophy with continuous oral oestrogen and progestogen *Obstetrics and Gynecology*, **65**, 496–9.

Maqueo, M. (1980). Vascular and perivascular changes in the endometrium of women using steroidal contraceptives. In *Endometrial bleeding and steroidal contraception* (ed. E. Diczfalusy, I.S. Fraser, and F.T.G. Webb), pp. 138–52. Pitman Press, Bath.

Maragoudakis, M.E., Missirlis, E., Karakiulakis, G.D., Sarmonica, M., Bastakis, M., and Tsopanoglou, N. (1993). Basement membrane biosynthesis as a target for developing inhibitors of angiogenesis with anti-tumour properties. *Kidney International*, **43**, 147–50.

Markee, J.E. (1940). Menstruation in intraocular endometrial transplants in the rhesus monkey. In *Contributions to embryology*. Carnegie Institute of Washington, **177**, 220–306.

Marsh, M., Butt, A.R., Riley, S.C., Rogers, P.A.W., Susil, B., Affandi, B., *et al.* (1995). Immunolocalization of endothelin and neutral endopeptidase in the endometrium of users of subdermally implanted levonorgestrel (Norplant®). *Human Reproduction*, **10**, 2584–9.

Martin, G.M., Timpl, R.T., and Kuhn, K. (1988). Basement membrane proteins: molecular structure and function. *Advances in Protein Chemistry*, **39**, 1–46.

Ober, W.B. (1970). Morphological changes in the uterus associated with steroid contraceptives and intrauterine contraceptive devices. *Acta Cytologica* (Baltimore), **14**, 156.

Odlind, V. and Fraser, I.S. (1990). Contraception and menstrual bleeding disturbances: a clinical overview. In *Contraception and mechanisms of endometrial bleeding* (ed. C. d'Arcangues, I.S. Fraser, J.R. Newton, and V. Odlind), pp. 5–31. Cambridge University Press.

Olive, D.L. and Schlaff, W.D. (1992). Amenorrhoea and breakthrough bleeding associated with contraceptive use. In *Steroid hormones and uterine bleeding* (ed. Nancy, J. Alexander, and Catherine d'Arcangues, Ch. 31, pp. 329–37). American Association for the Advancement of Science, Washington DC.

Palmer, J.A., Lau, T., Hickey, M., Simbar, M., and Rogers, P.A.W. (1996). Immunohistochemical study of endometrial microvascular basement membrane components in women using Norplant. *Human Reproduction*, **11**, 2142–50.

Perrot-Applanat, M., Groyer-Pickard, M.T., Garcia, E., Lorenzo, F., and Milgrom, E. (1988). Immunocytochemical demonstration of estrogen and progesterone receptors in muscle cells of uterine arteries in rabbits and humans. *Endocrinology*, **123**, 1511–19.

Roberts, D.K., Parmley, T.H., Walker, N.J., and Horbelt, D.V. (1992). Ultrastructure of the microvasculature in the human endometrium throughout the normal menstrual cycle. *American Journal of Obstetrics and Gynecology*, **166**, 1393–406.

Rogers, P.A.W., Au, C.L., and Affandi, B. (1993). Endometrial microvascular density during the normal menstrual cycle and following exposure to long-term levonorgestrel. *Human Reproduction*, **8**, 1396–404.

Rogers, W.H., Matrisian, L.M., Giudice, L.C., Dsupin, B., Cannon, P., Svitek, C., *et al.* (1994). Patterns of matrix metalloproteinases expression in cycling endometrium imply differential functions and regulation by steroid hormones. *Journal of Clinical Investigation*, **94** 946–53.

Said, S., Sadek, W., Rocca, M., Koetsawang, S., Kiriwak, O., Fiya-Anank, M. *et al.* (1996). Clinical evaluation of the therapeutic effectiveness of ethinyl oestradiol and oestrone sulphate on prolonged bleeding in women using depot medroxyprogesterone acetate for contraception. *Human Reproduction*, **11**, Supplement 2, 1–13.

Shaw, S.T., Jr, Macauley, L.K., Aznar, R., Gonzalez-Angulo, A., and Roy, S. (1981). Effects of a progesterone releasing intrauterine contraceptive device on endometrial blood vessels: a morphometric study. *American Journal of Obstetrics and Gynecology*, **141**, 821–7.

Sivin, I. (1994). Contraception with Norplant implants. *Human Reproduction*, **9**, 1818–26.

Sixma, J., Christiaens, G.C.M.L., and Haspels, A.A. (1980). The sequence of haemostatic events in the endometrium during normal menstruation. In *Endometrial bleeding and steroidal contraception* (ed. E. Diczfalusy, I.S. Fraser, and F.T.G. Webb), pp. 86–96. Pitman Press, Bath.

Snijders, M.P.M.L., de Goeij, A.F.P.M., Debets-Te Baerts, M.J.C., Rousch, M.J.M., Koudstaal, J., and Bosman F.T. (1992). Immunocytochemical analysis of oestrogen receptors and progesterone receptors in the human uterus throughout the menstrual cycle and after the menopause. *Journal of Reproduction and Fertility*, **94**, 363–71.

Snowden, R. and Christiaen, B. (1983). *Patterns and perception of menstruation*, Croom Helm, London.

Song, J.Y., Markham, R., Russell, P., Wong, T., Young, L., and Fraser, I.S. (1995). The effect of high dose medium and long-term progestogen exposure on endometrial vessels. *Human Reproduction*, **10**, 797–800.

Tabibzadeh, S.S. and Poubouridis, D. (1990). Expression of leukocyte adhesion molecules in human endometrium. *American Journal of Clinical Pathology*, **93**, 183–8.

Tawia, S.A., Beaton, L.A., and Rogers, P.A.W. (1993). Immunolocalisation of the cellular adhesion molecules, ICAM-1 and PECAM in human endometrium through the normal menstrual cycle. *Human Reproduction*, **8**, 175–81.

Tropey, N., Wylie, C.C., and Heasman, J. (1992). Function of maternal cytokeratin in Xenopus development. *Nature*, **357**, 413–15.

White, J.O., Sullivan, M.H.F., Patel, L., Croxtall, C., d'Arcangues, C., Belsey, E.M., and Elder, M.G. (1991). Prostaglandin production in human endometrium following continuous exposure to low-dose levonorgestrel released from a vaginal ring. *Contraception*, **43**, 401–12.

Witjaksono, J., Lau, T.M., Affandi, B. and Rogers, P.A.W. (1996). Effects of estrogen treatment of the endometrium of Norplant users. *Human Reproduction*, **11**, Supplement 2, 109–14..

Wonodiresko, S., Au, C.L., Hadisputra, W., Affandi, B., and Rogers, P.A.W. (1993). Cytokeratins 8, 18 and 19 in endometrial epithelial cells during the normal menstrual cycle and in women receiving Norplant. *Contraception*, **48**, 481–93.

32 Hormone replacement therapy and disturbances of bleeding: mechanisms and management

David F. Archer

Background

Menopause has recently become a significant issue as the life expectancy of the female population increases. The average age of menopause in the United States is 52 years, with an average life expectancy to age 82. The majority of women in the world do not receive hormone replacement therapy following menopause. In fact, hormone replacement therapy as a treatment for post-menopausal women has only come into vogue in the developed world since the middle of the 1960s.

Following menopause, with its concomitant reduction in levels of ovarian oestrogen and progesterone, the endometrial lining becomes atrophic and loses height with sparse glands and a thin non-active stroma. Uterine size also reduces in the post-menopausal period. These two findings are directly related to the withdrawal of oestrogen stimulation. From a clinical standpoint, the uterine lining in the post-menopausal woman is stable and there is limited activity of glands and stroma as reflected in the absence of glandular and stromal mitoses.

No further uterine bleeding should occur in post-menopausal women who do not use hormone replacement therapy. In fact, for post-menopausal women who are not receiving hormone replacement therapy, vaginal bleeding should be a cause of concern and prompt evaluation by a clinical care giver. The reason for this is that in the older woman, there is a continuing increase in the incidence of cancer of the genital tract, specifically cancer of the cervix and uterine endometrium. Both of these cancers (or more rarely cancers of the ovary, Fallopian tube, and vagina) may present as vaginal bleeding. It is obvious that the annual Papanicolaou smear should be used as a preventive health care strategy for screening for cancer of the cervix. There are no current practical methods available for screening for endometrial cancer. At one time it was advocated that all women who were being considered as candidates for hormone replacement therapy undergo a screening endometrial biopsy to rule out hyperplasias or neoplasias. It is apparent that this is a cumbersome approach with a low yield. In fact, the incidence of adenocarcinoma of the endometrium is relatively low and estimated to be one case per 1000 women per year (Archer *et al.* 1991). Utilization of the endometrial biopsy to screen a population of women who had either no bleeding or a minimal degree of irregular bleeding yielded only five cases of atypia out of 800 women and only one case of cancer (Archer *et al.* 1991).

In the early 1980s it was advocated that a progestogen challenge test be utilized to interdict the development of cystic hyperplasia (Gambrell *et al.* 1980). The rationale behind this test was that as long as there were low levels of endogenous oestrogen, women would experience withdrawal bleeding following the administration of the oral progestotional agent. By using this clinical test, hyperplasias would be interdicted and absence of withdrawal bleeding would indicate hypoestrogenicity (Gambrell *et al.* 1980). This test has not continued to have any significant utilization principally due to the fact that most women either opt immediately for no treatment or go on to hormone replacement therapy. At this time the only need for prescribing cyclic exogenous progestogen would be for those women who are experiencing irregular and excessive bleeding during the perimenopausal transition.

Hormonal and menstrual changes in the perimenopause reflect an increasing occurrence of anovulation (Burger *et al.* 1995; Santoro *et al.* 1996). Menstrual cycles in perimenopausal women become longer in interval with an increase in the amount of bleeding probably secondary to the increasing occurrence of anovulation. Because of the prolonged oestrogen stimulation without progesterone secretion simple cystic hyperplasia occurs in about 5 per cent of cases (Archer *et al.* 1991). The current prognosis for simple endometrial hyperplasia is one of a low incidence (< 1 per cent) of progression to more severe conditions (Kurman *et al.* 1985). Atypical adenomatous hyperplasia, on the other hand, has been observed to progress to adenocarcinoma of the uterus in 29 per cent of cases (Kurman *et al.* 1985). It becomes obvious that simple cystic hyperplasia, although it does raise a concern, should not be construed as an indication for aggressive therapy such as a hysterectomy. The reason for this is that simple endometrial hyperplasia does not occur to any extent (< 1.0 per cent) with the use of concomitant exogenous progestogen (Gibbons *et al.* 1986; Moyer *et al.* 1993; Woodruff and Pickar 1994; The Writing Group for the PEPI Trial 1996*a*).

It is well known that in post-menopausal women who are not using hormone replacement therapy reinitiation of vaginal bleeding requires further investigation. Diagnostic procedures used to evaluate spontaneous uterine bleeding in post-menopausal women are outlined below:

- endometrial aspiration biopsy
- transvaginal ultrasound
- sonohysterography
- hysteroscopy
- dilatation and curettage.

A diagnostic dilatation and curettage (D&C) usually performed under general anaesthesia has been the hallmark of gynaecological investigation (Grimes 1982). The accuracy of diagnostic D&C for excluding endometrial cancer is felt to be high (MacKenzie and Bibby 1978; Grimes 1982). The D&C has been used as the standard to evaluate other techniques of endometrial assessment. Endometrial sampling using a variety of simple aspiration devices has gained popularity for its convenience, low cost, and sensitivity and specificity. Thus the assessment of irregular uterine bleeding in post-menopausal women has moved from a surgical inpatient evaluation to an ambulatory outpatient facility.

Ancillary procedures to investigate further the endometrial changes in the post-menopausal woman who is experiencing uterine bleeding have involved transvaginal ultrasound for assessment of the endometrial lining of the uterus (Goldstein *et al.* 1990; Varner *et al.* 1991; Goldstein 1993; Sladkevicius *et al.* 1994; Karlsson *et al.* 1995). This technique has been advocated as a non-invasive means to determine the thickness of the lining of the uterus as well as to document any evidence of intrauterine abnormalities (see Chapter 21).

The ultrasound evaluation of the endometrium highlights the fact that post-menopausal uterine bleeding may occur even with an unstimulated or atrophic endometrium (Nasri and Coast 1989; Nasri *et al.* 1991). An endometrial thickness of less than 5 mm by transvaginal ultrasound has been utilized as a cut-off point below which further diagnostic intervention is not deemed necessary. Even this arbitrary value has been shown to have ethnic differences (Tsuda *et al.* 1995). The concern is that small, early cancers may be missed, arguing for the continued use of endometrial sampling. Since sensitivity of ultrasound or endometrial biopsy never reaches one hundred per cent, reinvestigation is warranted based on clinical findings of continued excessive uterine bleeding.

Management of post-menopausal bleeding

Spontaneous vaginal bleeding in a post-menopausal woman not associated with hormone replacement therapy deserves complete evaluation. Although endometrial abnormalities could be suspected, other problems in the lower genital tract such as cervical or vaginal neoplasia must be excluded. As part of the evaluation process for vaginal bleeding a Papanicolaou smear and endometrial assessment are required.

Endometrial assessment

An endometrial biopsy is the easiest and most practical method to evaluate the endometrial cavity. Use of an endometrial aspiration sampling device can be as sensitive and specific as a formal dilatation and curettage (Grimes 1982; Larson *et al.* 1995). Since the endometrial biopsy is performed in the outpatient ambulatory care setting, costs are significantly less than those incurred with anaesthesia and an operating room. Endometrial biopsy has a relatively high degree of accuracy in making a diagnosis (Holst *et al.* 1983). Persistent uterine bleeding is an indication for further diagnostic studies as described below.

Ultrasound evaluation of the endometrial cavity

Two techniques are currently used. The first is a simple transvaginal ultrasound (TVUS), with assessment of the endometrial thickness, uterine size and shape, and adnexal structures. The TVUS can rule out significant adnexal pathology. It is also of help in diagnosing intramural uterine myomas. The second technique, described below, is sonohysterography. The major use of TVUS is in evaluating endometrial thickness. Endometrial thickness of less than 5 to 6 mm has rarely been reported to be associated with significant endometrial pathology (Nasri and Coast 1989). Thus, this test, which is less invasive than an endometrial biopsy, has been used as a screening procedure for women with post-menopausal bleeding (Goldstein *et al.* 1990; Granberg *et al.* 1991). Persistent or recurrent uterine bleeding even with a thin endometrium should be an indication for an endometrial biopsy.

Hysteroscopy

Hysteroscopy is best utilized for evaluating persistent bleeding where the endometrial biopsy reports an inadequate amount of endometrium or atrophic endometrial tissue (Nagele *et al.*

1996*a*). Endometrial polyps or small foci of adenocarcinoma can be missed by the endometrial biopsy and TVUS. Hysteroscopy is not generally a first line diagnostic procedure. Rather, it is best utilized as a back-up procedure for problem cases with recurrent or persistent bleeding (Nagele *et al.* 1996*b*).

Dilatation and curettage under anaesthesia

This procedure is best used for patients with cervical stenosis, and those who have at least adenomatous hyperplasia on endometrial biopsy (Grimes 1982; Holst *et al.* 1983). Systematic evaluation of the uterine cavity is required in patients with adenomatous endometrial hyperplasia with or without atypia. Hysteroscopy can be combined with this procedure to enhance the diagnostic process by directly visualizing the uterine cavity and endometrium (Larson *et al.* 1995).

Sonohysterography

A relatively recent procedure, sonohysterography allows the introduction of sterile fluid into the uterine cavity during a TVUS evaluation (Syrop and Sahakian 1992; Goldstein 1993; Parsons and Lense 1993). The technique can be used to identify polyps and other intrauterine pathology that might have been missed by blind endometrial biopsy. There is probably limited utility of this procedure for screening of women with post-menopausal bleeding. It can be used adjunctively to TVUS or hysteroscopy.

A comprehensive organized approach to post-menopausal bleeding requires an evaluation of the adnexa, uterus, cervix, and vagina by the techniques listed above to rule out carcinoma. No significant abnormalities are found in over 50 per cent of evaluations for post-menopausal bleeding. This in itself is reassuring, but should not be used as a rationale for a less than complete evaluation of the reproductive tract.

The utilization of hormone replacement therapy

Over the past several years there has been an increasing interest in the utilization of hormone replacement therapy (oestrogen and progestogen) in post-menopausal women. The reason for this advocacy has been the accumulated evidence that the use of exogenous oestrogen reduces the risk of cardiovascular events and prevents loss of bone (Manolio *et al.* 1993; Marcus *et al.* 1994; Lobo 1995, The Writing Group for the PEPI Trial 1995; 1996*b*; Speroff *et al.* 1996; Ettinger *et al.* 1996). Progestogen is added to prevent the development of endometrial hyperplasias and adenocarcinoma in women with a uterus. In the United States, it appears that only 15 to 20 per cent of women who initiate hormone replacement therapy will still be using it at the end of one year (Ravnikar 1987). The reasons for discontinuation are often not clearly identified, but common problems are breast tenderness, weight gain, and symptoms attributed to the progestogen such as moodiness, bloating, and oedema (Gelfand *et al.* 1989). Of all the symptoms, perhaps the one that is most correlated to the discontinuation of hormone replacement therapy is the re-institution of uterine bleeding (Ravnikar 1987; Hahn 1989). For this reason, various treatment regimens have been utilized to reduce or eliminate uterine bleeding in the post-menopausal woman. These treatment regimens are described in the following section and listed below:

(1) oestrogen daily (oral or transdermal);

(2) oestrogen daily with 12–14 days of a progestogen (cyclic or sequential therapy);

(3) oestrogen and progestogen daily (continuous combined therapy);

(4) oestrogen and progestogen daily for five days out of seven;

(5) oestrogen daily with intermittent progestogen (three days on and three days off repetitively – cyclophasic);

(6) oestrogen daily and 14 days of a progestogen every three months (long interval);

(7) oestrogen daily and an intrauterine delivery system (progesterone or levonorgestrel).

Administration of oestrogen alone

The use of oestrogen alone for replacement therapy (ERT) is indicated for those women who have previously undergone hysterectomy. The justification for this statement is the fact that oestrogen treatment results in an incidence of endometrial cystic hyperplasia of approximately 20 per cent at one year and 33 per cent at the end of three years in controlled clinical trials (Woodruff and Pickar 1994; The Writing Group for the PEPI Trial 1996*a*). Unopposed oestrogen has been found to increase the risk of adenocarcinoma of the endometrium significantly (Herrington and Weiss 1993). The addition of a progestogen to the oestrogen replacement therapy reduces the incidence of endometrial hyperplasia and adenocarcinoma but does not completely eliminate them (Herrington and Weiss 1993; Woodruff and Pickar 1994; The Writing Group for the PEPI Trial 1996*a*). It was presumed at one time that intermittent interruption of the consequent withdrawal bleeding would preclude the development of uterine endometrial cancer. This has not been shown to be the case. Therefore the use of ERT in women with a uterus requires an annual evaluation of the endometrium. At the present state of our knowledge, this endometrial evaluation should not be that of a screening ultrasound evaluation. Rather it should be one that assesses the endometrium by annual histology.

Women who are treated with ERT by either transdermal, oral, or vaginal administration appear to have a comparable degree of risk for endometrial hyperplasia and/or irregular bleeding (Whitehead *et al.* 1990; Woodruff and Pickar 1994). In fact the incidence of irregular uterine bleeding in women using oestrogen only is relatively low (< 25 per cent) (Archer *et al.* 1994*a*). Why the incidence of bleeding is so low is unknown. It is apparent that the longer the duration of oestrogen administration, the more likely women are to bleed (Archer *et al.* 1994*a*). It should be pointed out that between 12 and 15 per cent of women on oestrogen alone at the end of one year (after what appears to have been an adequate amount of hormone replacement) have evidence of unstimulated (atrophic) endometrium. The reason for this variation is also unknown, but it has been reported that the primate experiences a comparable reduction in endometrial thickness/endometrial atrophy with continued oestrogen replacement alone.

Estrogen and progestogen replacement therapy (HRT)

Because of the increased risk of endometrial hyperplasia and the potential for endometrial adenocarcinoma, it has been recommended that post-menopausal women who have a uterus and are candidates for hormone replacement therapy should receive both an oestrogen and a progestogen (HRT). The addition of a cyclic progestogen to the oestrogen regimen has resulted in the reinitiation of uterine bleeding in approximately 85 per cent of women (Whitehead *et al.* 1990; Clisham *et al.* 1992, Archer *et al.* 1994*a*). Several regimens have been designed to reduce the incidence of uterine bleeding. Oestrogen has been used continually with an oral progestogen for 14 days every three months (Ettinger *et al.* 1994); with progestogen therapy for three days off and three days on (Casper and Chapdelaine 1993); with progestogen daily as continuous combined therapy (Staland 1981); and in conjunction with an intrauterine delivery system (Andersson *et al.* 1992; Archer *et al.* 1994*b*).

Cyclic HRT

The utilization of oestrogen plus progestogen therapy began with a sequential administration of the progestogen that initially was given for seven days but has currently been increased to approximately 14 days of administration. The oestrogen component was originally given from days 1 through 25 with seven days off in an attempt to mimic the menstrual cycle. The addition of the progestogen for the last seven days of treatment led to inadequate protection of the endometrium resulting in a significant incidence of hyperplasia (Patterson *et al.* 1980; Whitehead *et al.* 1982). The progestogen was then increased to a minimum of 10 days to reduce the occurrence of endometrial hyperplasia (Padwick *et al.* 1986). Exogenous progestogen was shown to inhibit or alter endometrial biochemical parameters of oestrogenicity, such as mitosis and oestrogen-responsive endometrial enzymes (Whitehead *et al.* 1981). Over the years HRT has evolved into a continuous administration of oestrogen with 12 to 14 days of a progestotional agent given cyclically during the calendar month. Women who have been treated in this fashion have received a variety of progestotional compounds at a variety of doses (Whitehead *et al.* 1990). Perhaps the most extensively evaluated progestogen regimen at the present time has been one using either 5 mg or 10 mg per day of medroxyprogesterone acetate (MPA) on a cyclic basis. In these studies, the incidence of endometrial hyperplasia has been less than 1 per cent (Byrjalsen *et al.* 1992; Woodruff and Pickar 1994; The Writing Group for the PEPI Trial 1996*a*). Unopposed oestrogen has been found to increase the risk of adenocarcinoma of the endometrium significantly (Herrington and Weiss 1993). The addition of a cyclic progestotional agent has resulted in the reinitiation of uterine bleeding in most women (Archer *et al.* 1994*a*). It should be pointed out that this uterine withdrawal bleeding is usually less than that which the woman had experienced during menstruation in her pre-menopausal years. The uterine bleeding occurs at a regular interval related to the use of the progestogen. Bleeding episodes are not associated with menstrual cramps although there can be some pre-menstrual-like symptoms such as bloating and headache (Gelfand *et al.* 1989).

At one time it was felt that those women who had the onset of uterine bleeding prior to the completion of at least 10 days of the progestotional agent were receiving an inadequate amount of the progestogen (Padwick *et al.* 1986). This was predicated on a lack of secretory endometrial changes. These data implied that there was failure to inhibit the oestrogenic effect on the endometrium. Subsequent investigations have not substantiated this finding (Sturdee *et al.* 1994). It is not uncommon to see women begin to experience a bleeding episode while they are only on days 9, 10, or 11 of the progestogen replacement therapy (Archer *et al.* 1994*a*). At the present time, no clear-cut guidelines exist as to whether or not these women should continue to take the progestogen for the full 12 to 14 days after the initiation of bleeding. It has been the impression of this author that the entire 12 to 14 days of progestogen therapy should be given. All data on endometrial hyperplasia at the present time are predicated on the fact that the women have taken the entire number of days of the prescribed progestogen.

Hormone replacement therapy with progestogen at increasing intervals

The reinitiation of uterine bleeding on a monthly basis occurs with a high incidence in women on cyclic therapy, and bleeding is not desired by most post-menopausal women (Hahn 1989; Archer *et al.* 1994*a*). For these reasons the use of a progestotional agent for 12 to 14 days every three months (90 days) has been investigated (Ettinger *et al.* 1994). In these women, there are fewer episodes of menstrual bleeding in a calendar year. The amount of bleeding during or after every three month progestogen use appeared to be of longer duration (8 vs 5 days) and more women reported a heavier flow (31 per cent vs 8 per cent) compared to the volunteer's pre-study experience (Ettinger *et al.* 1994). A significant number of women were found to have unscheduled bleeding when the longer interval was compared to monthly sequential progestogen therapy (16 per cent vs 7 per cent). Insufficient information is available to recommend this treatment option at the present time although the incidence of hyperplasias of the endometrium was reported to be low (1.5 per cent).

Cyclic oestrogen and progestogen on a weekly basis

There is only one report of utilizing a combination of oestrogen and progestogen for five days, Monday through Friday, and then off for two days (Mishell *et al.* 1991). The study reported no uterine bleeding but the numbers were small ($n = 15$). There have been no reports by other investigators confirming this approach. There appears to be little advantage of this technique over continuous-combined therapy, unless the true incidence of uterine bleeding is as low as was reported in the pilot study.

Hormone replacement therapy (continuous-combined)

The concurrent administration of both an oestrogen and a progestogen was reported to be highly effective as a means to reduce the reinitiation of uterine bleeding during hormone replacement therapy (Staland 1981). Over the past 16 years a variety of oestrogens and progestogens have been used in what is called the continuous-combined manner (Hillard *et al.* 1992; Archer *et al.* 1994*a*; Udoff *et al.* 1995). The utilization of the continuous-combined technique has been reported to have an increased incidence of unanticipated irregular uterine bleeding during the first four to six months of treatment. A recent meta-analysis of these data indicated a reduction in the occurrence of uterine bleeding with continuation of the medication (Udoff *et al.* 1995). The use of conjugated oestrogens with medroxyprogesterone acetate as continuous-combined therapy has been studied in a large number of women in two major trials (Archer *et al.* 1994*a*; The Writing Group for the PEPI Trial 1995). The two reports found the incidence of endometrial hyperplasia and cancer to be less than 1 per cent (Woodruff and Pickar 1994; The Writing Group for the PEPI Trial 1996*a*). The incidence of uterine bleeding was 54 per cent at the beginning of treatment with 2.5 mg and 5 mg of medroxyprogesterone acetate respectively (Archer *et al.* 1994*a*). The occurrence of irregular bleeding declined with continued therapy, and after six months, over 70 per cent of individuals did not experience any uterine bleeding in the next six-month period (Marslew *et al.* 1991; Archer *et al.* 1994*a*; Udoff *et al.* 1995). In fact, it appears that continuous-combined HRT can maintain the lack of uterine bleeding for an indefinite period (Leather *et al.* 1991). Resumption of uterine bleeding after more than a six-month period of no bleeding should be viewed as a problem and appropriate diagnostic studies should be undertaken. Use of TVUS or endometrial biopsy in these women should be based on clinical assessment of the amount and duration of bleeding episode(s). Light spotting may require only reassurance and TVUS, but profuse bleeding should be investigated aggressively.

Interrupted continuous-combined (cyclophasic) therapy

An interesting approach has been continuous oestrogen with interrupted progestogen, termed cyclophasic (Casper and Chapdelaine 1993). Continuous oestrogen treatment has a progestogen administered for three days, stopped for three days, and then readministered for three days and continued in this interrupted pattern. The rationale behind the use of this treatment modality is that oestrogen will stabilize the endometrium and prevent bleeding. The addition of the progestogen inhibits oestrogen receptors, reduces their number, and inhibits mitotic activity of the cell. The progestogen is stopped before the endometrium destabilizes enough to bleed. The only report in the literature used piperazine oestrone sulphfate 0.75 mg daily and norethindrone 0.35 mg. There was no evidence of hyperplasia and a minimal incidence of endometrial bleeding after six months in the 40 volunteers (Casper and Chapdelaine 1993).

Utilization of oral oestrogen and an intrauterine delivery system for progestogen

A means of circumventing some of the side-effects associated with oral progestogens has been the utilization of an oral oestrogen and an intrauterine delivery system with a progesterone/progestogen-releasing intrauterine device (Shoupe *et al.* 1991; Archer *et al.* 1994*b*). Only a small number of volunteers has been studied, but the available data imply that this could be an attractive alternative (Archer *et al.* 1994*b*). There was a significant decline in uterine bleeding after the first three months, with several women reporting no bleeding at all.

The levonorgestrel-releasing intrauterine system (LNG-IUS) was initially used for contraception, for menorrhagia, and in perimenopausal women to control heavy bleeding (Andersson *et al.* 1992). Currently the use of the LNG-IUS in post-menopausal women has been studied in combination with either oral, transdermal, or subcutaneous oestrogen. In all instances, the intrauterine delivery system appeared to decrease the frequency and amount of uterine bleeding (Archer *et al.* 1994*b*; Raudaskoski *et al.* 1995; Suhonen *et al.* 1995*a*, *b*). There have not been any direct comparisons with oral cyclic or continuous-combined therapy.

Both progesterone and levonorgestrel intrauterine delivery systems have been shown to have an increased occurrence of irregular uterine bleeding during the first three months following insertion with a gradual decrease to no bleeding with continued utilization of the devices during follow-up of 12 to 24 months. The clinical assessment of an intrauterine delivery system for this purpose is in its beginning stages. More information will be needed to further delineate the incidence of irregular bleeding as well as the acceptability of this approach in perimenopausal and post-menopausal women.

Management of the reinitiation of uterine bleeding in post-menopausal women receiving hormone replacement therapy

Oestrogen-alone treatment

Management of women on oestrogen alone who develop irregular or prolonged bleeding is obvious. Women with a uterus should not usually be given unopposed oestrogen. Women with a uterus who, for whatever reasons, are treated with oestrogen alone require an endometrial assessment (endometrial biopsy) on a yearly basis because of the potential increase in the incidence of endometrial hyperplasia. The appropriate therapy after the biopsy will be based on the histological findings. Appropriate therapy for cystic hyperplasia is the addition of progestogen to the treatment regimen in either a cyclic or a continuous-combined approach. Cyclic progestogen therapy as a treatment does reduce the incidence of hyperplasia to almost zero (The Writing Group for the PEPI Trial 1996*a*). Further observation and intervention is predicated on the resulting change in the uterine bleeding pattern. Recurrent excessive and irregular bleeding is an indication for a repeat endometrial biopsy. The preferred treatment of adenomatous hyperplasia with atypia or adenocarcinoma of the endometrium is hysterectomy.

Cyclic progestogen replacement with continuous oestrogen

Management of women on cyclic hormone replacement therapy who experience irregular or profuse bleeding is difficult. This is because there are no clear-cut answers. Counselling in advance should emphasize to the woman that reinitiation of uterine bleeding is to be anticipated. Obviously, bleeding that is related to the utilization of the progestogen and its withdrawal is to be construed as 'normal'. Prolonged heavy bleeding or erratic bleeding not related to the progestogen should be an indication for further assessment.

Transvaginal ultrasound, sonohysterography, endometrial biopsy, or hysteroscopy can all be used for assessing these patients. Many of these women will be found to have an endometrial polyp or uterine myoma. Removal of an endometrial polyp can result in improvement in the bleeding pattern. Observation only is recommended for uterine myomas, since the current clinical findings do not support a growth in uterine myomas with HRT.

Obviously the need to exclude any type of endometrial atypia is important. Histological assessment of the endometrium using an endometrial biopsy is the current standard. Appropriate intervention is predicated on the findings of the clinical investigation. Increasing the dose of progestogen can be considered if the patient was on a low-dose regimen to begin with, and the endometrium showed a proliferative pattern. Although this treatment may be appropriate, there are no data indicating that this will successfully reduce the amount of the uterine bleeding.

Continuous-combined oestrogen and progestogen

Irregular or nuisance bleeding within the first six to seven months of treatment with continuous-combined hormone replacement therapy is to be anticipated and should be considered as relatively normal. None of the reports to date have indicated any evidence of endometrial hyperplasia in this group of women. Therefore, it is felt that only those women who have prolonged and/or profuse bleeding should have an endometrial biopsy performed. Transvaginal ultrasound or sonohysterography could be utilized. The expected outcome is to find a thin endometrial lining by ultrasound assessment reflecting an atrophic (suppressed) endometrium. It should be pointed out that it is still possible for a small adenocarcinoma to exist and remain unidentified despite the appearance of a thin endometrial echo using this technique.

Treatment for irregular bleeding in women on continuous-combined therapy

Return to cyclic therapy

Therapy is controversial for those women who are experiencing a sufficient amount of uterine bleeding to be construed as more than nuisance value. One option is to stop continuous-combined treatment and go back to cyclic therapy. This allows the individual to have a predictable withdrawal bleeding episode.

Increase the dose of the progestotional agent

A second option is to increase the dose of the progestotional agent. Currently, in the United States, a combination of conjugated oestrogen (0.625 mg) and medroxyprogesterone acetate (2.5 mg) has been approved by the Food and Drug Administration. In the published clinical study, women who used the combination of 0.625 mg conjugated oestrogen and 5 mg medroxyprogesterone acetate had a lower incidence of uterine bleeding after six months of treatment. The difference between the two medroxprogesterone acetate doses was statistically significant after six months of therapy (Archer *et al.* 1994*a*). Therefore, one could argue theoretically that increasing the dose of the progestogen could result in a reduction in the amount and incidence of uterine bleeding. The physician should consider this option in an attempt to reduce the bleeding and maintain compliance with the HRT regimen.

Reduce the oestrogen dosage

Another alternative that has no reported experience would be to reduce the amount of oestrogen in the treatment medication. Theoretically this would reduce the number of progesterone receptors. By analogy, this hypothesis proposes that progestogens in some manner initiate uterine bleeding. The administration of continuous oestrogen and progestogen replacement to castrated rhesus monkeys resulted in a 12 per cent incidence of uterine bleeding. Addition of an antiprogestin (RU486) reduced the incidence of uterine bleeding to 3 per cent in this animal model (Williams *et al.* 1994). Comparable data are not available for the human. The incidence of uterine bleeding is relatively low in women on oestrogen-only treatment (Archer *et al.* 1994*a*). The addition of a progestogen, either as sequential or continuous treatment, results in the reinitiation of uterine bleeding (Whitehead *et al.* 1990). These data imply that the progestogen alters the endometrium in some fashion, resulting in the uterine bleeding.

Stop progestogen therapy for one to two months

The last option is to stop the progestogen entirely for a brief period and leave the woman on oestrogen alone. This option is viable if used for a short time and should result in the cessation of uterine bleeding. Recommencement of the progestogen will involve counselling regarding the potential resumption of uterine bleeding. This author prefers returning to cyclic therapy and then restarting continuous combined treatment after four to six months. The reason for this approach is to attempt to interdict all uterine bleeding without stopping the HRT.

Management of bleeding with an intrauterine delivery system

Management of women who are experiencing irregular bleeding in the presence of replacement oestrogen and the intrauterine delivery of progesterone or levonorgestrel has not yet been assessed. Although bleeding does occur in these women, the appropriate treatment for managing the bleeding has not been determined. Since oestrogen has been shown to be effective in stopping bleeding, an increase in the oestrogen dose for four to six weeks is recommended at this time, although the high levels of progestogen in the endometrium may prevent an oestrogen effect in some women.

Summary

The motivation of both the patient and the physician to use and prescribe hormone replacement therapy can be severely tested if the individual begins to experience erratic uterine bleeding. Even highly motivated women can become disenchanted with the inability to control the uterine bleeding. Concerns on the part of the physician regarding the development of endometrial cancer or endometrial hyperplasias are legitimate.

The post-menopausal woman with iatrogenic uterine bleeding requires extensive counselling and management by the physician who may need to try several alternative treatments to achieve total cessation of uterine bleeding (continuous-combined therapy) or regular uterine bleeding (cyclic or sequential therapy). Extra time and effort is needed because of the frustration of a trial-and-error approach to the bleeding problem. This reflects our lack of understanding of the mechanisms involved in uterine bleeding, both in normal cycling women as well as in those on HRT. The easiest way out of the dilemma of iatrogenic uterine bleeding is to stop all hormones. Although this approach results in the cessation of uterine bleeding, it abrogates the rationale for the medical use of HRT in post-menopausal women. Because of this, the physician should explore all therapeutic options prior to discontinuing HRT. This results in continued counselling and an increased time commitment for these patients. Several therapeutic options exist, as detailed above, for managing the uterine bleeding. The physician's knowledge and willingness to commit the appropriate time is needed in order to be successful in this regard.

References

Andersson, K., Mattson, L.A., Rybo, G., and Stadberg, E. (1992). Intrauterine release of levonorgestrel – a new way of adding progestogen in hormone replacement therapy. *Obstetrics and Gynecology*, **79**, 963–7.

Archer, D.F., McIntyre-Seltman, K., Wilborn, W.W. Jr., Dowling, E.A., Cone, F., Creasy, G.W., and Kafrissen M.E. (1991). Endometrial morphology in asymptomatic postmenopausal women. *American Journal of Obstetrics and Gynecology*, **165**, 317–22.

Archer, D.F., Pickar, J.H., and Bottiglioni, F. (1994*a*). Bleeding patterns in postmenopausal women taking continuous combined or sequential regimes of conjugated estrogens with medroxyprogesterone acetate. *American Journal of Obstetrics and Gynecology*, **83**, 686–92.

Archer, D.F., Viniegra-Sibal, A., Hsiu, J.-G., Seltman, H.J., Muesing, R., and Ross B. (1994*b*). Endometrial histology, uterine bleeding, and metabolic changes in postmenopausal women using a progesterone-releasing intrauterine device and oral conjugated estrogens for hormone replacement therapy. *Menopause*, **1**, 109–16.

Burger, H.G., Dudley, E.C., Hopper, J.L., Shelley, J.M., Green, A., Smith, A. *et al.* (1995). The endocrinology of the menopausal transition: a cross-sectional study of a population-based sample. *Journal of Clinical Endocrinology and Metabolism*, **80**, 3537–45.

Byrjalsen, I., Thormann, L., Meinecke, B., Riis, B.J., and Christiansen, C. (1992). Sequential estrogen and progestogen therapy: assessment of progestational effects on the postmenopausal endometrium. *Obstetrics and Gynecology*, **79**, 523–8.

Casper, R.F. and Chapdelaine, A. (1993). Estrogen and interrupted progestin: a new concept for menopausal hormone replacement therapy. *American Journal of Obsterics and Gynecology*, **168**, 1188–96.

Clisham, P.R., Cedars, M.I., Greendale, G., Fu, Y.S., Gambone, J., and Judd, H.L. (1992). Long-term transdermal estradiol therapy: effects on endometrial histology and bleeding patterns. *Obstetrics annd Gynecology*, **79**, 196–201.

Ettinger, B., Selby, J., Citron, J.T., Vangessel, A., Ettinger, V., and Hendrickson, M. (1994). Cyclic hormone replacement therapy using quarterly progestin. *Obstetrics and Gynecology*, **83**, 693–700.

Ettinger, B., Friedman, G.D., Bush, T., and Quesenberry, C.P. Jr. (1996). Reduced mortality associated with long-term postmenopausal estrogen therapy. *Obstetrics and Gynecology*, **87**, 6–12.

Gambrell, R.D. Jr., Massey, F.M., Castenda, T.A., Ugenes, A.J., Ricci, C.A., and Wright, J.M. (1980). Use of the progestogen challenge test to reduce the risk of endometrial cancer. *Obstetrics and Gynecology*, **55**, 732–8.

Gelfand, M.M., Ferenczy, A., and Bergeron, C. (1989). Endometrial response to oestrogen–androgen stimulation. In *Menopause: evaluation, treatment, and health concerns* (ed. C.B. Hammond F.P., Haseltine and I. Schiff), pp. 29–40. Alan R. Liss, New York.

Gibbons, W.E., Moyer, D.L., Lobo, R.A., Roy, S., and Mishell, D.R. (1986). Biochemical and histologic effects of sequential estrogen/progestin therapy on the endometrium of post-menopausal women. *American Journal of Obstetrics and Gynecology*, **154**, 456–61.

Goldstein, S.R. (1993). Use of ultrasonhysterography for triage of perimenopausal patients with unexplained uterine bleeding. *American Journal of Obstetrics and Gynecology*, **170**, 565–70.

Goldstein, S.R., Nachtigall, M., Snyder. J.R., and Nachtigall, L. (1990). Endometrial assessment by vaginal ultrasonography before endometrial sampling in patients with postmenopausal bleeding. *American Journal of Obstetrics and Gynecology*, **163**, 119–23.

Granberg, S., Wikland, M., Karlsson, B., Norstrom, A., and Friberg, L.-G. (1991). Endometrial thickness as measured by endovaginal ultrasonography for identifying endometrial abnormality. *American Journal of Obstetrics and Gynecology*, **164**, 47–52.

Grimes, D.A. (1982). Diagnostic dilation and curettage: a reappraisal. *American Journal of Obstetrics and Gynecology*, **142**, 1–6.

Hahn, R.G. (1989). Compliance considerations with estrogen replacement: withdrawal bleeding and other factors. *American Journal of Obstetrics and Gynecology*, **161**, 1854–8.

Herrington, L.J. and Weiss, N.S. (1993). Postmenopausal unopposed estrogens. Characteristics of use in relation to the risk of endometrial carcinoma. *Annals of Epidemiology*, **3**, 308–18.

Hillard, T.C., Siddle, N.C., Whitehead, M.I., Fraser, I.D., and Pryse-Davies, J. (1992). Continuous combined conjugated equine estrogen–progestogen therapy: effects of medroxyprogesterone acetate and norethindrone acetate on bleeding patterns and endometrial histologic diagnosis. *American Journal of Obstetrics and Gynecology*, **167**, 1–7.

Holst, J., Koskela, O., and Von Shoultz, B. (1983). Endometrial findings following curettage in 2018 women according to age and indications. *Annals Chirurgiae Gynaecologiae*, **72**, 274–7.

Karlsson, B., Granberg, S., Wikland, M., Ylöstalo, P., Torvid, K., Marsal, K., and Valentin, L. (1995). Transvaginal ultrasonography of the endometrium in women with postmenopausal bleeding – a Nordic multicenter study. *American Journal of Obstetrics and Gynecology*, **172**, 1488–93.

Kurman, R.J., Kaminski, P.F., and Norris, H.J. (1985). The behavior of endometrial hyperplasia. A long-term study of 'untreated' hyperplasia in 170 patients. *Cancer*, **56**, 403–12.

Larson, D.M., Johnson, K.K., Broste, S.K., Krawisz, B.R., and Kresl, J.J. (1995). Comparison of D&C and office endometrial biopsy in predicting final histopathologic grade in endometrial cancer. *Obstetrics Gynecology*, **86**, 38–42.

Leather, A.T., Savvas, M., and Studd, J.W. (1991). Endometrial histology and bleeding patterns after 8 years of continuous combined estrogen and progestogen therapy in postmenopausal women. *Obstetrics and Gynecology*, **78**, 1008–10.

Lobo, R.A. (1995). Benefits and risks of estrogen replacement therapy. *American Journal of Obstetrics and Gynecology*, **173**, 982–9.

MacKenzie, I.Z. and Bibby, J.G. (1978). Critical assessment of dilation and curettage in 1029 women. *Lancet*, **ii**, 566–8.

Manolio, T.A., Furberg, C.D., Shemanski, L., Tracy, R.P., Peaty, B.M., O'Leary, D.H. *et al.* (1993). Associations of postmenopausal estrogen use with cardiovascular disease and its risk factors in older women. The CHS Collaborative Research Group. *Circulation*, **88**, 2163–71.

Marcus, R., Greendale, G., Blunt, B.A., Bush, T.L., Sherman, S., Sherwin, R. *et al.* (1994). Correlates of bone mineral density in the postmenopausal estrogen/progestin interventions trial. *Journal of Bone Mineral Research*, **9**, 1467–76.

Marslew, U., Riis, B.J., and Christiansen, C. (1991). Bleeding patterns during continuous combined estrogen–progestogen therapy. *American Journal of Obstetrics and Gynecology*, **164**, 1163–8.

Mishell, D.R. Jr, Shoupe, D., Moyer, D.L., Roy, S., and Page, M.A. (1991). Postmenopausal hormone replacement with a combination estrogen–progestin regimen for five days per week. *Journal of Reproductive Medicine*, **36**, 351–5.

Moyer, D., deLignieres, B., Driguez, P., and Pez, J.P. (1993). Prevention of endometrial hyperplasia by progesterone during long-term estradiol replacement: influence of bleeding pattern and secretory changes. *Fertility and Sterility*, **59**, 992–7.

Nagele, F., O'Connor, H., Davies, A., Badawy, A., Mohamed, H., and Magos, A. (1996*a*). Outpatient diagnostic hysteroscopies. *Obstetrics and Gynecology*, **88**, 87–92.

Nagele, F., O'Connor, H., Baskett, T.F., Davies, A., Mohammed, H., and Magos, A.L. (1996*b*). Hysteroscopy in women with abnormal uterine bleeding on hormone replacement therapy: a comparison with postmenopausal bleeding. *Fertility and Sterility*, **65**, 1145–50.

Nasri, M.N. and Coast, G.J. (1989). Correlation of ultrasound findings and endometrial histopathology in postmenopausal women. *British Journal of Obstetrics and Gynaecology*, **96**, 1333–7.

Nasri, M.N., Shepherd, J.H., Setchell, M.E., Lowe, D.G., and Chard, T. (1991). The role of vaginal scan in measurement of endometrial thickness in postmenopausal women. *British Journal of Obstetrics and Gynaecology*, **98**, 470–5.

Padwick, M.L., Pryse-Davies, J., and Whitehead, M.I. (1986). A simple method for determining the optimal dosage of progestin in postmenopausal women receiving estrogens. *New England Journal of Medicine*, **315**, 930–4.

Parsons, A.K. and Lense, J.J. (1993). Sonohysterography for endometrial abnormalities: preliminary results. *Journal of Clinical Ultrasound*, **21**, 87–95.

Patterson, M.E., Wade-Evans, T., Sturdee, D.W., Thom, M.H., and Studd, J.W. (1980). Endometrial disease after treatment with oestrogens and progestogens in the climacteric. *British Medical Journal*, **280**, 822–4.

Raudaskoski, T.H., Lahti, E.I., Kauppila, A.J., Apaja-Sarkkinen, M.A., and Laatikainen, T.J. (1995). Transdermal estrogen with a levonorgestrel-releasing intrauterine device for climacteric complaints: clinical and endometrial responses. *American Journal of Obstetrics and Gynecology*, **172**, 114–19.

Ravnikar, V. (1987). Compliance with hormone therapy. *American Journal of Obstetrics and Gynecology*, **156**, 1332–4.

Santoro, N., Brown, J.R., Adel, T., and Skurnick, J.H. (1996). Characterization of reproductive hormonal dynamics in the perimenopause. *Journal of Clinical Endocrinology and Metabolism*, **81**, 1495–501.

Shoupe, D., Meme, D., Mezrow, G., and Lobo, R.A. (1991). Prevention of endometrial hyperplasia in postmenopausal women with intrauterine progesterone. (Letter to the editor). *New England Journal of Medicine*, **325**, 1811–12.

Sladkevicius, P., Valentin, L., and Marsal, K. (1994). Endometrial thickness and Doppler velocimetry of the uterine arteries as discriminators of endometrial status in women with postmenopausal bleeding: a comparative study. *American Journal of Obstetrics and Gynecology*, **171**, 722–8.

Speroff, L., Rowan, M.S., Symons, J., Genant, H., and Wilborn, W. (1996). The comparative effect on bone density, endometrium, and lipids of continuous hormones as replacement therapy. The Chart Study. *Journal of the American Medical Association*, **276**, 1397–403.

Staland, B. (1981). Continuous treatment with natural oestrogens and progestogens. A method of avoid endometrial stimulation. *Maturitas*, **3**, 145–56.

Sturdee, D.W., Barlow, D.H., Ulrich, L.G., Wells, M., Gydesen, H., Campbell, M., *et al.* (1994). Is the timing of withdrawal bleeding a guide to endometrial safety during sequential oestrogen-progestagen replacement therapy? *Lancet*, **344**, 979–82.

Suhonen, S.P., Allonen, H.O., and Lähteenmäki, P. (1995*a*). Sustained-release estradiol implants and a levonorgestrel-releasing intrauterine device in hormone replacement therapy. *American Journal of Obstetrics and Gynecology*, **172**, 562–7.

Suhonen, S.P., Holmström, T., Allonen, H.O., and Läteenmäki, P. (1995*b*). Intrauterine and subdermal progestin administration in postmenopausal hormone replacement therapy. *Fertility and Sterility*, **63**, 336–42.

Syrop, C. and Sahakian, V. (1992). Transvaginal sonographic detection of endometrial polyps with fluid contrast augmentation. *Obstetrics and Gynecology*, **79**, 1041–3.

The Writing Group for the PEPI Trial (1995). Effects of estrogen or estrogen/progestin regimens on heart disease risk factors in postmenopausal women. The postmenopausal estrogen/progestin interventions PEPI trial. *Journal of the American Medical Association*, **273**, 199–208.

The Writing Group for the PEPI Trial. (1996*a*). Effects of hormone replacement therapy on endometrial histology in postmenopausal women. The postmenopausal estrogen/progestin interventions PEPI trial. *Journal of the American Medical Association*, **275**, 370–5.

The Writing Group for the PEPI Trial (1996*b*). Effects of hormone therapy on bone mineral density. The postmenopausal estrogen/progestin intervention PEPI trial. *Journal of the American Medical Association*, **276**, 1389–96.

Tsuda, H., Kawabata, M., Kawabata, K., Yamamoto, K., Hidaka, A., Umesaki, N., and Ogita, S. (1995). Differences between occidental and oriental postmenopausal women in cutoff level of endometrial thickness for endometrial cancer screening by vaginal scan. *American Journal of Obstetrics and Gynecology*, **172**, 1494–5.

Udoff, L., Langenberg, P., and Adashi, E.Y. (1995). Combined continuous hormone replacement therapy: a critical review. *Obstetrics and Gynecology*, **86**, 306–16.

Varner, R.E., Sparks, J.M., Cameron, C.D., Roberts, L.L., and Soong, S.J. (1991). Transvaginal sonography of the endometrium in postmenopausal women. *Obstetrics and Gynecology*, **78**, 195–9.

Whitehead, M.I., Townsend, P.T., Pryse-Davies, J., Ryder, T.A., and King, R.J. (1981). Effects of estrogens and progestins on the biochemistry and morphology of the postmenopausal endometrium. *New England Journal of Medicine*, **305**, 1599–605.

Whitehead, M.I., Townsend, P.T., Pryse-Davies, J., Ryder, T., Lane, G., Siddle, N., and King, R.J. (1982). Actions of progestins on the morphology and biochemistry of the endometrium of postmenopausal women receiving low-dose estrogen therapy. *American Journal of Obstetrics and Gynecology* **142**, 791–5.

Whitehead, M.I., Hillard, T.C., and Crook, D. (1990). The role and use of progestogens. *Obstetrics and Gynecology*, **75**, 59S–76S.

Williams, R.F., Chwalisz, K., Kim, S., Hsiu, J.G., and Hodgen, G.D. (1994). Intermittent antiprogestin reduces unscheduled (breakthrough) bleeding during estrogen–progestin hormonal therapy in ovariectomized monkeys. Scientific Program and Abstracts, 41st Annual Meeting, The Society for Gynecologic Investigation, Chicago Abstract P-8, p. 198.

Woodruff, J.D. and Pickar, J.H. (1994). Incidence of endometrial hyperplasia in postmenopausal women taking conjugated estrogens (premarin) with medroxyprogesterone acetate or conjugated estrogens alone. The menopause study group. *American Journal of Obstetrics and Gynecology*, **172**, 1213–23.

Index

Where several pages are indicated, the figures in **bold** represent a section devoted to the topic.

The manufacturer's authorised representative in the EU for product safety is Oxford University Press España S.A. of El Parque Empresarial San Fernando de Henares, Avenida de Castilla, 2 - 28830 Madrid (www.oup.es/en or product.safety@oup.com). OUP España S.A. also acts as importer into Spain of products made by the manufacturer.
Printed and bound by CPI Group (UK) Ltd, Croydon, CR0 4YY
14/09/2026
02216284-0013